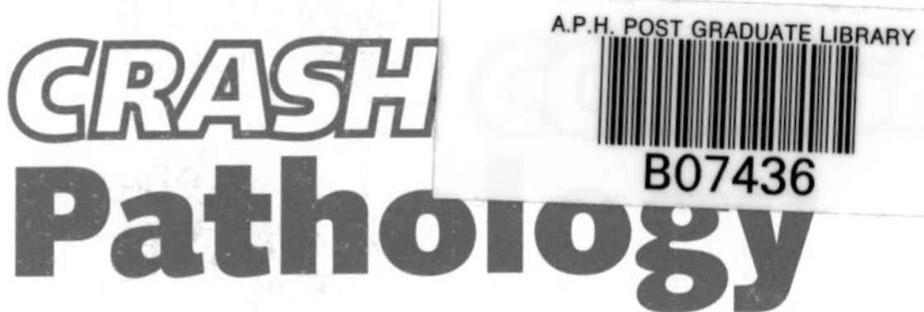

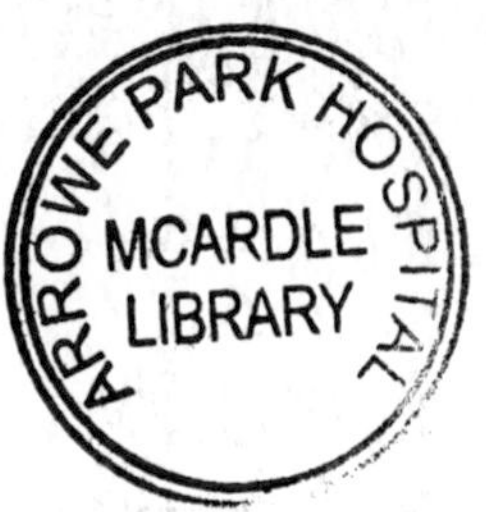

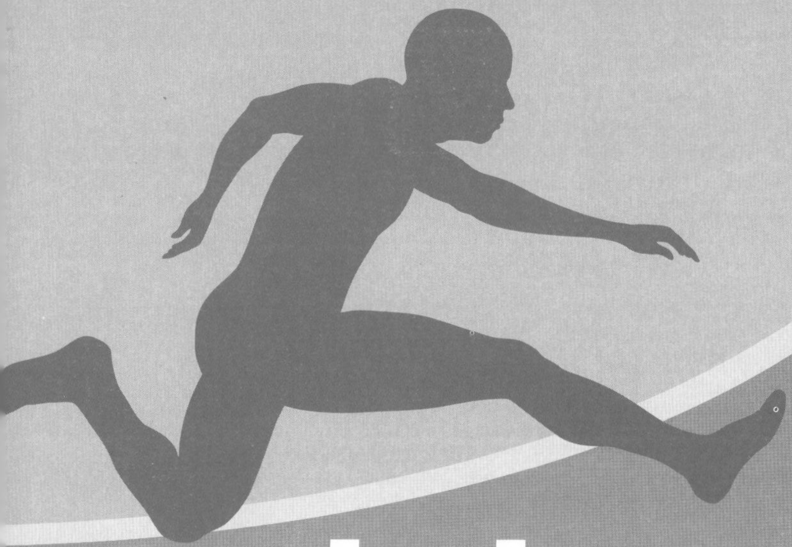

Pathology

James L. Fishback, MD
Associate Professor of Pathology
University of Kansas School of Medicine
Kansas City, Kansas

UK edition authors
Daniel O'Connor and Bethan Goodman Jones

UK series editor
Dan Horton-Szar

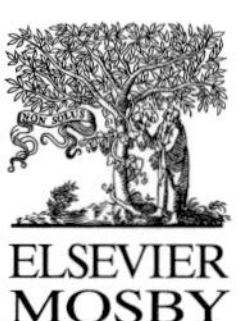

ELSEVIER
MOSBY

ELSEVIER
MOSBY

1600 John F. Kennedy Blvd. Ste 1800
Philadelphia, PA 19103-2899

CRASH COURSE: PATHOLOGY ISBN 0-323-03308-3

Notice

Knowledge and best practice in this field are constantly changing. As new research and experience broaden our knowledge, changes in practice, treatment and drug therapy may become necessary or appropriate. Readers are advised to check the most current information provided (i) on procedures featured or (ii) by the manufacturer of each product to be administered, to verifty the recommended dose or formula, the method and duration of administration, and contraindications. It is the responsibility of the practitioner, relying on their own experience and knowledge of the patient, to make diagnoses, to determine dosages and the best treatment for each individual patient, and to take all appropriate safety precautions. To the fullest extent of the law, neither the Publisher nor the Author assumes any liability for any injury and/or damage to persons or property arising out or related to any use of the material contained in this book.

First Edition 1999. Second Edition 2002.

Library of Congress Cataloging-in-Publication Data

Fishback, James L.
Pathology/James L. Fishback—1st ed.
p. ; cm.—(Crash course)
Includes index.
ISBN 0-323-03308-3
1. Pathology. I. Title. II. Series.
[DNLM: 1. Pathology. QZ 4 F532p 2005]
RB111.F54 2005
616.07—dc22 2004063168

Acquisitions Editor: Alex Stibbe
Project Development Manager: Stan Ward
Publishing Services Manager: David Saltzberg
Designer: Andy Chapman
Cover Design: Richard Tibbets
Illustration Manager: Mick Ruddy

Printed in China

Last digit is the print number: 9 8 7 6 5 4 3 2 1

Preface

Like other titles in the *Crash Course* series, *Crash Course Pathology* offers a straightforward approach to a complex field of study. Part I outlines the principles of pathology, including chapters about cancer, inflammation and tissue damage, and infectious disease. Part II offers a more focused examination of pathology as it relates to the major systems of the body. Numerous figures and tables throughout the book help to explain complicated concepts and disorders, and boxed "hints" point to crucial information that every student must know.

Since this book is indeed a "crash course," most students will derive the greatest benefit by using it in concert with a general textbook in pathology, such *as Robbins Basic Pathology* (2004), or with a good pathology atlas. It is important for students to read further about topics that they do not understand well. Only then can they master the most important principles and concepts of their field.

Lastly, to students past and present, I hope that this book can make your personal journey through medical school a little easier and more enjoyable than mine turned out to be!

James L. Fishback, MD

Acknowledgments

This book is not really mine, in a sense, as I was simply asked to "Americanize" the British edition by Dan O'Connor and Rosemary Walker. Hopefully, not too much of my Kansas City accent will show through, and the results will be readable by students on both coasts!

I would like to thank my department chair, Patricia Thomas, MD, for encouraging me to follow my inclinations toward medical education and for giving me the time to work on my teaching and writing skills. I also thank my parents for encouraging me in my pursuit of a medical education, especially when it was not entirely clear that I was going to make it. Lastly, I thank my wife, Meg, for hanging in there during my absence in the late war. I knew I wasn't in Kansas any more, but just thinking of her made me certain that I was going to make it home.

Figure acknowledgment

Figures 2.4, 2.6, 2.7, 5.19, 6.17, 10.2, 12.24, and 14.14 adapted with permission from *General and Systematic Pathology*, 3rd edn, edited by Professor J.C.E. Underwood. Churchill Livingstone, Edinburgh, 2000.

Contents

PRINCIPLES OF PATHOLOGY

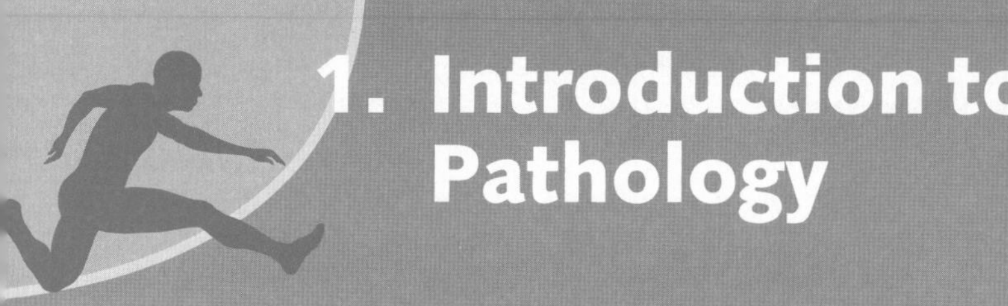

1. Introduction to Pathology

Disease

A disease is an alteration from the normal function/structure of an organ or system, which manifests as a characteristic set of signs and symptoms.

Pathology

Pathology is the scientific study of disease. It is concerned with the causes and effects of disease, and the functional and structural changes that occur. Changes at the molecular and cellular level correlate with the clinical manifestations of the disease.

Understanding the processes of disease assists in the accurate recognition, diagnosis, and treatment of diseases.

Divisions of pathology

Pathology is traditionally subdivided into five main clinical disciplines. The divisions are:

- Histopathology—the study of histological abnormalities of diseased cells and tissues.
- Hematology—the study of primary diseases of the blood, and the secondary effects of other diseases on the blood.
- Chemical pathology—the study of biochemical abnormalities associated with disease.
- Microbiology—the study of infectious diseases and the organisms that cause them.
- Immunopathology—the study of diseases caused by a disturbance of immune function.

Classification of disease

The causes of disease are numerous and diverse. For convenience, diseases are often classified as either congenital or acquired disorders. Congenital diseases are present from birth, whereas acquired disorders are incurred as a result of factors originating in the external environment.

Causes of disease are easily remembered by the mnemonic **VINDICATES:**

V = Vascular (e.g., atherosclerosis, thrombosis)
I = Infectious (e.g., viral, bacterial)
N = Neoplastic (both benign and malignant tumors)
D = Drugs or toxins
I = Inflammatory/idiopathic
C = Congenital (genetic or epigenetic)
A = Autoimmune (e.g., lupus, rheumatoid arthritis)
T = Trauma or environmental (e.g., heat, cold, vitamin deficiencies, nutrition)
E = Endocrine/metabolic (e.g., diabetes)
S = Something else

However, many if not most diseases are due to a combination of causes, and they are therefore said to have a multifactorial etiology.

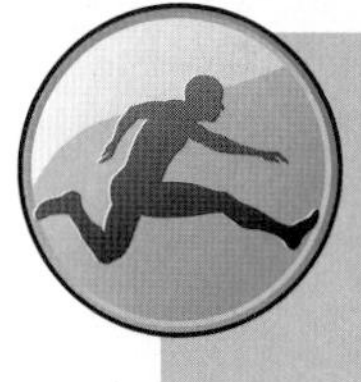

It is important to have a logical and methodical approach to disease description. Fig. 1.1 illustrates the features of disease.

How pathology is covered in this book

Part I: Principles of pathology

The number of tissue responses that underlie all diseases is limited. These responses are known as basic pathological responses. The first part of this book describes the principles of these in relation to our advancing knowledge of the molecular sciences.

Part II: Systemic pathology

As well as an understanding of the basic pathological responses, it is also necessary to understand how they affect individual tissues and organs. The second part of this book describes the common pathology of the specific diseases as they affect individual organs or organ systems. This approach is termed systematic pathology, and it is illustrated by clinical examples of disease.

Characteristics of disease	
Characteristic	**Explanation**
Definition	A clear, concise and accurate description
Incidence	Number of new cases of disease occurring in a population of a defined size during a defined period
Prevalence	Number of cases of disease to be found in a defined population at a stated time
Etiology	Cause of disease
Pathogenesis	Mechanism by which a disease is caused
Morphology	Form and structural changes
Complications and sequelae	Secondary consequences of disease
Treatment	Treatment regimens, effectiveness and side effects
Prognosis	Expected outcome of the disease

Fig. 1.1 Features of disease include definition, etiology, pathogenesis, treatment, and prognosis.

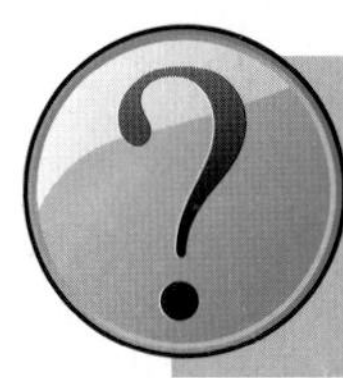

- Define pathology.
- What are the divisions of pathology?
- What are the characteristics of a disease?
- Define congenital and acquired disorders.

2. Cancer

Definitions and nomenclature

Definitions

Tumor

Strictly speaking, tumor is Latin for "swelling." In everyday usage, however, a tumor can be defined as an abnormal mass of tissue resulting from autonomous disordered growth that persists after the initiating stimulus has been removed. A tumor results from genetic alteration and deregulated growth control mechanisms.

Tumors are:

- Progressive—they are independent of normal growth control, and they continue to grow regardless of requirements, and in the absence of any external stimuli.
- Purposeless—abnormal mass serves no useful purpose.
- Parasitic—endogenous in origin but draw nourishment from the body while contributing nothing to its function.

All tumors have the suffix "–oma," by convention.

Other related definitions are:

- Neoplasm (i.e., new growth)—synonymous with tumor.
- Neoplasia—the process of tumor growth.
- Cancer—a malignant neoplasm.
- Anaplastic neoplasm—a very poorly differentiated neoplasm.

Dysplasia

Dysplasia is the disordered development of cells resulting in an alteration in their size, shape, and organization. It may be reversible, but is also known to precede neoplasia. For example, a tissue that can show dysplasia is the squamous epithelium of the uterine cervix following human papilloma virus (HPV) infection. This is referred to as cervical intra-epithelial neoplasia (CIN) and three grades are observed. CIN I is mildly dysplasic; CIN II is moderately dysplasic; and CIN III is severely dysplasic.

Metaplasia

Metaplasia is the change from one type of differentiated tissue to another, usually in response to an irritating stimulus, e.g., a change from mucus-secreting epithelium to stratified squamous epithelium in the bronchial mucosa, due to irritation associated with cigarette smoking. Metaplasia is reversible, and it often represents an adaptive response to environmental stress.

Benign versus malignant

Tumors are classified as either benign or malignant according to their appearance and behavior (Fig. 2.1). Benign tumors are localized neoplasms that do not invade the surrounding tissues or metastasize to other organs. Malignant tumors are capable of invasion and spread to distant organs. This distinction is crucial in the clinic, because metastases from malignant tumors are associated with significant morbidity and mortality.

Nomenclature of tumors

Tumor nomenclature (Fig. 2.2) is based on histological and behavior patterns. Histology provides information about the type of cell from which the tumor has arisen, while behavior provides information as to whether the cell is benign or malignant.

A few simple rules to follow:

- –oma: suffix for tumors. But there are some non-neoplastic "–omas" (e.g., granuloma).
- Carcinomas: malignant tumors of epithelial (ectoderm or endoderm) origin; prefixed by tissue of origin.
- –sarcomas: suffix for malignant tumors of connective tissue (mesoderm) origin.

Characteristics of benign versus malignant tumors	
Benign	**Malignant**
Localized	Metastatic spread
No invasion	Invasion of normal structures
No metastases	Metastases
Relatively slow growth rate	Relatively rapid growth rate
Good differentiation	Poorly differentiated
Few mitoses	Many mitoses
Normal nuclear chromatin	Increased nuclear chromatin
Uniform size cells	Cells and nuclei vary in size
Exophytic growth	Endophytic growth
Compression of normal tissue	Invasion and destruction of normal tissue

Fig. 2.1 Characteristics of benign versus malignant tumors. Note that metastasis is the only absolute distinguishing feature between benign and malignant neoplasms.

Classification of carcinomas

Carcinomas are malignant tumors of epithelial tissue. Carcinomas of non-glandular epithelium are prefixed by the name of the epithelial cell type. Malignant tumors of glandular epithelium are termed adenocarcinomas.

Carcinoma in situ

This is an epithelial neoplasm that has all the cellular features associated with malignancy, but which has not yet invaded through the epithelial basement membrane. The in situ phase may progress, or it may last for several years before invasion commences.

Intra-epithelial neoplasia

This covers the spectrum of changes short of invasive carcinoma:

- Mild dysplasia.
- Moderate dysplasia.
- Severe dysplasia/carcinoma in situ.

Important tumor nomenclature		
Histological type	**Benign**	**Malignant**
Epithelial		
Glandular	Adenoma	Adenocarcinoma
Non-glandular	Papilloma	Carcinoma
Connective tissue		
Adipose	Lipoma	Liposarcoma
Cartilage	Chondroma	Chondrosarcoma
Bone	Osteoma	Osteosarcoma
Smooth muscle	Leiomyoma	Leiomyosarcoma
Voluntary muscle	Rhabdomyoma	Rhabdomyosarcoma
Blood vessels	Angioma	Angiosarcoma
Nerve	Neurofibroma	Neurofibrosarcoma
Nerve sheath	Neurilemmoma	Neurilemmosarcoma
Glial cells	Glioma	Malignant glioma
Others		
Hemopoietic	Polyclonal leukocytosis	Leukemia
Lymphoreticular	Polyclonal lymphocytosis	Lymphoma
Melanocytes	Nevus	Malignant melanoma
Germinal cell	Benign teratoma	Malignant teratoma

Fig. 2.2 Examples of tumor nomenclature.

These three categories are clearly illustrated by the example of CIN.

Invasive carcinoma

This is an epithelial neoplasm that invades through the basement membrane. The tumor gains access to the vascular supply and lymphatics, and it will often metastasize to distant tissues.

Epidemiological aspects of cancer

Cancer in the U.S.

As a cause of mortality in the U.S., cancer is the second biggest killer (after cardiovascular disease). Its incidence (Fig. 2.3) is as follows:

- Almost 1 in 3 of the population will develop cancer during their lifetime.
- Almost 1 in 4 of the population will die of cancer.
- Incidence of cancer deaths increases with increasing age.
- Incidence of cancer varies between males and females.

Cancer worldwide

The incidence of different cancers varies from country to country, and this variation provides clues to the causes of the cancers.

For example, in Japan, gastric carcinoma is 30 times more common than in the U.S., whereas pancreatic cancer is much rarer. However, migration of a subset of the Japanese population to different geographical areas (e.g., U.S., U.K.) alters the incidences of these diseases within that population to a rate resembling that of the host country.

These findings suggest that environmental factors (such as diet and occupational, social, and geographic effects) rather than genetic causes account for most of the observed differences between countries.

Molecular basis of cancer

Oncogenes and tumor suppressor genes (anti-oncogenes)

Cell proliferation and division are usually tightly regulated by two sets of opposing functioning genes. These are the growth promoting genes—called proto-oncogenes—and the negative cell cycle regulators—called tumor suppressor genes (TSGs). Abnormal activation of proto-oncogenes and loss of function of tumor suppressor genes may lead to the transformation of a normal cell into a cancer cell.

Proto-oncogenes

Proto-oncogenes are genes that are expressed in normal cells. These genes code for oncoproteins, which positively regulate cell growth and differentiation (growth factors, transcription factors,

Ten leading types of cancer in the U.S.

Estimated new cases*		Estimated deaths	
Men	**Women**	**Men**	**Women**
Prostate (33%)	Breast (32%)	Lung and bronchus (32%)	Lung and bronchus (25%)
Lung and bronchus (13%)	Lung and bronchus (12%)	Prostate (10%)	Breast (15%)
Colon and rectum (11%)	Colon and rectum (11%)	Colon and rectum (10%)	Colon and rectum (10%)
Urinary bladder (6%)	Uterine corpus (6%)	Pancreas (5%)	Ovary (6%)
Melanoma of the skin (4%)	Ovary (4%)	Leukemia (5%)	Pancreas (6%)
Non-Hodgkin lymphoma (4%)	Non-Hodgkin lymphoma (4%)	Non-Hodgkin lymphoma (4%)	Leukemia (4%)
Kidney (3%)	Melanoma of the skin (4%)	Esophagus (4%)	Non-Hodgkin lymphoma (3%)
Leukemia (3%)	Thyroid (3%)	Liver (3%)	Uterine corpus (3%)
Oral cavity (3%)	Pancreas (2%)	Urinary bladder (3%)	Multiple myeloma (2%)
Pancreas (2%)	Urinary bladder (2%)	Kidney (3%)	Brain (2%)
All other sites (18%)	All other sites (20%)	All other sites (21%)	All other sites (24%)

Note: *Excludes basal and squamous cell skin cancers and in-situ carcinomas except urinary bladder.

Source: American Cancer Society, Surveillance Research, 2004.

Fig. 2.3 Incidence and mortality of common cancers in men and women in the U.S.

and receptor molecules). In healthy cells, transcription of these genes is tightly controlled. Inappropriate expression of oncoproteins leads to abnormal cell growth and survival. Normally functioning proto-oncogenes can be activated into cancer-causing oncogenes in two ways:

- A mutation can produce an oncoprotein that is functionally altered and abnormally active. For example, intracellular signalling is affected by the hyperactive mutant *ras* protein.
- A normal oncoprotein can be produced in abnormally large quantities because of enhanced gene amplification (the *myc* oncogene in neuroblastomas) or enhanced transcription (formation of the Philadelphia chromosome from a translocation between chromosomes 9 and 22).

Oncogenes can be classified according to the function of the gene product. Oncogenes include genes which express:

- Nuclear binding proteins (e.g., *c-myc*).
- Tyrosine kinase proteins (e.g., *src*).
- Growth factors (e.g., platelet derived growth factor (PDGF)).
- Receptors for growth factors (e.g., c-*erb*B-2/HER-2 which is related to epidermal growth factor receptor (EGFR)).
- GTP- binding proteins (e.g., *ras*).

Expression of abnormal oncogene products corresponds to the behavior and appearance of transformed cells. These include:

- Independence from the requirement of extrinsic growth factors.
- Production of proteases which assist tissue invasion.
- Reduced cell cohesiveness which assist metastasis.
- Ability to grow at higher cell densities.
- Abnormal cellular orientation.
- Increased plasma membrane and cellular motility.

Tumor suppressor genes

Tumor suppressor genes (e.g., p53 and Rb1) encode proteins that prevent or suppress the growth of tumors. Inactivation of TSGs results in increased susceptibility to cancer formation. Genetically increased susceptibility to cancer formation was first proposed by Knudson who studied the childhood retinal cancer retinoblastoma. In some cases, the tumors are bilateral and familial, but in other cases they are unilateral and sporadic. He proposed that familial retinoblastoma resulted in a high risk of bilateral eye tumors because of the predisposition to cancer from a germline mutation in one copy of the RB1 gene. Therefore, only one further mutation was required for tumor formation. In contrast, sporadic retinoblastoma occurs in patients who have an initially fully functioning RB1 gene. These tumors are rare and unilateral because two somatic mutations are required. This has been coined the "two hit" hypothesis.

Examples of dysfunctional TSGs involved in human cancers are:

- APC implicated in colorectal tumors and located on chromosome 5q.
- NF1 implicated in neurofibrosarcoma and located on chromosome 17q.
- RB1 implicated in retinoblastoma and located on chromosome 13q.
- BRCA1 implicated in breast and ovarian cancer and located on chromosome 17q.
- p53 implicated in many tumors and located on chromosome 17p.

Loss of function of TSGs or their protein products can result in uncontrolled neoplastic cell growth. TSGs can lose their normal function by a variety of mechanisms:

- Mutations (hereditary or acquired).
- Binding of normal TSG protein to proteins encoded by viral genes, e.g., human papilloma virus proteins E6/E7.
- Complexing of normal TSG protein to mutant TSG protein in heterozygous cells.

TSGs function by maintaining the integrity of the genome through arrested cell growth and repair of DNA damage. They also function to promote cell suicide or apoptosis in cells with sustained DNA damage. One of the most studied TSGs is the p53 gene located at 17p—termed "the guardian of the genome." It is mutated or functionally altered in over 50% of all human cancers. In addition a familial inherited mutation is found in Li–Fraumeni syndrome. Affected individuals have an increased predisposition to several tumor types. The TSG p53 can recognize damaged DNA and can respond either through cell cycle growth arrest at the G_1 check point or through the initiation of apoptosis.

Cellular proliferation is tightly regulated by two sets of opposed function genes. Proto-oncogenes are growth-promoting genes, and tumor suppressor genes are growth-suppressing genes. Deregulated function of proto-oncogenes and tumor suppressor genes leads to cell transformation and tumorigenesis.

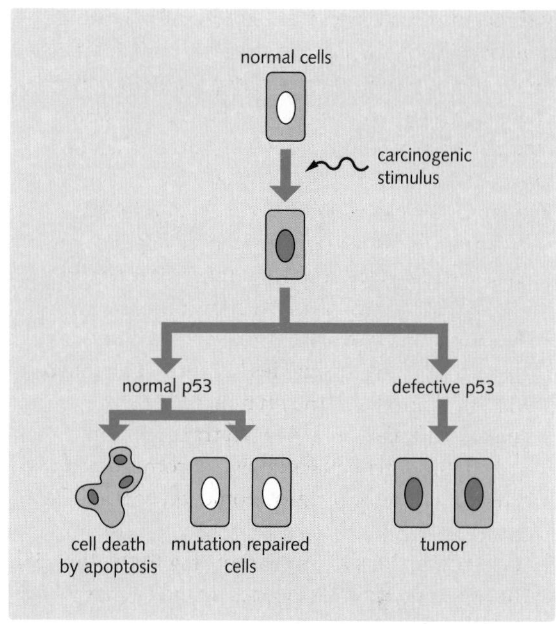

Fig. 2.4 Role of p53 in cells with damaged DNA. Cells either undergo G_1 arrest and DNA repair, or cell death by apoptosis. (Adapted from Underwood, 2000.)

Apoptosis

The importance of apoptosis has only been fully appreciated since the early 1990s. Apoptosis (programmed cell death) is an active process whereby a single cell initiates its own death under normal physiological conditions. Apoptosis occurs physiologically in tissue modelling, embryogenesis, and the regulation of the immune system. It is often deregulated in tumors. There are a number of different mechanisms for the activation of apoptotic pathways and many of these are altered during the process of tumorigenesis. The final common pathway is the activation of the interleukin-2 converting enzymes (ICE) and the expression of genes for cytoplasmic proteases, transglutaminases, and endonucleases. Death signals converge on the mitochondria. Morphologically the cell is characterized by loss of cell surface markings, cell shrinkage, nuclear chromatin condensation (internucleosomal cleavage), and the formation of apoptotic bodies, which are eventually phagocytosed by adjacent cells.

The advantage of pathological apoptosis is that the mutated cell is destroyed before it can perpetuate itself, thus preventing potential tumor formation. For example, the p53 tumor suppressor gene protein product recognizes DNA damage caused by ultraviolet (UV) irradiation, and it activates apoptotic cell death pathways before the cell can divide and proliferate (Fig. 2.4).

Genes and proteins involved in the process of apoptosis include the death receptor and ligand families, cell cycle related genes, the Bcl-2 family, the caspase family, and the caspase substrates.

Multistage model of tumor progression

Tumorigenesis is a multistage process that results from accumulated mutation. Tumors arise from single cells, which proliferate to form a clone of cells with identical abnormalities. As tumors develop, they undergo further somatic mutations, which cause abnormalities in other oncogenes and/or tumor suppressor genes. These additional mutations result in cells that are genetically different from each other, but which are part of the same tumor—this is heterogeneity.

Fast-growing, less-differentiated cells take over, and these eliminate the slower-growing, better-differentiated cells.

Chemotherapy may kill the majority of tumor cells. However, tumor cells that are resistant to chemotherapy will survive and be selected for (because of ablation of competing, non-resistant cells), resulting in the regrowth of a tumor resistant to chemotherapy (Fig. 2.5).

The progressive nature of tumorigenesis is clearly illustrated in Vogelstein's model of the development of colonic cancer. The accumulation over time of mutations in oncogenes such as Ki-*ras* and loss of

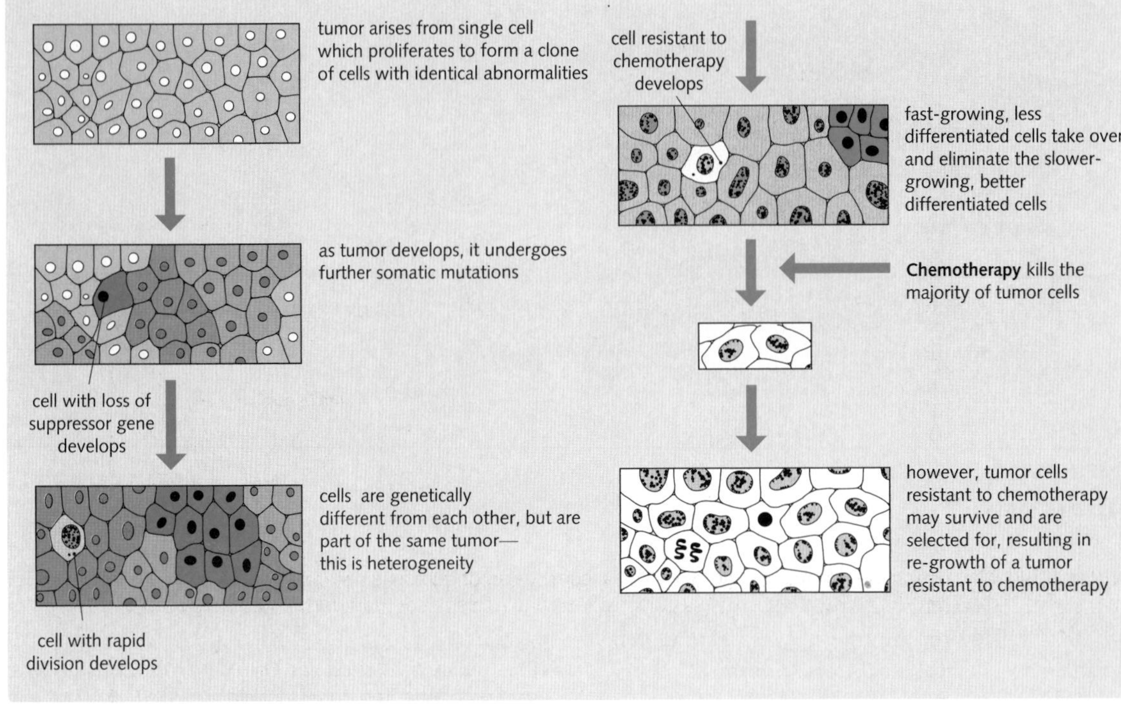

Fig. 2.5 Tumor progression and genetic heterogeneity.

function mutations in tumor suppressor genes such as APC results in the formation of colon carcinoma (Fig. 2.6).

Tumor growth

Kinetics of tumor growth and angiogenesis

Angiogenesis is an important physiological process in normal embryogenesis, the female reproductive cycle, and wound healing. However, pathological angiogenesis is a key player in many disorders, and this includes cancer. This is because a solid tumor cannot grow beyond a few millimeters in diameter without a blood supply to maintain nutrient and oxygen provision and remove metabolic waste.

In normal cells, angiogenesis is a tightly-controlled, highly-regulated mechanism. In contrast, tumor cells can release pro-angiogenic factors, which induce vascular proliferation. This is sometimes called the angiogenic switch. The angiogenic switch results in the production of pro-angiogenic molecules such as vascular endothelial growth factor (VEGF).

Eventually, the tumor may outgrow its blood supply, and areas of necrosis may appear, resulting in slower growth but a more malignant phenotype (Fig. 2.7). This is because only the strongest cells survive the hypoxic conditions.

Mechanisms and pathways of invasion and metastasis

Invasion

The ability to metastasize is the only absolute criterion for malignancy. Invading malignant cells have the following properties:

- Abnormal or increased cellular motility—due to loss of contact inhibition.
- Altered cellular adhesion—due to changes in surface adhesion molecules.
- Increased secretion of proteolytic enzymes, e.g., metalloproteinases.

Metalloproteinases, such as collagenases and gelatinases, are the most important enzymes in neoplastic invasion. These enzymes digest the surrounding connective tissue thus aiding invasion.

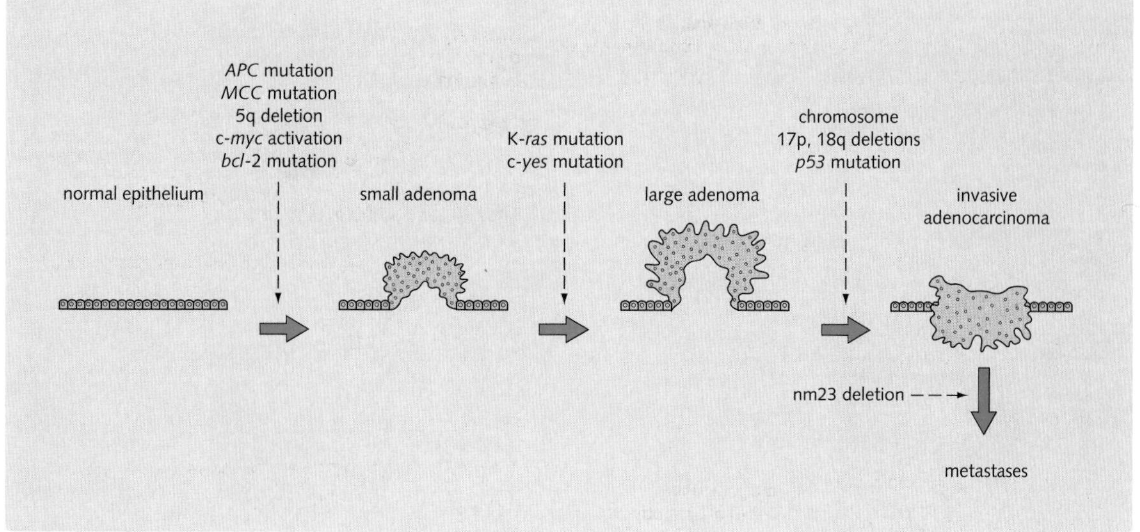

Fig. 2.6 Multi-step development of colonic cancer. The accumulation of genetic mutations corresponds to the altered behavior of the tumor cells. (APC, adenomatous polyposis coli; MCC, mutated in colorectal cancer.) (Adapted from Underwood, 2000.)

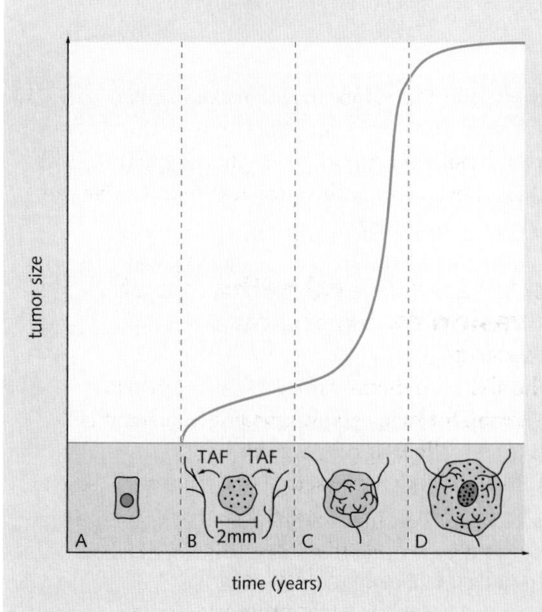

Fig. 2.7 Kinetics of tumor growth and angiogenesis. (A) Transformed cell. (B) Avascular tumor nodule. (C) Vascularized tumor. (D) Vascularized tumor with central necrosis. (TAF, tumor angiogenic factors.) (Adapted from Underwood, 2000.)

Metastasis

Metastasis is the process whereby malignant cells spread from their site of origin—primary tumor—to distant sites and grow to secondary tumors.

Total mass of secondary tumors usually exceeds that of the primary lesion. Only a proportion of neoplastic cells in a malignant tumor are able to metastasize. It is sometimes impossible to find the primary lesion in some cancer patients who present with extensive secondary metastases.

In order to metastasize, neoplastic cells undergo the following sequence of events:

- Detachment of tumor cells from neighboring cells.
- Invasion of surrounding connective tissue.
- Intravasation into blood/lymphatic vessels.
- Evasion of the host's defense mechanisms.
- Adherence to endothelium at a distant site.
- Extravasation of cells from vessel lumen into surrounding tissue.

Following extravasation, the malignant cells proliferate and secrete more angiogenic growth factors for vascularization. Hence, a new tumor is formed. However, not all cancer cells will grow at all distant sites. This is the seed and soil effect—conditions must be appropriate for cell proliferation.

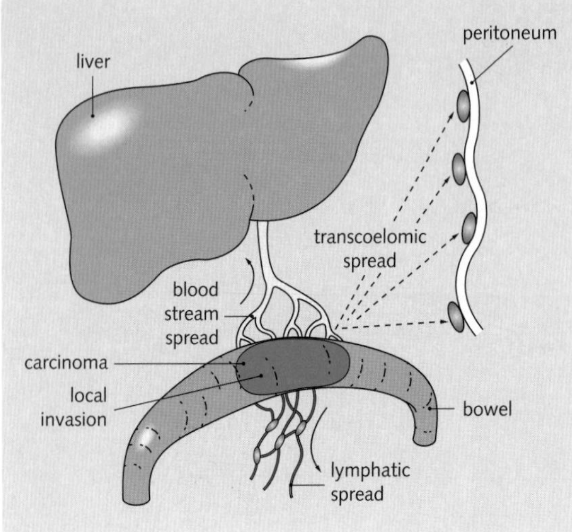

Fig. 2.8 Routes of metastasis exemplified by a carcinoma of the bowel, i.e., via the bloodstream, via the lymphatic spread, through peritoneal cavities, and via local invasion.

Main routes of metastasis

There are four main routes of metastasis (Fig. 2.8):

- Local invasion—most common pattern of spread of malignant tumors is by direct growth into adjacent tissues.
- Lymphatic spread—forms secondary tumors in lymph nodes.
- Bloodborne spread—cells enter the bloodstream and form secondary tumors in organs perfused by blood that has drained from a tumor. Common tumors that spread to bone by the blood are bronchus, breast, thyroid, kidney, and prostate.
- Transcoelomic spread—in pleural, pericardial, and peritoneal cavities.

Routes of metastasis are the lymphatics, local invasion, coelomic spaces, and vascular spread. Clinically, it is important to know the tumors that spread to bone via the blood. These are cancers of the bronchus, breast, thyroid, kidney, and prostate.

Examples of chemical carcinogens

Chemical compound	Cancer type
Indirect carcinogens	
Polycyclic hydrocarbons • soot [benzo(a)pyrene; dibenzanthracene] • tobacco smoke	 Skin, colon Lung, bladder, oral cavity, larynx, esophagus
Aromatic amines • benzidine, 2-naphthylamine	 Bladder
Nitrosamines • chemotherapeutic agents • cyclophosphamide, chlorambucil, thiotepa, busulphan	 Esophagus, stomach Leukemias
Vinyl chloride	Liver (angiosarcoma)
Aflatoxins	Liver
Unknown mechanisms	
Heavy metals • nickel, cadmium, chromium • arsenic	 Lung Skin

Fig. 2.9 Examples of chemical carcinogens.

Carcinogenic agents

Carcinogens are substances known to cause an increased incidence of cancer.

Carcinogens can exert their effect by either genetic mechanisms (i.e., causing DNA alteration—this is the majority of carcinogens) or epigenetic mechanisms (i.e., acting on the protein product of growth regulating genes).

Chemical carcinogens

Most chemical carcinogens are procarcinogens, and they require metabolic conversion into active carcinogens (ultimate carcinogens). Some carcinogens act directly to induce cellular damage. Examples of chemical carcinogens are given in Fig. 2.9.

Stages of chemical carcinogenesis

The progressive model of carcinogenesis (Fig. 2.10) is based on observations on the effects of chemical carcinogens on laboratory animals. This model proposes three main stages of carcinogenesis:

- Initiation—induction of a genetic alteration in oncogene or tumor suppressor gene.

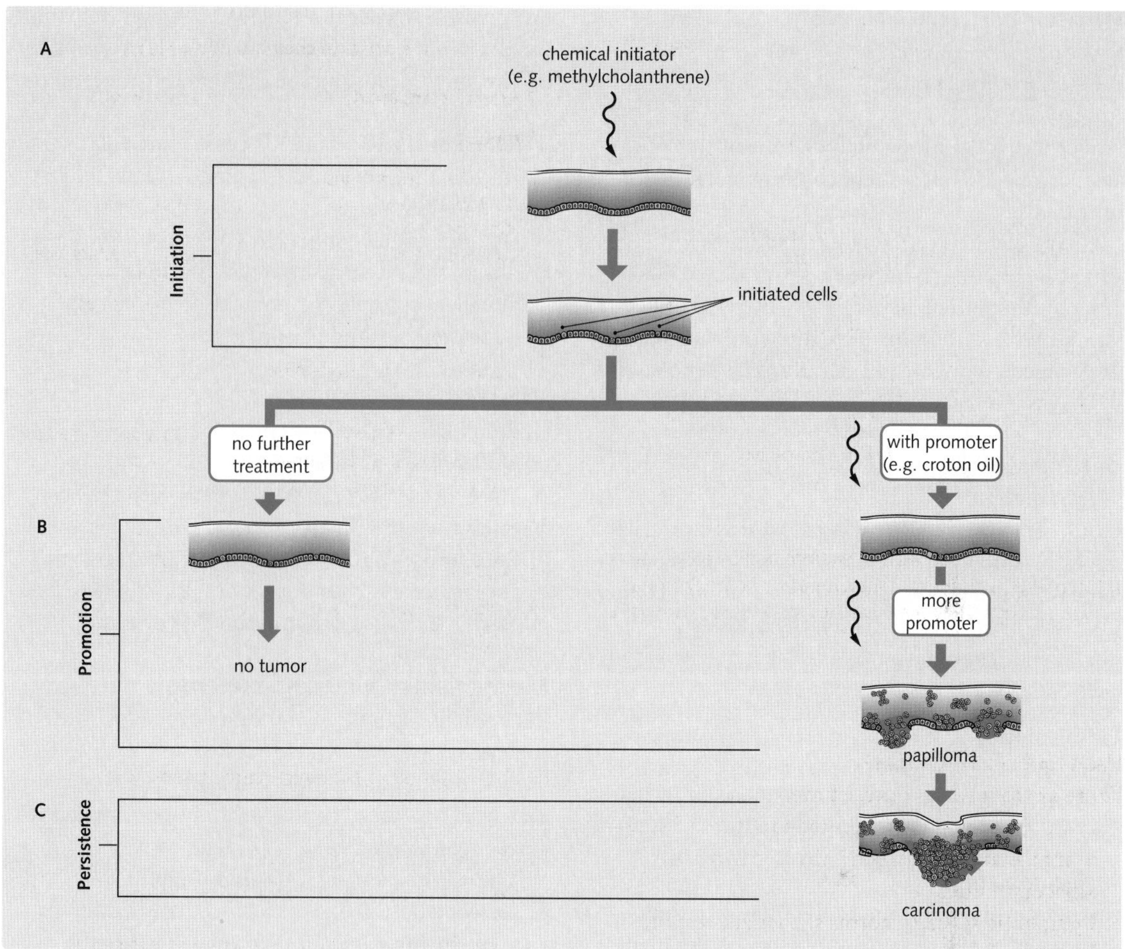

Fig. 2.10 Stages of chemical carcinogenesis. (A) Initiation: induction of genetic changes in cells that results in neoplastic potential. (B) Promotion: induction of cellular proliferation in the initiated cell. (C) Persistence: proliferating tumor cells no longer require the presence of initiators or promoters. Tumor cells exhibit autonomous growth.

- Promotion—a stimulus for proliferation of initiated cell; this may be an external agent or a further random mutational genetic abnormality.
- Persistence—stage where proliferation of tumor cells becomes autonomous, i.e., it no longer requires the presence of initiators or promoters.

Stages of chemical carcinogenesis are initiation, promotion, and persistence. The classic example of initiation and promotion are the effects of methylcholanthrene and croton oil.

Radiation

Radiation can be:

- Ionizing—natural radiation, therapeutic radiation, and nuclear radiation.
- Non-ionizing—UV radiation.

Radiation can result in DNA damage in two ways:

- Directly—causing strand breaks, base alterations, and cross-linking of DNA.
- Indirectly—ionization of H_2O with formation of reactive oxygen free radicals, which interact with and damage DNA.

Ultraviolet radiation

UV radiation is associated with many different kinds of skin cancer, particularly:

- Squamous cell carcinoma.
- Basal cell carcinoma.
- Malignant melanoma.

Skin cancer is the most common type of cancer in the U.S. and U.K. It is more common in fair-skinned individuals.

Ultraviolet light is thought to induce the formation of linkages between pyrimidine bases on DNA molecule. The risk is greatly increased in patients with xeroderma pigmentosum, which is a rare congenital disease characterized by deficiency of DNA repair enzymes.

Ionizing radiation

X-ray radiation

Radiotherapy can cause cancer as well as curing it! It is associated with radiation-induced malignant neoplasms, usually sarcomas. These tumors occur months or years after radiation therapy, e.g., in the lungs, central nervous system (CNS), bones, kidneys, and liver.

Radioisotopes

Radioactive iodine, used to treat thyroid disease, is associated with increased risk of cancer development 15–25 years post treatment.

Nuclear radiation

Survivors of the Hiroshima and Nagasaki atomic bombs, and of the Chernobyl nuclear power plant accident, have a greatly increased incidence of cancer including leukemia and carcinoma of breast, lung, and thyroid.

DNA repair mechanisms and their failure

DNA is the cellular constituent most sensitive to radiation. Fortunately, cells have DNA repair mechanisms that deal with DNA damage. Repair is usually rapid, but sometimes damage is irreparable and major chromosomal and chromatid alterations occur.

Repair of single-stranded breaks, particularly in rapidly dividing cells, is error prone and introduces single base mutations.

Double-stranded cleavage leads to chromosome breakage, and attempts to repair multiple breaks lead to inappropriate recombination events, e.g., translocation or interstitial deletion.

Viruses

Certain DNA viruses and retroviruses (Fig. 2.11) can cause neoplasia, as follows:

- DNA viruses insert DNA directly into the host genome.
- Retroviruses have reverse transcriptase enzyme to produce a DNA copy of viral RNA. The DNA copy is then inserted into the host genome.

Mechanism of viral carcinogenesis

Inserted viral genes may be viral oncogenes themselves (v-*onc*), whose expression may lead to uncontrolled proliferation, or inserted viral genes may be activators or repressors of important cell cycle regulating genes.

The mechanism of viral carcinogenesis is understood best in one of the most studied tumor viruses, the human papilloma virus. This double stranded DNA virus has a tropism for squamous epithelium and subtypes 16 and 18 are implicated in cervical carcinoma. The viral genome incorporates into the host DNA and expresses the E6 oncoprotein, which inactivates the tumor suppressor protein p53. In addition expression of the E7 oncoprotein inactivates the tumor suppressor protein

Examples of oncogenic human viruses

Type	Virus	Tumor type
Retroviruses	Human T cell leukemia virus (HTLV)	T cell leukemia
	Human immunodeficiency virus (HIV)	AIDS-related lymphomas
DNA viruses	Human papillomavirus	Skin papilloma (common wart) Cervical carcinoma
	Epstein–Barr virus	Carcinoma of the nasopharynx Burkitt's lymphoma
	Hepatitis B virus	Hepatocellular carcinoma

Fig. 2.11 Examples of oncogenic human viruses.

RB1. These oncoproteins together with other factors result in CIN.

Host defenses against cancer

Some tumors are known to stimulate both innate (passive) and adaptive immunological reactions in the host.

Innate immunity

Activation of macrophages and natural killer cells can prevent growth of some tumors in vitro. Some tumors activate complement via the alternative pathway.

Adaptive immunity

Humoral

Antibodies may have a protective role, and they are more likely to be effective against free cells (e.g., leukemia or metastasizing tumors) than those in solid lumps.

Cell-mediated immunity

Cell-mediated immunity is involved in recognition and monitoring of cells progressing toward malignancy. Therefore, cells that become significantly different to be recognized as "foreign" may be eliminated by the immune system. This is particularly true of those tumors with a suspected viral etiology. The importance of immune surveillance in the prevention of cancer is clearly illustrated in immunocompromised patients. For example, lymphomas associated with Epstein–Barr virus can present 4–7 years post-immunosuppressive therapy following organ transplant.

In addition, cytotoxic T cells are thought to play a role in tumor regression. Infiltration of some tumors by lymphocytes and macrophages is associated with better prognosis.

Despite many immune mechanisms known to be active against tumor cells, most tumors are not distinguishable from normal host cells, and so they are not easily detected by the immune system. There are many factors that determine whether cancer cells survive, persist, and result in death. This includes the nature of the tumor and the host response.

The importance of the immune system in anticancer activity is clearly demonstrated in immunocompromised patients who have an increased susceptibility to tumor formation. This is especially true of tumors with a viral etiology.

Clinical cancer pathology

Tumor markers are increasingly being used for prognostic and management decision processes. These are products derived from the tumor that can be found in the blood and used for diagnosis, assessing response to treatment, and detecting recurrence. Examples include the CA 125 ovarian tumor marker, the prostate specific antigen (PSA) marker in prostate carcinoma, and the α-fetoprotein in testicular teratoma. Pathology reports of resected tumors contain macroscopic and microscopic descriptions that give information about the size and type of a cancer, local invasion, and lymph node metastasis. The grade of a tumor is based on morphological study (proliferation, differentiation, pleomorphism) and indicates tumor differentiation, or likelihood of metastasis. Staging is used to determine how advanced a tumor is clinically. For example, colorectal tumors can be staged by the Dukes classification (A–C/D). The TNM (tumor size, lymph node spread, metastasis formation) system is used to stage many tumors. For an example of the TNM system refer to p. 93 for the staging of lung cancer.

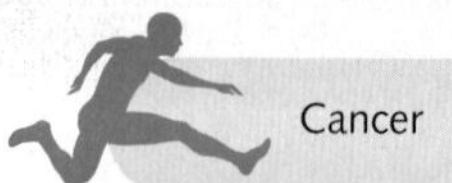

- Define tumor.
- Define dysplasia and metaplasia.
- List the types of benign and malignant tumors.
- Explain the behavioral and structural differences between malignant and benign tumors.
- What are the three most common cancers in males and females?
- How have geographic and environmental factors influenced the prevalence of various types of tumor?
- What are proto-oncogenes and tumor suppressor genes?
- Why is apoptosis important in tumorigenesis?
- Describe the process of tumor growth and angiogenesis, invasion, and metastasis.
- Describe the host defenses against cancer.

3. Inflammation, Tissue Damage, and Repair

Inflammation

Definition
Inflammation is the response of living tissues to cellular injury. It involves both innate and adaptive immune mechanisms.

Purpose
The purpose of inflammation is to localize and eliminate the causative agent, limit tissue injury, and restore tissue to normality.

Inflammation can be divided into two types: acute and chronic. The division of inflammation is based on the time course and cellular components involved. These categories are not mutually exclusive, and some overlap exists (Fig. 3.1).

Causes of acute inflammation
The causes of acute inflammation are:

Physical agents (e.g., trauma, heat, cold, ultraviolet light, radiation).

Irritant and corrosive chemical substances (e.g., acids, alkalis).

Microbial infections (e.g., pyogenic bacteria).

Immune-mediated hypersensitivity reactions (e.g., immune-mediated vasculitis, seasonal allergic rhinitis (hay fever)).

Tissue necrosis (e.g., ischemia resulting in a myocardial infarction).

Causes of chronic inflammation
Chronic inflammation usually develops as a primary response to:

- Microorganisms resistant to phagocytosis or intracellular killing mechanisms (e.g., tuberculosis (TB), leprosy).
- Foreign bodies—endogenous (bone, adipose tissue, uric acid crystals) or exogenous (silica, suture materials, implanted prostheses).
- Some autoimmune diseases (e.g., Hashimoto's thyroiditis, rheumatoid arthritis, contact hypersensitivity reactions).
- Primary granulomatous diseases—Crohn's disease, sarcoidosis.

Chronic inflammation can occur secondary to acute inflammation due to the persistence of the causative agent. Fig. 3.2 shows the sequelae of inflammation.

Acute inflammation

Classic signs of acute inflammation
The classic signs of acute inflammation are:

- Redness (rubor).
- Heat (calor).
- Swelling (tumor).
- Pain (dolor).
- Loss of function (functio laesa).

These classic signs are caused by a rapidly developing vascular response and cellular events characteristic of acute inflammation.

The main function of these events is to bring elements of the immune system to the site of injury and prevent further tissue damage.

Vascular response

Widespread vasodilation (hyperemia)
Normally, blood flow to the capillary bed is limited by the precapillary sphincters. In acute inflammation, a phase of vasodilatation occurs when the arterioles and precapillary sphincters relax. This results in increased blood flow to the injured area and increased hydrostatic pressure.

Increased vascular permeability
Endothelial intracellular proteins, such as actin, contract under the influence of chemical inflammatory mediators, such as histamine, bradykinin, nitric oxide, and leukotriene B4. Endothelial contraction results in:

- Increased fenestrations (i.e., transient gaps) between endothelial cells.
- Increased permeability of vessels to plasma proteins.

Proteins leak out of the plasma into the interstitial spaces, leading to a decrease in the plasma oncotic

Comparison of acute and chronic inflammation		
	Acute inflammation	**Chronic inflammation**
Response	Immediate reaction of tissue to injury	Persisting reactions of tissue to injury
Onset	Rapid	Slow response
Immunity	Innate	Cell-mediated
Predominant cell type	Neutrophil	Lymphocytes, plasma cells, macrophages
Duration	Hours–weeks	Weeks/months/years
Vascular response	Prominent	Less important

Fig. 3.1 Comparison of acute and chronic inflammation. Note that the acute and chronic categories are not mutually exclusive.

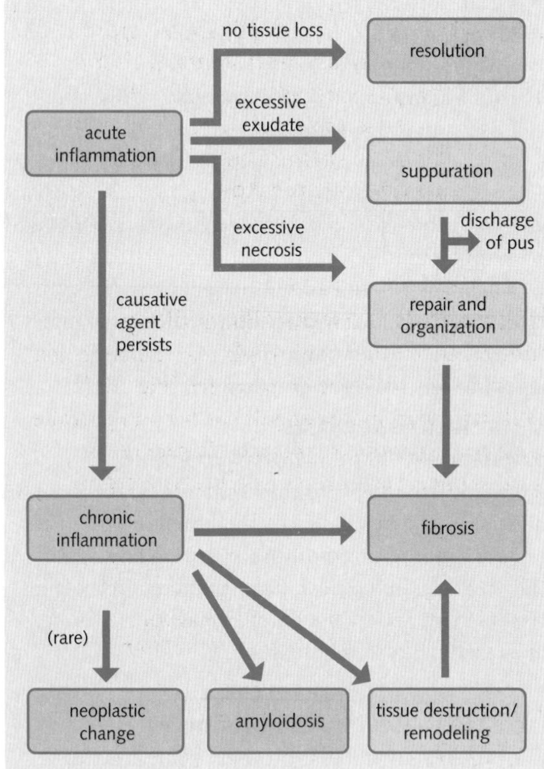

Fig. 3.2 Sequelae of inflammation.

pressure. The protein rich fluid is an exudate. The protein present in the exudate includes immunoglobulins, and coagulation factors.

Inflammatory edema

The combined increase in hydrostatic pressure (from hyperemia) and the decreased oncotic pressure (from leakage of proteins into interstitial spaces) causes net fluid movement from plasma into tissues; this is inflammatory edema. As a result, blood viscosity is increased and blood flow rate is decreased.

Advantages of inflammatory edema

Fluid increase in the damaged tissue dilutes and modifies the action of toxins. Protein levels increase in the tissue—these include protective antibodies and fibrin. Nonspecific antibodies act as opsonins for neutrophil-mediated phagocytosis and function to neutralize toxins. The formation of a fibrin net acts as a scaffold for inflammatory cells, preventing the spread of microorganisms. Circulation of the exudate into the lymphatic system assists in the development of a specific heightened immune response.

Cellular events

Neutrophils pass between endothelial cell junctions and invade damaged tissue to combat the effects of injury.

There are four stages (Fig. 3.3):

1. Margination of neutrophils to the plasmatic zone (Fig. 3.4). This is assisted by the slowing of the blood (blood cells flow nearer to the vessel wall in the plasmatic zone than the axial stream).
2. Adhesion of neutrophils ("pavementing")—leucocytes adhere to the vascular endothelium at sites of acute inflammation. Increased adhesion results from the interaction of paired molecules on the leukocyte and endothelial cell surface (i.e., β_2-integrin and ICAM-1).
3. Emigration of neutrophils—leukocytes pass between the endothelial cell junctions by amoeboid movement through the venule wall into tissue spaces (diapedesis).

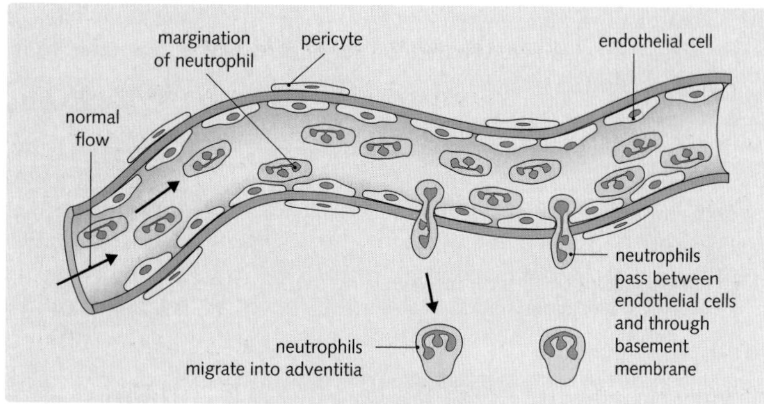

Fig. 3.3 Cellular events in acute inflammation. Neutrophils are the predominant cell type of acute inflammation. They reach the injured tissues by margination, adhesion, and emigration.

increased plasma viscosity (due to loss of intravascular fluid) → decreased blood flow → cells fall out of axial stream into plasmatic zone (margination)

Fig. 3.4 Mechanism of margination of neutrophil polymorphs.

The predominant cell type of acute inflammation is the neutrophil. Lymphocytes, plasma cells, and macrophages are the cells found in chronic inflammation.

4. Chemotaxis of neutrophils—neutrophils are attracted toward, and possibly activated by, chemical substances (chemotaxins) released at sites of tissue injury. These chemotaxins are thought to be leukotrienes, complement components, and bacterial products.

Phagocytosis and intracellular killing

At the site of injury, neutrophils and monocytes ingest debris and foreign particles (Fig. 3.5). Cellular pseudopodia engulf the foreign particle and fuse to produce a phagocytic vacuole or phagosome. Phagocytosis is often assisted by

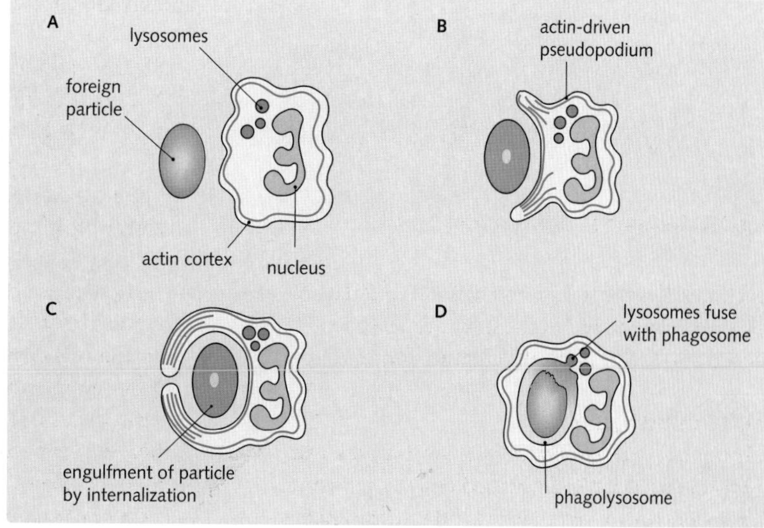

Fig. 3.5 Phagocytosis of foreign particle by leucocyte. (A) Attachment of foreign particle. (B) Pseudopodia engulfing particle. (C, D) Incorporation within the cell in a vacuole called a phagosome.

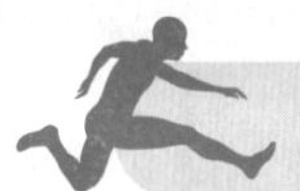

opsonization of the microorganism with immunoglobulins and complement components.

Following phagocytosis, leukocytes attempt to destroy phagocytosed material by:

- Discharge of lysosomal enzymes into the phagosome.
- Oxygen-dependent mechanisms such as H_2O_2, O_2^-, $\cdot OH$.
- Oxygen-independent mechanisms such as lactoferrin, lysozyme, and hydrolases.

Chemical mediators of inflammation

There are several different inflammatory mediator systems, all of which interact together to produce inflammation, but no single chemical mediator can be responsible for any single feature of inflammatory response.

Regulatory mechanisms exist in all mediator systems.

The complement system

This is a cascading sequence of serum proteins, made up of more than 20 proteins; the activated product of one protein activates another (Figs 3.6 and 3.7). The complement system can be activated in four ways during the acute inflammatory response.

- Necrotic cells release enzymes capable of activating complement.
- Antibody–antigen complexes activate complement through the classical pathway.
- Gram-negative bacterial endotoxins activate complement through the alternative pathway.
- Products of the kinin and fibrinolytic systems activate complement.

Kinins

Kinins are small vasoactive peptides (about 10 amino acids). Bradykinin is the most well known, and it exerts its effects by increasing vascular permeability

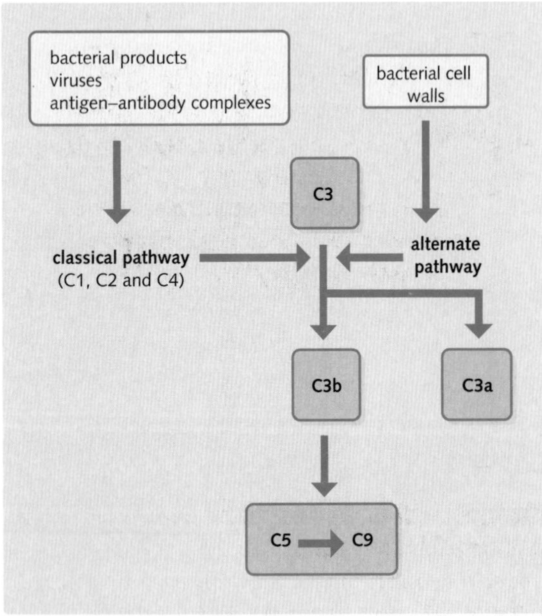

Fig. 3.6 Simplified version of the complement cascade showing how the activated product of one protein activates another.

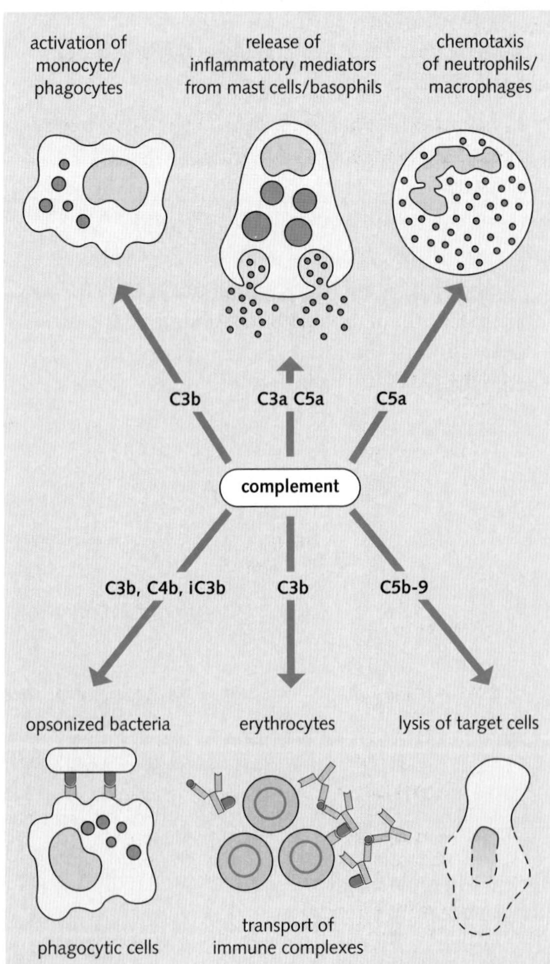

Fig. 3.7 The major functions of the complement system.

and producing pain. Both effects are cardinal features of acute inflammation.

The kinin system is activated by activated coagulation factor XII.

Arachidonic acid, prostaglandins, and leukotrienes

During acute inflammation, the membrane phospholipids of neutrophils and mast cells are metabolized to form prostaglandins and leukotrienes (Fig. 3.8).

The anti-inflammatory action of drugs (e.g., glucocorticoids, aspirin, and aspirin-like drugs) is attributable to their ability to inhibit prostaglandin production.

Platelet activation factors

Platelet activation factors are released from mast cells and neutrophils during degranulation. They have the following effects:

- Induce platelet aggregation and degranulation.
- Increase vascular permeability.
- Induce leukocyte adhesion to the endothelium.
- Stimulate synthesis of arachidonic acid derivatives.

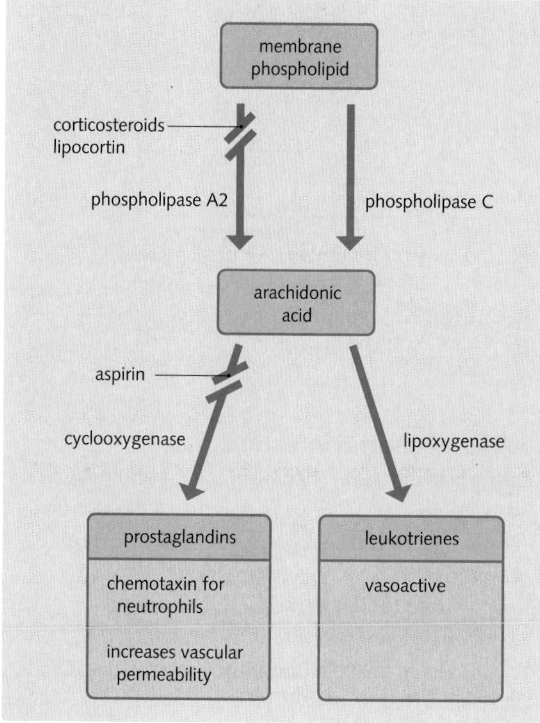

Fig. 3.8 Formation of arachidonic acid and its metabolites.

Cytokines

Cytokines are a family of chemical messengers released by activated T lymphocytes and macrophages, e.g., interleukin-1 (IL-1), interleukin-8 (IL-8) and tumor necrosis factor α (TNFα). They act over short distances (autocrine and/or paracrine) by binding specific receptors on target cell surfaces. They include:

- Lymphokines—cytokines produced by lymphocytes.
- Monokines—cytokines produced by monocytes/macrophages.
- Interleukins—cytokines which act between leukocytes (more than 15 types).
- Interferons—inhibit replication of viruses within cells and activate macrophages and natural killer (NK) cells.
- Growth factors.
- Tumor necrosis factors—kill tumor cells, but also stimulate adipose and muscle catabolism leading to weight loss.

Acute-phase proteins

Proteins whose serum level dramatically increases during inflammation are called acute-phase proteins. These proteins are produced by the liver and induced by circulating levels of IL-1 (e.g., the C-reactive protein).

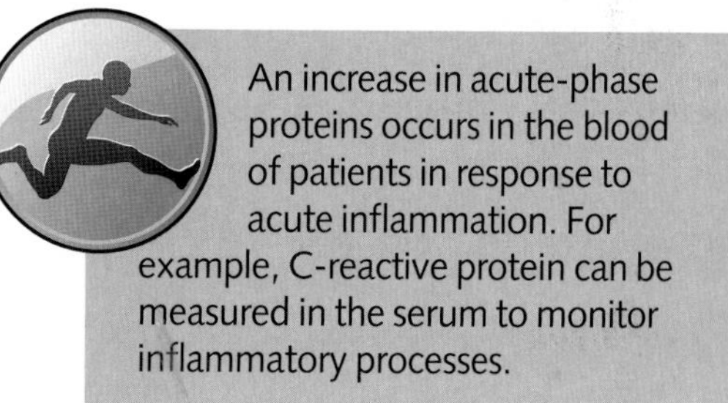

An increase in acute-phase proteins occurs in the blood of patients in response to acute inflammation. For example, C-reactive protein can be measured in the serum to monitor inflammatory processes.

Chronic inflammation

Mononuclear infiltration and granulation tissue

The cells involved in chronic inflammation are shown in Fig. 3.9. The site of chronic inflammation is dominated by:

- Lymphocytes.
- Plasma cells (for antibody production).

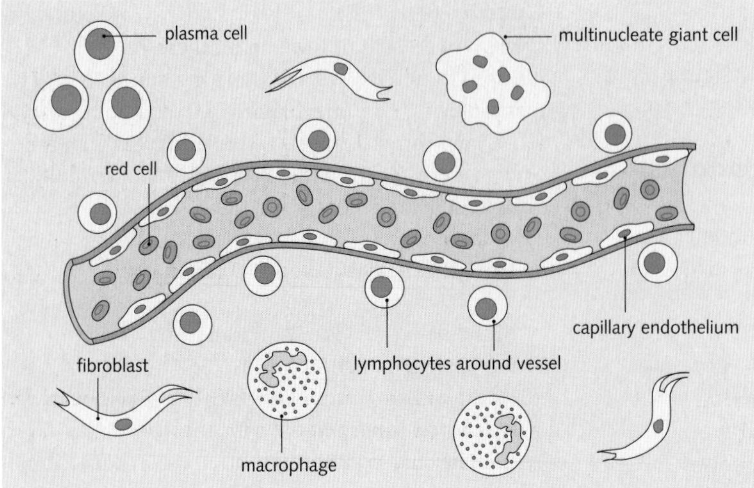

Fig. 3.9 Cells involved in chronic inflammation are lymphocytes, plasma cells, and macrophages. Intercellular communication exists between these cell types.

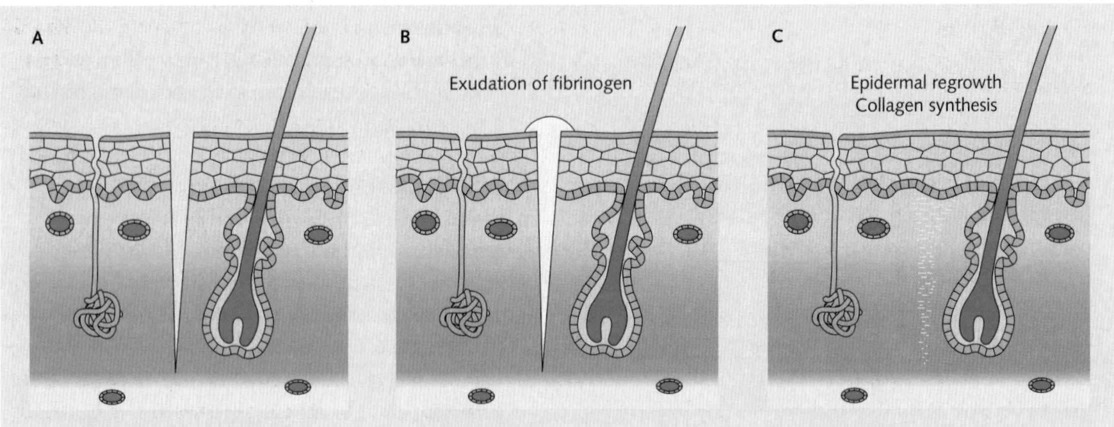

Fig. 3.10 Skin incision healed by first intention. (A) Incision. (B) Weak fibrin join. (C) Strong collagen join.

- Macrophages (for phagocytosis). Some macrophages fuse to form multinucleate giant cells.

Damaged tissue is gradually removed by macrophages. It is slowly replaced by granulation tissue, which consists of new capillaries and new connective tissue formed from fibroblasts and the collagen that they secrete.

Wound healing

The ultimate consequence of tissue injury depends on many factors. For example, only labile or stable cells can be replaced. Permanent cells such as nerve cells have little or no effective regeneration ability. In addition, complex tissue architecture may not be replaced. The process of wound healing in the skin depends on the size of the injury, and it occurs by two mechanisms.

Healing by first intention

Apposed wound margins are joined by fibrin deposition, which is subsequently replaced by collagen and covered by epidermal growth (Fig. 3.10), e.g., surgical incision wound.

Healing by second intention

Healing by second intention (Fig. 3.11) involves the following:

- Wound margins are unapposed, due to extensive tissue damage.
- Tissue defect fills with granulation tissue.
- Epithelial regeneration to cover surface.
- Granulation tissue eventually contracts, resulting in scar formation (due to the action of myofibroblasts, specialized fibroblasts capable of contraction).

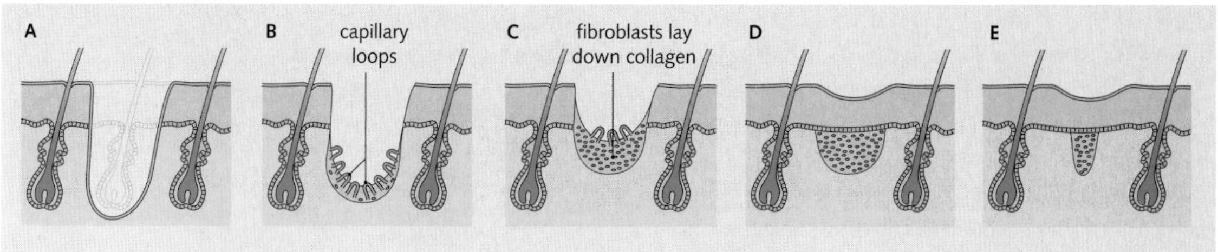

Fig. 3.11 Skin wound repaired by second intention. (A) Loss of tissue. (B) Granulation tissue. (C) Organization. (D) Early fibrous scar. (E) Scar contraction.

Wounds are healed by either first or second intention healing processes. The type of healing process depends on the extent of tissue damage:

- Minimal tissue loss—involves healing by first intention.
- Extensive tissue loss—involves healing by second intention.

Scar formation

Myofibroblasts within granulation tissue are attached to one another and to adjacent extracellular matrix. Their contraction draws together the surrounding matrix and thus reduces the size of the defect.

Patterns of inflammation

Fibrinous inflammation

Fibrinous inflammation is the deposition of increased amounts of fibrin on the tissue's surface, e.g., in acute pleurisy secondary to acute lobar pneumonia. Presence of fibrin tends to inhibit resolution.

Suppurative inflammation

Suppurative inflammation is characterized by the production of pus. It is usually caused by infection with pyogenic bacteria such as *Staphylococcus aureus* and *Streptococcus pyogenes*. Pus becomes surrounded by a "pyogenic membrane" of sprouting capillaries, neutrophils, and fibroblasts.

There are two types of suppurative inflammation: superficial (e.g., a boil) and deep-seated (e.g., an abscess within tissue).

Hemorrhagic inflammation

If damage is severe, blood vessels within the area may rupture (e.g., hemorrhagic pneumonia, meningococcal septicemia).

Granulomatous inflammation

Granulomatous inflammation is a form of chronic inflammation in which modified macrophages (epithelioid histiocytes) aggregate to form small clusters or granulomas surrounded by lymphoid cells. It usually occurs in response to the presence of indigestible particulate matter within macrophages. Causes of granulomatous inflammation include:

- Microorganisms resistant to intracellular killing mechanisms (e.g., *Mycobacterium tuberculosis* and *M. leprae*).
- Foreign bodies—endogenous (e.g., bone, adipose tissue, uric acid crystals); exogenous (e.g., silica, suture materials, implanted prostheses).
- Idiopathic (e.g., in Crohn's disease and sarcoidosis).

Granulomas are aggregates of epithelioid (pink, like epithelial cells) histiocytes, but commonly they contain multinucleate giant cells—Langhans' giant cell, foreign body giant cell, and Touton giant cell—formed either from the fusion of many macrophages or by nuclear division without cytoplasmic separation.

Commonly confused terms. A granuloma is an aggregation of epithelioid histiocytes, and it is a feature of some chronic inflammatory diseases. Granulation tissue is a combination of capillary loops and fibroblasts, and it is a wound-healing phenomenon.

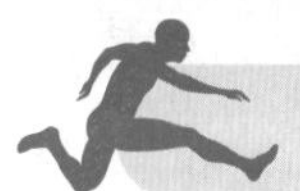

Ulceration

Ulcers are formed when the surface of an organ or tissue is lost because of necrosis and replaced by inflammatory tissue. The most common sites are the alimentary canal and the skin.

Chronic ulceration is a balance between tissue damage (e.g., by gastric acid) and tissue repair by the body's healing response (i.e., the chronic inflammatory response).

Systemic effects of inflammation

Both acute and chronic inflammation can produce a number of systemic effects including:

- Pyrexia; polymorphs and macrophages produce pyrogens, which act on the hypothalamus.
- Constitutional symptoms—malaise, nausea, and anorexia.
- Weight loss—occurs in severe chronic inflammation such as TB.
- Reactive hyperplasia of the mononuclear phagocyte system—enlargement of local and systemic lymph nodes.
- Hematological changes—increased erythrocyte sedimentation rate and leukocytosis.

Tissue necrosis

Cell death

Cells may be damaged either reversibly (sublethal damage) or irreversibly (lethal damage) (Fig. 3.12). The type of damage depends on:

- Nature and duration of injury.
- Type of cells affected.
- Regenerative ability of tissues.

Note that there are no absolute ultrastructural criteria by which reversible and irreversibly cellular injury may be distinguished, and that there is a continuum from reversibly injured cell through to irreversibly necrotically damaged cell.

Necrosis

Necrosis is the death of cells or tissues that are still part of the living organism. Necrosis is a pathological process following cellular injury, which results in an inflammatory response following loss of the integrity of the plasma membrane.

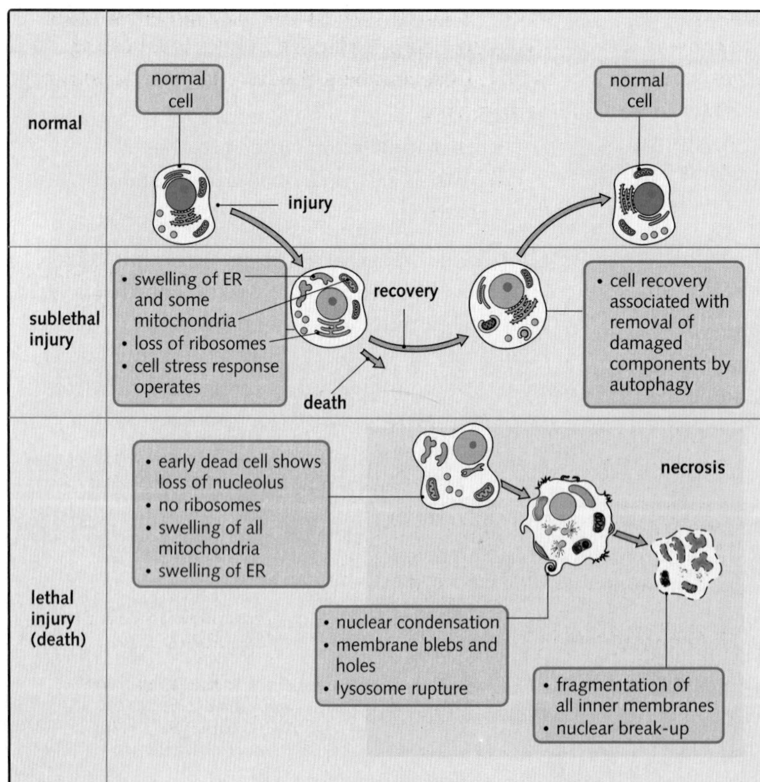

Fig. 3.12 Relationships between sublethal and lethal cell damage. Sublethal damage can be repaired and the cell survives. Lethal cell damage is irreversible and results in cell death. Types of cellular injury include mechanical trauma, loss of membrane integrity, inhibition of metabolic pathways, DNA damage, and deficiency of essential metabolites.

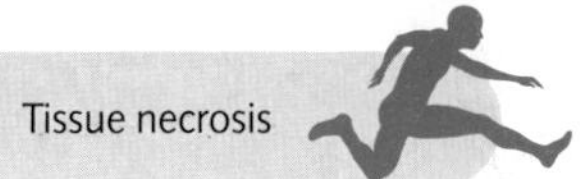

Regardless of the cause of cell death, necrosis is the result of:

- Depletion of intracellular energy systems.
- Disruption of cytoplasmic organelles.
- Liberation of intracellular enzymes.
- Production of oxygen free radicals.
- Disintegration of nucleus.
- Alterations and failure of the plasma membrane.
- Alteration in ionic transport mechanisms.
- Increased permeability of membrane phospholipids.
- Physical disruption of the plasma membrane, which can seen under the light microscope.

Mechanisms of cell death

The initiating mechanisms of cell death depend on the type of injury and are summarized in Fig. 3.13.

Histological types of necrosis

Coagulative necrosis

This is the most common form of necrosis, characteristically occurring in the heart, kidney, and spleen, but it may occur in most tissues.

Dead tissue is initially swollen and firm, but later it becomes soft as a result of digestion by macrophages. Dead cells retain "ghost" outlines, and the necrotic area is highly eosinophilic.

It usually evokes an inflammatory response; damaged tissue is removed by phagocytosis and repaired or regenerated.

Liquefactive necrosis

This characteristically occurs in the brain due to minimal supporting stroma. Necrotic neural tissue undergoes near total liquefaction, and a glial reaction occurs around the periphery with eventual cyst formation.

Caseous necrosis (caseation)

This is commonly seen in TB. Histologically, the complete loss of normal tissue architecture is replaced by amorphous, granular, and eosinophilic debris. There are variable amounts of fat and an appearance reminiscent of cheese, hence the term caseation.

Gangrene

Necrotic tissue produced by coagulative necrosis is invaded by putrefactive organisms, notably clostridia. The tissue appears green or black because of the breakdown of hemoglobin. This is known as "wet" gangrene.

Dry gangrene

An example is ischemic necrosis of the toes, which is common in diabetic people with gradual arterial occlusion. The putrefactive process is very slow, and the small numbers of putrefactive organisms are insignificant.

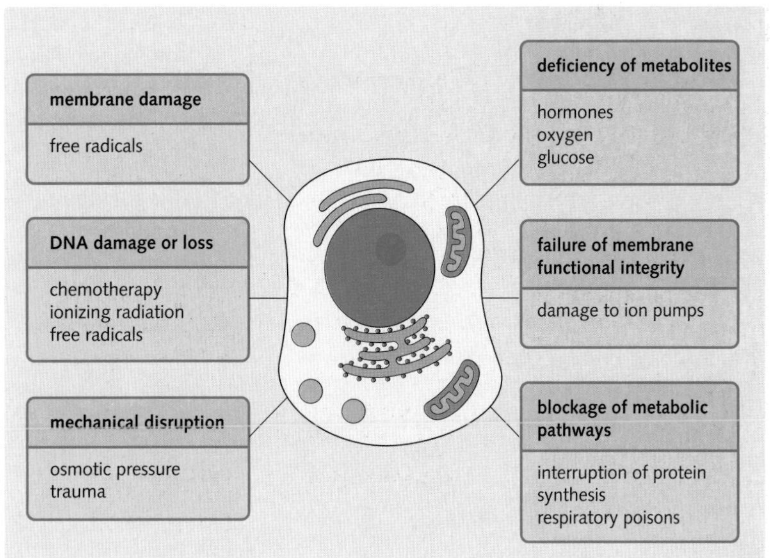

Fig. 3.13 Mechanisms of cell death. Various cell and tissue types are differentially susceptible to various injurious agents (e.g., the cellular response to ischemia).

Gas gangrene

This is a primary infection of necrotic tissue by *Clostridium perfringens* resulting in putrefactive necrosis and the formation of methane gas by the bacteria. Surgical debridement is required.

Fibrinoid necrosis

This occurs in malignant hypertension, where increased arterial pressure results in necrosis of the smooth muscle wall of the artery. Plasma leaks into the media with consequent deposition of fibrin, hence fibrinoid necrosis. The histological appearance of the vessel wall is strongly eosinophilic.

Fat necrosis

Adipose tissue damage may be due to:

- Direct trauma—release of triglycerides following trauma elicits a rapid inflammatory response. Necrotic fat cells are phagocytosed by neutrophils and macrophages, which ultimately results in fibrosis.
- Enzymatic lipolysis—in acute pancreatitis, lipases liberated from damaged acini act on fat cells in the peritoneal cavity as depicted in Fig. 3.14.

Insoluble calcium salts appear as whitish chalky areas scattered within otherwise normal adipose tissue.

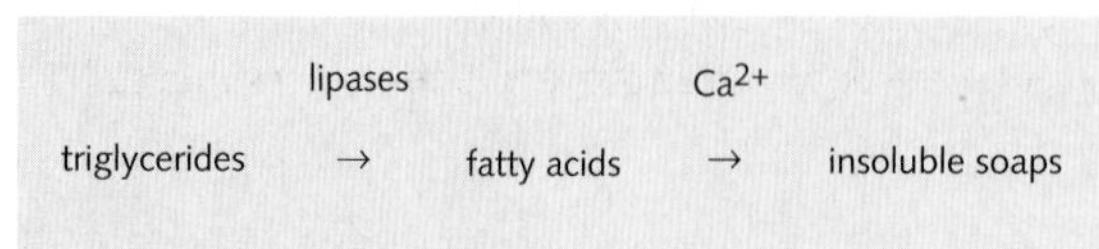

Fig. 3.14 Enzymatic lipolysis.

Apoptosis

Apoptosis is an energy-dependent mechanism of cell death for the deletion of unwanted individual cells; it is also known as "programmed cell death." Inhibition of apoptosis results in cell accumulation, e.g., neoplasia, whereas increased apoptosis results in cell loss (e.g., atrophy).

Apoptosis can be either physiological (i.e., associated with the maintenance of organ size in adults and organ development and remodelling in the embryo) or pathological (i.e., in response to irrepairable DNA damage, thereby permitting the perpetuation of a genetically abnormal cell).

A key point. Apoptosis is an energy-dependent process that results in individual cell death, usually without an inflammatory response. This is in contrast to necrosis, an energy-independent process that involves the death of many cells and may cause inflammation.

Stages of apoptosis

The process of apoptosis occurs in the following four stages:

Priming

This is the synthesis of enzymes needed to cause cell dissolution, e.g., proteases and nucleases. There are no structural cellular changes.

Enzyme activation

Endonucleases cleave chromatin, resulting in DNA fragmentation. Proteases degrade the cytoskeleton, resulting in cell shrinkage. The plasma membrane and organelles remain intact.

Fragmentation of the cell

The cell is fragmented into apoptotic bodies. Each fragment contains viable mitochondria and intact organelles. The presence of intact plasma membranes around apoptotic bodies explains the absence of any inflammatory response.

Phagocytosis

Apoptotic fragments are phagocytosed and destroyed by adjacent cells. Surrounding cells then move together to fill vacant space.

A comparison of cell death by apoptosis and necrosis is given in Fig. 3.15.

Fig. 3.15 Comparison of cell death by necrosis and apoptosis.

Comparison of cell death by necrosis and apoptosis

Feature	Necrosis	Apoptosis
Induction	Pathological conditions	Pathological or physiological conditions
Number of cells	Groups of cells	Single cells
Plasma membrane	Loss of membrane integrity	Membrane remains intact
Morphology	Cell swelling and lysis	Cell shrinkage and fragmentation, formation of characteristic apoptotic bodies
Inflammation	Inflammatory response	No inflammatory response
Fate of cells	Phagocytosed by neutrophils and macrophages	Phagocytosed by neighboring cells
Biochemical mechanism	Energy-independent Loss of ion homeostasis	Energy-dependent Endonuclease activity

- Describe the mechanisms of acute inflammation: vascular response and cellular events.
- What are the chemical mediators of inflammation?
- Describe the mechanisms of chronic inflammation.
- Briefly describe wound healing by primary and secondary intention, and scar formation.
- What are the patterns of inflammation seen in TB infection, acute pleurisy and *Staphylococcus aureus* infection?
- What are the key differences between acute and chronic inflammation?
- Tissue necrosis—describe the mechanisms of cell death, the differences between sublethal and lethal cell injury.
- What are the histological types of necrosis?
- Compare and contrast necrosis and apoptosis.
- Distinguish between granuloma and granulation tissue.

4. Infectious Disease

General principles of infection

Infection and colonization

Infectious diseases are a common cause of morbidity and mortality. The prevalence of infectious diseases varies considerably between developed and developing nations. The burden of specific diseases depends on the quality of the drinking water, sanitation, health-care system, and social and climatic conditions.

Infection is the invasion and proliferation of microorganisms in the tissues of the body. This usually follows the successful breach of host barriers and immune defense mechanisms.

Infectious agents can be transmitted in the following ways:

- Human to human (horizontal and vertical transmission, i.e., person to person or mother to fetus).
- Animal to human (zoonoses).
- Environment to human (airborne, water, fomites).
- Medical institution to patient (nosocomial).

Following invasion, infective organisms can spread to distant tissue sites by:

- Local spread.
- Lymphatic spread.
- Hematogenous spread.
- Dissemination in the tissue fluid.
- Neural spread.

Colonization is the inhabitation of the external body surfaces—the skin, gastrointestinal (GI) tract, external genitalia, and vagina—by microorganisms. This generally occurs soon after birth. These organisms may invade and cause infection (disease).

Koch's postulates

To establish that a given disease has an infective cause, the postulates stated by the German bacteriologist Robert Koch (1843–1910) must be fulfilled. These are:

- The infectious agent should be found in all cases of the disease, and in parts of the body affected by the disease.
- The infectious agent associated with the disease can be isolated from the lesions of an infected person and grown in artificial culture media.
- The cultivated infectious agent can reproduce the disease upon inoculation of a member of the same species.

Be aware that there are certain diseases to which one or more of these criteria cannot be applied but which can still be confidently attributed to a particular organism. For example, *Treponema pallidum* is the cause of syphilis, but it cannot be grown in artificial culture.

Pathogens and commensals

Pathogens are microorganisms that have mechanisms to invade and cause infection. Commensals are those microorganisms that constitute the normal flora of a healthy body. They do not normally cause disease, and they are often advantageous to the host by the production of nutrients such as B_{12} and by the exclusion of harmful bacteria. For example, the normal commensal flora of the gut prevent the colonization by pathogenic bacteria.

The distinction between commensals and pathogens is not absolute. Many commensals are potential pathogens; that is, they are harmless only so long as they are kept at bay by the host's defense mechanisms.

Other microorganism characteristics

Pathogenicity

Pathogenicity is the capacity of a particular microorganism to cause disease.

Virulence

Virulence is the degree of pathogenicity of a microorganism measured by the severity of the ensuing

Classification of major pathogens					
	Viruses	**Bacteria**	**Fungi**	**Protozoa**	**Helminths and ectoparasites**
Size	20–300nm	0.1–5µm	2–10µm	2–100µm	0.5–35cm
Pro- or eukaryote	Neither	Prokaryote	Eukaryote	Eukaryote	Eukaryote
Nucleic acid	DNA or RNA	DNA + RNA	DNA + RNA	DNA + RNA	DNA + RNA
Replication	Intracellular	Intra- and/or extracellular	Intra- and/or extracellular	Intra- and/or extracellular	Extracellular
External cell wall	No	Yes (usually): peptidoglycan	Yes: right chitin	No	No
Reproduction	Assembly	Binary fission	Binary fission and sexually	Binary fission and sexually	Sexually

Fig. 4.1 Classification of major pathogens.

infection. Microorganisms are said to be highly virulent if a small number of microbes can cause severe disease.

Opportunistic infection

Opportunistic infection is an infection by organisms of low pathogenicity, usually due to impaired host immune responses. Opportunistic infections are common in immunocompromised patients such as those with a primary or second immunodeficiency (e.g., children with SCID, patients infected with human immunodeficiency virus (HIV), and transplant patients using immunosuppressive drugs such as cyclosporin A).

Deficiency of specific immune defenses predisposes individuals to characteristic patterns of infection. For example the T cell-deficient disease, DiGeorge syndrome, results in chronic viral, fungal, and intracellular bacterial infections.

Categories of infectious agent

The main infectious agents of man are the viruses, bacteria, fungi, protozoa, helminths, and ectoparasites. Figure 4.1 shows the classification of the major pathogens.

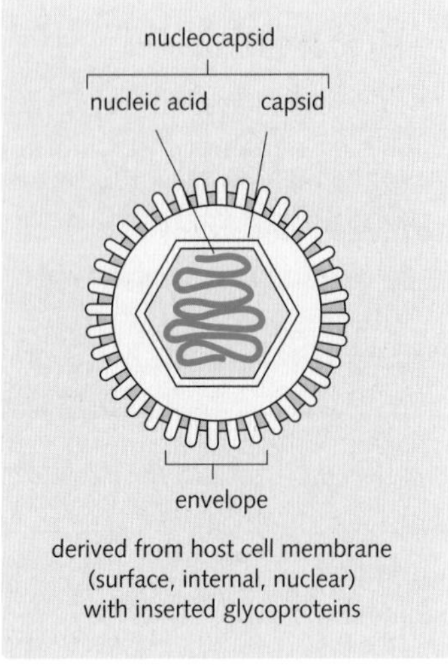

Fig. 4.2 Structure of an enveloped virus.

Viruses

Viruses carry nucleic acids, but they lack synthetic machinery, therefore, they can only replicate within the host cell, i.e., they are obligate intracellular parasites (Fig. 4.2).

Viruses have the following characteristics:

- They consist of a nucleic acid core and protein coat (capsid), which together constitute the nucleocapsid.
- Some, but not all, viruses are enveloped by the membrane of host cell origin.
- Morphology is icosahedral, helical, or complex.
- Classification is usually based on type of nucleic acid (Fig. 4.3).

Fig. 4.3 Classification of viruses based on nucleic acid type.

Classification of viruses based on nucleic acid type		
Virus type	**Mode of replication**	**Examples**
DNA viruses	Utilize host cell polymerases for mRNA synthesis Can remain in infected cell and establish persistent infections (latent, immortalizing viruses)	Herpes simplex virus Varicella-zoster virus Adenovirus Papillomavirus
RNA viruses	Encode their own replicative enzymes for formation of more mRNA (Host enzymes cannot replicate RNA)	Measles virus Mumps virus Influenza virus Rabies virus Poliovirus
Retroviruses (RNA)	Contain "reverse transcriptase" enzyme for production of viral DNA Viral DNA is inserted into host genome	HIV I and II HTLV I and II

Pathogenesis of cell injury

Viruses produce tissue injury by:

- Direct cytopathic effect.
- Induction of an immune response.
- Incorporation of viral genes into the host genome.

The harmful effects of viral infections include cell death, acute and chronic tissue damage, triggering of an autoimmune response, and transformation of cells to form tumors.

Virus infections can be detected by a variety of methods:

- Direct detection of the virus by electron microscopy.
- Observed specific cellular cytopathic effects (CPE).
- Detection of viral proteins by immunofluorescence techniques.
- Detection of host produced antiviral antibodies by enzyme-linked immunosorbent assay (ELISA).
- Detection of viral nucleic acid by polymerase chain reaction (PCR).

Bacteria

Bacteria are prokaryotes with a single circular DNA chromosome. Bacteria are divided into two broad groups—gram-positive and gram-negative—based on their reaction to the Gram stain (a staining procedure used with light microscopy).

Differential staining is obtained because of inherent differences in the structures of bacteria's cell walls. Not all bacteria stain using the Gram method. For example, *Mycobacterium tuberculosis* requires the use of a special staining technique—acid-fast stain.

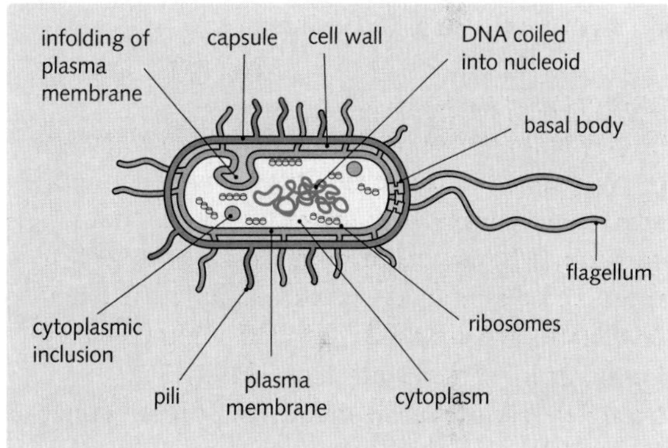

Fig. 4.4 Generalized structure of a bacterium.

Further classification is based on practical characteristics (i.e., size, shape, respiration and reproduction, and the analysis of biochemical and immunological criteria). A generalized structure of a bacterium is shown in Fig. 4.4, and an example of the characteristics used to classify bacteria is shown in Fig. 4.5.

Pathogenic effects of bacteria are due to endotoxin and exotoxin release. These toxins produce acute and chronic inflammation and tissue damage.

Bacterial infections can be diagnosed from a number of different samples obtained from the

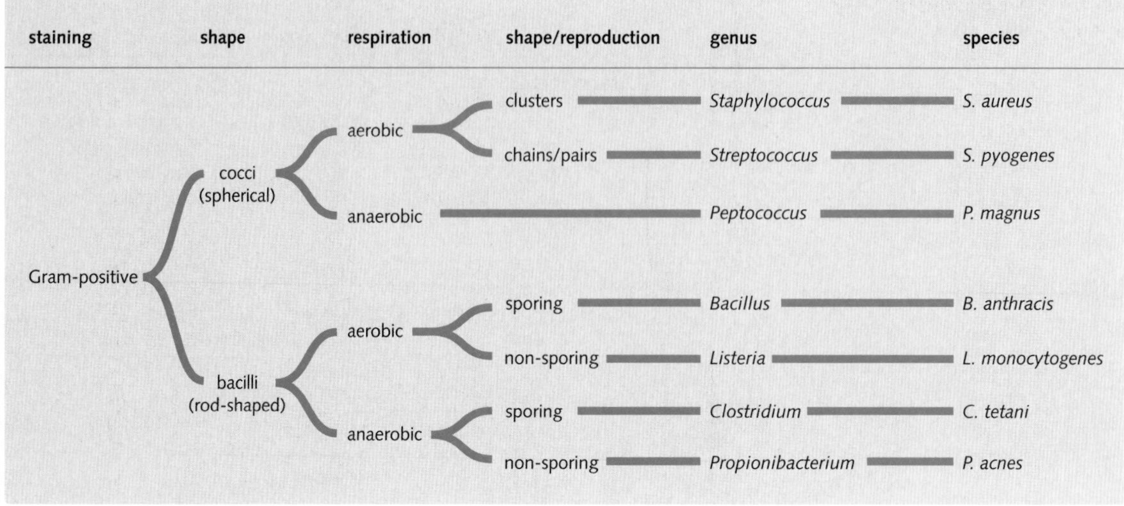

Fig. 4.5 The characteristics used to classify bacteria, using Gram-positive bacteria as an example.

Classification of fungi		
Yeast-like form	**Hyphal form**	**Dimorphic form**
single, rounded cells multiply by budding, e.g., *Candida albicans*, *Cryptococcus neoformans*	branching filaments interlaced to make mycelium or mould produce spores hyphae may be several hundred mm in length, e.g., *Aspergillus fumigatus*, dermatophytes	can assume either yeast or hyphal form depending on environment, e.g., *Histoplasma capsulatum*, *Blastomyces dermatitidis*

Fig. 4.6 Classification of fungi.

patient. These include blood, feces, urine, cerebral spinal fluid, and tissue taken from infected wounds. Samples will generally be cultured to determine the species of bacteria and their resistance to an array of antibiotics.

Fungi

Fungi are unicellular, multicellular or multinucleate organisms (Fig. 4.6). They are eukaryotes, but contain ergosterol instead of cholesterol in their plasma membranes.

Fungi have a well-defined cell wall composed of polysaccharides and chitin; they can be moulds, yeasts, or dimorphic.

Fungal infections are either superficial (e.g., involving the skin, hair, nails, and mucus membranes) or systemic (e.g., involving the lungs, brain, or heart). Such opportunistic fungi as *Aspergillus*, *Candida*,

Fig. 4.7 Main divisions of protozoa.

Main divisions of protozoa			
Sporozoa	**Flagellates**	**Amoebae**	**Ciliates**
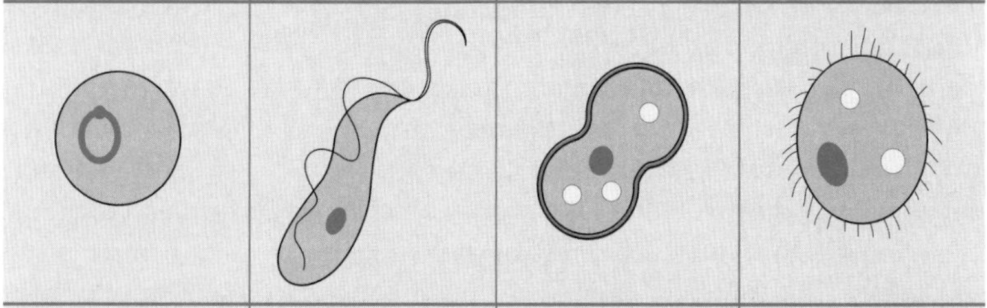			
all are intracellular parasites, e.g., Plasmodium in red blood cells	move by beating one or more flagella, e.g., Trypanosoma	move by extending pseudopodia; they have no fixed shape, e.g., Entamoeba	move by beating many cilia, e.g., Balantidium

Fig. 4.8 Main groups of helminths (parasitic worms).

Main groups of helminths (parasitic worms)		
Nematodes (roundworms)	**Cestodes (tapeworms)**	**Trematodes (flukes)**
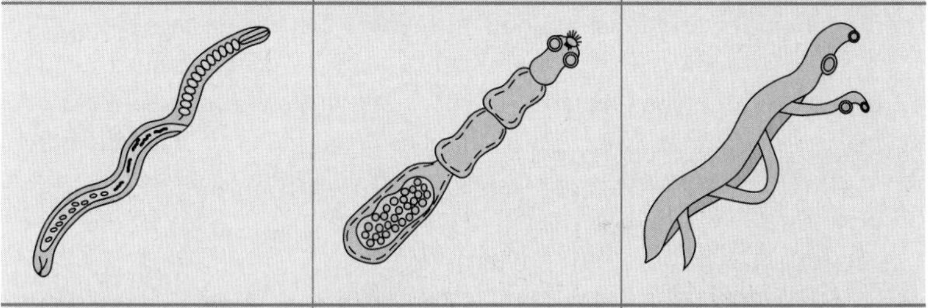		
resistant cuticle; longitudinal muscles; complete digestive system; separate sexed reproductive system, e.g., *Ascaris lumbricoides*, *Strongyloides stercoralis*	cellular epithelium; no digestive system; all hermaphrodites, e.g., *Taenia solium*, *Echinococcus granulosus*	cellular epithelium; circular and longitudinal muscles; incomplete digestive system; mostly hermaphrodites, e.g., *Schistosoma*

and *Cryptococcus* may infect immunocompromised hosts.

Mycotoxins are toxins produced by some fungi. For example, *Aspergillus flavus* proliferates on food stored in warm humid conditions and produces the mycotoxin, aflatoxin. Ingestion of food contaminated with aflatoxins in humans causes an increased risk of hepatocellular carcinoma.

Skin scrapings and tissue biopsies are often the specimens used to try and diagnose mycoses.

Protozoa

Protozoa are unicellular eukaryotes that may develop into cysts in harsh environmental conditions. The main divisions of protozoa are shown in Fig. 4.7. The most important protozoal disease worldwide is malaria, which is caused by the *Plasmodium* species.

Identification of protozoa often occurs by microscopy of patient specimens. Specimens include feces, blood, and tissue. Culture methods are not routinely applied for identification purposes.

Helminths and ectoparasites

Helminths are a group of parasitic worms, as shown in Fig. 4.8. Ectoparasites (e.g., bed bugs, crab louse, fleas, etc.) are parasites that live on the outer surfaces of the host.

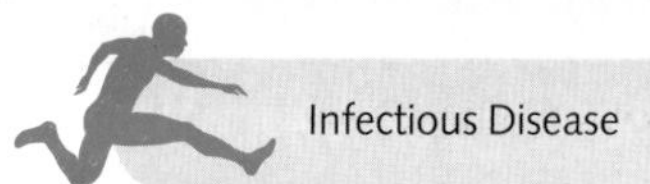

Microscopy of patient specimens (feces, blood, tissue) allows the identification of most helminths and ectoparasites.

Prions

Prions are an abnormal isoform of a normal host protein. Prions are not microorganisms but are "infectious" proteins that are highly resistant to decontamination methods such as standard autoclaving or disinfectants. They were formerly classified as "slow viruses" because of their long incubation time. Humans express normal prion proteins, but their function is largely unknown. However, if an abnormal prion protein is inoculated into a normal host, conformational changes are induced in the normal host prions (prp), resulting in their conversion to abnormal host prions (prp*).

These abnormal host proteins then induce further conformational changes in remaining normal host prions. Thus, the original inoculated prion protein is able to catalyse a chain reaction in which host proteins become conformationally abnormal. Interestingly, there is no evidence of inflammation, immune reaction, or cytokine release in the infected host.

The net result is the formation of amyloid plaques of prion protein in the CNS. These plaques result in vacuolar spongiform degeneration of neuronal processes with neuronal loss and glial proliferation.

In humans, two forms of prion protein disease exist—kuru ("laughing death") and Creutzfeldt–Jakob disease—which are always fatal, usually within 6 months. The degenerative neurological disease Creutzfeldt–Jakob disease (new variant form) occurs in people under the age of 50. The consumption of offal contaminated with bovine spongiform encephalopathy (BSE, "Mad Cow") has recently been implicated in its etiology.

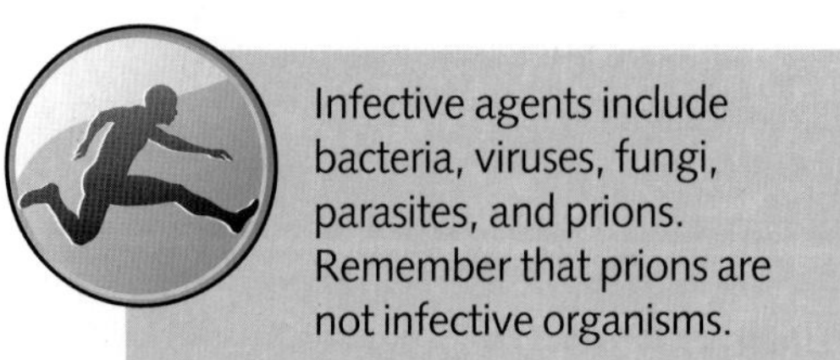

Infective agents include bacteria, viruses, fungi, parasites, and prions. Remember that prions are not infective organisms.

Mechanisms of pathogenicity

Host defenses and routes of entry

The majority of infectious agents encountered by an individual are prevented from entering the body by a variety of biochemical and physical barriers (Fig. 4.9). For example, anatomical barriers such as the skin, mucus membranes, GI tract, and genitourinary tract provide a physical environment of unfavorable growth conditions for bacteria.

Further host defense is provided by the innate and adaptive immune mechanisms. Innate immunity consists of non-specific mechanisms that contribute to resistance and recovery from infection. Innate immunity includes soluble proteins (complement, acute phase proteins), immune cells (macrophages, neutrophils, NK cells) and receptors (Toll-like receptors). Adaptive immunity is specific and includes cellular immunity (cytotoxic and helper T cells) and humoral immunity (B cells). Adaptive immunity is characterized by antigen specificity and clonal proliferation. In addition, the generation of immunological memory initiates a heightened response to subsequent antigen exposure.

However, despite these defenses, pathogenic microorganisms possess efficient mechanisms for attaching to, and often penetrating, the body surfaces where they proliferate and disseminate. If they are to be transmitted to a fresh host, the microorganisms must also exit from the body.

The different routes of entry and exit of microorganisms are outlined in Fig. 4.10.

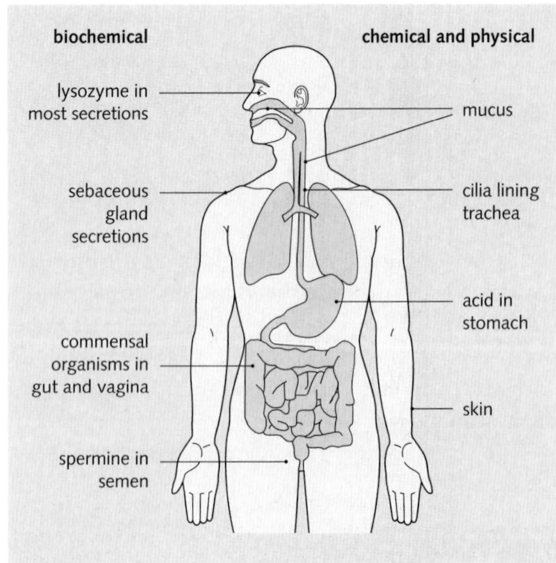

Fig. 4.9 Exterior host defenses.

Virus infections

Viral replication cycles

Figure 4.11 outlines two types of viral replication cycles.

DNA viruses have their own DNA, and they use the host's cellular machinery to make more DNA, protein, and glycoprotein. These are then reassembled into new virus particles prior to release from the cell.

RNA retroviruses first make viral DNA using viral "reverse transcriptase." Viral DNA is then inserted into the host genome prior to its transcription to form mRNA. Viral RNA is in turn translated into viral protein, which is packaged together with the RNA into new virus particles and released.

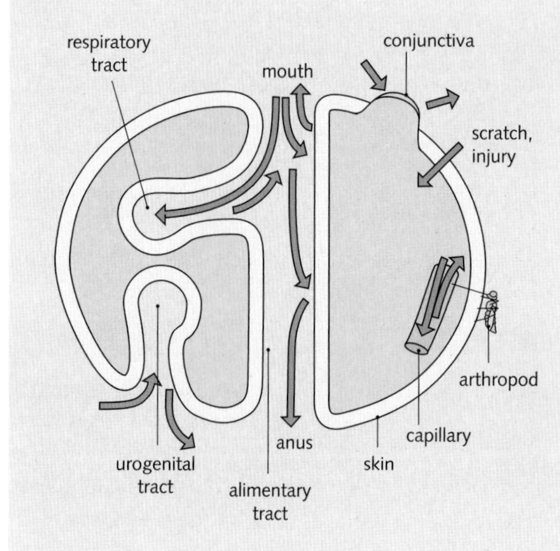

Fig. 4.10 Routes of entry and exit of microorganisms.

Release of new virus particles

Cell lysis (cytolysis)

Nonenveloped viruses (e.g., adenoviruses) are released directly into the extracellular environment by lysis of the host cell; their mode of release results in the death of the cell.

Budding

Enveloped viruses (e.g., HIV and herpesvirus) are released by "budding" from the host cell membrane, thus:

- Nucleocapsid proteins are inserted into the host cell membrane.
- Modified area of host cell membrane extends out from cell surface, and is pinched off (i.e., budded) from the host cell enclosing the new viral particle.
- Mechanism does not cause the death of the cell, and so viral replication can continue.

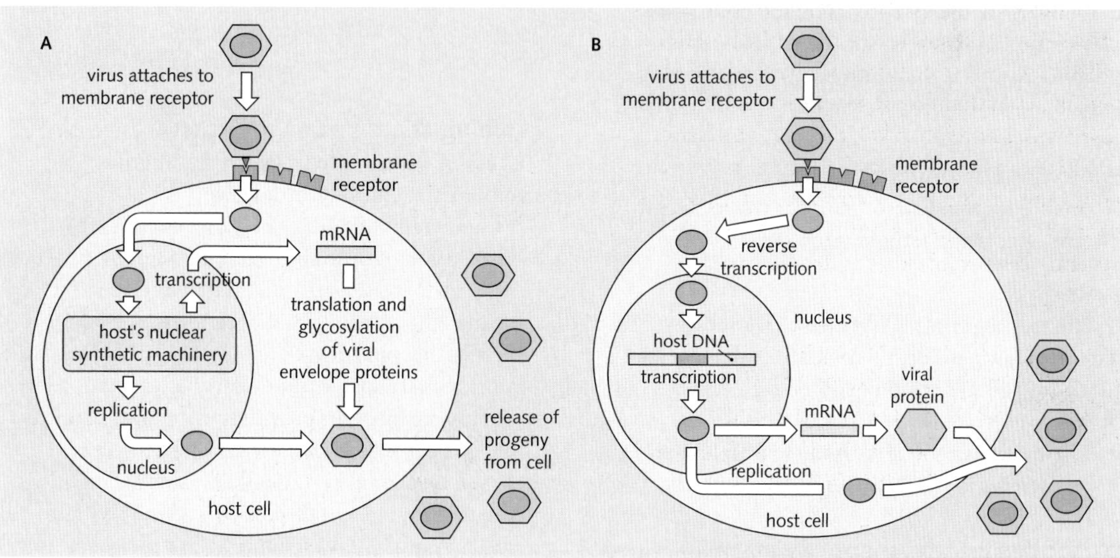

Fig. 4.11 Viral replication cycles. (A) DNA virus—DNA viruses have their own DNA. The viruses use the host's cellular machinery to make more DNA, protein, and glycoprotein. These are then reassembled into new virus particles prior to release from the cell. (B) RNA retrovirus—RNA retroviruses first make viral DNA using viral "reverse transcriptase." Viral DNA is then inserted into the host genome prior to its transcription to form mRNA. Viral RNA is in turn translated into viral protein, which is packaged together with the RNA into new virus particles and released.

Immune reaction to virally infected cells

Cytotoxic T cells kill virally infected cells as follows:

- Virally infected cells express viral peptides bound to MHC class I on their cell surfaces.
- Cytotoxic T cells (T_C) recognize viral antigen via the T cell receptor.
- T_C cells secrete cytolysins, which results in the lysis of the virally infected cells.

NK cells can do the same, but less effectively. The activity of these cells is enhanced by interferons produced by T_C and T_H cells. Interferons also prevent adjacent cells from becoming infected by intercellular viral transport.

Bacterial infections

Adherence

Certain bacteria are able to adhere specifically to epithelial cells by means of pili (also called fimbriae), which are slender processes on the surfaces of some bacteria. Pili are coated with recognition molecules called adhesins. Specific interactions between adhesins of pili and molecules on the surface epithelial cells enable the bacterium to adhere to the host cell membranes.

Pili are more common in Gram-negative bacteria, although a few Gram-positive bacteria also possess them. Recent research has shown that some individuals are more susceptible to certain types of infection. It has been suggested that certain polymorphisms in cell surface glycoproteins result in increased binding with the bacteria adhesins.

Exotoxins and endotoxins

Toxins are responsible for many of the local and distant effects of bacterial infection.

Exotoxins

Exotoxins are proteins secreted externally by bacteria which are highly toxic to the host. The modes of action of some exotoxins are considered below:

- Enzymatic lysis (e.g., α-toxin (phospholipase C) of *Clostridium perfringens* breaks down host cell membranes).
- Pore forming (e.g., α-toxin of *Staphylococcus aureus* disrupts host cell membrane by pore formation).
- Inhibiting protein synthesis (e.g., diphtheria toxin).
- G protein hyperactivating (e.g., cholera toxin).
- Affecting synaptic transmission at neuromuscular junctions (e.g., tetanus and botulinum toxins).

Treating exotoxin with formaldehyde or high temperatures can denature the toxin, forming toxoids, which can be useful for vaccination.

Endotoxins

Endotoxins are integral parts of bacterial cell walls, normally released only when the bacterium dies. They are typically lipopolysaccharides contained within the cell walls of Gram-negative bacteria.

These endotoxins induce toxic effects due to their potent activation of:

- The complement cascade, causing inflammatory damage.
- The coagulation cascade, causing disseminated intravascular coagulation.
- Tumor necrosis factor and IL-1 released from leukocytes, causing fever.

In overwhelming infections, the patient is said to suffer from endotoxic shock with fever, hypotension, and cardiac and renal failure.

Aggressins

Aggressins are bacterially produced enzymes that act predominantly in the local tissue environment. Aggressins include enzymes such as coagulase, streptokinase, and collagenases. These enzymes facilitate the growth and proliferation of the bacteria.

Avoiding death by phagocytosis

Successful parasites have evolved numerous ingenious antiphagocytic devices:

- Phagocyte killing (e.g., via exotoxin release).
- Prevention of opsonization. The microbe produces protein that prevents interaction between opsonizing antibody and phagocyte.
- Preventing phagocyte contact. Some bacteria have an external capsule of polysaccharide, which gives a slimy surface and provides protection against phagocytosis (e.g., *Streptococcus pneumoniae*).
- Protection against intracellular death. This allows the microorganism to survive within the phagocyte as follows: inhibition of phagosome and lysosome fusion (e.g., mycobacteria), escape of microbe from phagolysosome into cytoplasm, resistance to killing by antioxidant production (e.g., mycobacteria, brucella, and *Salmonella typhi*).

Antibiotic resistance and plasmids

Many bacteria are resistant to antibiotics. Resistance is conferred by genes that encode bacterial enzymes that block the effect of an antibiotic. These genes are not usually contained within the bacterial genome, but rather they are contained within extrachromosomal DNA termed "plasmids." These plasmids are capable of self-replication and they can be transferred from bacterium to bacterium.

Antibiotic-susceptible bacteria (those lacking plasmid conferring antibiotic resistance) can acquire plasmids from resistant bacteria and so gain antibiotic resistance. These newly resistant forms are then differentially selected under antibiotic treatment, the non-resistant bacteria being deleted from the population.

Mechanisms of antibiotic resistance include:

- Prevention of the drug entering the bacteria.
- Enzyme inactivation.
- Alteration of the target site.
- Efflux resistance where the antibiotic is pumped out of the bacteria.

Hospital-acquired infection (nosocomial infection) occurs in up to 10% of uninfected admitted patients. It is thought to be the direct cause of 5000 deaths per year, and it contributes to a further 15,000 deaths. An important antibiotic resistant bacteria is methicillin-resistant *S. aureus* (MRSA), which is a common cause of hospital associated sepsis.

Resistance to antibiotics can be transferred between bacteria by conjugation, transduction, and transformation.

Inflammatory responses to infection

Suppurative polymorphonuclear inflammation

This is characterized by the production of pus, such as in a boil, which is usually caused by infection with pyogenic bacteria (e.g., *Staphylococcus aureus, Streptococcus pyogenes*).

Chronic inflammation and scarring

This is caused by persisting reactions of tissue to injury, and it occurs over weeks, months, or even years. The cell-mediated immune response is characterized by lymphocytes, plasma cells, and macrophages.

Granulomatous mononuclear inflammation

This is a form of chronic inflammation in which modified macrophages—epithelioid cells—aggregate to form small clusters or granulomas surrounded by lymphoid cells. It occurs in response to the presence of microorganisms within macrophages that are resistant to intracellular cell killing (e.g., *Mycobacterium tuberculosis* or *M. leprae*).

Necrotizing inflammation

Gangrene

In gangrene, necrotic tissue is invaded by putrefactive organisms, notably clostridia. Tissue appears green or black because of the breakdown of hemoglobin.

- Define infection, colonization, pathogen, and commensals.
- What are the criteria for Koch's postulates of disease?
- What are the categories of infectious agents, their key features, and main differences?
- How are viral infections diagnosed?
- What type of infectious agent are prions?
- Describe the host's defences against invasion and microbial routes of entry.
- Describe the mechanisms of viral infection and pathogenicity, and the immune responses of the host.
- What are endotoxins and exotoxins?
- Describe the mechanisms of bacterial antibiotic resistance.
- Outline the inflammatory responses to infection.

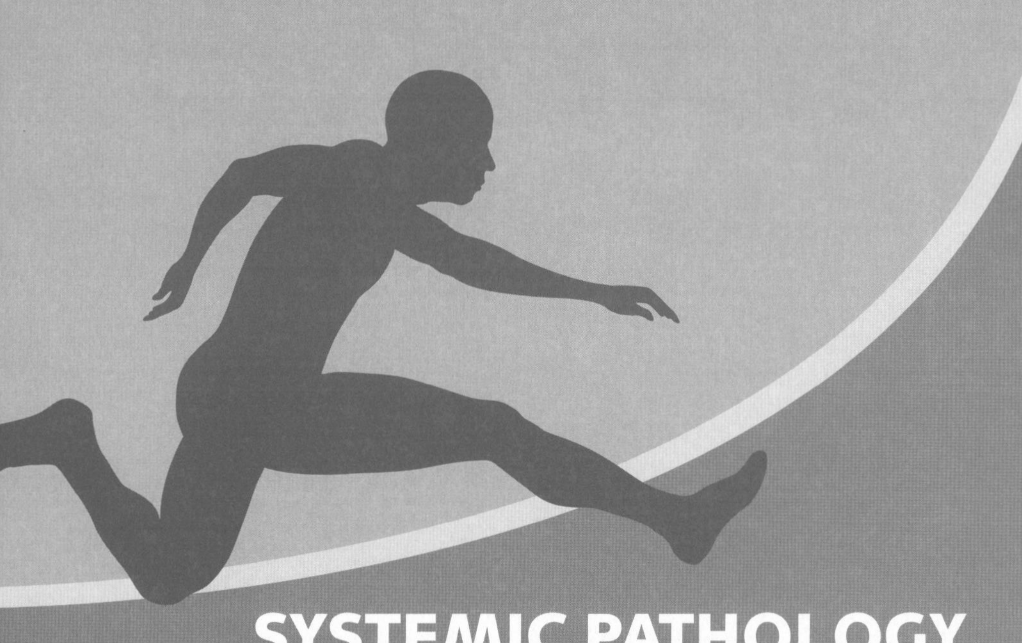

SYSTEMIC PATHOLOGY

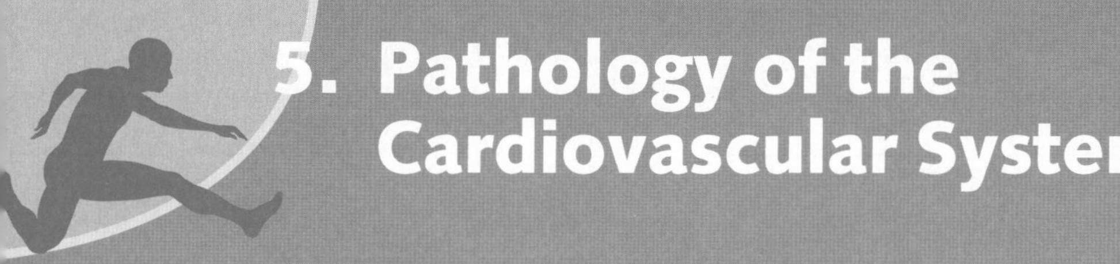

5. Pathology of the Cardiovascular System

Congenital abnormalities of the heart

Overview

Congenital heart abnormalities are relatively common, affecting about 8 per 1000 live births.

Causes

Sporadic

These are the majority of cases. No teratogenic factors can be identified.

Maternal factors

There is an increased incidence associated with certain maternal factors, including:

- Maternal rubella infections.
- Chronic alcohol abuse.
- Intrauterine radiation.
- Drugs such as thalidomide.

These factors are of greatest importance between the fourth and ninth week after conception.

Genetic or chromosomal abnormalities

These are associated with an increased incidence of congenital heart malformations. An example of this is Down syndrome.

Clinical features

Most cardiac abnormalities become apparent at or shortly after birth usually by some manifestation of heart failure such as cyanosis, breathlessness, feeding difficulties, or a failure to thrive.

Types

Congenital heart defects may be divided into two main groups depending on whether the lesions cause:

- Abnormal shunting of blood between the two sides of the heart—either left-to-right shunts, which are more common because of higher pressure in the left side of the heart; or right-to-left shunts caused by an increased resistance to blood moving on from the right side of the heart.
- Obstruction to blood flow.

Left-to-right shunts

These are malformations that result in the shunting of blood from the left side of the heart to the right; they are the most common group of congenital heart abnormalities. Shunting is from left to right because of the higher pressures in the left side of the heart. These defects are not associated with clinical cyanosis as the blood does not bypass the lungs.

Figure 5.1 lists the prevalence of left-to-right shunts.

Ventricular septal defect

This defect of the interventricular septum is the most common cardiac abnormality, accounting for approximately 25–30% of all cases of congenital heart disease (Fig. 5.2). The interventricular septum can be divided into a membranous (fibrous) portion and a muscular portion.

Most congenital defects are perimembranous, i.e., occurring at the junction of the membranous and muscular portions.

There are small and large defects:

- Small defects—often confined to the tiny membranous area.
- Larger defects—also involve the muscular wall of the septum.

The size and site of the defect determines the extent of shunting of the blood from left to right. Defects may present as cardiac failure in infants, or as a murmur in older children or adults.

Physical signs include:

- Pansystolic murmur: caused by flow from the high-pressure left ventricle to the low-pressure right ventricle during systole.
- Tachypnea.
- Indrawing of the lower ribs on inspiration.

Management—Small defects need no treatment and often close spontaneously. Larger defects are associated with persistent cardiac failure, and so need surgical repair.

Atrial septal defect

This is a common congenital heart defect, affecting females more than males by 2:1. There is a defect of

Prevalence of left-to-right shunts	
Type	**% of all CHD abnormalities**
Ventricular septal defect	25–30
Atrial septal defect	10–15
Patent ductus arteriosus	10
Atrioventricular septal defect	5

Fig. 5.1 Prevalence of left-to-right shunts. (CHD, congenital heart disease.)

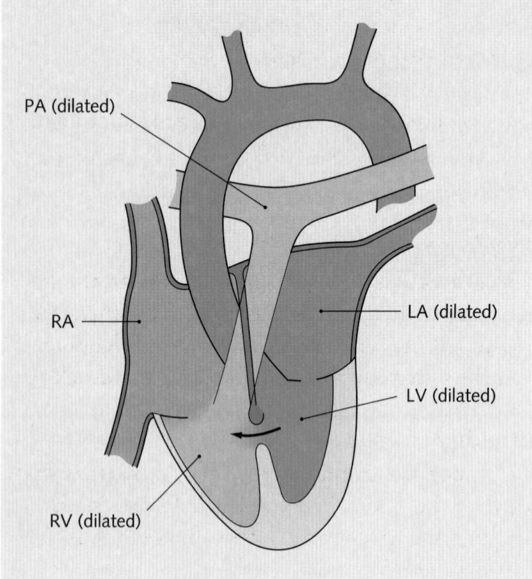

Fig. 5.2 Ventricular septal defect. Larger defects involve the septal muscle but smaller defects may be confined to the maladie de Roger (tiny membranous region).

the interatrial septum causing chronic shunting to the right with gradual enlargement of the right side of the heart and of the pulmonary arteries (Fig. 5.3). The lesion is usually located at the level of the fossa ovalis, which is incompletely closed (ostium secundum defect).

Clinical features—Most children are free of symptoms for many years and the condition is often detected at routine clinical examination or following a chest radiograph. Some children present with dyspnea, chest infections, cardiac failure, or arrhythmia (e.g., atrial fibrillation).

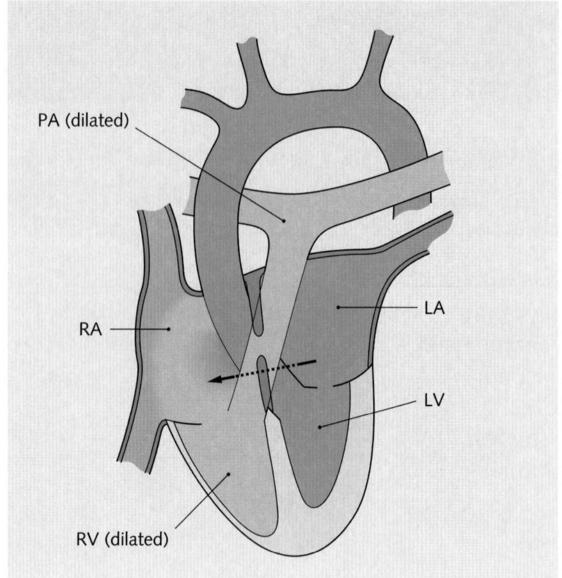

Fig. 5.3 Atrial septal defect. The defect is usually located at the level of the fossa ovalis.

The characteristic physical signs are the result of the volume overload of the right ventricle, as follows:

- Systolic flow murmur over the pulmonary valve.
- Wide splitting of the second heart sound: caused by the delayed closure of the pulmonary valve, which is a result of the increased stroke volume and right bundle branch block.
- Diastolic rumbling murmur due to the increased flow across the tricuspid valve.

Atrial septal defects should be closed surgically. Untreated, right ventricular hypertrophy and pulmonary hypertension inevitably develop, and shunt reversal may eventually occur.

Long-term prognosis following surgical intervention is excellent unless pulmonary hypertension has developed. Pulmonary hypertension and shunt reversal are contraindications to surgery.

Patent ductus arteriosus

This is persistence of an embryological connection between the aorta and the pulmonary trunk (or left main pulmonary artery), as shown in Fig. 5.4. Patent (open) ductus arteriosus occurs in about 10% of all cases of congenital heart disease, affecting females more than males. There is a recognized association with maternal rubella.

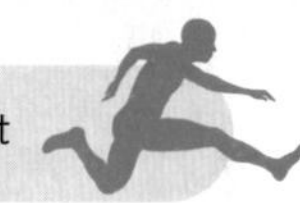

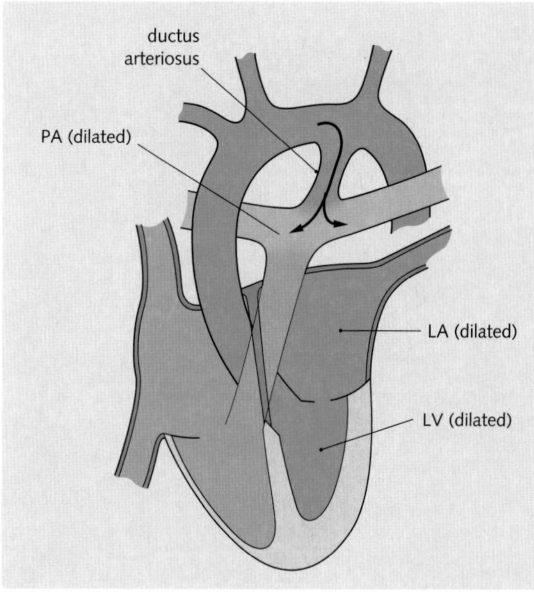

Fig. 5.4 Patent ductus arteriosus. Persistence of the duct is more common in females, and it is associated with maternal rubella.

Understanding the embryonic development of the heart assists in the understanding of congenital abnormalities. For example, the involvement of the septum primum and septum secundum in the development of atrial septal defects.

Embryology

In intrauterine life, the ductus arteriosus allows oxygenated placental blood to flow from the pulmonary artery to the aorta, thereby bypassing the lungs.

At birth, the pulmonary vascular resistance declines, blood is diverted to the lungs for oxygenation and the ductus arteriosus closes within the first few days of life.

However, if the ductus remains patent, blood is continually shunted from the aorta to the pulmonary artery, and as much as 50% of the left ventricular output may be recirculated through the lungs, with a consequent increase in the work of the heart.

Clinical features—The symptoms are proportional to the size of the left-to-right shunt. Small shunts are asymptomatic, whereas larger shunts produce retarded growth and development, with eventual cardiac failure. A continuous "machinery" murmur can be heard, which is loudest at the time of the second heart sound.

A patent ductus arteriosus usually requires surgical treatment in childhood.

Atrioventricular septal defect

This is a septal defect with both an atrial and a ventricular component caused by failure of the endocardial cushions to fuse together. An atrioventricular canal persists resulting in a single heart chamber partially separated by abnormal valve leaflets. This defect is often seen in infants with Down's syndrome.

Right-to-left shunts

Defects leading to permanent right-to-left shunts are less common than left-to-right shunts. The result of a right-to-left shunt is that blood bypasses the lungs to enter the systemic circulation. Cyanosis may develop.

Tetralogy of Fallot

This is the most common cause of cyanosis in infancy (<1 year), occurring in about 1 in 2000 live births. The abnormality consists of four (hence "tetra-") defects (Fig. 5.5):

- Ventricular septal defect.
- Overriding aorta, which sits astride the ventricular septal defect so that it receives blood from both right and left ventricles.
- Pulmonary stenosis, which is usually due to thickening of the subvalvar muscle in the pulmonary outflow tract but sometimes associated with fused stenotic valve cusps.
- Right ventricular hypertrophy.

Etiopathogenesis—Defects are caused by the abnormal embryological development of the bulbar septum, which normally separates the ascending aorta from the pulmonary artery and which aligns and fuses with the interventricular septum.

Pulmonary stenosis leads to inadequate perfusion of the lungs, and the overriding aorta receives blood from both the right and left ventricles. The net result

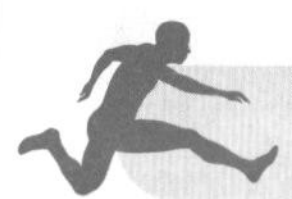

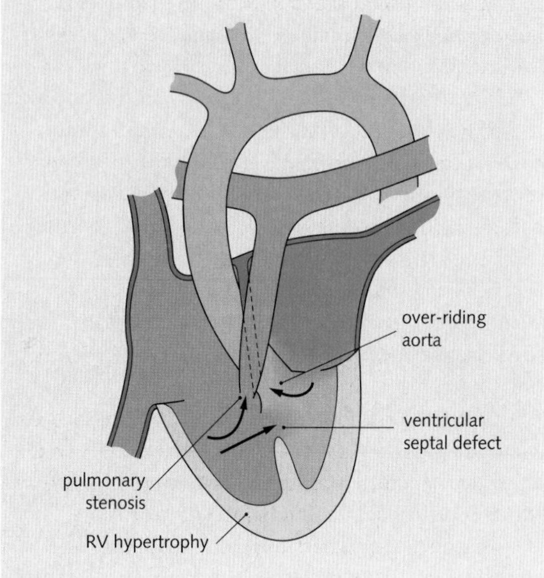

Fig. 5.5 Tetralogy of Fallot is an important cause of right-to-left shunting.

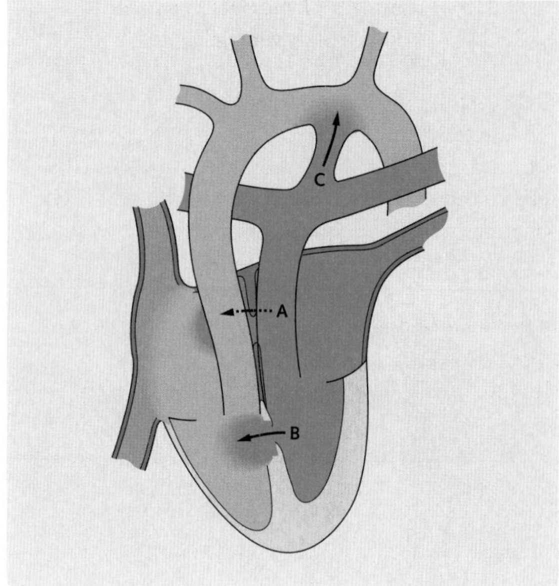

Fig. 5.6 Transposition of the great vessels. Survival is possible only if other shunts are present at either the atrial (A), ventricular (B), or ductus (C) level.

is that the systemic circulation contains deoxygenated blood, causing cyanosis in affected individuals.

Clinical features are:

- Cyanosis—especially after feeding or a crying attack. In older children cyanosis causes stunting of growth, digital clubbing, and polycythemia. Some children characteristically obtain relief by squatting after exertion.
- Loud ejection systolic murmur—either from ventricular septal defect or pulmonary stenosis.

Before the advent of surgical treatment, most patients died well before adult life. Most cases are now surgically corrected by closing the ventricular septal defect, rechannelling the flow into the aorta from the left ventricle only, and relieving the pulmonary stenosis. Complications include bacterial endocarditis, and consequent cerebral infarction or brain abscess.

Transposition of the great vessels

This is a complex malformation in which connections between the right and left ventricle, aorta, and pulmonary artery are disordered—the aorta emanating from the right ventricle, and the pulmonary artery arising from the left (Fig. 5.6).

Postnatal survival is possible only if there is one or more of the following:

- Atrial septal defect.
- Ventricular septal defect.
- Patent ductus arteriosus.

Surgical correction is possible.

Persistent truncus arteriosus

Both the aorta and pulmonary artery develop from a single tube—the truncus arteriosus. Persistence of the truncus is caused by failure of the conotruncal ridges to fuse and to descend toward the ventricles. The result is that the pulmonary artery arises some distance above the origin of the undivided truncus.

Persistent truncus is always accompanied by a defective interventricular septum since the ridges also participate in the formation of the interventricular septum. The undivided truncus, therefore, overrides both ventricles and receives blood from both sides.

Tricuspid atresia

This rare disorder is caused by an absent tricuspid orifice. The defect is always associated with:

- Patent foramen ovale.
- Ventricular septal defect.

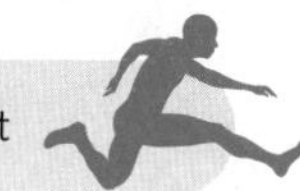

- Underdevelopment of the right ventricle.
- Hypertrophy of the left ventricle.

Blood is shunted first from the right atrium to the left, and then a small proportion is shunted from the left ventricle to the right through ventricular septal defect. Some of the deoxygenated blood enters the systemic circulation resulting in cyanosis.

Surgical correction may be possible.

Total anomalous pulmonary venous connection

Here, pulmonary veins do not open into the left atrium but into either the right atrium, systemic veins, or both. There is always an atrial septal defect resulting in right-to-left shunting with mixing of saturated and desaturated blood in the atria.

The increased pulmonary flow leads to pulmonary vascular disease.

Obstructive congenital defects

Coarctation of the aorta

This is a stenotic narrowing of the aorta, usually located at, or just beyond, the site of the ductus arteriosus (Fig. 5.7). About 50% of affected individuals have an associated bicuspid aortic valve.

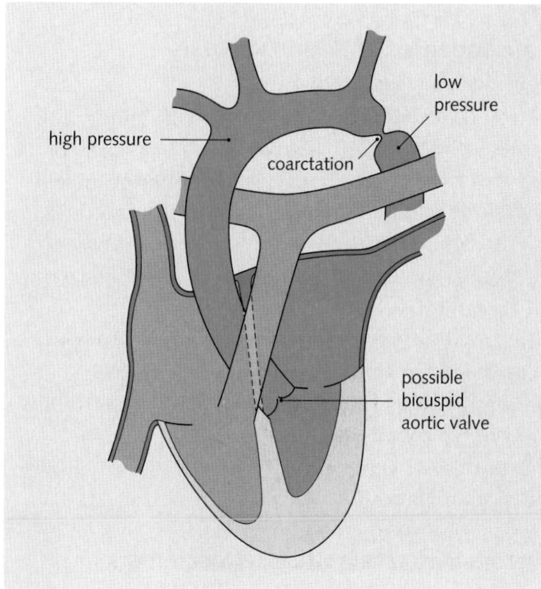

Fig. 5.7 Coarctation of the aorta. Signs and symptoms depend largely on the size of the narrowing.

This defect accounts for up to 5% of all forms of congenital heart disease, and it affects 1 in 4000 live births, male incidence being greater than female by 2:1.

Clinical features—Stricture produces:

- Hypertension proximal to the stenosis, leading to symptoms such as headache and dizziness.
- Hypotension distal to the stenosis, leading to generalized weakness and poor peripheral circulation.

Characteristically, the blood pressure is raised in the upper body but is normal or low in the legs:

- Upper body—abnormally large arterial pulsations may be seen in the neck, and severe hypertension leads to the development of collateral circulations involving pericapsular and intercostal arteries, which become dilated and tortuous, and may be visible or even palpable in older children and adults.
- Lower body—femoral pulses are weak and delayed.

A systolic murmur may sometimes be heard posteriorly over the coarctation. An ejection systolic murmur may be present in the aortic area due to the bicuspid valve.

Pathological complications—In untreated severe cases death may occur in several ways:

- Left ventricular failure, following prolonged hypertension.
- Dissection of the aorta, particularly in patients with associated bicuspid aortic valves.
- Bacterial endocarditis, usually at the site of aortic constriction.
- Cerebral hemorrhage.

A rare variant is the so-called "infantile preductal coarctation," in which there is stenosis of a long segment of the aorta between the left subclavian artery origin and the ductus arteriosus, which remains patent. Systemic circulation to the lower part of the body often depends on a right-to-left shunt through the patent ductus, causing peripheral cyanosis.

Pulmonary artery stenosis or atresia with intact ventricular septum

This presents as a narrowing (stenosis) or fusion (atresia) of the trunk of the pulmonary artery. In atretic cases, the patent foramen ovale forms the only outlet for blood from the right side of the heart. The ductus arteriosus is always patent and represents the only access route to the pulmonary circulation.

Aortic stenosis and atresia

Semilunar aortic valves are stenosed or even atretic. If fusion is complete, the aorta, left ventricle, and left atrium are markedly underdeveloped. This is usually accompanied by an open ductus arteriosus which delivers blood into the aorta. The condition is associated with severe cyanosis.

Figure 5.8 gives a summary of congenital cardiac malformations.

Summary of congenital cardiac malformations

Left-to-right shunts
- ventricular septal defect
- atrial septal defect
- patent ductus arteriosus
- atrioventricular septal defect

Right-to-left shunts
- tetralogy of Fallot
- transposition of the great arteries
- persistent truncus arteriosus
- total anomalous venous connection

Obstructive congenital defects
- coarctation of the aorta
- pulmonary artery stenosis/atresia
- aortic stenosis/atresia

Fig. 5.8 Summary of congenital cardiac malformations.

Atherosclerosis, hypertension, and ischemic heart disease

Definitions and concepts

Arteriosclerosis

This is an imprecise term meaning thickening and loss of elasticity of the arteries caused by any condition.

Atherosclerosis

This is the most common form of arteriosclerosis and is defined below. Atherosclerotic lesions are called atheromas.

The terms "arteriosclerosis" and "atherosclerosis" are often confused. They are not synonymous, and they should not be used interchangeably. Arteriosclerosis is hardening or loss of elasticity of the arteries from any cause, whereas atherosclerosis implies hardening or loss of elasticity due to atheroma.

Most common types of arteriosclerosis

There are many types of arteriosclerosis; three of the most common are outlined below.

Atherosclerosis

A degenerative disease, this involves the intima of large- and medium-sized arteries.

Mönckeberg's medial calcific sclerosis

This degenerative disease affects the media of medium-sized muscular arteries, particularly in the limbs. Calcification of the vessels occurs, but the lumen is not decreased.

Arteriolosclerosis (arteriolar sclerosis)

With thickening of the walls of small arteries and arterioles in response to systemic hypertension, this particularly affects the kidneys, pancreas, gall bladder, small intestine, adrenals, and retina.

Consequences of arteriosclerosis

The consequences are:

- Vessel thickening → narrowing of lumen → poor tissue perfusion.
- Inelasticity of vessels → predisposition to vessel rupture and hemorrhage.
- Alterations in vascular endothelium → increased predisposition to thrombosis.

Arteriosclerosis contributes to the high frequency of cardiac (myocardial infarction, angina pectoris), cerebral (stroke, transient ischemic attack), colonic (malabsorption, ischemic colitis) and peripheral (intermittent claudication, rest pain) diseases in the elderly population.

Factors that accelerate arteriosclerosis

Arteriosclerotic changes, in a mild form, represent the response of the arterial wall to wear and tear, progressing gradually with age. However, certain

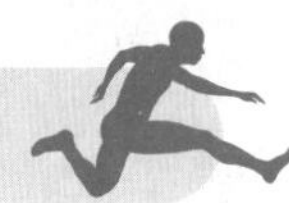

diseases are known to accelerate and aggravate arteriosclerosis (e.g., hypertension and diabetes).

Atherosclerosis

A degenerative disease of large- and medium-sized arteries (but not veins), this is characterized by the focal accumulation of lipid-rich material in the intima of arteries and associated cellular reactions. Although essentially a disease of the tunica intima, atherosclerosis also has an impact on the structure and function of the underlying tunica media.

Atherosclerotic lesions are found to some extent in virtually every adult over the age of 40 as well as in many younger individuals. Its consequences account for half of all deaths in the Western world.

Commonly affected arteries are:

- Aorta (especially the abdominal aorta).
- Coronary arteries.
- Cerebral arteries.
- Common iliac/femoral arteries.

Atherosclerosis is rare in the arteries of the upper limb and in the pulmonary arteries (unless pulmonary hypertension is also present).

Epidemiological studies have identified risk factors associated with atheroma development. These can be broadly classified into:

- Constitutional risk factors, i.e., risk factors inherent to an individual.
- Hard risk factors: direct association with atherosclerosis.
- Soft risk factors: direct association with ischemic heart disease → indirect association with atherosclerosis.

Constitutional risk factors are:

- Age—atherosclerotic lesions increase in number with increasing age.
- Gender—up to the age of 55, males have a higher incidence than females by 2:1, due to the protective effect of estrogens; over 55 years the male to female ratio is equal.
- Familial traits—familial increase in predisposition is often associated with familial hyperlipidemia.
- Race—wide interracial variations exist in the incidence of atheroma, but this may be due to dietary differences. The condition is relatively uncommon in China, Japan, and Africa.

Hard risk factors lead to an increased severity of atherosclerosis:

- Hypercholesterolemia increased serum levels of cholesterol or low density lipoprotein (LDL)—usually diet-dependent but may also occur as a result of some forms of familial hypercholesterolemia. For example, mutation of apoprotein B100 gene on chromosome 2 results in high levels of circulating LDLs. Lipoproteins that contain the apoprotein B100 have been implicated in the transport of cholesterol into artery walls. Polymorphisms in apoprotein E have been linked to polygenic hypercholesterolemia. These patients do not have a familial hypercholesterolemia but have raised serum cholesterol levels. Screening for such individuals is becoming of increasing importance.
- Hypertension—increased blood pressure, especially diastolic blood pressure.
- Diabetes mellitus—probably an effect of hypercholesterolemia.
- Cigarette smoking—there is a strong link between smoking and deaths from coronary artery disease; the mechanism is unclear.

Soft risk factors lead to an increased incidence of ischemic heart disease:

- Lack of exercise—exercise decreases the incidence of sudden death from ischemic heart disease but it is not clear whether it reduces atherosclerosis formation.
- Obesity—this may be a reflection of diet and resultant hyperlipidemia.
- Stress and personality traits—linked to deaths from ischemic heart disease.

Pathogenesis

Pathogenesis of the characteristic lipid plaques, which appear in atherosclerosis, is uncertain; several hypotheses have been proposed:

- Response to injury hypothesis.
- Thrombogenic hypothesis.
- Clonal proliferation hypothesis.
- Lipid infiltration/insudation hypothesis.

Response to injury hypothesis

This is the most widely accepted hypothesis, and it proposes that the first step in formation of the atheromatous plaque, is chronic, low-grade endothelial injury.

Endothelial injury may itself be induced by:

- Cigarette smoking.
- Hypertension.

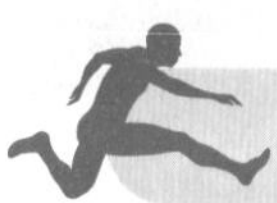

- Hyperlipidemia: direct endothelial damage; promotion of platelet attachment.

Stages of development in atherosclerosis

Atherosclerotic plaques (atheromas) develop as follows:

1. Endothelial injury results in platelet adhesion to damaged endothelium; diffusion of plasma proteins (including LDL) into the intima of arteries; migration of monocytes into the intima of arteries.
2. Platelets release platelet-derived growth factor (PDGF), leading to a proliferation of intimal smooth muscle cells (myointimal cells).
3. Myointimal cells deposit excess collagen and elastin in the intima.
4. Macrophages phagocytose LDL and then release free lipid.

The stages of plaque development are shown in Fig. 5.9. Fig. 5.10 provides a summary of the events involved in the pathogenesis.

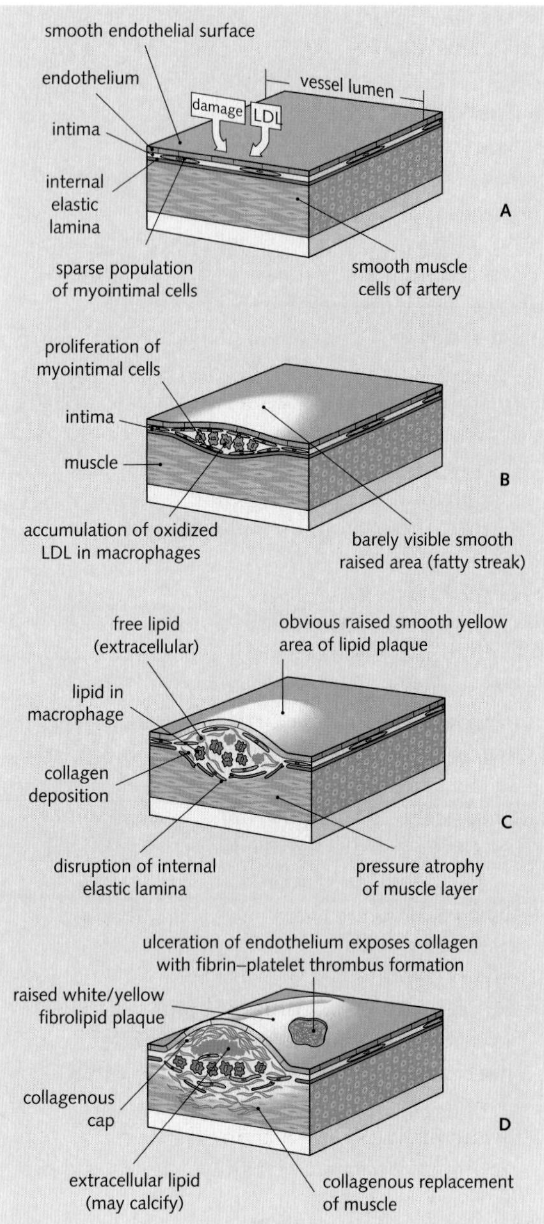

Fig. 5.9 Atheroma formation. (A) Endothelial injury—Allows entry of cholesterol-rich, low-density lipoproteins (LDLs) into the intima. (B) "Fatty streaks"—Barely visible pale bulges form as a result of phagocytosis and accumulation of lipid by intimal macrophages. (C) Lipid plaques—Raised, yellow lesions within the intima consisting of free lipid released by macrophages, and collagen deposited by myointimal cells. (D) Fibrolipid plaques—increased collagen deposition → dense fibrous plaque → pressure atrophy of the underlying media and elastic lamina → weakening of the arterial wall. The endothelium often ulcerates, allowing platelet aggregation and thrombosis.

Other hypotheses of pathogenesis

Thrombogenic hypothesis

This suggests that pathogenesis progresses as follows:

- Repeated episodes of mural thrombosis.
- Organization of thrombi produces elevated plaques.
- Lipid is thought to be derived from platelet membranes and/or leukocytes stimulated to proliferate by PDGFs.
- Not proven by studies.

Clonal proliferation hypothesis

This suggests that pathogenesis progresses as follows:

- Primary event is smooth muscle proliferation.
- Endothelial injury is a secondary phenomenon.
- Clonal proliferation of smooth muscle in plaques.

Lipid infiltration/insudation hypothesis

This suggests that pathogenesis progresses as follows:

- Increased uptake of LDL from plasma.
- LDL in intima are then chemically oxidized to act as toxic, proinflammatory, and chemotactic factors.

Management of atherosclerosis

Atherosclerosis can be managed by the following:

- Reduction or avoidance of risk factors (e.g., treat hypertension, stop smoking, regular exercise).

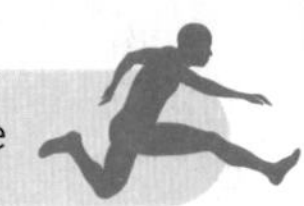

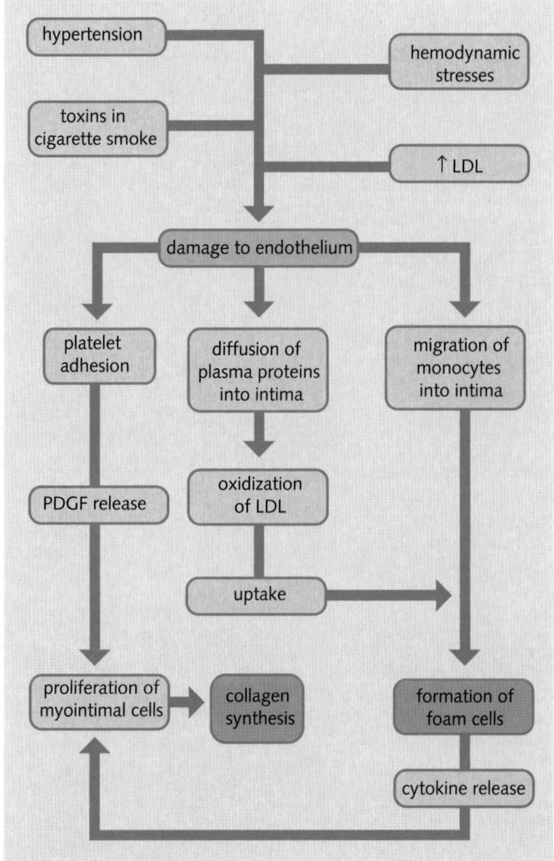

Fig. 5.10 Summary of events involved in pathogenesis.

- Antihyperlipidemic drugs to lower serum lipid and cholesterol (e.g., statins inhibit HMG CoA reductase required for hepatic cholesterol synthesis).
- Anticoagulants (e.g., aspirin to prevent thrombotic complications).

Mönckeberg's medial calcific sclerosis

This is a degenerative disease affecting the media of medium-sized muscular arteries, particularly in the limbs. Vessel walls become calcified, appearing tortuous and hard but with no associated decrease in lumen diameter (pipe-stem arteries). The disorder does not by itself produce ischemia.

Hypertension

Elevated blood pressure is an important and treatable cause of cardiac failure, and it is a major risk factor for atherosclerosis and cerebral hemorrhage. Any increase in blood pressure is associated with an increased risk of disease. Consequently, there are no thresholds below which a person has no risk of developing disease in which blood pressure is implicated as a pathogenic factor. Definitions of hypertension are, therefore, arbitrary.

Functional or operational definition

Hypertension is a sustained rise of the systemic blood pressure above 160mmHg systolic and/or above 95mmHg diastolic.

Borderline hypertension is 140–160mmHg systolic and/or 90–95mmHg diastolic.

Etiological classification

Hypertension can be classified into two main types according to its etiology (Fig. 5.11):

- Primary (essential or idiopathic) hypertension—elevation of blood pressure with age but with no apparent cause; this accounts for 90% of all cases. A key feature is an increase in total peripheral vascular resistance.
- Secondary hypertension—elevated blood pressure due to an identifiable cause; this accounts for 10% of hypertension. Examples include renal hypertension, endocrine causes, and coarctation of the aorta.

Pathological classification

Hypertension can also be classified according to the clinical course of disease:

- Benign hypertension—stable elevation of blood pressure over many years.
- Malignant (accelerated) hypertension—dramatic elevation of blood pressure over a short period of time.

Benign hypertension

Here, vessel changes develop gradually in response to a persistent stable elevated blood pressure; it affects males more than females. Histologically, it is characterized by:

- Hypertrophy and thickening of muscular media.
- Thickening of elastic lamina.
- Fibroelastic thickening of intima.
- Hyaline deposition in arteriole walls (hyaline arteriolosclerosis).

The effects are:

- Reduced size of vessel lumen leads to tissue ischemia.

Causes of hypertension	
Primary hypertension: unknown etiology but probably multifactorial involving...	
Genetic predisposition	Strong familial association
Socio-economic factors	Related to social deprivation
Dietary factors	Obesity, high salt intake, high alcohol, caffeine intake
Hormonal factors	Abnormalities in renin-angiotensin-aldosterone system
Neurological factors	Excessive sympathetic nervous system activity
Secondary hypertension: secondary to...	
Renal disease	Parenchymal disease, e.g., chronic pyelonephritis, glomerulonephritis, polycystic kidneys, amyloidosis Vascular disease, e.g., stenosis of renal artery
Adrenal disorders	Pheochromocytoma, Cushing's syndrome, Conn's syndrome (primary hyperaldosteronism), congenital adrenal hyperplasia
Other endocrine disorders	Thyrotoxicosis, hypothyroidism, acromegaly, hyperparathyroidism, diabetes with renal involvement
Cardiovascular disorders	Coarctation of the aorta, arteriovenous fistulae and shunts
Drugs	e.g., Oral contraceptives, anabolic steroids, corticosteroids, adrenaline and related sympatheticomimetic drugs
Pregnancy	±Pre-eclampsia

Fig. 5.11 Causes of hypertension are divided into primary and secondary etiological factors.

- Increased rigidity leads to limited capacity for expansion and constriction.
- Increased fragility of vessels leads to an increased risk of hemorrhage (especially cerebral).

After many years of benign progression, 5% of such patients enter an accelerated malignant phase.

Malignant hypertension

Here, there are acute destructive changes occurring in the walls of small arteries when blood pressure rises suddenly and markedly. There are two main effects: necrosis of the vessel wall (i.e., fibrinoid necrosis of vessels) and infiltration of necrotic media by fibrin (i.e., fibrinoid necrosis of vessels).

Destructive changes lead to cessation of blood flow through the small vessels with multiple foci of tissue necrosis, e.g., in the glomeruli of the kidney.

See Fig. 5.12 for a table of the features of malignant and benign hypertension.

Complications and effects of hypertension

Vascular effects

Hypertension accelerates atherosclerosis, and it causes thickening of the media of muscular arteries, particularly the smaller arteries and arterioles.

The normal flow of protein into the vessel wall is increased resulting in intramural protein deposition termed hyaline in benign hypertension, and fibrinoid in malignant hypertension:

- Hyaline deposition—a common feature of aging arteries; refers to the homogeneous appearance of vessel walls due to infiltration by plasma proteins.
- Fibrinoid deposition—a combination of fibrin with necrosis of the vessel wall.

Heart

The left ventricle undergoes hypertrophy resulting from the increased workload, causing increased susceptibility to spontaneous arrhythmias. Ischemic

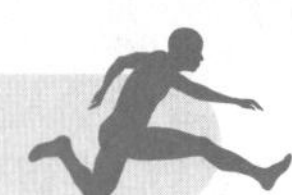

Features of benign and malignant hypertension		
	Benign	**Malignant**
Incidence	Very common (at least 5% of U.S. population)	Rare
Age	Begins at <45 years but prolonged into 6th and 7th decades	Young adults (25–35 years)
Gender	Females > males	Females = males
Etiology	Majority of cases due to primary hypertension	Majority of cases secondary to renal disease (few cases arise out of benign essential hypertension)
Disease progression	Very slow (many years)	Rapid (months to 1–2 years)
Blood pressure	Very slow rise diastolic = 90–120mmHg	Rapid rise Diastolic ≥120mmHg
Arterial changes	Potentiates atheroma → accelerated arteriosclerosis	Intimal fibrous thickening → accelerated arteriosclerosis
Arteriole changes	Hyaline thickening with narrowed lumen	Fibrinoid necrosis of vessel wall Lumen occluded by thrombus Affects mainly kidney and abdominal viscera

Fig. 5.12 Features of benign and malignant hypertension.

Complications and effects of hypertension		
	Benign	**Malignant**
Vessles	Hyaline deposition due to infiltration by plasma proteins	Fibrinoid deposition due to combination of fibrin deposition and necrosis of vessel wall
Heart	Hypertrophy of left ventricle → ↑ susceptibility to spontaneous arrhythmias Heart failure in 60% of cases Ischemic heart disease	Hypertrophy of left ventricle → ↑ susceptibility to spontaneous arrhythmias Focal myocardial necrosis Acute heart failure Ischemic heart disease
Brain	Cerebral hemorrhage	Encephalopathy (fits and loss of consciousness) due to cerebral edema Cerebral hemorrhage
Kidney	Nephrosclerosis, but not usually serious	Severe renal damage; death in uremia
Other organs	No significant damage	Focal necrosis, e.g., perforation of gut

Fig. 5.13 Complications and effects of hypertension.

heart disease due to accelerated atherosclerosis is a common complication of hypertension.

Brain

Intracerebral hemorrhage is a frequent cause of death in hypertension. Small vessel damage within the cerebral hemispheres results in the development of microinfarcts, which form hypertensive lacunae, i.e., small areas of brain destruction filled with fluid.

Kidneys

Arteriolosclerosis leads to progressive ischemia of the nephrons and chronic renal failure. This is termed benign hypertensive nephrosclerosis, and it is a common cause of chronic renal failure in the middle-aged and elderly population.

See Fig. 5.13 for a table of the complications and effects of hypertension.

Pulmonary hypertension

Definition and causes

This is defined as pulmonary arterial pressure in excess of 30mmHg. See Fig. 5.14 for a list of the causes.

Effects of pulmonary hypertension

With acute onset, there is a massive transudation of fluid from the pulmonary capillaries into the alveoli, leading to shortness of breath and expectoration of bloodstained, watery fluid.

Chronic onset has three effects:

- Hyperplastic arteriosclerosis—muscular hypertrophy, intimal fibrosis, and dilatation of the pulmonary arteries.
- Necrotizing arteriolitis—increased pressure within the pulmonary arteries causes weakening of the vessel wall with repeated episodes of hemorrhage into the alveolar spaces, which contain hemosiderin-laden macrophages.
- Cor pulmonale—right ventricular hypertrophy and dysfunction as a result of increased workload.

Effects of diabetes mellitus on the vessels

Diabetics suffer from an increased severity of atherosclerosis and capillary microangiopathy, in which small vessel wall thickening is attributed to a marked expansion of the basement membrane termed hyaline arteriolosclerosis.

Vessel damage is complex, and it is probably due to the increased plasma levels of cholesterol and triglycerides. Biochemically there is abnormal glycosylation of protein within the vessel wall. Clinical sequelae of diabetic vessel damage are described in detail in Chapter 9; they include diabetic retinopathy, diabetic glomerulosclerosis, and peripheral neuropathy.

Ischemic heart disease

Ischemic heart disease (IHD) is a condition caused by a reduction or cessation of the blood supply to the myocardium (myocardial ischemia). This is usually as a result of atherosclerosis, although in rare cases it may be caused by coronary embolism, arteritis, or ostial obstruction. The left ventricle is more prone to ischemia because of its greater bulk and work requirement, and its higher oxygen demand.

IHD is the most common type of cardiac disease and a leading cause of death in the Western world accounting for about 30% of all male deaths and 23% of all female deaths. Risk factors for the development of ischemic heart disease are the same as those for the development of atherosclerosis.

Effects

IHD results in four main syndromes:

- Stable angina (chronic manifestation).
- Unstable angina (acute manifestation).

Causes of pulmonary hypertension

Mechanism	Example
Precapillary causes • increased pulmonary blood flow	Left-to-right shunts, e.g., atrial septal defects, ventricular septal defects
Capillary causes • destruction of lung capillary bed	Emphysema Interstitial fibrosis of lungs
• mechanical arterial occlusion	Recurrent pulmonary emboli
• alveolar hypoxia causing pulmonary vasoconstriction	High altitude Obesity Chronic obstructive airways disease
Postcapillary causes • pulmonary venous congestion	Mitral valve disease, e.g., stenosis Chronic left ventricular failure
Idiopathic causes • primary pulmonary hypertension	Rare disease of young women due to increased tone in pulmonary vessels → progressive vascular changes and death

Fig. 5.14 Causes of pulmonary hypertension.

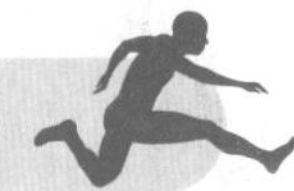

- Myocardial infarction (acute manifestation).
- Sudden cardiac death (acute manifestation).

Angina pectoris

Angina pectoris is episodic chest pain caused by ischemia of the myocardium (i.e., ischemic heart disease) following exercise. Ischemia is usually the result of stenosis of one or more of the coronary arteries resulting in reduced blood flow to the myocardium.

Stenosis of the coronary arteries is typically the result of atherosclerosis, and these atheromatous plaques may be one of two types:

- Eccentric—fibrolipid plaques affecting only one side of the wall of a coronary artery. Improvement of flow at the site of such plaques may be achieved by the use of vasodilator drugs. These drugs, such as glyceryl trinitrate, produce relaxation of the unaffected part of the vessel wall.
- Concentric—collagenous plaques affecting the whole of the arterial wall circumference. As the whole wall is abnormal, drug therapy cannot improve flow over a narrowed segment.

Cardiac referred pain

Pain of angina (and myocardial infarction) commonly radiates from the substernal and left pectoral regions to the left shoulder and the medial aspect of the left arm; this is known as cardiac referred pain.

Afferent fibers of the heart, and sensory fibers of affected cutaneous zones, enter the same spinal cord segments (T1 to T4/T5 on the left side) and ascend in the central nervous system (CNS) along a common pathway. The brain is unable to discern the origin of the pain; hence the phenomenon of cardiac referred pain.

Less commonly, pain radiates to the right shoulder and arm, with or without concomitant pain on the left side.

Types of angina

Stable angina

This is a predictable angina that occurs at a fixed level of exercise, as a result of an increased demand in myocardial work, usually in the presence of impaired perfusion by blood. It is caused by a fixed arterial obstruction, which limits any increase in coronary blood flow. Pain can usually be relieved by one or two minutes of rest. A stenosis of at least 75% of the lumen of the arteries is required to produce angina on exercise.

Unstable angina

Unstable anginal pain is unpredictable and not related to exercise. It reflects reversible ischemia due to variable luminal stenosis of some segments of the coronary arteries—dynamic stenosis.

The condition may be caused by either variations in vasomotor tone in segments markedly stenosed by eccentric plaques, or by active fissuring or rupture of plaques with intimal surface thrombus deposition, microembolization, and occlusion.

> Stable angina is predictable (i.e., it occurs at a fixed level of exercise), and it is caused by a fixed arterial obstruction.
> Unstable angina is unpredictable (i.e., it is unrelated to exercise), and it is caused by a variable luminal stenosis of the coronary arteries.
> Prinzmetal's angina is also unpredictable, and this is caused by coronary artery spasm.

Prinzmetal's angina (vasospastic angina)

This is angina at rest caused by an increase in the coronary vasomotor tone. The mechanism for coronary spasm is unknown. The disorder may occur in non-atheromatous arteries (where an increase in tone must be extreme to produce angina) or in atheromatous arteries (where even physiological changes in tone may produce a critical reduction in blood flow).

Prinzmetal's angina is particularly common in the early morning. Attacks are usually self-limiting and, although pain may be severe, they rarely lead on to myocardial infarction.

Management of angina

Angina can be managed as follows:

- Avoidance of risk factors for atherosclerosis (see p. 47).
- Drug therapy is a combination therapy with nitrates, β-blockers, and Ca^{2+} channel blockers.

- Surgery—coronary angioplasty or coronary artery bypass is indicated when there are signs of progressive coronary occlusion. Such changes may lead to the development of a myocardial infarction. This is especially true of patients presenting with unstable angina.

Myocardial infarction

Myocardial infarction (MI) is necrosis of the myocardium as a result of severe ischemia. MI is extremely common, accounting for 10–15% of all deaths and about 60% of sudden unexpected deaths. It typically affects the middle-aged, between 50 and 60 years, but 10% occur in 35–50 year olds. MI affects males more than premenopausal women (by 5:1), but there is an increasing incidence in women postmenopausally.

Clinical features are chest pain accompanied by breathlessness, vomiting, and collapse or syncope. Pain occurs in the same sites as angina, but it is usually more severe and lasts for longer.

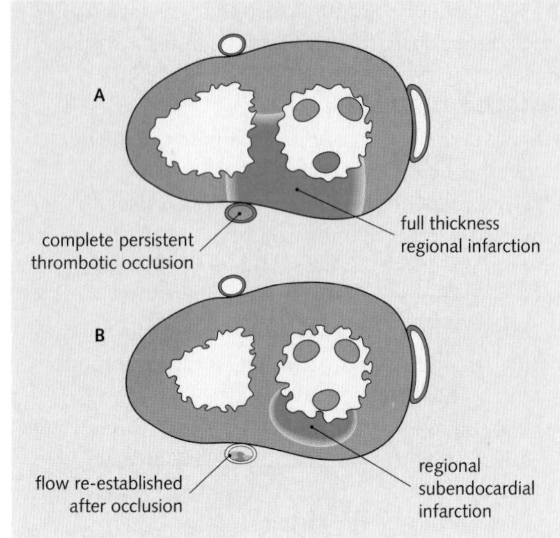

Fig. 5.15 Patterns of regional myocardial infarction (MI). (A) Transmural or full thickness infarct. (B) Regional subendocardial infarct.

Types

There are two main types of MI:

- Regional (90% of cases)—infarction occurs in the territory supplied by one major common artery.
- Diffuse (10% of cases)—relates to problems of overall myocardial perfusion rather than to thrombotic occlusion in any one artery.

Regional myocardial infarction

This involves only one segment of the ventricular wall. The cause of infarction is nearly always thrombus formation on a complicated atheromatous plaque.

Patterns of regional MI (Fig. 5.15):

- Full thickness infarct or transmural infarct, due to complete occlusion of an artery (no collateral supply).
- Subendocardial infarct, due to lysis of thrombus or due to collateral supply.

Diffuse myocardial infarction

General hypoperfusion of the main coronary arteries usually as a result of an episode of hypotension causes a critical reduction in flow in arteries already affected by high-grade atherosclerotic stenoses.

The pattern of diffuse MI differs from that of regional MI in that there is circumferential necrosis of the subendocardial zone (the region at the end of the arterial perfusion zone) resulting from failure of perfusion.

Site of myocardial infarction and vessel involvement

The site of regional MI depends on which vessel is involved, as shown in Fig. 5.16. The majority of infarcts affect the left ventricle and septal region; infarction of the right ventricle is relatively rare.

Histological changes following myocardial infarction

MI comprises necrosis and acute inflammation. The necrotic tissue is gradually replaced by a collagenous scar. The entire process from coagulative necrosis to scar formation takes 6–8 weeks, the macroscopic and microscopic appearances of the infarct changing with time (Fig. 5.17). The extensive necrosis of cardiac muscle is associated with the release of cardiac enzymes and proteins that can be used as clinical markers for a MI event. Examples include creatinine kinase (CK-MB cardiac isoform), lactic dehydrogenase and troponin T.

Sequelae of myocardial infarction

The effects and sequelae of MI are variable, and they can be classified into:

- Immediate effects: sudden cardiac death (described below).
- Short-term complications: occurring in the first 2 weeks post MI.
- Long-term complications.

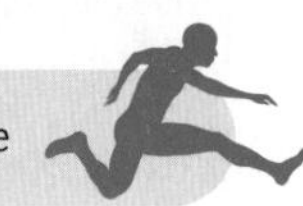

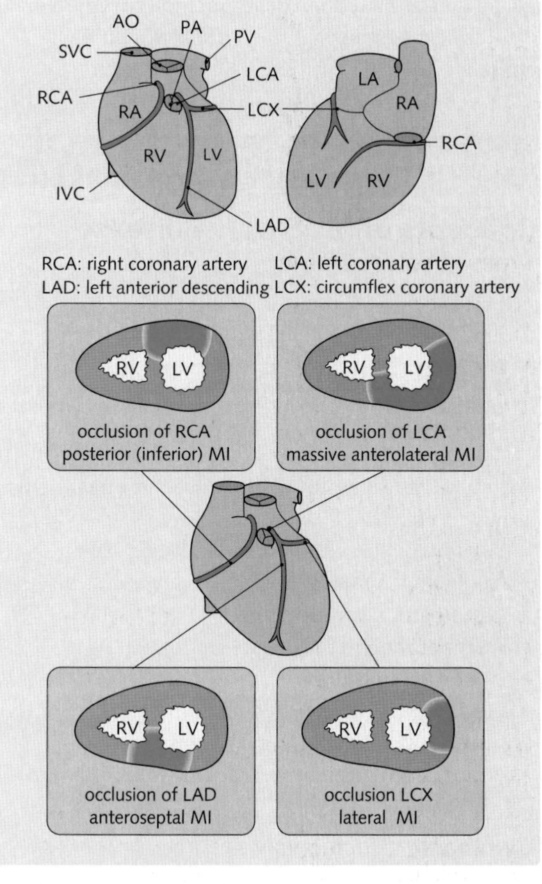

Fig. 5.16 Site of myocardial infarction (MI) and vessel involvement.

Morphological changes occurring post MI		
time	**macroscopic appearance**	**microscopic appearance**
0–12 hours	not visible	infarcted muscle appears uncolored on staining with nitroblue tetrazolium due to loss of oxidative enzymes; non-infarcted muscle stains blue
12–24 hours	pale with blotchy discoloration	infarcted muscle is brightly eosinophilic with intercellular edema
24–72 hours	dead area appears soft and pale with a slight yellow color	infarcted area excites an acute inflammatory response neutrophils infiltrate between dead cardiac muscle fibres
3–10 days	hyperemic border develops around the yellow dead muscle	organization of infarcted area replacement with vascular granulation tissue
weeks to months	white scar	progressive collagen deposition infarct is replaced by a collagenous scar

Fig. 5.17 Morphological changes occurring post myocardial infarction (MI).

Short-term complications

There are six short-term complications:

- Arrhythmias—due to the involvement of conduction tissue, leading to ventricular fibrillation, atrial fibrillation, heart block, and sinus bradycardia.
- Left ventricular failure—this is common with large areas of infarction; the necrotic wall softens in organization leading to cardiac dilatation.
- Rupture, which can be:
  - External (majority)—blood bursts through the external wall into the pericardial cavity (hemopericardium); the sudden rise in intrapericardial cavity pressure prevents cardiac filling (cardiac tamponade), leading to rapid death.
  - Internal (rarely)—intracardiac rupture through the septum leads to acquired septal defect causing a left-to-right shunt and the development of left ventricular failure.
- Papillary muscle dysfunction—when one or more valve leaflets are unable to close during systole there is mitral valve incompetence.
- Mural thrombosis—on the inflamed endocardium over the area of infarction; there is a high risk of embolization producing infarction of various organs (e.g., cerebral, renal, splenic, mesenteric, and lower limbs).
- Acute pericarditis—caused by inflammation over the infarct surface.

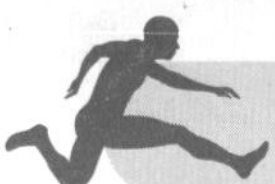

Long-term complications

There are four long-term complications:

- Chronic intractable left-heart failure—resulting from inadequate left ventricular pumping action; common when the infarct is extensive and full thickness.
- Ventricular aneurysm (in 10% of long-term survivors)—gradual distension of the weakened fibrotic part of the left ventricular wall with thrombus formation, embolism or severe functional deficit.
- Recurrent MI—risk of developing a further episode due to underlying coronary artery insufficiency.
- Dressler's syndrome—a form of autoimmune-mediated pericarditis associated with a high erythrocyte sedimentation ratio (ESR); develops in a very small number of cases after infarction.

Management is by investigations, i.e., electrocardiogram (ECG), chest X-ray (excluding aortic dissection), blood (increased ESR, cardiac enzymes), and treatment is as follows:

Oxygen to overcome lowered Po_2.

- Analgesia—morphine, diamorphine with antiemetics.
- Nitrates: sublingual glyceryl nitrates.
- Fibrinolytic therapy—should be considered within the first 12 hours post infarction (e.g., streptokinase, tissue plasminogen activator).
- Anticoagulation to prevent thromboembolic complications from prolonged immobilization (e.g., heparin).
- Beta antagonist such as metoprolol.
- ACE inhibitors for patients with heart failure.
- Bed rest for the first 24–48 hours on the coronary care unit.

Sudden cardiac death

Sudden cardiac death is the most important immediate consequence of myocardial ischemia, and it is usually due to ventricular fibrillation.

Arrhythmias causing ventricular fibrillation may be a result of:

- Previous ischemic heart disease, e.g., angina or previous infarction; cardiac arrhythmias can arise from muscle adjacent to an area of old scarring.
- Acute myocardial ischemia, which, due to a new thrombotic event, may precipitate arrhythmia.

Other causes of sudden death include ruptured or dissecting aneurysms of the aorta and pulmonary emboli.

Disorders of the heart valves

Concepts of heart valve disease

Types of valve disorder

Value disorders can be:

- Stenosis—narrowing or abnormal rigidity of a valve.
- Regurgitation (or incompetence)—failure of a valve to close fully.

Both types may coexist in one valve but one type is usually dominant.

Factors that may cause heart valve damage:

- Congenital abnormality.
- Postinflammatory scarring.
- Degeneration with aging.
- Dilatation of the valve ring.
- Degeneration of collagenous support tissue of the valve.
- Acute destruction by necrotizing inflammation.

Commonly affected valves

The mitral and aortic valves are the most frequently affected, the tricuspid and pulmonary valves only infrequently.

Fig. 5.18 gives an outline of the major causes and basic features of acquired valve disease.

Abnormalities of flow and their effects

Diseased valves often cause regurgitant jets of blood, with concomitant development of endocardial lesions opposite the jet's site. These lesions (jet lesions) are typically seen on the septum opposite the aortic valve.

Degenerative valve disease

Calcific aortic stenosis

There are two types:

- Degenerative calcific aortic valve stenosis—calcification of the aortic valve associated with increasing age; typically affects the elderly.
- Bicuspid calcific aortic valve stenosis—calcification of the congenital bicuspid aortic valve; quite common, usually manifesting by 40–50 years of age.

Major causes and basic features of acquired valve disease			
Valve lesion	**Causes**	**Effects**	**Physical findings**
Mitral stenosis	Rheumatic	Left-sided cardiac failure with predisposition to atrial thrombosis Left atrial hypertrophy and dilatation leads to: • pulmonary vascular congestion • pulmonary hypertension • right ventricular hypertrophy • "nutmeg liver" and congested kidneys	Loud S_1 Opening snap Diastolic rumble
Mitral regurgitation	Acute: • papillary muscle dysfunction • cusp damage by endocarditis Chronic: • postinflammatory scarring, commonly rheumatic • left ventricular dilatation • floppy mitral valve syndrome	Acute: • pulmonary edema Chronic: • left ventricle hypertrophy and dilatation • giant left atrium • progressive left-sided cardiac failure develops with time	Pansystolic murmur Widely split S_2
Aortic stenosis	Calcification of congenital bicuspid aortic valve Rheumatic Senile calcific degeneration	Early: • asymptomatic but with slowly progressive left ventricular hypertrophy Late: • left ventricular failure • low cardiac output → breathlessness • coronary artery insufficiency → angina • cerebrovascular insufficiency → syncope • sudden death	Systolic ejection murmur reaching peak intensity in mid- or late systole
Aortic regurgitation	Rheumatic Endocarditis Senile calcification Aortic root dilatation	Left ventricular hypertrophy Progressive left ventricular failure	Diastolic murmur Wide pulse pressure Collapsing pulse

Fig. 5.18 Major causes and basic features of acquired valve disease.

In both types, the valves become thick and fibrotic with a fusion of the commissures. Large nodular masses of calcium may be found subendothelially within the sinuses of Valsalva behind the aortic cusps.

Effects

There are two effects:

- Aortic stenosis (i.e., thickening and fusion of valves) → decreased valve lumen → reduced systolic flow.
- Aortic regurgitation: increased rigidity of valves → failure to close properly → backflow into the left ventricle during diastole.

Stenosis and regurgitation result in left ventricular hypertrophy, coronary insufficiency, and syncope or sudden death due to acute heart failure.

Mitral annular calcification

This is "wear and tear" of the mitral valve with calcification of the valve leaflets. Massive calcification can immobilize the valve and predispose to the development of either thrombosis or bacterial endocarditis.

Myxomatous degeneration of the mitral valve ("floppy valve syndrome")

This is the idiopathic prolapse of the mitral valve leaflets. The leaflets are thickened and redundant, containing large amounts of mucopolysaccharides and abnormal collagen. It most commonly involves the posterior mitral leaflet, which is soft and bulges upwards into the atrium during systole. The net result is mild valvular incompetence and an increased risk of rupture of one of the chordae, which may lead to severe valvular incompetence.

Rheumatic heart disease

Rheumatic fever is an immune disorder that follows 2–3 weeks after a streptococcal infection, usually tonsillitis or pharyngitis.

Epidemiology

This disease occurs mainly in children aged 5–15 years, and it was once prevalent in Europe and in the U.S. Its incidence has decreased in the developed world, and it is now most frequently seen in parts of central Africa, the Middle East, and India. It is associated with poor nutrition and overcrowding.

Pathogenesis

Susceptible individuals develop antibodies to antigens produced by specific strains of streptococci; these antibodies then cross-react with host antigens. The disease is a systemic disorder affecting:

- Heart—pericarditis, myocarditis, and endocarditis (collectively known as pancarditis).
- Joints—polyarthritis.
- Skin—subcutaneous nodules and erythema marginatum.
- Arteries—arteritis.

The most important target organ is the heart. Repeated attacks of rheumatic fever lead to progressive fibrosis of the endocardium and valves, which is the main cause of chronic scarring of the valves.

Aschoff's nodules

These are areas of degenerate collagen surrounded by activated histiocytic cells and lymphoid cells. Lesions stimulate fibroblast proliferation and lead to scarring.

Acute rheumatic heart disease

In the acute phase, rheumatic fever causes a pancarditis, the components of which are:

- Rheumatic pericarditis—acute inflammation of the pericardium.
- Rheumatic myocarditis—mild inflammation with occasional muscle fibre necrosis.
- Rheumatic endocarditis—mitral valves are most prone to the development of severe lesions.

Chronic rheumatic heart disease

The main morbidity of rheumatic fever is the long-term effects of the immune damage causing chronic scarring of valves. Chronic valvular heart disease develops in about 50% of those affected by rheumatic fever with carditis. Lesions may develop after 10–20 years in Western countries, but much earlier in developing countries.

Pathogenesis

Endocardial valvular damage from the acute phase heals by progressive fibrosis. Valve leaflets and chordae tendineae become thickened, fibrotic, and shrunken, often with fusion to their partners, and there is frequent secondary deposition of calcium.

Once damage has developed, the altered hemodynamic stresses extend the damage even in the absence of continued autoimmune processes.

Infective endocarditis

This is an acute or subacute disease resulting from infection of a focal area of the endocardium. It can affect almost any age, but it is increasing in incidence in the elderly population. Predisposing factors include genitourinary infection, diabetes, tooth extraction, pressure sores, and surgical procedures. It is more common in males than females (3:1).

> Patients with valvular disease are at risk of developing infective endocarditits from even the most minor surgical or dental procedures. It is, therefore, important to prophylatically treat such patients with high doses of antibiotics to prevent bacteremia.

Morphological features

The characteristic lesions of endocarditis are termed vegetations, and they are formed from deposits of platelets, fibrin, and bacteria. The mechanism of formation is outlined in Fig. 5.19. Research suggests that vegetations may form in areas of high-pressure gradients, for example at an incompetent valve.

Almost all vegetation occurs on valve leaflets or chordae tendinae. The size varies from a small nodule to a large mass that may occlude the valve orifice. The mitral and aortic valves are the most commonly affected.

Causative organisms

Bacteria

The two groups of bacteria are:

- Pathogens—*Staphylococcus aureus*, β-hemolytic streptococci, pneumococci, meningococci, *Escherichia coli*, etc.
- Low-grade pathogens—Viridans streptococci, *S. fecalis*, *Staph. epidermidis*, *Hemophilus*, *Brucella*, mycobacteria, and various Gram-negative organisms.

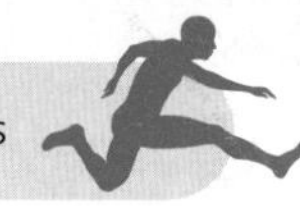

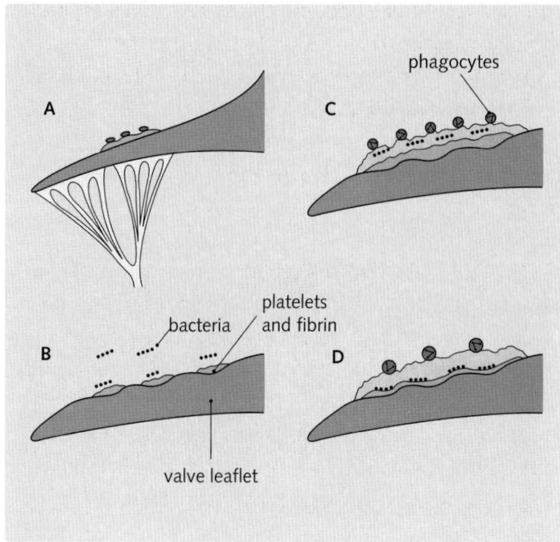

Fig. 5.19 Pathogenesis of vegetation formation in infective endocarditis. (A) Abnormality on endocardium of valve leaflet is coated with small deposits of platelets and fibrin (thrombus). (B) Circulating bacteria or fungi colonize the platelet thrombus. (C, D) Further layers of platelets and fibrin are deposited, and the microorganisms proliferate in the superficial layer of the vegetation. They are separated from blood by a thin layer of fibrinous material, which protects against immune destruction but allows diffusion of nutrients. (Adapted from Underwood, 2000.)

Fungi

Fungi such as *Candida*, *Aspergillus*, etc., may cause endocarditis, particularly in drug addicts, the immunosuppressed, or those with valve prostheses.

The type of causative organism responsible depends on whether the affected valve is structurally normal or abnormal.

Infection of structurally normal valves

Infective organisms are pathogenic and directly invade the valve causing rapid destruction. This is commonly seen in intravenous drug addicts, after open heart surgery, and following septicemia from other causes.

Infection of structurally abnormal heart valves

Infective organisms are of low pathogenicity, and derived from normal commensal organisms of the skin, mouth, urinary tract, and gut. Following trivial episodes of bacteremia, organisms become enmeshed in platelet aggregates on the surface of the abnormal endocardium, growing to cause persistent infection. The main underlying abnormalities in this group are:

- Congenital bicuspid aortic valves.
- Postinflammatory scarring.
- Mitral valve prolapse syndrome.
- Prosthetic valves.

The incidence has increased in Western countries in recent years, mainly as a result of patients surviving with structurally abnormal hearts and heart valves.

Types of infective endocarditis

Acute

The cause is usually a virulent organism, such as *Staphylococcus aureus*, but it may affect either normal or abnormal heart valves.

The bacteria proliferate in the valve causing necrosis and the generation of thrombotic vegetations.

Consequently, there is destruction of valve leaflets with perforation and acute disturbance of valve function leading to acute heart failure.

Prognosis—Disease is rapidly progressive and often fatal.

Subacute

The cause here is, typically, low virulence organisms, such as Viridans streptococci, infecting structurally abnormal valves, or partially treated endocarditis.

The bacteria proliferate slowly in the thrombotic vegetation on damaged valve surfaces. Gradual valve destruction occurs, stimulating further thrombus formation with the potential for systemic embolization.

Clinical features of endocarditis

The main clinical features of endocarditis are:

- Systemic symptoms: fever, weight loss, and malaise due to cytokine generation from low-grade infection.
- Skin petechiae and microhemorrhages in the retina and skin, particularly around the fingernails (splinter hemorrhages), caused by the deposition of immune complexes (antibodies react with antigen of the infecting organism) in small vessels; they also cause a form of glomerulonephritis.
- Clubbing of fingers (cause unknown).

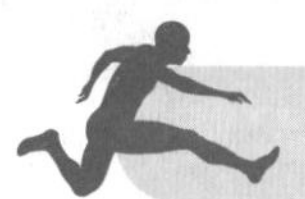

- Splenomegaly and anemia due to persistent bacteremia.

Sequelae

The sequelae are as follows:

- Valvular regurgitation due to gradual destruction of valves leading to cardiac failure.
- Perivalvular abscesses following extension of the infection into the valve ring and myocardium, producing sinuses, fistulae, septal defects, and abnormalities of conduction.
- Mycotic aneurysms: infection of the muscular wall of a medium-sized artery caused by embolisms to the vasa vasorum.
- Multi-organ infarction: small emboli of infected thrombotic material enter the systemic circulation producing infarction of many organs especially the brain, spleen, and kidneys. Infarcted organs may in turn become infected by organisms within the occluding thrombus.

Complications of infective endocarditis are summarized in Fig. 5.20.

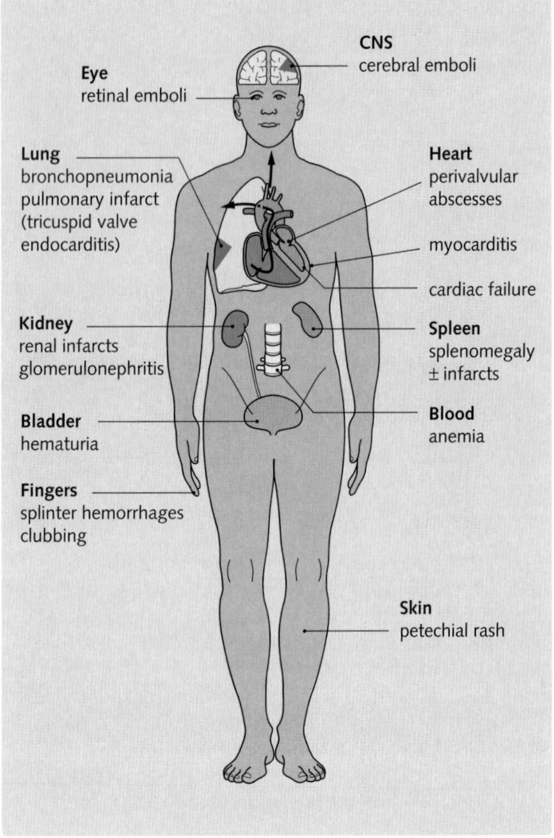

Fig. 5.20 Complications of infective endocarditis.

Nonbacterial thrombotic (marantic) endocarditis

Nonbacterial thrombotic endocarditis is inflammation of the valves with the formation of sterile thrombotic vegetations (marantic vegetations) on the closure lines of valve cusps. It occurs in severely debilitated patients with serious systemic disease.

Endocarditis of systemic lupus erythematosus (Libman–Sacks disease)

Thrombotic vegetations complicate systemic lupus erythematosus (SLE). This is seen in 50% or more of fatal cases of SLE. Valvular changes rarely give rise to any appreciable functional deficiency, but thrombotic material can fragment and cause embolic infarction.

Carcinoid heart disease

Carcinoid syndrome is caused by excess 5-hydroxytryptamine secretion by a carcinoid tumor (usually of the small intestine which has metastasized to the liver), and can result in endocardial fibrosis of the tricuspid and pulmonary valves, in turn resulting in stenosis or incompetence.

Complications of artificial heart valves

Prosthetic valve diseases

The prosthetic value diseases are:

- Thrombosis leading to valve obstruction or embolism.
- Valve failure due to mechanical breakage of the prosthesis, or tissue calcification and cusp rupture of bioprosthesis.
- Infective endocarditis from turbulence and prosthetic material; its incidence is 1–2% per year.
- Paravalvular leak—caused by poor surgical technique, or due to poor quality tissues (e.g., calcium, active infective endocarditis).
- Obstructive gradients—valve may be too small, or there may be tissue ingrowth of the pannus on to the valve ring.
- Hemolysis and, rarely, jaundice.

Precautions necessary to avoid complications of artificial heart valves

The precautions are lifelong anticoagulation, and prophylactic antibiotic therapy to protect against infective endocarditis.

Diseases of the myocardium

Concepts of myocardial disease

Cardiomyopathy

This is a group of disorders in which the structural or functional abnormality primarily affects the myocardium. It should only be considered if all other potential causes of myocardial impairment have been excluded (e.g., hypertension, valvular, or coronary artery disease).

Effects of cardiomyopathy

Cardiomyopathies usually cause progressive development of cardiac failure. The time scale varies according to the cause of the disease, occurring over weeks or years. In some instances, sudden cardiac death is the first manifestation of disease.

The terms "cardiomyopathy" and "myocarditis" are frequently confused. Myocarditis refers to inflammation of the myocardium and is a cause of secondary cardiomyopathy, but it is not synonymous with cardiomyopathy.

Classification

Cardiomyopathies can be grouped into two types according to etiology:

- Primary idiopathic cardiomyopathies (etiology unknown).
- Secondary cardiomyopathies (also known as specific heart muscle diseases): diseases of the heart muscle associated with or caused by a systemic disease.

Primary idiopathic cardiomyopathy

Primary cardiomyopathies follow three main patterns according to the dysfunction of the myocardium: dilated, hypertrophic obstructive, or restrictive.

Dilated (congestive) cardiomyopathy

These are abnormalities of the myocardium causing poor systolic contraction. They are characterized by:

- Dilatation of the ventricles.
- Thin, stretched chamber walls.
- Hypocontractile muscle.

Etiology is usually unidentifiable, but the condition occasionally represents end-stage myocardial damage for known causes including viral myocarditis and other forms of secondary cardiomyopathies.

Hypertrophic cardiomyopathy

A familial condition resulting in hyperkinetic systolic function with marked reduction in systolic volume and difficulty in diastolic filling. This is characterized by:

- Gross hypertrophy of the heart walls, particularly affecting the interventricular septum.
- Loss of the normal parallel orientation of hypertrophied muscle fibers—disorganized branching.

This condition may present in young adults and juveniles with sudden unexplained death on exertion (hypertrophic obstructive cardiomyopathy, HOCM). Less dramatic presentations include angina and breathlessness on exertion in a young person or repeated fainting attacks.

Restrictive cardiomyopathy

Abnormal stiffness of the myocardium results in impaired ventricular filling. The stiffness is caused by infiltration of the myocardium, for example:

- Amyloid in amyloidosis.
- Fibrosis in endomyocardial fibrosis (fibrosis of thrombotic material deposited on the endocardial surfaces).
- Hemochromatosis.

The condition causes high atrial pressures resulting in atrial hypertrophy → atrial dilatation → atrial fibrillation.

Secondary cardiomyopathies

Myocarditis

This rare disease is characterized by the presence of inflammatory cells in the myocardium.

Etiology

The vast majority of cases of myocarditis are either infectious or immune-mediated.

The infectious causes are:

- Viruses—viral infection is the commonest cause of myocarditis in the U.S. Coxsackie virus is the commonest culprit. Other agents include influenza, echovirus, HIV, CMV, poliomyelitis or mumps virus.
- Bacteria—direct infection (with chlamydia, rickettsia or pyogenic bacteria) or indirect toxin-mediated damage (e.g., diphtheria or typhoid).
- Fungi.
- Protozoa—toxoplasmosis; Chagas' disease due to *Trypanosoma cruzi*.
- Helminths.

The immune-mediated causes are:

- Poststreptococcal (e.g., acute rheumatic fever).
- Postviral.
- SLE.
- Drug hypersensitivity, e.g., sulphonamides, doxorubicin, cyclophosphamide.
- Transplant rejection.

Other less common causes include sarcoidosis (see Chapter 6) and giant cell myocarditis, an acute fulminating form of fatal acute myocarditis.

Other secondary cardiomyopathies

Other causes of secondary cardiomyopathies are listed in Fig. 5.21.

Etiology of secondary cardiomyopathies	
Causes	**Example**
Infection and inflammation	Myocarditis
Multisystem disease	Diabetes Amyloidosis Thyroid dysfunction Hemochromatosis
Toxic and metabolic disturbances	Alcohol Catecholamines Drugs, e.g., Adriamycin
Primary muscle disorders	Muscular dystrophy Mitochondrial cytopathy

Fig. 5.21 Etiology of secondary cardiomyopathies.

Neoplasms of the heart

Tumors of the heart are extremely rare. Examples include:

- Myxoma—a benign tumor of stellate cells, typically arising from the endocardium.
- Connective tissue tumors such as lipomas.
- Malignant tumors such as rhabdomyosarcomas.
- Metastatic or local spread tumors.

Diseases of the pericardium

Accumulation of fluid in the pericardial sac

Pericardial effusion

This is the accumulation of fluid within the pericardial cavity. Effusions may be:

- Serous—transudate with low protein content (<2g/100mL) and usually containing only very scanty mesothelial cells, caused by heart failure, hypoalbuminemia, or myxedema.
- Serosanguinous—exudate with high protein content (>3g/100mL) occurring with infection, uremia, neoplasia, or connective tissue disorders.
- Chylous—accumulation of lymphatic fluid occurring in the presence of lymphatic obstruction of pericardial drainage, most commonly due to neoplasms and tuberculosis.

Remember the "Five I's" of possible causes of pericarditis: infarctive, infective, injury, invasive, immunological.

The etiology is of two types: inflammatory (e.g., acute pericarditis) and noninflammatory. Noninflammatory has the following characteristics:

- ↑ Capillary permeability (e.g., severe hypothyroidism).
- ↑ Capillary hydrostatic pressure (e.g., congestive heart failure).
- ↓ Plasma oncotic pressure (e.g., cirrhosis and the nephrotic syndrome).

Pathophysiology—Large amounts of fluid eventually interfere with the heart's action.

Clinical effects depend on the increase in pressure within the pericardium which, in turn, depends on:

- Volume of effusion: the greater the volume the greater the increase in internal pressure.
- Rate at which the fluid accumulates. Sudden increase → marked elevation of pressure → severe cardiac chamber compression. Slow effusion (over weeks to months) → pericardium stretches → no elevation of pressure.
- Compliance characteristics of the pericardium: even small effusions may cause marked elevation of pressure if there is stiffness of the pericardium (e.g., in the presence of tumor or fibrosis).

The condition is often asymptomatic, but it may present with a dull constant ache in the left side of the chest. Unlike ischemic cardiac pain, it is accentuated by inspiration, by movement, and by lying flat.

Hemopericardium

This is the accumulation of blood in the pericardial sac. For its etiology see Fig. 5.22, where the causes of hemopericardium are outlined. In most cases, death occurs rapidly due to the sudden rise in intrapericardial cavity pressure, which prevents cardiac filling (cardiac tamponade)—as little as 200–300mL commonly being sufficient.

Cardiac tamponade

In this condition, fluid (of any kind) accumulates under high pressure compressing the cardiac chambers to such an extent that filling of the heart is severely limited.

Etiology of hemopericardium	
Causes	**Example**
Rupture of heart	Traumatic, e.g., stab wound Spontaneous, e.g., myocardial infarct
Rupture of intrapericardial portion of aorta	Dissecting aneurysm Syphilitic aneurysm Traumatic
Hemorrhagic tendencies	Purpura Scurvy Hypoprothrombinemia Anticoagulant therapy

Fig. 5.22 Etiology of hemopericardium.

Diagnosis

The physical signs are:

- Sinus tachycardia.
- Increased jugular venous pulse (often with a further rise on inspiration).
- Decreased systemic blood pressure (producing shock in severe cases).
- Cyclical decrease in systolic blood pressure during each inspiration—pulsus paradoxus.

Investigations include echocardiography (which shows the presence of pericardial effusion with right ventricular diastolic collapse) and cardiac catheterization combined with pericardiocentesis.

The management of cardiac tamponade depends on the extent of hemodynamic compromise. Severe cases may be rapidly fatal and require relief by emergency paracentesis; less critical cases require formal surgical drainage.

Electromechanical dissociation

Electromechanical dissociation (EMD) is a condition in which electrical activity is normal or near normal on ECG, but there is no effective cardiac output. It is associated with a poor prognosis as it is often due to cardiac rupture, which is rarely amenable to treatment. However, treatable causes of EMD should not be overlooked and these include:

- Cardiac tamponade.
- Hypovolemia.
- Pneumothorax.
- Pulmonary embolism.

Pericarditis

Pericarditis—i.e., inflammation of the pericardium—is the main disorder of the pericardium. The condition is often complicated by the development of an effusion.

Acute pericarditis

In acute pericarditis both pericardial surfaces (visceral and parietal layers) are coated with a fibrin-rich acute inflammatory exudate. The loss of smoothness leads to the clinical sign of a friction rub. The causes of acute pericarditis are listed in Fig. 5.23.

Etiology of acute pericarditis	
Infarction	Myocardial infarction: local pericarditis over infarct is the most common cause of pericarditis
Infective	Viral infections: second most common cause, usually clinically mild, rarely requiring hospital treatment Pyogenic: e.g., staphylococci, streptococci, hemophilus septicemia or pneumonia Tuberculosis: spread to pericardium from tuberculous lymph nodes in mediastinum; now rare
Injury	Postoperative: following open heart surgery Pericarditis is diffuse, involving entire pericardial surface Heals by fibrosis → obliteration of pericardial cavity
Invasive	Malignant pericarditis: usually due to infiltration of pericardium by local spread from a primary bronchial tumor; less commonly the cause is blood-borne metastases from a distant site, e.g., malignant melanoma
Immunologic	Immune pericarditis: associated with rheumatic fever or may present in patient with systemic autoimmune disease, e.g., SLE, rheumatoid disease

Fig. 5.23 Etiology of acute pericarditis.

Variants can be:

- Serous, nonbacterial inflammation: the exudate is a clear, straw-colored and protein-rich fluid.
- Serofibrinous or fibrinous occurs with MI; the exudate contains plasma protein, including fibrinogen.
- Suppurative (or purulent) pericarditis associated with pyogenic bacterial infection; serosal surfaces are erythematous and coated with thick creamy pus.
- Hemorrhagic: blood is mixed with inflammatory exudate.
- Caseous, fibrinous exudate with granulation tissue and areas of caseation caused by tuberculosis.

Clinical features

The clinical features of acute pericarditis are:

- Pleuritic chest pain.
- Fever.
- Pericardial friction rub.
- ECG abnormalities.

Chronic pericarditis

Adhesive pericarditis

Although fibrinous pericarditis may resolve completely, it occasionally results in fibrinous adhesions or even in complete obliteration of the pericardial sac.

Constrictive pericarditis

Gross fibrosis and calcification of the pericardium cause restriction of ventricular filling and interference with ventricular systole. The heart is effectively encased in a solid shell and filling is impaired. Calcification may extend into the myocardium, producing impaired myocardial contraction.

This condition often follows tuberculous pericarditis, but it can also complicate invasive pericarditis, hemopericardium, viral pericarditis, rheumatoid arthritis, and purulent pericarditis.

Clinical features

In chronic pericarditis, the fibrous tissue impairs venous return resulting in symptoms and signs of systemic venous congestion, namely raised jugular venous pressure, enlarged liver, and ascites.

Rheumatic disease of the pericardium

Rheumatic disease of the pericardium is an acute form of pericarditis occurring with generalized pancarditis following streptococcal infection (see p. 57).

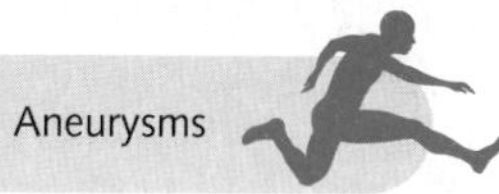

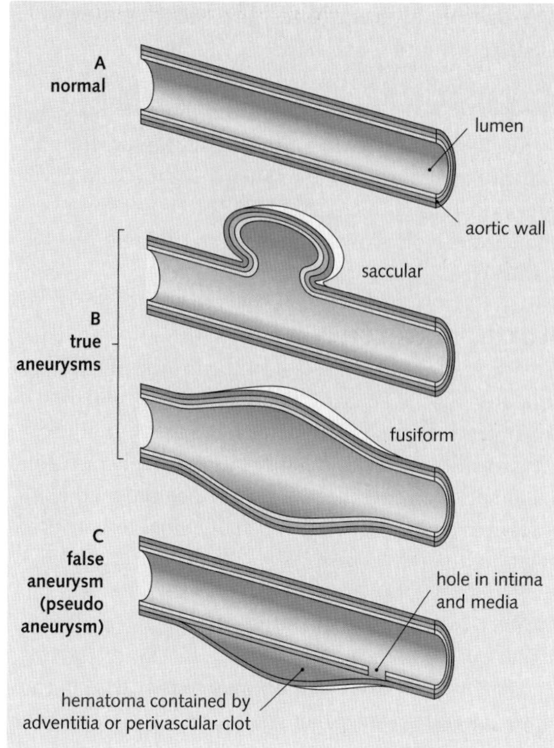

Fig. 5.24 Aortic aneurysms. (A) Normal. (B) True aneurysms. (C) False aneurysm (pseudo-aneurysm).

Aneurysms

Definitions and concepts

Aneurysm

An aneurysm is an abnormal localized, permanent, dilatation of an artery. Types of aneurysm are shown in Fig. 5.24:

- True aneurysms: the wall is formed by one or more layers of the affected vessel. These can be saccular or fusiform.
- False aneurysms: the wall is formed by connective tissue which is not a part of vessel; usually due to traumatic or infective rupture of vessel forming a blood-filled space limited by surrounding tissue (usually an organized hematoma).

True aneurysm morphology

Saccular aneurysms take the form of globular sacs, whereas fusiform aneurysms are spindle shaped due to long segments of the vessel wall being affected around the whole circumference.

Main causes of aneurysms

Any abnormality that weakens the media may produce an aneurysm:

- Atherosclerosis is the most common cause, typically affecting the abdominal aorta causing thinning and fibrous replacement of media.
- Cystic medial degeneration: focal degeneration of media with the formation of small cyst-like spaces filled with mucopolysaccharide. Etiology may be idiopathic or associated with connective tissue diseases, e.g., Marfan's syndrome, and Ehlers–Danlos syndrome.

The condition is generally confined to the aorta and the origins of its major branches. Extensive disease leads to dissecting aneurysm. These diseases include:

- Infectious aortitis, such as syphilitic aortitis (rare, typically affecting the ascending and transverse portions of the aortic arch and causing inflammatory destruction of the media with fibrous replacement), and mycotic aneurysms (small saccular dilatations with destruction of the wall caused by bacteria in infected thrombus).
- Vasculitic syndromes (see p. 67): inflammation of the vessels caused by immune complex deposition or cell-mediated immune reactions of the arterial wall leading to a weakening of the vessel wall then aneurysmal dilatations.
- Congenital aneurysms.

Pathogenesis

The majority of aneurysms occur because of a weakening of the arterial wall with loss of elasticity and contractability. Stretching of the weakened wall is gradually progressive due to hemodynamic pressure forces producing an increased thinning of the wall until eventual rupture occurs.

The build-up of layers of thrombus within the lumen of the aneurysmal sac is protective, but not usually sufficient to repair the defect and reconstitute a normal lumen to the artery.

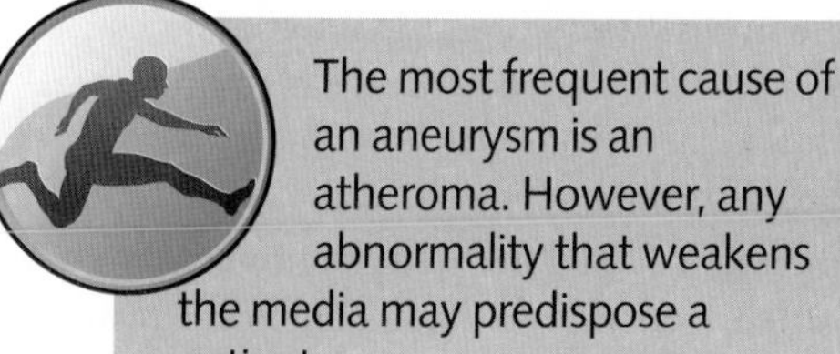

The most frequent cause of an aneurysm is an atheroma. However, any abnormality that weakens the media may predispose a patient.

Main complications

The main complications of aneurysms are rupture with critical hemorrhage and predisposition to thrombosis.

Abdominal aortic aneurysms

Abdominal aortic aneurysms (AAAs) are more common in men, especially over 60 years of age.

Etiology—Atherosclerosis is the most common cause of abdominal aneurysms. However, they may also arise as a result of inflammation (vasculitis) or infection (mycotic aneurysms).

Site—The majority are situated below the origin of the renal arteries and are thus amenable to resection and replacement by graft.

Morphology—Atherosclerotic aneurysms produce a fusiform dilatation of the wall.

Symptoms and signs

The majority of AAAs are asymptomatic, but occasionally patients are aware of a pulsatile mass. It is often first suspected because of aortic dilatation observed on radiographs, especially if the walls of aneurysm are calcified. It may also come to attention by careful palpation during physical examination. AAAs can be detected by ultrasound examination and the value of this investigation for screening purposes is currently being evaluated.

Symptoms may occur because of compression of neighboring structures by the expanding aneurysm; for example, erosion of the vertebrae by a large abdominal aneurysm may cause back pain.

Confirmation of an AAA is achieved by ultrasonography computed tomography (CT), magnetic resonance imaging (MRI), or arteriography.

Consequences

Rupture is the most devastating consequence, and it is often fatal. This may occur suddenly without warning or, alternatively, may slowly leak into the vessel wall resulting in pain and local tenderness.

Hemorrhage may occur into the retroperitoneal space, abdominal cavity or erode into the intestines resulting in massive gastrointestinal bleeding.

Prognostic factors

Fifty per cent of all abdominal aortic aneurysms that are more than 6cm in transverse diameter rupture within 2 years if not surgically resected. Aneurysms less than 6cm across may also rupture, albeit less frequently.

Mortalities of emergency and elective surgery

Elective surgical repair has a much lower mortality than emergency surgery for rupture and it is, therefore, recommended for most abdominal aortic aneurysms greater than 5cm in diameter, or those expanding in diameter at a rate exceeding 1cm per year. Mortality for surgical repair of abdominal aneurysms is also lower than that of thoracic aneurysms.

Aortic dissection

An aortic dissection is a tear in the intima of the aorta followed by the entry of blood into media with separation of a "flap" of intima from the rest of the aortic wall. A false lumen is created, usually between the inner two thirds and outer third of the medial thickness giving the appearance of a double-barrelled aorta.

Types of dissecting aneurysms

There are two types:

- Type A (67% of dissecting aneurysms) arise in the ascending aorta with or without extension into the descending aorta.
- Type B (33% of dissecting aneurysms) are confined to the descending aorta, distal to the origin of the left subclavian artery.

Epidemiology—Dissecting aneurysms occur most commonly in people between 50 and 70 years old, affecting males more than females by 2:1.

It is usually the result of cystic medial degeneration (see p. 65). Predisposing factors are:

- Hypertension.
- Connective tissue disorders (e.g., Marfan's syndrome).
- Pregnancy.
- Congenital abnormalities of the aortic valve.

Consequences

The false lumen inevitably ruptures, either:

- Externally—external rupture leads to massive fatal bleed into the thoracic cavity, or, less commonly, the pericardial sac, pleural cavity, or abdomen.
- Internally—rarely, blood tracks back into the lumen by rupturing through the inner media and intima forming a double-channelled aorta.

The clinical features are characterized by:

- Severe pain: sudden onset in the chest and back, often arising between the shoulder blades.

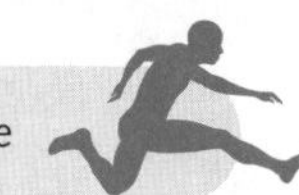

- Hypertension.
- Asymmetry of brachial, carotid, or femoral pulses.
- Broadening of the upper mediastinum on chest radiography.
- Distortion of the aortic "knuckle" (but not invariably) on chest radiography.
- Commonly, left-sided pleural effusion.

Diagnosis is by CT or angiography.

Management depends on which type occurs:

- Type A requires emergency surgical repair under cardiopulmonary bypass.
- Type B requires control of hypertension with bedrest; surgical intervention may be needed if there is evidence of leakage, or of renal or bowel ischemia.

Prognosis—This condition is fatal without treatment: 25% die within 24 hours, 50% within the week, and almost all by one year.

Syphilitic (luetic) aneurysms

Tertiary syphilis is now rare in the Western world. However, cardiovascular complications of untreated syphilis manifest one to three decades after the initial infection, and they include:

- Inflammation of the arterial media (aortitis), primarily of the ascending aorta.
- Aneurysm formation due to deterioration of elastic fibres and weakening of the media.
- Aortic regurgitation: dilatation of the aortic root weakens aortic valve support.
- Narrowing of the coronary artery ostia by inflammation and aortic intimal proliferation leading to an increased rise of myocardial ischemia.

These complications are now rare due to the early administration of antibiotic therapy.

Inflammatory and neoplastic vascular disease

Concepts and classification

Vasculitides

This is a group of disorders characterized by inflammation of the blood vessel walls (vasculitis). Vasculitis can affect capillaries, venules, arterioles, arteries, and, occasionally, large veins.

Effect

The effects are:

- Mild cases—transient damage to the vessel wall that produces leakage of red blood cells.
- Severe cases—irreversible vessel wall destruction resulting in ischemia and organ damage with associated systemic disturbances.

Classification

Vasculitis can be classified either according to the size of the vessel affected (Fig. 5.25) or according to the pathogenesis of the inflammation (Fig. 5.26).

Mechanisms of pathogenesis

Idiopathic The etiology is unknown, but the disorders (Fig. 5.26) are as follows:

- Giant cell arteritis (see below).
- Scleroderma (systemic sclerosis)—vascular changes are similar to those of benign or malignant hypertension, but only about 25% of patients are hypertensive. The condition is associated with progressive subcutaneous fibrosis leading to a marked tightening of the skin of the arms and hands; there are no effective treatments.
- Takayasu's (pulseless) disease—a rare inflammatory disorder of the aorta and its proximal branches, typically affecting young or middle-aged females. The condition is characterized by severe necrotizing inflammation of all layers of affected vessel walls with fibrous replacement of muscle and a reduction of lumen.

Classification of vasculitis according to size of affected vessel

Size of vessel	Disorders
Large, medium and small	Syphilitic aortitis Takayasu's disease Giant cell arteritis Kawasaki's disease Rheumatoid disease
Medium and small	Wegener's granulomatosis Polyarteritis nodosa Buerger's disease SLE
Small	Small vessel disease of arterioles, capillaries, and venules Henoch-Schönlein purpura

Fig. 5.25 Classification of vasculitis according to the size of the affected vessel.

Classification of vasculitis by pathogenesis	
Pathogenesis	**Disorders**
Idiopathic	Giant cell arteritis Scleroderma (systemic sclerosis) Takayasu's (pulseless) disease Kawasaki's disease Buerger's disease
Immune-mediated	Polyarteritis nodosa Wegener's granulomatosis Rheumatoid vasculitis SLE Henoch–Schönlein purpura
Infectious	Syphilitic aortitis Bacterial aortitis

Fig. 5.26 Classification of vasculitis by pathogenesis.

It presents clinically with hypertension or ischemic symptoms of the arms, with loss of arm pulses.

- Kawasaki's disease—a disease of infants that affects the main aortic branch arteries particularly the coronary arteries; characterized by medial fibroblastic thickening and, sometimes, aneurysm formation.
- Buerger's disease (thromboangitis obliterans)—a rare disease with a strong association with smoking. The condition mainly affects the small arteries of the arms and lower leg which show intimal fibrosis, thrombus formation, and adventitial tissue changes affecting adjacent veins and nerves. Clinically, peripheral gangrene develops in the fingers and toes; the disease is progressive and amputations are often required.

Immune-mediated vasculitis Pathogenesis is due to immune complex formation between antigens and antibodies. Immune complexes become trapped in venule walls and activated complement produces a local, acute inflammatory response with neutrophil chemotaxis. Neutrophils release enzymes that destroy the vessel wall.

There are two main types:

- Hypersensitivity (neutrophilic) vasculitis: the most common pattern affecting capillaries and venules; usually manifests as a skin rash, often as a result of an allergy to a drug or occasionally arising as an allergic rash in viremia or bacteremia. It also occurs in Henoch–Schönlein purpura, serum sickness, and cryoglobulinemia.
- Multiorgan autoimmune diseases, such as SLE and rheumatoid disease (mainly affects the aorta).

Autoantibodies that react against neutrophils can be detected in 90% of patients with Wegener's granulomatosis and in other types of vasculitis. Identification of these antibodies in serum is used in diagnostic evaluation of patients with possible vasculitis.

Infectious vasculitis These disorders (Fig. 5.26) include:

- Syphilitic aortitis—tertiary manifestation of syphilis typically affecting the ascending and transverse portions of the aortic arch causing inflammatory destruction of media with fibrous replacement.
- Other infections—bacteria in infected thrombi can cause destruction of vessel walls with the development of small saccular dilatations and mycotic aneurysms.

Giant cell (temporal) arteritis

Giant cell arteritis is a systemic disease that mainly involves arteries in the head and neck region, particularly the temporal arteries (hence the alternative name of temporal arteritis).

Epidemiology—The disease is relatively common, affecting 10 per 100,000 per year in the general population. Incidence increases with age, and it is rare in people under 50 years; it affects females more than males by 2:1.

Etiology—An idiopathic disease with associations with certain types of HLA.

The microscopic appearance of vessels is as follows:

- Thickened nodular vessel wall.
- Necrosis of inner media and gradual replacement with fibrosis.
- Fragmentation of internal elastic lamina.
- Inflammatory cell infiltration: mainly T lymphocytes but also histiocytes and giant cells (hence the name).
- Often complicated by thrombosis.

Clinical features—Patients have ill-defined symptoms of:

- Malaise.
- Tiredness.
- Severe headaches.
- An association with polymyalgia rheumatica.

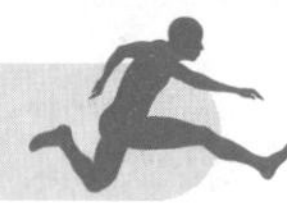

Investigations characteristically reveal high ESR and hyperglobulinemia. Diagnosis is made by biopsy of the temporal artery with histological investigation. Management is with corticosteroid therapy to control the disease.

Polyarteritis nodosa

This systemic disease is characterized by inflammatory necrosis of the walls of small and medium-sized arteries. Although the disease is systemic, it causes patchy and focal inflammation with only parts of some arteries being involved.

Epidemiology—A rare disease (about 5–10 per million per year in most populations), but it can occur in all age groups; males more than females by 2:1.

Etiology—The cause is unknown but the presence of antineutrophil cytoplasmic antibodies suggests an autoimmune pathogenesis. There is also an association with chronic hepatitis B virus antigenemia.

Pathogenesis—Inflammatory destruction results in the loss of the normal architecture of the vessel wall with necrosis of muscle cells and destruction of the elastic lamina. Healing occurs with fibrous replacement of the muscular media. Extensive damage to the intima predisposes to thrombosis, which is often followed by vessel occlusion and infarction of target tissue.

Microscopically, the artery wall shows:

- Inflammatory cell infiltration: neutrophils and eosinophils are most numerous.
- Fibrinoid necrosis of segments of artery wall.
- Thrombosis, which is common.

Clinical features include systemic features of inflammation (fever, weight loss, myalgia, and muscle wasting) and the effects of vessel occlusion producing small areas of infarction. Tissues most seriously affected are the kidneys, heart, GI tract, liver, CNS, peripheral nerves, skeletal muscle, and skin.

Diagnosis is by:

- Blood: neutrophilia and raised ESR.
- Antineutrophil cytoplasmic antibodies (ANCA) which are present in most cases.
- Tissue biopsy, usually of a kidney or asymptomatic muscle.

The prognosis depends on the intensity and pattern of organ involvement; 30% of patients develop renal failure and hypertensive complications.

Management is by cyclophosphamide with corticosteroids, which has significantly improved the outcome. Antihypertensive drugs reduce morbidity from hypertensive complications.

Neoplastic vascular disease

Benign

Hemangiomas

Hemangiomas are common developmental malformations composed of dilated vascular spaces derived from blood vessels.

There are three types of hemangioma:

- Capillary hemangiomas (strawberry nevi), which are composed of small, capillary-like vessels.
- Cavernous hemangiomas, which are composed of cavernous, endothelial-lined spaces (vein-like vessels).
- Sclerosing hemangiomas, which are fibrous nodules containing iron pigment produced as a result of fibrosis or sclerosis of a capillary hemangioma.

> Hemangiomas are not "'true" tumors, but they are often grouped with neoplasms because they appear as localized tissue masses. They are more accurately described as hamartomas, i.e., non-neoplastic overgrowths of tissue.

Telangiectasias

Dilatations of capillaries are often seen in the elderly and those with irradiated skin or liver failure (spider naevi). Vessels are dilated but histologically normal.

Malignant

Kaposi's sarcoma

Kaposi's sarcoma (KS) is a malignant tumor that is thought to be derived from lymphatic endothelial cells; it is rapidly becoming more important and common. There are four patterns of disease:

- Endemic KS (seen in Africa) is highly malignant in children (through lymphatic spread) with a more indolent course in adults (through blood spread).
- Classic KS is a rare, low-grade, malignant tumor of the skin that develops in the lower limbs of elderly

Predisposing factors of varicose veins
Defective support of vessel wall • familial tendency: in approx. 40% of all cases • gender: significantly increased incidence in females • obesity: adipose tissue = poor venous support; muscle = good venous support • age: degenerative changes in surrounding tissues and decreased activity of muscles → loss of venous support
Increased venous pressure • standing occupations: increased incidence in occupations involving prolonged standing (venous pressure is greatest on standing) • pregnancy • intravascular thrombosis • tumor masses pressing on veins (e.g., uterine fibroids and ovarian tumors) • garters and other constrictions

Fig. 5.27 Predisposing factors of varicose veins.

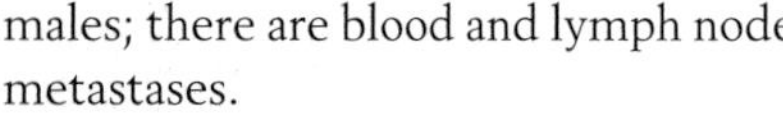

males; there are blood and lymph node metastases.

- KS in therapeutic immunosuppression, which resembles classic KS.
- Epidemic KS is a highly malignant tumor of the skin seen in patients with acquired immune deficiency syndrome (AIDS); spreads to lymph nodes and the visceral organs.

Angiosarcoma

A malignant tumor of blood vessel endothelium. This most commonly occurs as a raised bluish-red patch on the face or scalp of elderly people. Progressive enlargement of the tumor is accompanied by ulceration and, later, metastasis to regional lymph nodes.

Diseases of the veins and lymphatics

Varicose veins

Varicose veins are persistently distended superficial veins in the lower limbs (long and short saphenous veins). They result from incompetent valves that allow the veins to become engorged with blood under the influence of gravity.

Epidemiology—The condition affects 10–20% of the general population at some age. There is an increasing incidence with age, and it is most common above 50. It affects females more than males by 4:1.

See Fig. 5.27 for the predisposing factors of varicose veins.

Anatomy of varicose veins—The superficial and deep venous plexuses of the lower limb are connected by perforating veins (Fig. 5.28).

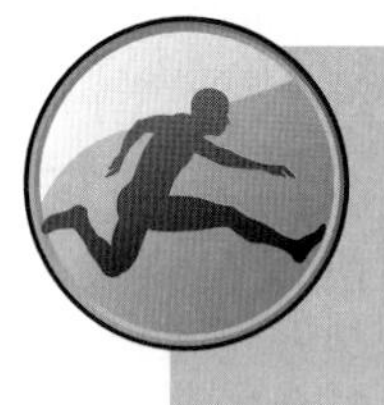

Varicose leg ulcers are a common clinical condition, and they are associated with chronic venous insufficiency.

Pathogenesis—The return of blood from the deep veins is aided by normal contraction of the calf and thigh muscles. If the valves in the perforating veins become incompetent, blood is forced from deep venous plexuses to superficial venous plexuses resulting in increased pressure in the superficial veins; this is a major factor in the development of varicosities.

Morphological changes

The morphological changes are:

- Increased pressure produces a dilatation of the lumen and an increased tension on vessel walls with compensatory hypertrophy of the muscle and elastic tissues.
- Prolonged increased pressure produces irregular atrophy of muscle and elastic lamina with fibrous replacement leading to stretched, tortuous veins with localized bulging.

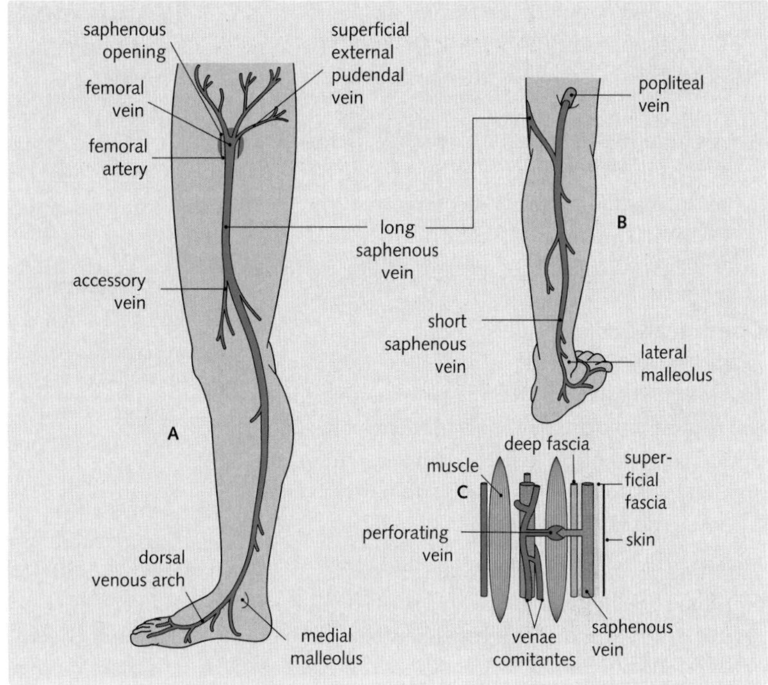

Fig. 5.28 Superficial veins of the right lower limb. (A) Long saphenous vein. (B) Short saphenous vein. (C) "Venous pump" showing valved perforating veins, which link deep and superficial veins.

Sequelae of varicose veins

The sequelae are:

- Edema (of lower limbs) due to increased hydrostatic pressure.
- Thromboembolism: thrombosis is a frequent complication.
- Dermatitis: varicose dermatitis with pigmentation due to hemosiderin deposition.
- Varicose ulcers: dermatitis may proceed to ulceration, which is very slow to heal. Usually on the medial aspect of the ankle or lower leg.

Thrombophlebitis and phlebothrombosis

Definitions

Thrombophlebitis is thrombosis initiated by inflammation of the vessel wall. Phlebothrombosis is inflammation of the vessel wall secondary to thrombosis of a noninflammatory origin (when a vein becomes thrombosed it evokes an inflammatory response). Thrombosis of a noninflammatory origin can occur because of abnormalities of the vessel wall, blood components, or blood flow. These three thrombus predisposing factors are referred to as Virchow's triad.

A histological differentiation between the two types is in most cases impossible.

Causes

Thrombosis can be caused by factors giving rise to stasis. For example:

- Cardiac failure.
- Pregnancy.
- Prolonged bed rest.
- Immobilization.
- Varicose veins.

Others factors that can cause thrombosis are direct injury or infection of the veins (e.g., trauma or intravenous cannulation) and hypercoagulable states such as anti-thrombin III deficiency and polycythemia. Smoking is also implicated as a predisposing risk factor to thrombosis.

Affected sites

The most commonly affected sites are:

- Deep leg veins (90% of cases) particularly the lower leg.
- Skull and dural sinuses.
- Portal venous tributaries.
- Pelvic veins.

Presentation

Presentation of both types is similar, with distention of the veins by laminated thrombus. Outcomes of thrombosis include:

- Lysis—dissolution of the thrombus by activated fibrinolytic system.
- Propagation—spread of the thrombus proximally in the veins.
- Organization—reparative process with ingrowth of fibroblasts.
- Recanalization—usually incomplete re-establishment of blood flow.
- Embolism—thrombus migrates to a distant site.

Complications

Acute

The most serious acute complication is embolism of the thrombus to the pulmonary arteries causing a pulmonary embolism (PE). Pulmonary embolisms are divided into massive, major, and minor events. These are discussed in detail on page 97.

Chronic

Chronic complications are aching pains due to varicose veins, venous congestion, edema, venous eczema, and ulceration.

Management of thrombotic events

High-risk patients should be identified and offered prophylaxis.

Treatment is aimed at preventing the propagation of the thrombus. Immediate treatment is anticoagulation by heparin and warfarin. Thrombolytic therapy is occasionally indicated for patients with large iliofemoral thrombosis.

Long-term treatment is by oral anticoagulants, mobilization, and graduated elastic stockings. In extreme cases a filter may be inserted in the vena cava.

Lymphangitis and lymphedema

Lymphangitis

Lymphangitis is inflammation of lymphatic channels draining any focus of infection. The channels are dilated and contain inflammatory cells. The condition may result in the spread of the infection in some cases (e.g., in tuberculosis).

Lymphedema

Lymphedema is edema of the tissues caused by obstruction of the lymphatics.

Causes

The causes of obstructive lymphedema are:

- Metastatic spread of tumors causing mechanical blockage.
- Surgical removal of nodes.
- Postirradiation fibrosis.
- Filariasis (elephantiasis): nematode infection of lymph nodes (most common culprit is *Wuchereria bancrofti*; transmitted to man by the bite of an infected mosquito).
- Post-inflammatory thrombosis and scarring, e.g., lymphogranuloma venereum.
- Primary lymphatic disorders (rare).

Effects

The effects of obstructive lymphedema are:

- Gross swelling.
- Increased predisposition to attacks of lymphangitis and ulceration.
- Severe cases result in thickening of skin and overgrowth of dermal connective tissues leading to elephantiasis.

- Name the congenital abnormalities that cause left-to-right shunts and right-to-left shunts.
- Define atherosclerosis, and list the risk factors implicated in its development.
- Describe the different types of hypertension.
- Describe the types of atheromatous plaques that occur in the coronary arteries.
- Name the sites of myocardial infarction and the vessel involved in each case.
- Describe the major causes and basic features of valve disease.
- Describe the pathogenesis of chronic rheumatic heart disease.
- Describe the etiology and pathogenesis of infective endocarditis.
- Define cardiomyopathy, and describe the types and basic features of primary and secondary cardiomyopathies.
- Define myocarditis, and explain its etiology.
- What is the most common primary heart tumor?
- Define cardiac tamponade, and describe the physical signs.
- List the causes of acute pericarditis, and describe the different types of inflammation.
- List the main causes of aneurysms.
- Describe the features of abdominal aortic aneurysms and aortic dissection.
- Define vasculitides, and explain the pathogenesis.
- Define varicose veins, and comment on the factors that predispose to their development.
- What is the difference between thrombophlebitis and phlebothrombosis?
- What are the causes and complications of inflammation and thrombosis of vessel walls?
- Describe the causes of lymphedema.

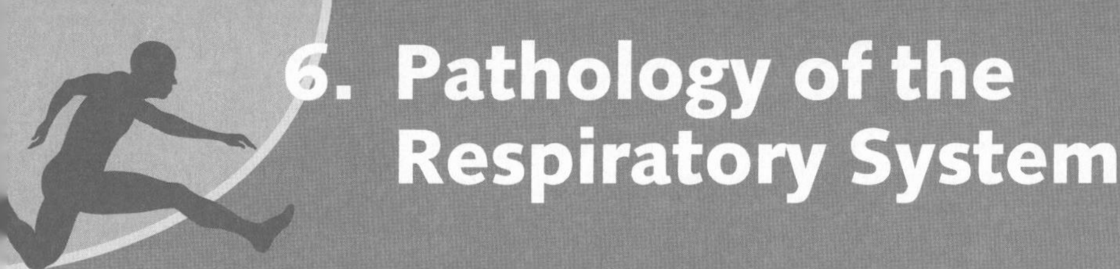

6. Pathology of the Respiratory System

Disorders of the upper respiratory tract

The nose and nasopharynx

Inflammatory conditions

Rhinitis

Rhinitis, inflammation of the nasal mucosa, is the most common nasal disorder seen in family practice. The condition may be either acute or chronic.

Acute rhinitis Etiology of acute rhinitis is either:

- Infective.
- Allergic.

Infectious rhinitis is usually of viral origin—for example, the common cold (rhinoviruses, respiratory syncytial virus, para-influenza viruses, coronaviruses) and influenza (influenza virus). Virally induced inflammation of surface epithelial cells is followed by exudation of fluid and mucus from the damaged surface ("runny nose"). Later, submucosal edema produces swelling, which may lead to a partial blockage of the nasal airways.

Allergic rhinitis ("hay fever") is a type I (IgE-mediated) hypersensitivity reaction to inhaled materials, such as grass and pollens, that produces a mixed serous–mucus exudate, and submucosal edema, leading to nasal blockage.

Chronic rhinitis Chronic rhinitis can be caused by either chronic infective inflammation or chronic allergic inflammation, and it may result in the development of nasal polyps.

Macroscopically, nasal polyps are typically smooth-surfaced, creamy, semi-translucent, ovoid masses.

Microscopically, they have edematous tissue with scattered infiltrate of chronic inflammatory cells including plasma cells. Eosinophils are often very numerous in allergic polyps.

Sinusitis (inflammation of the sinuses)

Acute sinusitis The most important type of sinus inflammation is acute maxillary sinusitis (ethmoidal and frontal sinusitis being less common).

Etiology—Usually secondary to acute rhinitis.

Pathogenesis—In acute rhinitis, there is usually associated inflammation of the sinus linings; swelling of the mucosa around the drainage foramen of the maxillary sinus in the nasal cavity may cause stasis of maxillary sinus secretions. Stasis predisposes to secondary bacterial infection with alteration of the static maxillary fluid from seromucous to purulent.

In severe cases, the infection may spread into the ethmoid and frontal sinuses with a risk of spread of infection to the meninges.

Chronic sinusitis This condition is characterized by chronically thickened and inflamed mucosa of the sinuses, and persistent fluid accumulation.

The condition may arise as a result of:

- Acute sinusitis from failure of drainage of acutely inflamed sinus.
- Chronic inhalation of irritant (e.g., cigarette smoke, industrial exposure).
- Nasal obstruction as a result of a severely deviated nasal septum or from the presence of nasal polyps.

Kartagener's syndrome This is a syndrome of bronchiectasis, sinusitis, and situs inversus (transposition of viscera). Each element of the triad is caused by abnormal ciliary function, due to a defect in the dynein arm of tubulin protein. The result is failure to clear mucus and bacteria.

Necrotizing lesions

Mucormycotic infections

This fulminant opportunistic fungal infection of the nose is usually the result of immune suppression or prolonged antibiotic therapy. It may be rapidly fatal unless treated promptly with systemic antifungals.

Wegener's granulomatosis

An autoimmune granulomatous vasculitis, this frequently presents with nasal lesions.

Lethal midline granuloma (lymphoma)

This is a condition presenting with progressive ulceration and destruction of the structures in the upper respiratory tract, i.e., the nose, nasopharynx, palate, and sinuses. It is thought to be a form of T cell lymphoma, and it is characterized histologically by the infiltration of small lymphocytes, plasma cells, blast cells, and atypical large lymphoid cells.

Untreated, death occurs from systemic disease caused by erosion of blood vessels, local infection, or the development of pneumonia.

Neoplasms

Nasopharyngeal angiofibroma

This rare benign tumor (also known as juvenile angiofibroma) occurs almost exclusively in males between 10 and 25 years old. The lesions are typically located in the nasopharynx rather than the nose, and, during puberty, that may mimic a malignant tumor in their rapid growth and tendency to erode bone. Ulceration and bleeding are common.

Inverted papilloma

A benign, endophytic (hence "inverted") tumor of adults, this is associated with human papillomavirus infection. It can be difficult to eradicate and may recur. Malignant transformation occurs in approximately 3%.

Plasmacytomas

This malignant tumor is composed of monoclonal plasma cells. It presents as a soft, hemorrhagic nasal/nasopharyngeal mass, which may progress to disseminated myeloma after many years.

Olfactory neuroblastoma

A rare nasal tumor presenting in the upper part of the nasal cavity, often as a hemorrhagic mass with evidence of bone destruction, it is typically slow growing, but it may recur after surgical removal. Metastases occur in about 20% of cases.

Nasopharyngeal carcinoma

This is a squamous or anaplastic carcinoma of the nasopharynx (part of pharynx that lies immediately behind the nasal cavities) with characteristic abundant lymphoid tissue in the stroma.

It is strongly associated with Epstein–Barr virus infection, the virus being demonstrable in tumor cells in most cases.

The tumors often remain small and undetected until metastasis to the lymph nodes in the neck has occurred. The vast majority of patients with nasopharyngeal carcinoma have lymph node metastases when they first present.

The prognosis is better with radiation therapy: the 5-year survival rate is 80% for localized disease and 50% for advanced disease.

The larynx

Inflammatory conditions

Acute laryngitis

This acute inflammation of the larynx may be infective (majority of cases), allergic, or irritative.

Infective laryngitis

This typically occurs secondary to either viral or bacterial upper respiratory tract infection involving the nose, sinuses, etc.

Allergic laryngitis

This follows inhalation or ingestion of an allergen.

Irritative laryngitis

This follows ingestion or inhalation of irritant gases or fluids (e.g., ammonia, cigarette smoke) or following irritation by mechanical factors, e.g., endotracheal intubation.

Sequelae of acute laryngitis

The sequelae are:

- Resolution: infective causes typically resolve without complications.
- Spread of infection may occur throughout the respiratory tract with the development of tracheobronchitis, bronchopneumonia or lung abscesses; it is more common in the elderly or debilitated due to a poor cough reflex.
- Airway obstruction: laryngeal edema can result in a life-threatening narrowing of the airway, especially in children (whose airways are narrower) suffering from *Hemophilus influenzae* epiglottitis or in cases of corrosive chemical ingestion.

Croup

Croup is acute inflammation and obstruction of the respiratory tract involving the larynx, trachea, and bronchi. It usually affects young children aged 6 months to 3 years.

Etiology—Typically caused by viral infection but secondary bacterial infection can occur.

The condition produces symptoms of laryngitis accompanied by signs of obstruction: harsh difficult breathing (stridor), a rising pulse rate, restlessness, and cyanosis.

Treatment is by reassurance and humidification of inspired air, which usually reverses the symptoms. In

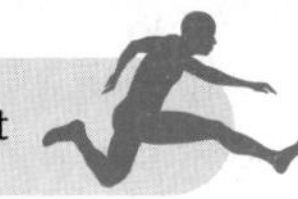

severe cases, the obstruction may require treatment by intubation or tracheostomy.

Chronic laryngitis

This is a chronic inflammation of the larynx, most commonly seen in heavy cigarette smokers. It may lead to a permanent thickening of the laryngeal mucosa and submucosa, particularly where there is associated excess production of keratin ("smoker's keratosis"), due to squamous metaplasia.

Overlying epidermis may also undergo keratotic thickening with dysplastic change in the basal layer; this is a predisposing factor in the development of squamous carcinoma.

Reactive nodules

Polyps

This common benign lesion is associated with upper respiratory tract infection or occurs after vocal abuse, e.g., shouting. It causes hoarseness that will not resolve until the polyp is removed.

Singer's nodules

These are smooth, round, minute nodules located at the nodal point (junction between the anterior third and posterior two thirds of the vocal cords). Nodules are especially common in singers and professional voice users, and they can alter the character of the voice even when only a few millimeters in diameter. They consist of edematous connective tissue with submucosal fibrosis covered by squamous epithelium.

Papilloma and papillomatosis

Papilloma Warty papillomas on the larynx are usually due to infection by the human papillomavirus (HPV 11 and 16). The lesions are usually solitary and confined to the vocal cords. Papilloma is clinically and histologically difficult to distinguish from early verrucous carcinomas (see below).

Juvenile laryngeal papillomatosis These multiple soft pink papillomas on the vocal cords are largely confined to children. Lesions often extend into other parts of the larynx, sometimes even down the trachea, and they have the histological features of florid viral warts. They are typically persistent and recurrent, such that eradication is difficult, often requiring repeated multiple excisions.

Squamous cell carcinoma of the larynx

This accounts for 1–2% of cancers with an incidence of 1–2 per 100,000 per year worldwide. It typically presents after 40 years of age, affecting males more than females (but the incidence is rising in females). The risk factors are smoking, radiation to head and neck, carcinoma in situ and keratosis (see above).

The affected sites are:

- Supraglottic region (30%); e.g., epiglottis, false cords, and ventricles.
- Glottic region (60%): true vocal cords and anterior and posterior commissures; best prognosis if detected early (early symptom being hoarseness).
- Subglottic region (10%): arising below the true vocal cords and above the first tracheal ring; poor prognosis if late presentation.

Macroscopically, they are ulcerated, diffuse, gray, solid, or papillary lesions.

Microscopically, the majority are well-differentiated, keratinizing squamous carcinomas; a minority are poorly differentiated with spindle cells.

Spread can be:

- Local—to adjacent laryngeal structures but often confined by laryngeal cartilages for a considerable time.
- Lymphatic—to regional lymph nodes.
- Hematogenous—occurs late if at all; lungs are the most common site.

The prognosis depends on location, extent of spread, and the presence of lymph node metastasis. The overall 5-year survival is as follows:

- Glottic tumors—80%.
- Supraglottic tumors—65%.
- Subglottic tumors—40%.

Verrucous carcinoma

This is a variant of laryngeal squamous cell carcinoma, often presenting as a large, warty, papillary tumor with all the clinical features of malignancy. It usually affects one or both of the true vocal cords, the lesions being composed of benign-looking squamous epithelium with hyperkeratosis. However, the tumor is locally destructive and it requires surgical removal to prevent fatal obstruction or laryngeal destruction. Metastasis is rare.

Disorders of the lungs

Atelectasis

This is a defective expansion and collapse of the lung. It may occur as a result of:

- Obstruction.
- Compression.
- Scarring.
- Surfactant loss.

Obstructive causes

Obstruction of the larger bronchial tubes leads to resorption of air from the lung distal to the obstruction. Causes of obstruction can be within the lung (retained secretions, inhaled foreign bodies, or bronchial cancer) or outside the lung (enlarged lymph nodes as in tuberculosis (TB) or lung cancer).

Patchy atelectasis describes the pattern of atelectasis associated with chronic obstructive airway diseases.

Compressive causes

Compressive atelectasis is the compression of the lung caused by the accumulation of fluid or air in the pleural cavity.

Scarring

Scarring of the lung may cause contraction of the parenchyma and lung collapse.

Surfactant loss

Surfactant loss can be either developmental or acquired and leads to a generalized failure of lung expansion, termed microatelectasis.

Consequences of atelectasis

The collapse of a lung has important clinical consequences as respiratory function will be disturbed. Expansion can be aided by physiotherapy and bronchoscopy-mediated removal of the obstructive/compressive cause. However, prolonged atelectasis becomes irreversible.

Chronic obstructive pulmonary disease

Differences between obstructive and restrictive lung diseases

Obstructive lung diseases

Obstructive lung diseases are those diseases in which there is obstruction to the *flow* of air within the lungs, although the lungs themselves may be hyperinflated. If obstruction is long term, then these conditions are collectively known as chronic obstructive pulmonary (or airway) diseases (i.e., COPD).

Restrictive lung diseases

Restrictive lung diseases are those diseases in which there is obstruction to the *expansion* of the lungs (e.g., due to fibrosis or edema) such that they can only take in a limited amount of air. In these diseases, although the lungs are often underinflated, the rate of air flow is unaffected. An example of a restrictive lung disease is pulmonary fibrosis. These diseases are covered in more detail later under "Diffuse interstitial diseases" on p. 94.

Both obstructive and restrictive lung diseases can cause significant respiratory impairment with a characteristic pattern of pulmonary function tests (Fig. 6.1 and Fig. 6.2).

Mechanisms

There are two main mechanisms by which airflow may be reduced in COPD, causing two different clinical pictures:

- Increased airway resistance, typically by a narrowing of the airways, e.g., chronic bronchitis,

Characteristic patterns of lung function tests in obstructive and restrictive lung disease

	Obstructive lung diseases	Restrictive lung diseases
Vital capacity (VC)	↓ or normal	↓↓
FEV_1	↓↓	↓
FEV_1/VC ratio	↓	Normal or ↑
Peak respiratory flow rate (PEFR)	↓	Normal

Fig. 6.1 Characteristic patterns of lung function tests in obstructive and restrictive lung diseases.

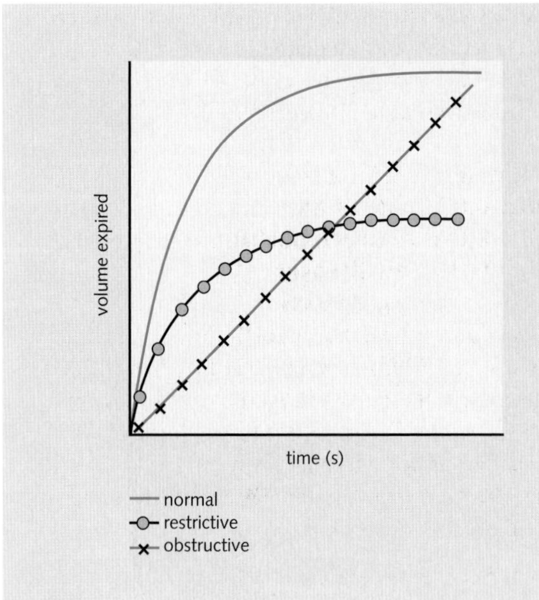

Fig. 6.2 Illustration of a normal, obstructive deficit, and restrictive deficit vitalography.

bronchiectasis, and asthma; this results in hypercapnia, hypoxemia, and cyanosis.
- Decreased outflow pressure due to loss of elastic recoil of the lungs, e.g., emphysema. However, in this case, compensatory hyperventilation leads to relatively normal levels of $Pa{CO_2}$ and $Pa{O_2}$ at rest.

Diagnosis and treatment

COPDs can be diagnosed with chest X-ray (which may show hyperinflation, flat hemidiaphragms, reduced peripheral vascular markings, and bullae) and lung function tests (Figs 6.1 and 6.2).

Treatment is by:
- Physiotherapy.
- Bronchodilators (e.g., salbutamol): there is often a reversible element to airway obstruction due to local bronchial irritation.
- Antibiotics for associated chronic bronchitis.

Note that the respiratory centers of some patients with COPD are relatively insensitive to CO_2, relying on hypoxic drive to maintain respiratory effort. It is, therefore, dangerous to give these patients supplemental oxygen without careful observation, as hypoventilation or apnea may result.

Emphysema

Emphysema is a permanent dilatation of any part of the air spaces distal to the terminal bronchiole with or without destruction of tissue but with no scarring. It is a common condition with increasing incidence with age, and it is more common in males than in females.

The etiology is unclear, but risk factors include cigarette smoking, atmospheric pollution, and a family history. It is thought to due to an imbalance of the protease/antiprotease system brought about by extrinsic toxins (see below).

Associations—The majority of cases are seen in conjunction with chronic bronchitis, but α_1-antitrypsin deficiency can be an inherited factor.

Pathogenesis

In normal individuals, extracellular proteases secreted into the lung by inflammatory cells are inhibited by protease-inhibitors (particularly α_1-antitrypsin). In emphysema, these inhibitors are either inactivated (e.g., by cigarette smoke) or absent, resulting in continued activity of the proteases with destruction of lung parenchyma (Fig. 6.3). Destruction of respiratory tissue leads to a loss of elastic recoil in the lungs and a decreased area available for gaseous exchange. About one third of lung capacity must be destroyed before clinical symptoms of emphysema appear.

Types of emphysema

There are several forms of emphysema, defined by the location of damage in the respiratory acinus (Fig. 6.4):
- Centrilobular: dilatation of the respiratory bronchioles at the center of acinus. It is most common in men and is closely associated with cigarette smoking. Lesions are most commonly found in the upper lobes.
- Panlobular: dilatation of the terminal alveoli and alveolar ducts, which later affects the respiratory bronchioles, thereby affecting the whole acinus. Typically affects the lower lobes.
- Paraseptal: involves air spaces at the periphery of lobules, typically adjacent to the pleura. Usually affects the upper lobes.
- Irregular: irregular involvement of the respiratory acinus, and almost always associated with scarring. It is thought to be caused by the trapping of air following lung fibrosis, and it is, therefore, commonly present around old, healed tuberculous scars at the lung apices.

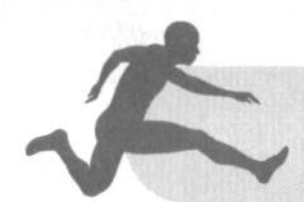

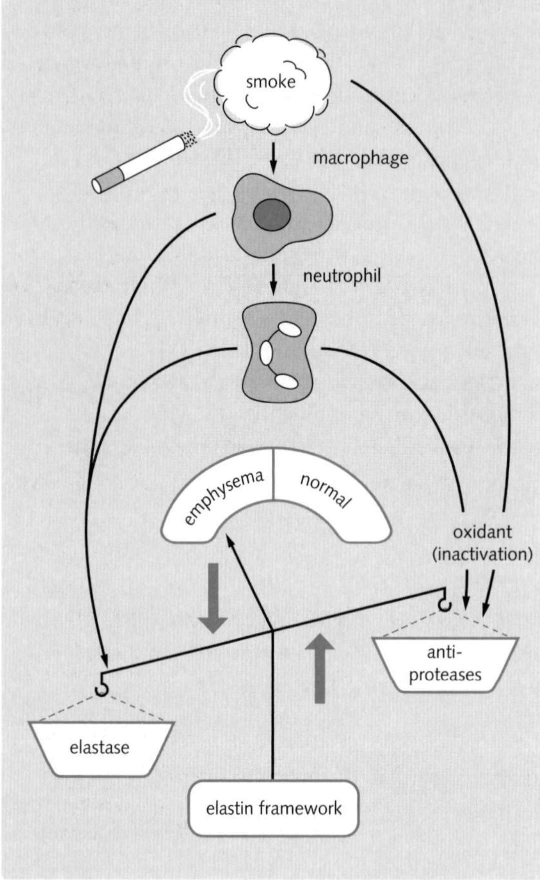

Fig. 6.3 Pathogenesis of emphysema. (Adapted from *The Lungs* by B. Corrin, Churchill Livingstone, 1990.)

Clinical features

These have two stages:

- Early stage—rapid respiratory rate enables individuals to maintain blood oxygenation, such that levels of $Pa\text{CO}_2$ and $Pa\text{O}_2$ are near normal. Patients are breathless but not cyanosed ("pink puffers"). However, on the slightest exertion patients become increasingly breathless and ultimately hypoxic (type 1 respiratory failure).
- Later stage—despite an increased respiratory rate, there is reduced oxygen uptake even at rest. A progressive decline in respiratory function ensues with the development of cyanosis, hypercapnia, and cor pulmonale (right heart failure).

The lungs are hyperinflated, the trachea is often descended (i.e., there is decreased distance between the thyroid cartilage and the sternal notch), and the

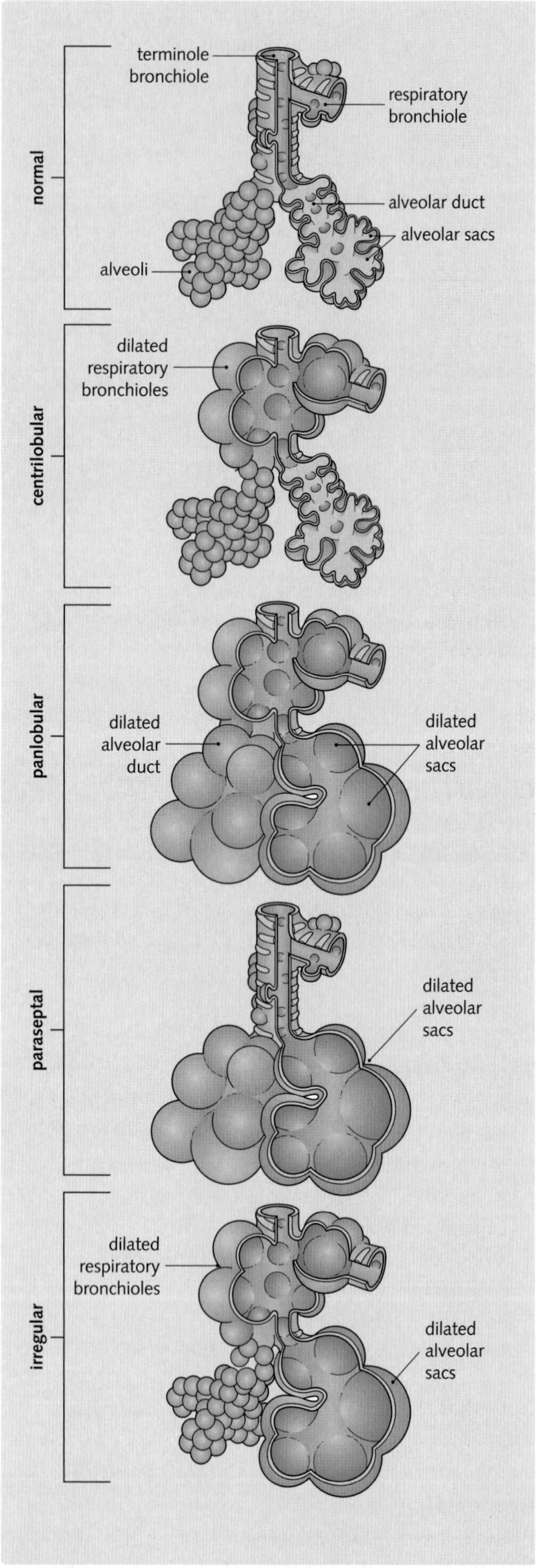

Fig. 6.4 Diagrams of the main types of emphysema.

accessory muscles may be hypertrophied. Associated chronic bronchitis may produce cough and sputum. Breath sounds are quiet especially over bullae, often with crepitations or wheezes.

Chronic bronchitis

Chronic bronchitis is defined as a cough productive of sputum on most days for 3 months of the year for at least two successive years. It typically affects middle-aged men, and most cases are due to cigarette smoking.

Pathogenesis

Constant irritation by cigarette smoke causes chronic inflammation of the respiratory bronchioles (bronchiolitis) and increased mucus secretion.

Hypersecretion of mucus is associated with hypertrophy and hyperplasia of the bronchial mucus-secreting glands. The Reid index gives the ratio of gland to wall thickness in the bronchus, and it is significantly increased in cases of chronic bronchitis.

Bronchiolar obstruction must be extensive and widespread to give clinical symptoms. Eventually, extensive mucus plugging leads to the clinical obstructive features of the disease with typical cough and sputum production.

Clinical features

These are:

- Early stages—chronic cough with sputum.
- Later stages—disease becomes progressively more severe, and it is accompanied by hypercapnia, hypoxemia, and cyanosis (often producing "blue bloaters"). Eventually right heart failure (cor pulmonale) or respiratory failure ensues.

The condition may be complicated by:

- Recurrent low-grade bronchial infections caused by bacteria such as *Hemophilus influenzae* and *Streptococcus pneumoniae*, or viruses such as respiratory syncytial virus and adenovirus.
- Squamous metaplasia: loss of ciliated cells as a result of squamous metaplasia can further exacerbate the problem.
- Malignancy: persistent injury by smoking may invoke dysplastic changes in metaplastic squamous epithelium, which may ultimately become malignant (squamous cell carcinoma of the bronchus).

Bronchial asthma

Bronchial asthma is an increased irritability of the bronchial tree with paroxysmal narrowing of the airways, which may reverse either spontaneously or after treatment with bronchodilators.

This is a common disorder, affecting around 10% of children and 5% of adults. Its incidence is thought to be rising, possibly due to environmental atmospheric pollution.

There are several known triggers of asthma:

- Allergy—a large number of allergens can precipitate asthma by inducing an IgE-mediated type 1 hypersensitivity reaction. Examples include pollen, house dust mites, animal dander, foods, and drugs.
- Infection—respiratory tract infection can trigger bronchoconstriction.
- Occupational exposure—some agents act as allergens, others by direct irritation of the airway.
- Drug-induced (e.g., β-antagonists and aspirin).
- Irritant gases (e.g., sulphur dioxide, nitric oxide, ozone in smog).
- Psychological stress can exacerbate attacks.
- Cold air.
- Exercise—especially in combination with cold air.

Asthma is associated with other atopic diseases such as eczema, hay fever, and some allergies.

Asthma can be classified into two categories, depending on whether there is an allergic basis to the disease:

- Extrinsic asthma (atopic): early onset asthma triggered by environmental allergens. Individuals often have a family history of allergic disorders. IgE levels are raised and an immediate type 1 hypersensitivity to the allergen is produced on skin challenge. This is the most common type of asthma.
- Intrinsic asthma (non-atopic): a late onset asthma often triggered by infection of the upper respiratory tract. IgE levels are normal, there is no family history of allergic disorders, and skin testing is negative.

However, there is often much overlap between the two types, and many patients do not fit neatly into any one type.

Pathogenesis—In both types of asthma, obstruction is caused by a combination of bronchospasm, edema, and mucus plugging. The exact mechanisms of intrinsic asthma are uncertain, but in the case of extrinsic (atopic) asthma a generalized airway hyperresponsiveness to bronchoconstrictor trigger factors is known to be central to the pathogenesis.

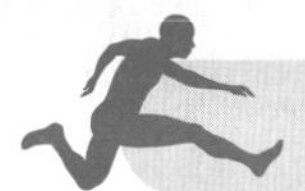

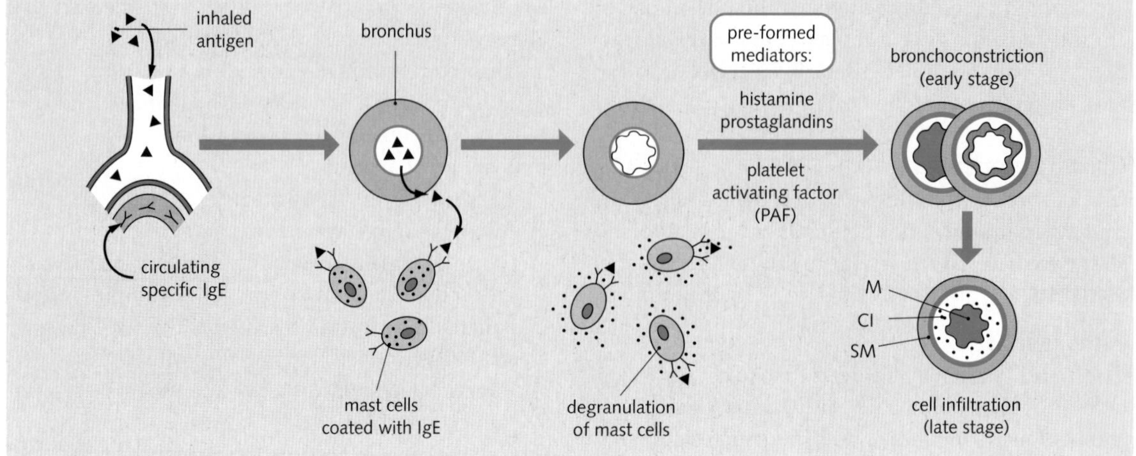

Fig. 6.5 Pathogenesis of the early and late stages of asthma. M, mucus; CI, cellular infiltration; SM, smooth muscle.

The three phases of extrinsic asthma

- Early (15–20 minutes): a rapid onset of bronchoconstriction caused by histamine release from mast cell degranulation. The allergen binds to IgE antibodies on the surface of mast cells causing cross-linking and degranulation (Fig. 6.5).
- Late (4–6 hours): a second wave of bronchoconstriction after recovery from the early phase. Inflammatory mediators released by mast cells during the early phase cause activation of macrophages and chemotaxis of polymorphs and eosinophils into the bronchial mucosa. These cells release inflammatory mediators causing a secondary wave of bronchoconstriction (Fig. 6.6).
- Prolonged hyperreactivity (over days): an exaggerated response of the airway on further re-exposure to the allergen or other bronchoconstrictor trigger factors over ensuing days. There is persistence of inflammatory cells within the bronchial wall leading to damage and loss of epithelial cells.

Structural changes

The main structural changes that take place in asthmatic airways are listed below and illustrated in Fig. 6.6:

- Immune cell infiltration: bronchial mucosa is infiltrated by eosinophils, mast cells, lymphoid cells, and macrophages.
- Mucosal edema: extravasation of plasma into submucosal tissues produces a narrowing of the airways.
- Mucus hypersecretion leads to plugging of airways.
- Hypertrophy of bronchial smooth muscle due to recurrent bronchoconstriction.
- Focal necrosis of the airway epithelium, caused by prolonged inflammation.
- Deposition of collagen beneath the bronchial epithelium in long-standing cases.
- Sputum contains Charcot–Leyden crystals (derived from eosinophil granules) and Curschmann's spirals (composed of mucus plugs from small airways).

Clinical features

Clinical features are as follows:

- Mild disease (majority of cases)—acute intermittent episodes of bronchospasm (wheezing, dyspnea, or coughing) are triggered by well-recognized causes.
- Moderate to severe disease (small percentage)—increasingly severe and increasingly irreversible asthma in middle or old age (chronic asthma); patients may present with signs of respiratory distress.
- Status asthmaticus—severe, acute disease that does not respond to drug therapy. Air entry may be inadequate to generate any wheeze (the silent chest is an ominous sign), and death may result from acute respiratory insufficiency.

The clinical signs of asthma include widespread, polyphonic, high-pitched wheezes. The affected

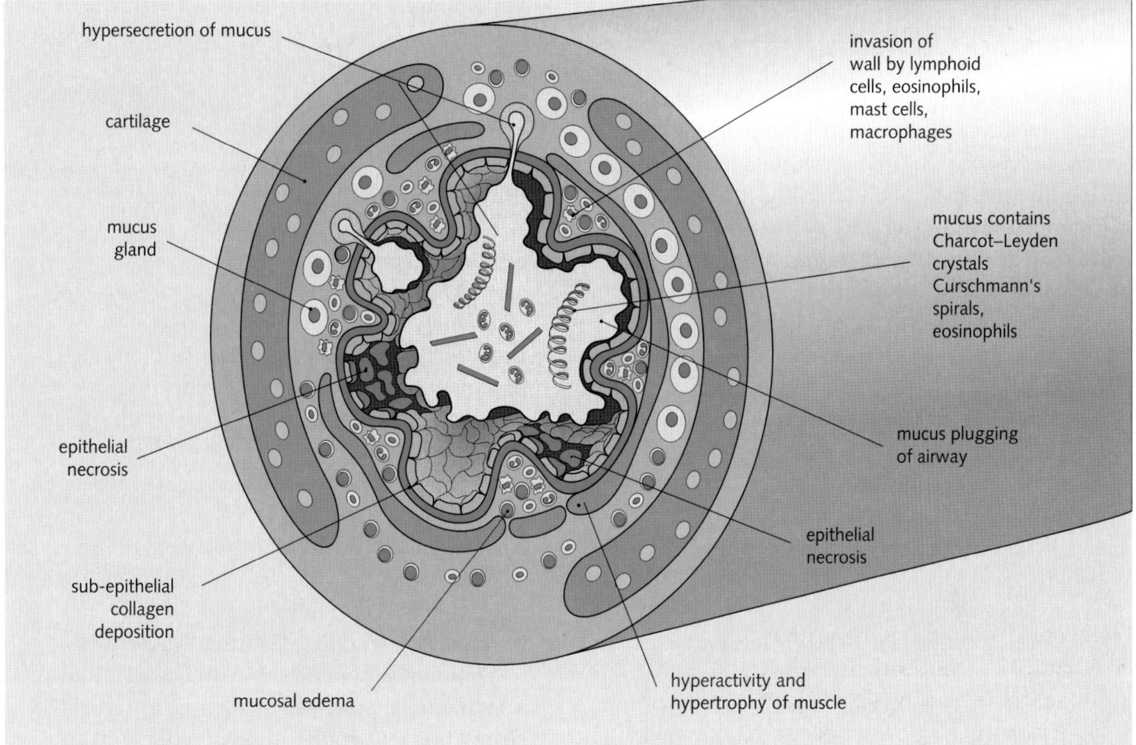

Fig. 6.6 Morphological changes in the airways in asthma.

airways are of varying size but mostly of small caliber. Barrel chest may be seen in cases of chronic asthma.

The main complication is cor pulmonale. Pulmonary vasoconstriction caused by chronic alveolar hypoventilation results in pulmonary hypertension leading to right ventricular hypertrophy.

The disease can usually be successfully controlled by drug therapy. Treatment includes the use of β_2-adrenoreceptor agonists, corticosteroids, aminophylline, anticholinergics, and cromoglycate.

Prognosis

The prognosis is:

- Remission—approximately 50% of cases of childhood asthma resolve spontaneously; remission in adult-onset asthma is less likely.
- Mortality—death occurs in approximately 0.2% of asthmatics. Mortality is usually (but not always) preceded by an acute attack, and about 50% are more than 65 years old.

Bronchiectasis

This is an irreversible dilatation of the bronchi or their branches. Its causes are:

- Congenital: cystic fibrosis and Kartagener's syndrome (bronchiectasis, dextrocardia, and sinusitis).
- Acquired: infection (especially whooping cough, pneumonia, or measles in childhood) and obstruction (either by an inhaled foreign body or by a growth).

Widened bronchi are more prone to infections, *Hemophilus influenzae* and *Pseudomonas aeruginosa* being the most common pathogens. Patients often cough up purulent sputum, which may contain blood.

Treatment consists of antibiotics for infections and physiotherapy to drain sputum.

Cystic fibrosis

Cystic fibrosis (CF) is a hereditary multisystem disease characterized by the production of abnormally thick mucus, and primarily affecting the lung and pancreas. It is the most common autosomal recessive disorder affecting 1 in 2000 newborns. Approximately 1 in 25 Caucasians are heterozygous carriers of the CF gene.

Pathogenesis

The mutated gene is found on chromosome 7 and encodes for a protein termed the cystic fibrosis transmembrane regulator (CFTR). The most common mutation is deletion of the phenylalanine residue at position 508. This protein normally enables the transport of chloride ions across cell membranes. In cystic fibrosis, defective CFTR results in impaired chloride transport, which prevents the release of sodium and water to liquefy mucus. The net result is the production of an extremely thick and viscous mucus by the exocrine glands.

Viscid mucus may cause obstruction of the following systems:

- Bronchi—abnormally viscid mucus cannot be cleared from the lungs.
- Intestine—causing meconium ileus in newborn babies.
- Pancreas—causing deficiency of the pancreatic enzymes, resulting in malabsorption and failure to thrive.

In the respiratory tract, the bronchi and bronchioles become obstructed by abnormally viscid mucus, which leads to four main problems:

- Infections: obstruction and stagnation of secretions leads to repeated bouts of infection, particularly with S. *aureus* and the mucoid form of *Pseudomonas*.
- Bronchiectasis: a frequent complication (see above).
- Hyperinflation of the lungs due to air trapping behind mucin plugs; increased risk of developing pneumothorax.
- Hypoxia, scarring, and destruction of the pulmonary vascular bed, leading to pulmonary hypertension and cor pulmonale.

Prognosis

The median age of survival is just over 30 years. However future treatment goals include the replacement of the defective gene using gene therapy strategies. Current therapy Includes physiotherapy to drain mucus secretions, antibiotics, and ultimately lung transplantation.

Infections of the lungs

Pneumonia is defined as the consolidation of lung tissue caused by the formation of an intra-alveolar inflammatory exudate as a result of a lung infection.

Pneumonia is the fifth most common cause of death in the U.S., and it is more common in the very young and elderly.

Predisposing factors

Although pneumonia frequently occurs in previously healthy individuals, it is also predisposed by the presence of debility and immobility:

- Suppressed cough reflex (e.g., in coma, anaesthesia, and neuromuscular junction (NMJ) disorders).
- Impaired mucociliary clearance (e.g., through cigarette smoke, irritant gases, viral diseases such as influenza, and genetic conditions such as immotile cilia).
- Pulmonary edema (e.g., due to right-sided cardiac failure).
- Impaired alveolar macrophages: alcohol, cigarette smoke, oxygen toxicity.
- Retention of secretions due to COPD.
- Immunosuppression (e.g., drugs (cytotoxics and immunosuppressives), AIDS, congenital immunodeficiencies, and leukemias).
- Drugs: previous course of broad-spectrum antibiotics or cytotoxics.
- Instrumentation: endotracheal intubation or mechanical ventilation.
- Prior viral respiratory tract infection.
- Other: prolonged hospitalization, general debility, immobility.

Remember INSPIRATION for the predisposing factors of pneumonia:
Immunosuppression
Neurological impairment of the cough reflex
Secretion retention
Pulmonary edema
Impaired mucociliary clearance
Respiratory tract infection (viral)
Antibiotics and cytotoxics
Tracheal instrumentation
Impaired alveolar macrophages
Other
Neoplasia

Classification

Pneumonia can be classified according to:

- Microbiology—causative organism may be bacterial, viral, fungal, or protozoal.
- Pattern of spread of infection—either lobar or bronchopneumonia.
- Clinical classification—according to circumstances surrounding the development of disease (e.g., community acquired, hospital acquired, disease of immunosuppression, and aspiration pneumonia).

Bacterial pneumonia

This is the most common type of pneumonia, accounting for 80–90% of cases.

Causative organisms

Knowledge of the circumstances in which a person develops pneumonia is a strong clue as to the likely organism causing the infection (Fig. 6.7).

The clinical features are fever, shortness of breath, cough, and sputum (occasionally with hemoptysis). There are signs of consolidation with bronchial breathing and/or coarse crackles.

> As a general rule of thumb, community-acquired pneumonia is usually caused by Gram-positive bacteria, whereas hospital-acquired pneumonias are mainly due to Gram-negative bacteria.

Bronchopneumonia

Infection is centered on the bronchi but with the extension of the inflammatory exudate into the alveoli, causing a patchy consolidation of the lung (lobular distribution). Bronchopneumonia is illustrated in Fig. 6.8.

The condition primarily affects the very young, very old, or debilitated patients.

The infecting organism depends on whether the infection is hospital or community acquired, but it is quite often of the hospital-acquired variety due to underlying disease.

Pathogenesis Patients develop retention of secretions which gravitate to dependent parts of the lungs and become infected, hence

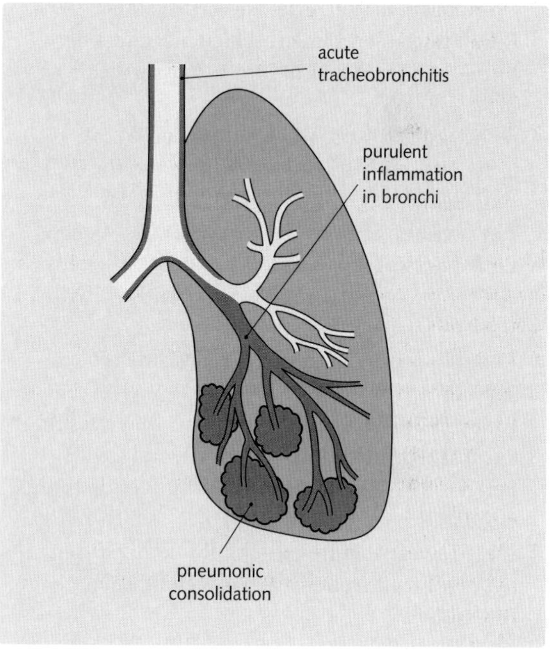

Fig. 6.8 Bronchopneumonia.

Common pathogenic bacteria in hospital- and community-acquired pneumonia	
Community-acquired infection	**Hospital-acquired infection**
Streptococcus pneumoniae (>60%) *Hemophilus influenzae* *Legionella pneumophilus* *Staphylococcus aureus* *Mycoplasma pneumoniae* *Chlamydia pneumoniae* *Chlamydia psittaci*	*Klebsiella* *Pseudomonas* *Escherichia coli* *Proteus* *Serratia* As well as organisms responsible for community-acquired pneumonia (but much less frequently)

Fig. 6.7 Common pathogenic bacteria in hospital- and community-acquired pneumonia.

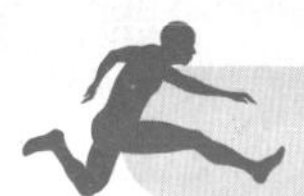

bronchopneumonia most commonly involves the lower lobes.

Macroscopically, it is usually bilateral with multiple areas of consolidation distributed around bronchi/bronchioles in dependent parts of the lung. Affected areas are firm and airless, and they have a dark red or grey appearance. Bronchial mucosa is inflamed and pus may be present in the more peripheral bronchi. Patchy collapse is associated with bronchial obstruction. Involvement of the pleura is common with purulent pleuritis.

Microscopically, there is acute inflammation of the bronchi and bronchioles with an acute inflammatory exudate present in the lumina and extending into the peribronchial alveoli.

Complications and sequelae are as follows:

- Resolution—complete resolution occurs only if treatment is instituted early, before the onset of structural damage.
- Bronchial damage—imperfect repair of the bronchial mucosa results in scarring of the bronchial wall, with increased predisposition to further infection and to bronchiectasis.
- Lung fibrosis—inflammatory exudate is often not completely absorbed but is organized with residual fibrous scarring.
- Lung abscesses—single or multiple areas of suppuration.
- Empyema—pus in the pleural cavity as a result of extension of infection into the pleural cavity.
- Pericarditis—direct extension of infection to the pericardium.
- Death—very common cause of death, particularly as a terminal manifestation of debilitating diseases.

Lobar pneumonia

This is a uniform consolidation of part of a lobe or of the whole lobe caused by infection (Fig. 6.9). The condition often affects otherwise healthy adults, primarily between the ages of 20 and 50 years old. Individuals living in poor social conditions and alcoholics who have reduced access to good medical care are particularly prone to this pattern of pneumonia, which is often caused by *Pneumococcus* or *Klebsiella* species.

Pathogenesis Encapsulated organisms gain entry to distal air spaces via the bronchi. Infection spreads rapidly through the alveolar spaces and bronchioles, causing acute inflammatory exudation into air spaces. Phagocytosis by alveolar macrophages is insufficient

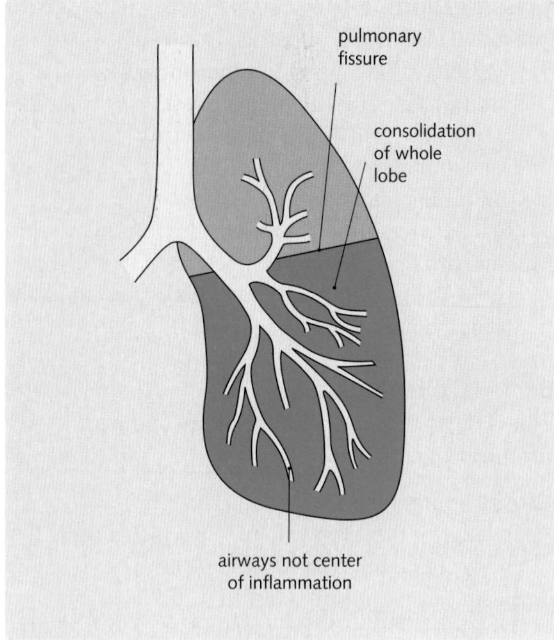

Fig. 6.9 Lobar pneumonia.

due to the encapsulation of *Klebsiella* and *S. pneumoniae*.

Macroscopically, the whole lobe becomes consolidated and airless.

Microscopically, the alveoli are filled with an acute inflammatory exudate, which is limited by the pulmonary fissures.

There are four pathological stages of lobar pneumonia:

- Congestion: outpouring of protein-rich exudate into the alveolae.
- Red hepatization: massive accumulation of polymorphs in the alveolar spaces.
- Gray hepatization: accumulation of fibrin in the lung spaces.
- Resolution: most patients recover with their lungs returning to normal structure and function.

Complications and sequelae are as follows:

- Lung fibrosis: inflammatory exudate is often not completely absorbed but is organized with residual fibrous scarring and permanent lung dysfunction.
- Bacteremia: bacterial dissemination of organisms can lead to septicemia with meningitis, arthritis, endocarditis or pyemic abscesses.
- Lung abscesses: single or multiple areas of suppuration.

- Empyema: pus in the pleural cavity as a result of extension of infection into the pleural cavity.
- Pleural effusion: non-infected effusion is common.
- Death.

Primary atypical pneumonia

This is an inflammation of the alveolar septa by inflammatory cells (acute interstitial pneumonitis) in the absence of any consolidation. Patients develop fever, dry cough, and dyspnea, but there are no signs of consolidation, hence the term "atypical" pneumonia. It may be caused by several factors, including infection by viruses, *Mycoplasma*, and *Chlamydia* and *Rickettsia*.

Viral pneumonia

This is a common cause of pneumonia in early childhood but is much less frequent in healthy adults. The majority of viral lung infections cause an atypical pneumonia, which is typically self-limiting (e.g., cytomegalovirus, measles, or varicella). However, in the immunocompromised host, these infections can prove fatal.

A minority of viruses cause a much more severe pattern of infection. The influenza viruses can cause an acute fulminating pneumonia with pulmonary hemorrhage; the clinical course may be rapidly fatal.

A common complication is secondary infection with pyogenic bacteria, which can transform a mild viral lung infection into a severe suppurative bronchopneumonia; this is particularly common in influenza.

Mycoplasma

Mycoplasma accounts for 15–20% of community-acquired pneumonia. It is more common in children between 5 and 15 years old, but more serious in adults. The organisms cause a low-grade, chronic, atypical pneumonia. It may result in pulmonary fibrosis.

Chlamydia and *rickettsia*

A number of chlamydial and rickettsial infections may be complicated by the development of pneumonia. Such infections include typhus, psittacosis and Q fever. Fatal cases are rare except in psittacosis.

Pulmonary tuberculosis

Pulmonary tuberculosis (TB) is a chronic granulomatous infection of the lung caused by *Mycobacterium tuberculosis*. It is uncommon in the U.S. and other developed countries (at about 7 per 100,000) but extremely common worldwide (up to 500 per 100,000 in parts of Africa), where it is a leading cause of death. In the U.S. it mainly affects older people, HIV-infected persons, and the immigrant population.

Spread is by various means:

- Inhalation of *M. tuberculosis* in the form of droplets (most common mode).
- Ingestion of contaminated food or milk.
- Inoculation of the skin.
- Transplacental spread (i.e., congenital TB).

The predisposing factors are:

- Close contact with infected individuals: increased risk for those living/working in crowded or unhygienic conditions, and for health-care workers.
- Immunosuppression: the very young, very old, immunosuppressive therapy (e.g., corticosteroids, cytotoxics) and other diseases of immunodeficiency, particularly AIDS.
- Malnourishment.
- Other diseases: pre-existing chronic lung disease (especially silicosis), diabetes mellitus, and alcoholism.

Pathogenesis

The destructive effects of infection are entirely due to the hypersensitivity reaction of the host directed against bacterial cell wall constituents. The following sequence of events occurs:

1. 0–10 days: mycobacteria excite a transient but marked acute inflammatory response. Neutrophils phagocytose the organisms but are unable to destroy them, as the cell walls are resistant to degradation. Instead, engulfed bacteria are drained into local lymph nodes.
2. After 10 days: development of a T cell-mediated immune response (type IV hypersensitivity reaction) to the bacillary cell wall constituents results in cytokine release, leading to activation of macrophages. Gradually a chronic inflammatory pattern develops, which is dominated by aggregates of macrophages called epithelioid cells, which form variable numbers of granulomas (see Chapter 3) with a central core of necrotic caseous tissue containing viable mycobacteria. Tuberculous granulomas are termed tubercles.

Macroscopically, the granulomas appear as pinhead-sized white or grayish foci (tubercles) in the tissues.

Microscopically, granulomas are the histological hallmark of TB infection. A granuloma consists of a central area of amorphous caseous necrosis, surrounded by three cellular layers. These include an inner layer of activated macrophages (epithelioid cells) with Langhans' giant cells, a middle layer of lymphocytes, and an outer layer of fibroblastic tissue that merges with surrounding structures and increases in amount with the age of the lesion.

The healing of a granuloma occurs slowly with progressive fibrosis and later calcification. The central necrotic area remains caseous for some time, and mycobacteria may remain viable indefinitely within a healed lesion. Reactivation results in secondary (or post primary) tuberculosis.

TB can be classified into two types, according to the pattern of infection:

- Primary infection: the first encounter with the organism, resulting in the development of a small parenchymal peripheral focus with a large response in the draining lymph nodes.
- Secondary infection: reactivation or reinfection of a previously infected individual, resulting in the development of a large, localized, parenchymal reaction but with minimal lymph node involvement.

Primary tuberculosis

The lung is by far the most common site of primary infection. Other sites include the pharynx, larynx, skin, and intestine.

Inhaled organisms proliferate in the alveoli at the periphery of the lung, often just beneath the pleura. This primary parenchymal tubercle is termed the Ghon focus. It is often associated with enlarged caseous hilar lymph nodes. The combination of lung and lymph node lesions together constitutes the primary complex or Ghon complex.

Primary tuberculosis will either resolve or progress as shown below.

Resolution This occurs in the majority of cases. The Ghon focus and caseating granulomas in the lymph nodes heal with fibrosis. The disease does not progress due to the confinement of organisms within a fibrotic shell. However, walled-off bacteria may remain viable within the healed primary complex (latent tuberculosis).

Progression In patients with poor immunity (and infants), the disease is progressive. There is a further spread of mycobacteria with continuing enlargement of the caseating granulomas in the lymph nodes (progressive primary TB). Enlarging nodes spread the infection by eroding into adjacent structures in two ways:

- Bronchus: erosion of an infected lymph node into a bronchus results in tuberculous bronchopneumonia (Fig. 6.10A). The bacilli pass down into the bronchi of one lung where infection can then spread into the opposite lung. There is further spread of infection into the bronchioles and alveoli with the development of extensive, confluent, caseating, granulomatous lesions. This condition is known as "galloping consumption" and it is usually rapidly fatal.
- Blood vessel: erosion of an infected lymph node into a blood vessel results in hematogenous spread of mycobacteria to many parts of the body, including the remainder of the lung, causing miliary tuberculosis (Fig. 6.10B).

Secondary tuberculosis

This occurs as a result of the reactivation of quiescent but viable mycobacteria in hosts with weakened immune responses, or as a result of reinfection by additional organisms.

Caseous granulomas typically develop in the apical segments of the lungs, spreading directly and locally but without lymph node lesions. The initiating apical lesion is often called an Assmann focus, and it is histologically similar to the Ghon focus.

Secondary tuberculosis will either resolve or spread as shown below.

Resolution Spontaneous healing with fibrosis and calcification occurs, though viable organisms may remain without producing any clinical symptoms.

Spread In adults with poor immune responses, secondary tuberculosis progresses locally with direct extension and continuing caseation. Further spread of mycobacteria produces various types of progressive tuberculosis:

- Apical cavitation fibrocaseous tuberculosis: a direct extension of the infection, and continuing caseation results in the formation of a large caseous mass surrounded by a thin cellular wall. If caseous material is expectorated, a cavity results. The lesion can heal at this stage, but it may spread further into the bronchi, bloodstream, or directly into the pleura.
- Tuberculous pneumonia (see above).

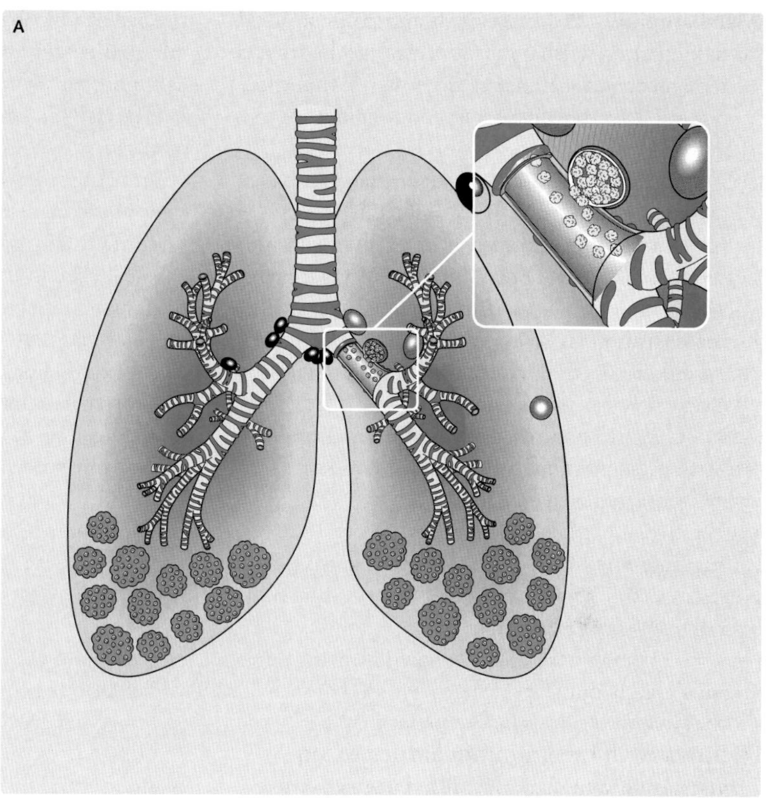

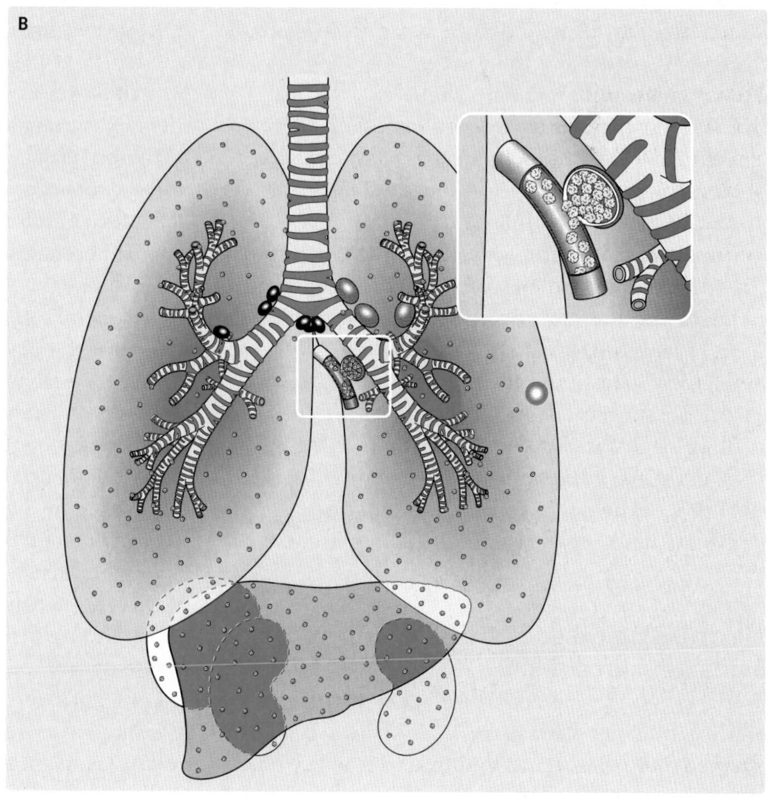

Fig. 6.10 Patterns of progressive pulmonary tuberculosis. (A) Tuberculous bronchopneumonia. (B) Miliary tuberculosis of the lung.

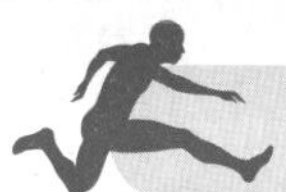

- Miliary tuberculosis: the disease becomes widely disseminated with numerous small granulomas in many organs. Common target tissues are the kidneys, liver, bone marrow, and meninges.

Complications are usually the result of extensive fibrosis involved in healing process:

- Pulmonary fibrosis: lung lesions typically heal with fibrosis, which may be extensive producing localized honeycombing. This is common in relapsing and progressive untreated disease.
- Pleural fibrosis with obliteration of the pleural space.
- Bronchiectasis: scarring of the bronchial walls can cause distal pulmonary collapse, secondary infection, and bronchiectasis.

Immunization with the BCG vaccine is common practice outside the U.S., leading to a positive skin test. Treatment of infected individuals involves long-term triple therapy with rifampicin, isoniazid, and ethambutol. Streptomycin may be added.

Pneumonia in the immunocompromised

The lungs of immunocompromised patients are extremely prone to disease by opportunistic infections—i.e., infections caused by microorganisms that are nonpathogenic to healthy, nonimmunocompromised individuals.

Common opportunistic agents include:

- Viruses—cytomegalovirus, *respiratory syncytial virus*, varicella-zoster virus, measles (see Primary Atypical Pneumonia, above).
- Fungi—both *Candida* and *Aspergillus* can cause widespread areas of necrosis with the formation of micro-abscesses containing characteristic hyphae; mortality is high.
- Protozoa—*Pneumocystis carinii* pneumonia (PCP) is common in AIDS patients, affecting 30–50% of cases. Alveoli are filled with a fine, foam-like material in which the minute bodies of the organism can be seen. This disease has a 30% mortality rate in patients with AIDS.

Neoplastic diseases of the lungs

Bronchogenic carcinoma

Bronchogenic carcinoma is the most common cause of death from neoplasia in the U.S. Males are affected more than females, but there is an increasing incidence in women. The peak incidence is between the ages of 40 and 70 years, reflecting the cumulative exposure to several potential causative carcinogens.

The risk factors include:

- Cigarette smoking: the earlier the age at which smoking starts and the more cigarettes smoked result in an increased risk. Cigarette smoke contains a large number of carcinogens (e.g., polycyclic hydrocarbons). There is a steady decline in risk if smoking stops.
- Occupational factors such as exposure to radioactive material, asbestos, nickel, chromium, iron oxides, and coal gas plants.
- Environmental factors such as radon (a natural radioactive gas in certain geographic areas).
- Pulmonary fibrosis: somewhat controversial, but there is an increase in lung adenocarcinoma in patients with lung fibrosis.

There are four main histological types of lung carcinoma:

- Squamous cell carcinoma—50%.
- Small cell carcinoma ("oat cell carcinoma")—20%.
- Adenocarcinoma (including bronchioalveolar carcinoma)—20%.
- Large cell anaplastic carcinoma—10%.

A small proportion of tumors are mixed adenocarcinoma/squamous carcinoma.

Tumors may be central (all types) or peripheral (mainly adenocarcinomas).

Central or hilar tumors (70%) arise in relation to the main bronchi extending into the bronchial lumen and invading the adjacent lung.

Peripheral tumors (30%) arise in peripheral airways or alveoli, often occurring in relation to scars and frequently extending to the pleural surface.

The route of spread is as follows:

- Local—central tumors invade locally either through the bronchial wall into the surrounding lung, or along the outside of the bronchi (peribronchial spread) to distant parts of the lung. Direct extension into pleura and adjacent mediastinal structures is a feature of advanced disease.
- Lymphatic spread—carcinomas spread to the ipsilateral and contralateral peribronchial and hilar lymph nodes. Compression of adjacent tissues by infiltrated nodes may then cause symptoms.

- Transcoelomic spread—tumor cells may seed within the pleural cavity, causing a malignant pleural effusion.
- Hematogenous spread—to the brain, bone, liver, and adrenal glands.

Histological types

Squamous cell carcinoma This is the most common type of lung cancer, which is thought to be derived from metaplastic squamous epithelium that develops to line the main bronchi as a result of exposure to agents such as cigarette smoke.

Tumors are typically central and close to the carina, frequently presenting with features related to bronchial obstruction. Compared with other types, they are relatively slow growing, and they may be resectable.

Histologically, the tumors show a range of differentiation from well-differentiated lesions producing lots of keratin, through to poorly differentiated lesions with only a few keratin-producing cells.

Small cell (oat cell) carcinoma These highly malignant tumors arise from the bronchial endocrine or APUD cells. They contain a few dense secretory granules that are also seen in greater numbers in bronchial carcinoid tumors. Therefore, small cell carcinoma is thought to represent a type of neuroendocrine tumor.

Due to their endocrine nature, this form of cancer can be associated with ectopic hormone production.

Macroscopically, these tumors are usually centrally located, and they are associated with a rapid rate of growth. Metastases are usually present at the time of diagnosis.

Microscopically, the cells are round to oval and have little cytoplasm. The nuclei are thought to resemble oat grains, hence the alternative name. In certain situations there can be diagnostic confusion with tumor of lymphoid cells.

Large cell anaplastic carcinoma This poorly differentiated tumor is thought to be of either squamous or adenocarcinoma origin. Lesions may be central or peripheral, and they are composed of large cells with nuclear pleomorphism and frequent giant cell forms. They have a poor prognosis and are frequently widely disseminated at the time of diagnosis.

Adenocarcinoma This tumor is derived from glandular cells, such as mucous goblet cells, Clara cells, or type II pneumocytes. A proportion of adenocarcinomas are thought to originate in areas of pre-existing lung scarring or fibrosis (scar cancers). Adenocarcinoma has the slowest rate of growth, and it differs from other types of lung cancer because it has an equal sex incidence. It can be linked to passive cigarette smoking and characteristically develops as a peripheral tumor.

There are four main histological patterns:

- Acinar: prominent gland-like spaces lined by columnar epithelium.
- Papillary: fronds of tumor on thin septa.
- Solid carcinoma with mucin production: poorly differentiated lesions.
- Bronchioalveolar carcinoma (see below).

Cigarette smoking is a known risk factor for the development of neoplastic diseases of the lung.

Clinical features of lung cancer

There are no early symptoms of lung cancer; it is usual for a lesion to have been growing for many years before clinical presentation. The presenting symptoms of lung cancer are outlined in Fig. 6.11 and they can be classified into:

- Pulmonary symptoms—most common types of presenting symptom including cough, dyspnea, chest pain and hemoptysis.
- Metastatic symptoms—metastatic spread is present in 70% of patients at presentation, and 30% of patients present with symptoms caused by metastatic disease.
- Local symptoms—local spread within the thorax can cause several clinical syndromes.
- Nonmetastatic extrapulmonary syndromes—lung cancer frequently causes systemic syndromes that are not associated with metastatic effects, and these may rarely be a presenting feature of disease.

Diagnosis is through clinical features (see above), imaging (chest X-ray and CT scans), and histological confirmation of the following:

- Bronchoscopy and biopsy: tumor biopsy obtained.
- Cytology of pleural effusion.

Clinicopathological features of lung cancer	
Cause	**Clinical features**
Pulmonary involvement	Cough (80%): infection distal to airway blocked by tumor Hemoptysis (70%): ulceration of tumor in bronchus Dyspnea (60%): local extension of tumor Chest pain (40%): involvement of pleura and/or chest wall Wheeze (15%): narrowing of airways Systemic features: weight loss, anorexia, and malaise
Local spread	Horner's syndrome: local invasion of cervical sympathetic ganglion Hoarseness: spread to the left hilar region may cause recurrent laryngeal nerve palsy Pain in T1 dermatome and wasting of intrinsic hand muscles: caused by brachial neuritis as a result of direct invasion of plexus by apical tumors (Pancoast tumor) Pericarditis: due to direct tumor invasion
Metastatic spread	Pathological fracture CNS symptoms (brain metastasis) Hepatomegaly or jaundice (liver metastasis)
Non-metastatic extrapulmonary syndromes	
Endocrine disturbances	Inappropriate ADH secretion: by small cell carcinoma and characterized by low sodium and plasma osmolality with high urine osmolality Ectopic ACTH secretion: caused by small cell carcinoma and associated with Cushing's syndrome Hypercalcemia: caused by secretion of parathyroid hormone-related peptide by a squamous cell carcinoma
Neurological syndromes	Peripheral sensory motor neuropathy Cerebellar degeneration causing ataxia Proximal myopathy Dermatomyositis Lambert-Eaton myasthenic syndrome: associated with small cell tumors
Hypertrophic pulmonary osteoarthropathy (HPOA)	Finger clubbing Swelling of wrists and ankles with periosteal new bone formation (seen in 2–3% of squamous cell carcinomas and adenocarcinomas)

Fig. 6.11 Clinicopathological features of lung cancer.

Prognosis and staging

Histological types and the stage of lung cancer determine the outcome and its likely response to treatment. Survival is better for early stage disease, except for small cell carcinoma (very early metastases).

The staging system used for lung cancer is shown in Fig. 6.12.

Treatment

Surgical intervention

Tumors are classified as either operable or inoperable according to the stage of the disease; only 10% of all lung tumors are considered operable at diagnosis. The key elements that offer a reasonable prospect of success with surgery include the following features:

- The tumor must be within a lobar bronchus or at least 2 cm distal to the carina.
- No direct extension to the chest wall, diaphragm, or pericardium.
- No involvement of the great vessels of the heart, trachea, esophagus, or vertebrae.
- No malignant pleural effusion.
- No contralateral nodal involvement.
- No distant metastases.

Of those patients who undergo tumor surgery, only 20% have successful resection of the tumor.

Radiotherapy and chemotherapy

Tumors are grouped into two categories according to differences in prognosis and response to radiotherapy and chemotherapy.

Fig. 6.12 TNM staging of lung cancer.

TNM staging of lung cancer		
Stage	**TNM group**	**Clinical**
Stage I	T1 N0 M0 T1 N1 M0	Tumor <3 cm; distal to origin of lobar bronchus (T1) With (N1) or without (N0) spread to ipsilateral hilar nodes No metastases (M0)
Stage II	T2 N0 M0 T2 N1 M0	Tumor >3 cm, 2 cm distal to the carina, which invades visceral pleural (T2) With (N1) or without (N0) spread to ipsilateral hilar nodes No metastases (M0)
Stage III	All T3/T4 cases All N3 cases All M1 cases	All tumors involving the carina; involving mediastinal structures (T3/T4) All tumors with spread to contralateral nodes (N3) All cases of metastases (M1)

Summary of histological types of lung cancers				
	Small cell	**Squamous**	**Large cell**	**Adenocarcinoma**
Relative incidence	20%	50%	10%	20%
Gender differences	Males > females	Males > females	Males > females	Males = females
Associated with cigarette smoking	Yes	Yes	Yes	No? (passive smoking)
Site	Centrally located	Centrally located	Centrally located	Peripherally located; often originating in areas of pre-existing lung scarring
Non-metastatic symptoms	ADH secretion Ectopic ACTH secretion Lambert-Eaton myasthenic syndrome	Hypercalcemia HPOA	—	HPOA
Rate of growth	Fast; metastases usually present at diagnosis	Slow growing; metastasizes late	Fast	Slowest growing

Fig. 6.13 Summary of histological types of lung cancers. (HPOA, hypertrophic pulmonary osteoarthropathy.)

Small cell lung carcinoma Small cell lung carcinoma (SCLC) is very sensitive to radiotherapy and chemotherapy, but the disease is usually extensive at diagnosis such that survival is still poor despite local control of tumor growth. Treatment offers good palliation of pain, cough, and dyspnea. Radiotherapy and combination chemotherapy cause complete local response in 30% of cases with a median survival of 11 months (compared with 3 months if untreated), and a 1-year survival of 45%.

Non-small cell lung carcinoma (squamous, large-cell, and adenocarcinoma) Inoperable cases of non-small cell lung carcinoma (NSCLC) may be treated with radiotherapy depending on clinical circumstances. The role of chemotherapy is limited. Overall prognosis is poor with only a 50% 2-year survival without spread, 10% with spread.

See Fig. 6.13 for a summary of histological types of lung cancers.

Bronchioalveolar carcinoma

This is a special type of adenocarcinoma derived from alveolar or bronchial epithelial cells (Clara cells and type II pneumocytes). There are two types:

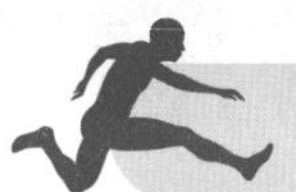

- Multifocal diffuse infiltrative tumors: replace areas of lung in a manner resembling pneumonic consolidation. Cells are tall, columnar, have few mitoses, and secrete mucin.
- Single, gray masses of tumor up to 10cm in diameter. Cells are cuboidal with hyperchromatic nuclei and mitoses, and form papillary structures; there is often no mucin secretion. In the absence of metastases, this subtype has a better prognosis than other forms of lung cancer.

Metastatic lung disease

Lung cancer metastases are found commonly in the lymph nodes, bone, brain, liver, and adrenals. All types of carcinoma of the lung spread by the four main routes of local spread, lymphatic spread, transcoelomic spread, and hematogenous spread.

Carcinoid tumors

These are neuroendocrine tumors of the lungs, representing about 5% of all pulmonary neoplasms. The majority of tumors are benign, although a minority have the potential for local recurrence or metastasis (atypical pulmonary neuroendocrine tumors).

In contrast to intestinal carcinoid tumors, most pulmonary lesions do not secrete 5-hydroxytryptamine.

Bronchial hamartomas

These common benign lesions composed of tissue are normally encountered in the lung. Most are 1–3cm in diameter and largely consist of cartilage, being firm and glistening white in appearance (often termed chondromas). Other elements are bronchial epithelium, fat, and muscle. Bronchial hamartomas are asymptomatic, and they are mainly discovered at postmortem examination.

Miscellaneous mesenchymal tumors

These tumors can be either benign (e.g., neurofibromas, lipomas) or malignant (sarcomas are extremely rare in the lung).

Diffuse interstitial diseases

Interstitial lung diseases are a group of noninfectious, nonmalignant disorders in which there is inflammation of the alveolar walls with a thickening of the interstitium between the alveoli, usually with fibrosis.

This is also known as alveolitis and often loosely referred to as pulmonary fibrosis.

Disorders can be classified into acute and chronic interstitial diseases as shown in Fig. 6.14.

Chronic pulmonary fibrosis

A progressive diffuse fibrosis of the lung interstitium occurring as a result of chronic interstitial disease.

Causes of chronic interstitial disease are listed in Fig. 6.14, and they can be classified into three etiological groups:

- Idiopathic (e.g., sarcoidosis and cryptogenic fibrosing alveolitis).
- Dust inhalation: inorganic dust (pneumoconioses, including coal miner's pneumoconiosis, silicosis, asbestosis) and organic dust (extrinsic allergic alveolitis, including farmer's lung and bird fancier's lung).
- Iatrogenic: drugs (e.g., nitrofurantoin, amiodarone and anticancer drugs—methotrexate, cyclophosphamide, and bleomycin) and radiation (see p. 99).

The initiating mechanism of interstitial inflammation depends on the etiology, but in all cases there is neutrophil migration, enlargement and desquamation of type I alveolar cells, and accumulation of fibroblasts.

Acute and chronic interstitial diseases of the lung	
Acute	Adult respiratory distress syndrome (ARDS) Drug and toxin reactions Acute radiation pneumonitis Diffuse intrapulmonary hemorrhage
Chronic	Pneumoconiosis Idiopathic fibrosing alveolitis Sarcoidosis Extrinsic allergic alveolitis Diffuse malignancies Connective tissue disease, e.g., rheumatoid disease, scleroderma, drug-induced pulmonary fibrosis Chronic pulmonary edema, e.g., as in mitral stenosis with raised pulmonary venous pressure Chronic radiation pneumonitis Rare disorders, e.g., alveolar proteinosis, histiocytosis

Fig. 6.14 Acute and chronic interstitial diseases of the lung.

Macroscopically, the lung is converted into a mass of cystic airspaces separated by areas of dense collagenous scarring. This characteristic appearance is termed "honeycomb lung" as the cut surface is said to resemble a honeycomb.

Microscopically, the cystic spaces are lined by flattened or cuboidal epithelium. The clinical feature of the early stage disease is a slowly increasing respiratory insufficiency due to reduced lung capacity and residual volume, reduced compliance, and reduced diffusion capacity.

The characteristic signs are dyspnea, cough, and finger clubbing. There is a restrictive pattern of lung function tests.

The pneumoconioses

This is a group of interstitial lung diseases resulting from chronic exposure to inorganic dust. The three most common types of pneumoconioses are coalworker's pneumoconiosis, silicosis, and asbestosis.

In the normal lung, inhaled dust is coughed out, or ingested by macrophages. However, if the dust is toxic to macrophages there is local inflammation, secretion of cytokines, and stimulation of fibrosis. The end result is a restrictive pattern of respiratory dysfunction.

Coalworker's pneumoconiosis

Coalworker's pneumoconiosis (CWP) is an interstitial lung disease caused by inhaling coal dust. It has four types of pathology:

- Simple coalworker's pneumoconiosis (macular CWP): This condition is not associated with any clinically significant impairment of respiratory function, despite focal aggregates of dust-laden macrophages.
- Complicated coalworker's pneumoconiosis (nodular CWP): there are nodular lesions, associated areas of scarring and signs of emphysema.
- Progressively massive fibrosis: large nodules and scarring results in severe respiratory impairment.
- Caplan's syndrome: associated with rheumatoid disease, where the nodules appear large, carbon-pigmented, and rheumatoid.

Silicosis

An interstitial lung disease, this is caused by the inhalation of quartz-containing dust (quartz being silicon dioxide), which is abundant in stone and sand.

It is associated with occupations involving slate mining, stone masonry, foundry and pottery work, tunnelling, quarrying, and coal mining through granite rocks.

Pathogenesis—Silicates are toxic to macrophages, which stimulate cytokine generation precipitating inflammation with fibrosis and nodule formation.

Tuberculosis is a common complication of silicosis (silicotuberculosis). This is thought to be due to impaired local defenses as a consequence of accumulated silica in macrophages.

Asbestosis

This interstitial lung disease is caused by the inhalation of asbestos, a fibrous silicate mineral that was widely used between 1890 and 1970. It is associated with occupations involving asbestos mining/processing, the building industry, insulating and fire resistant material, and shipyard and ship's engine room work.

There are two main forms of asbestos:

- Serpentine asbestos (including white asbestos): this is the most common form; fibers persist in the lung for a limited time.
- Amphibole asbestos (including blue and brown asbestos): fibers persist in the lung for many years, and they are the main cause of malignant mesothelioma.

Risk of disease depends on the duration and intensity of exposure, and the type of asbestos (short fibers are less pathogenic).

The characteristics of asbestosis are:

- There is usually a latent period of 25 years before clinical symptoms become evident.
- Interstitial fibrosis is maximal at lung bases, and asbestos bodies may be seen histologically. Asbestos bodies are fibers coated in acid mucopolysaccharides and hemosiderin.
- The disease progresses with an increasing restrictive defect associated with interstitial fibrosis.
- Pulmonary hypertension and cor pulmonale develop in the late stages.

Sarcoidosis

Sarcoidosis is a multisystem disease of unknown etiology characterized by the presence of histiocytic and giant cell granulomatous inflammatory reaction primarily affecting the lymph nodes and lungs.

Maximum incidence is in people between 30 and 40 years of age, affecting females more than males.

Other affected sites are the skin, eyes, liver, spleen, nervous system, phalanges, parotid glands, and (rarely) the heart.

The pathogenesis is unknown but thought to involve the type IV hypersensitivity reaction. The disease seems to be less common in smokers.

Histology shows noncaseating histiocytic granulomas in the lung interstitium. Patients with lung involvement present with slowly progressive dyspnea and cough and are found to have lung shadowing on chest radiograph with enlargement of the hilar lymph nodes.

Diagnosis—Subcutaneous injection of sarcoid tissue homogenate induces granulomas in affected patients (the Kveim test).

Other interstitial lung diseases

Other interstitial lung diseases are:

- Idiopathic pulmonary fibrosis (cryptogenic fibrosing alveolitis)—chronic fibrosis of the lung interstitium with type II pneumocyte hyperplasia.
- Goodpasture's syndrome—a diffuse pulmonary hemorrhagic syndrome caused by complement activation following autoantibody binding to the basement membrane.
- Idiopathic pulmonary hemosiderosis—a rare condition with type II pneumocyte hyperplasia.
- Rheumatoid disease—the lung and pleura are affected in 10–15% of patients.
- Extrinsic allergic alveolitis—immune mediated interstitial granulomatous inflammation caused by inhalation of organic agents (type III and type IV hypersensitivity). Examples include farmer's lung and pigeon fancier's lung.

Diseases of vascular origin

Pulmonary congestion and edema

Pulmonary edema is defined as an increase in extravascular fluid in the alveolar walls (pulmonary interstitium), which, if severe, subsequently affects the alveolar spaces.

Pathogenesis

Normally, a balance exists between hydrostatic pressure and colloid osmotic (oncotic) pressure such that only a small amount of fluid passes into the interstitium. This fluid is drained from the lung via lymphatic channels.

In pulmonary edema, the amount of fluid passing into the lungs exceeds the lymphatic drainage capacity such that there is an accumulation of fluid within the interstitium. This increases the stiffness of the lungs, giving rise to a subjective sensation of dyspnea.

Macroscopically, the lungs are heavy and congested. In fatal cases, fluid flows from the cut surfaces, and it can often be seen in the large airways.

Microscopically, the interstitium is widened, the capillaries are congested and the alveoli are filled with proteinaceous fluid.

Clinical features and causes

Clinical features of hypoxic respiratory failure may result due to a combination of ventilation/perfusion imbalance caused by fluid in the alveoli, and airway narrowing from the accumulation of peribronchial fluid.

Pulmonary edema can result from:

- Altered hemodynamic forces: increased hydrostatic pressure; decreased oncotic pressure.
- Injury to the alveolar capillary wall.
- Blockage of lymphatic drainage.

Hemodynamic pulmonary edema

Increased capillary hydrostatic pressure

This is the most common cause of pulmonary edema, and it may be the result of:

- Left ventricular heart failure (e.g., due to cases of myocardial infarction, aortic valve disease, mitral regurgitation, and tachyarrhythmias).
- Pulmonary venous hypertension (e.g., due to mitral stenosis).
- Constrictive pericarditis or pericardial effusions.
- Fluid overload: excess infusion of crystalloid solutes.

In chronic left heart failure, prolonged increased hydrostatic pressure can lead to rupture of capillaries with leakage of red cells into the interstitium and alveoli. Macrophages of the interstitium and alveoli phagocytose hemoglobin and accumulate iron pigment. These cells are often termed "heart failure cells."

Decreased plasma osmotic pressure

This is seen in hypoproteinemia. Etiology is:

- Malnutrition.
- Nephrotic syndrome.
- Hepatic failure.
- Intravenous infusion of hypotonic solutes.

Pulmonary edema due to alveolar capillary injury

Diffuse alveolar damage causes an increased permeability of alveolar capillary membrane leading to pulmonary edema, hemorrhage, cell necrosis, and hyaline membrane formation. These types of damage are seen in adult respiratory distress syndrome (see below).

Blockage of lymphatic drainage

Lymphatic obstruction prevents drainage of fluid to lymphatic channels. Obstruction may be caused by tumor emboli in lymphangitis carcinomatosa.

Adult respiratory distress syndrome

Adult respiratory distress syndrome (ARDS) is an acute restrictive lung disease characterized by pulmonary exudation and edema with widespread systemic metabolic derangements.

Many conditions predispose to ARDS, most commonly systemic sepsis and severe trauma. The causes are listed in Fig. 6.15.

The exact pathogenesis is unknown in many cases, but events that take place in the lung in ARDS are termed diffuse alveolar damage, and they occur in two phases: an acute exudative phase (destruction of alveolar lining cells) and a late organization phase (cell proliferation and fibrosis).

In severe cases of ARDS, cytokines liberated from the lung vascular bed can enter the systemic circulation, and these may cause systemic endothelial activation with neutrophil activation leading to multiorgan failure.

Fig. 6.16 shows the main events and outcomes in ARDS.

Embolism, hemorrhage, and infarction

Pulmonary embolism

Pulmonary embolism (PE) is the occlusion of a pulmonary artery, most commonly by

Causes of ARDS	
Cause	**Clinical features**
Blood-bome	Major trauma, especially associated with raised intracranial pressure Septicemia Major burns Disseminated intravascular coagulation Massive blood transfusion Amniotic fluid embolism Acute pancreatitis Cardiac surgery with bypass Antitumor chemotherapy Paraquat poisoning
Air-borne	Pulmonary aspiration of gastric contents Inhalation of toxic fumes or smoke Near drowning Pneumonia from many causes requiring ventilation

Fig. 6.15 Causes of adult respiratory distress syndrome (ARDS).

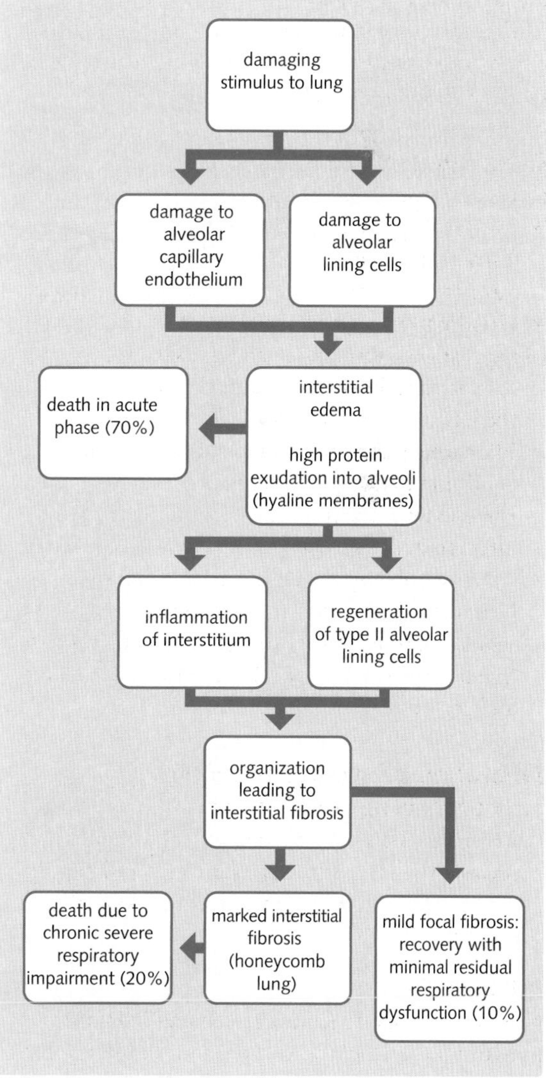

Fig. 6.16 Main events and outcomes in adult respiratory distress syndrome.

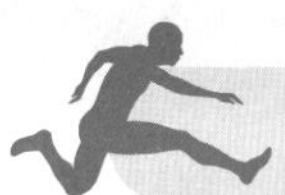

thromboemboli originating in the systemic veins (Fig. 6.17). The condition accounts for 1% of all hospital deaths, but this rises to 30% in patients with severe burns or trauma.

The vast majority of cases are caused by emboli arising from thrombosis of the deep leg veins (calf, popliteal, femoral, and iliac veins). Conditions predisposing to leg vein thrombosis are outlined in Chapter 5, p. 71.

The consequences of PE are pulmonary hypertension (which puts a strain on the right side of the heart) and infarction of the lung (which occurs in only about 10% of cases of PE, as dual circulation protects against ischemic necrosis).

Clinical features The effect of PE depends on the extent of the pulmonary vasculature blockage and the time scale involved:

- Massive PE (5% of cases) is a sudden blockage of more than 60% of the pulmonary vasculature, resulting in electromechanical dissociation of the heart, i.e., the heart continues to beat but there is no output as pulmonary vascular resistance is too high. This results in cardiovascular collapse and rapid death. One example is a saddle embolus at the bifurcation of the left and right pulmonary arteries.
- Major PE (10% of cases) is a blockage of the middle-sized pulmonary arteries. These patients commonly experience breathlessness. Lung infarction develops in about 10% of such cases, and it can lead to hemoptysis and, if adjacent to the pleura, pleuritic chest pain. If untreated, patients may develop a subsequent massive thromboembolism.
- Minor PE (85% of cases) is a blockage of the small peripheral vessels by small emboli. Patients may be asymptomatic or may experience breathlessness and pleuritic chest pain as a result of small infarcts. As with major pulmonary embolism, patients may develop a subsequent massive thromboembolism if untreated.
- Recurrent minor PE (minority) is a blockage of the many small peripheral arteries over a period of many months by recurrent small emboli. The condition can lead to the obliteration of the vascular bed with the development of pulmonary hypertension and right heart strain.

Prevention and treatment Pulmonary thromboembolism is the most common preventable cause of death in hospital patients. Prevention involves:

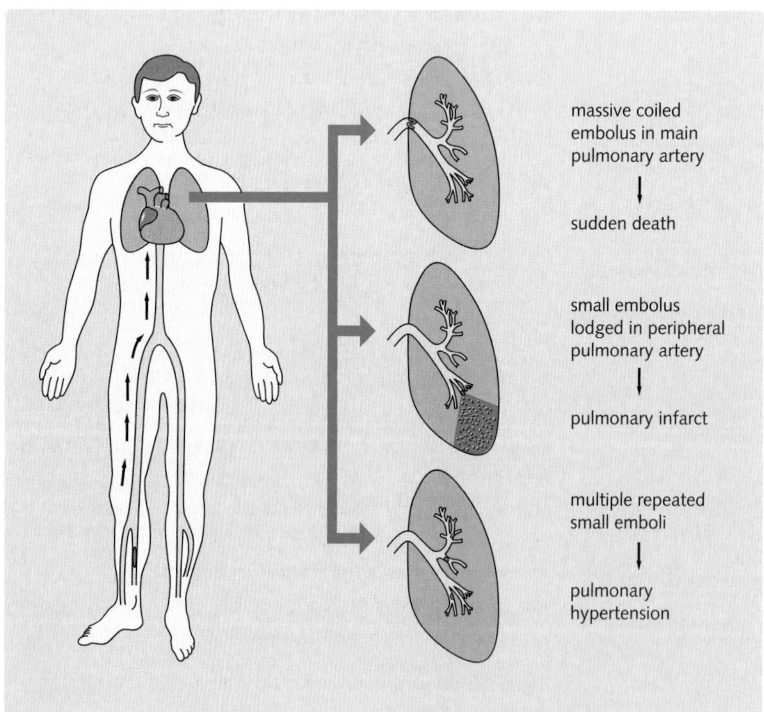

Fig. 6.17 Pulmonary thromboembolism. (Adapted from Underwood, 2000.)

- Mobilizing early following surgery.
- Antiembolic stocking.
- Heparin prophylaxis.

Treatment is with oxygen, analgesia, and anticoagulation therapy (heparin, warfarin).

Nonthrombotic emboli

These are rare, but include:

- Fat, following a bone fracture.
- Amniotic fluid during labor.
- Air (post trauma or post surgery).
- Decompression sickness, as in deep sea divers ("the bends" or caisson disease). Rapid decompression releases nitrogen bubbles, which cause problems in the CNS and bones, and can produce functional obstruction of the pulmonary vessels.
- Foreign bodies.
- Tumor embolism: renal or bronchial cell carcinoma.

Pulmonary infarction

Infarction of lung tissue is usually associated with embolism.

The lower lobes are involved in 75% of cases. Macroscopically, pulmonary infarcts are typically hemorrhagic (because of blood entering from the bronchial circulation) and wedge shaped, and there is often an associated pleural reaction, which causes chest pain. With time, the infarct becomes organized to form a fibrous scar.

Microscopically, there is extravasation of blood into the necrotic lung.

Common sequelae include:

- Pulmonary dysfunction due to the loss of lung tissue.
- Pulmonary vascular obstruction leading to cor pulmonale.
- Pleurisy and pleural effusion.
- Healing, with fibrous scarring.
- Septic infarction due to either a primary septic embolism or secondary infection, leading to abscess formation.

Pulmonary hypertension and vascular sclerosis

This is increased arterial pressure of the lung vasculature, the main causes of which are listed in Fig. 6.14, the most important being:

- Chronic obstructive airways disease.
- Interstitial fibrosis of the lungs.
- Chronic pulmonary venous congestion.

Pulmonary hypertension causes irreversible structural changes to:

- Pulmonary vasculature—medial hypertrophy of the muscular arteries (increased smooth muscle) and pulmonary veins (arterialization); occlusion of the pulmonary arteries caused by intimal proliferation.
- Lungs—interstitial fibrosis.
- Right side of the heart—increased workload of the right side of the heart causes ultimate development of right heart failure (cor pulmonale).

The clinical effects are breathlessness and the symptoms and signs of right-sided cardiac failure.

Diseases of iatrogenic origin

Drug-induced lung disease

There are many drugs available on the market that have pulmonary side effects. A few examples are given below.

Chronic pulmonary fibrosis can be caused by cancer drugs and amiodarone.

Asthma can by induced by aspirin (though the mechanism is unknown) and certain β-blockers (by bronchoconstriction caused by an antagonistic effect on β_2-receptors of bronchial smooth muscle).

Complication of radiotherapy

Acute radiation pneumonitis

Excessive exposure to radiation causes diffuse alveolar damage, and is an established cause of ARDS.

Chronic radiation pneumonitis

Less severe exposure occurring over a longer period of time results in progressive pulmonary fibrosis with the typical restrictive defect of pulmonary function.

Lung transplants

Heart–lung transplants are usually carried out for cardiac problems associated with pulmonary vascular hypertension.

Single lung transplants may be carried out for cystic fibrosis or pulmonary fibrosis. To avoid rejection, all transplant patients require immunosuppression for life.

Disorders of the pleura

Inflammatory pleural effusions

Serofibrinous pleuritis

This acute inflammation of the pleura is accompanied by an accumulation of high protein fluid (>30g protein/L; exudate) containing fibrinogen/fibrin between the pleural surfaces.

The condition is commonly due to infection, infarction, or tumor.

Pathogenesis

Effusion is the result of movement of fluid through damaged vessel walls.

Effusion is typically unilateral, with the pleural surface covered by a fibrinous exudate. The fluid consists of a straw-colored fibrinous fluid containing mesothelial cells, lymphocytes, and polymorphs. In neoplastic diseases, malignant cells can also be identified within the pleural fluid.

Sequelae

Common sequelae include:

- Atelectasis: compression of the lungs causes pulmonary collapse and respiratory impairment.
- Adhesions: formation of fibrous adhesions between the visceral and parietal pleura.
- Fibrosis: obliteration of the pleural space by fibrosis, which is common in long-standing effusions.
- Empyema (see below).

Suppurative pleuritis (empyema)

This is an acute inflammation of the pleura with accumulation of pus in the pleural cavity. Typically caused by pulmonary infection (e.g., pneumonia, tuberculosis, lung abscess), it can also result as a complication of thoracic surgery or penetrating chest wall injury.

Common sequelae include septicemia (hematogenous spread of infection to other organs) and atelectasis (lung collapse as a result of compression).

Hemorrhagic pleuritis

This acute inflammation of the pleura with the accumulation of a blood-stained exudate, is often caused by tumor or pulmonary infarcts.

Noninflammatory pleural effusions

Hydrothorax

This collection of low protein fluid (<30g protein/L; transudate) is due to the movement of excess fluid through normal vessel walls. Common causes are:

- Cardiac failure (most common): increased hydrostatic pressure in pulmonary hypertension.
- Hypoalbuminemia: decreased oncotic pressure.

Effusions are usually bilateral, and the pleural surface appears normal. Fluid is straw-colored and it contains occasional lymphocytes and mesothelial cells.

The condition can cause pulmonary collapse (compression of the lungs causing respiratory impairment) or it may resolve completely (resorption of fluid on correction of the cause with no structural alterations).

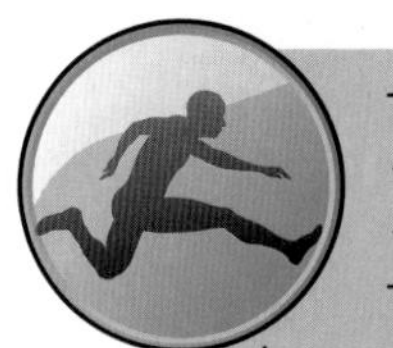

The difference between "transudate" and "exudate" is important. Transudates are characterized by a low-protein content (e.g., hydrothorax) in contrast to exudates, which have a high-protein content (serofibrinous pleuritis).

Hemothorax

Bleeding into the chest is called hemothorax. It is most commonly the result of:

- Trauma, especially with rib fractures.
- Surgery.
- Pulmonary infarction.
- Spontaneous rupture of diseased arteries (e.g., atheromatous and dissecting aortic aneurysm).

If blood remains within the pleural cavity, the result is organization and pleural fibrosis.

Chylothorax

The accumulation of chyle within the pleural cavity, caused by a leakage of chyle from the thoracic duct, is typically the result of malignant infiltration, surgery, or trauma; this is known as chylothorax.

Pneumothorax

This is the presence of air in the pleural cavity, the causes are described in Fig. 6.18.

Spontaneous pneumothorax can be either primary (of unknown cause occurring in otherwise healthy

Causes of pneumothorax		
Cause	**Type**	**Clinical features**
Spontaneous	Primary	Idiopathic rupture of pulmonary "bleb"; most common in thin young males
	Secondary	COPD: emphysema, chronic bronchitis and asthma Pneumonia Cystic fibrosis Whooping cough Pleural malignancy
Traumatic	Chest injury	Penetrating chest wounds Rib fractures Esophageal rupture
	Iatrogenic	Subclavian cannulation Positive pressure artificial ventilation Pleural aspiration Esophageal perforation during endoscopy Lung biopsy

Fig. 6.18 Causes of pneumothorax.

individuals) or secondary (i.e., secondary to lung disease).

Traumatic pneumothorax is a result of chest injury or is iatrogenic.

Complications of pneumothorax include:

- Atelectasis—lung collapse due to compression of the underlying lung.
- Tension pneumothorax—progressive increase in air pressure within the pleural cavity, causing massive collapse of the affected lung, mediastinal shift, and compression of the contralateral lung producing life-threatening respiratory insufficiency. The condition occurs as a result of a valve-like mechanism at the point at which air enters the pleural cavity. Air that enters the cavity in inspiration is unable to escape during expiration.

Neoplasms of the pleura

Pleural fibroma

This is a benign tumor of submesothelial connective tissue. The causes are unknown but there is no association with asbestos. The tumor is well-circumscribed, localized, and attached to the pleural surface by a pedicle. Histologically, it is composed of fibroblast-like cells with abundant collagen fibers.

Metastatic neoplasms

These are the commonest pleural tumors, most frequently arising from the lungs, breast, or ovary, but they can arise from any malignant tumor. They are usually associated with a high-protein exudate (see above).

Malignant mesothelioma

This primary neoplasm of the pleura is extremely rare, except following occupational asbestos exposure in workers of the ship building industry, etc. There is a latent interval between disease presentation and exposure to asbestos of up to 50 years. Fibers of crocidolite (blue asbestos) and amosite (brown asbestos) are implicated in the etiology. These asbestos fibers become trapped in the lung following inhalation, and they are particularly resistant to macrophage and neutrophil destruction.

Macroscopically, the tumors are highly malignant, and they spread locally around the pleural cavity and pericardium. However, hematogenous/lymphatic metastasis is rare.

Microscopically, mesotheliomas have spindle cells and glandular patterns.

Clinical features include chest pain and breathlessness, and there are commonly recurrent or persistent pleural effusions.

Prognosis—Poor. Death is usually within 10 months of diagnosis.

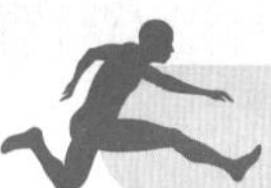

- What are the causes of acute and chronic rhinitis?
- Name the necrotizing lesions that may affect the nose and nasopharynx.
- What are the clinical features of nasopharyngeal tumors?
- List the causes of acute laryngitis.
- Define croup.
- Describe the pathology of squamous cell carcinoma of the larynx.
- Explain the differences between obstructive and restrictive lung diseases, and describe the characteristic patterns of lung function tests.
- Describe the pathogenesis and morphological features of extrinsic (atopic) asthma.
- Define pneumonia, and explain the difference between the broncho- and lobar types.
- What are the pathological features of tuberculosis?
- Describe the histological types of carcinoma of the bronchus.
- Name the acute and chronic interstitial lung diseases.
- Describe the morphological features of chronic pulmonary fibrosis.
- What are the three most common types of pneumoconiosis?
- Discuss pulmonary embolism.
- Explain the differences between serofibrinous pleuritis and hydrothorax.
- Name the common causes of an exudative pleural effusion.
- Name the common causes of a transudate pleural effusion.
- Classify the causes of pneumothorax.
- What is a tension pneumothorax?
- Describe the neoplasms that can affect the pleura.

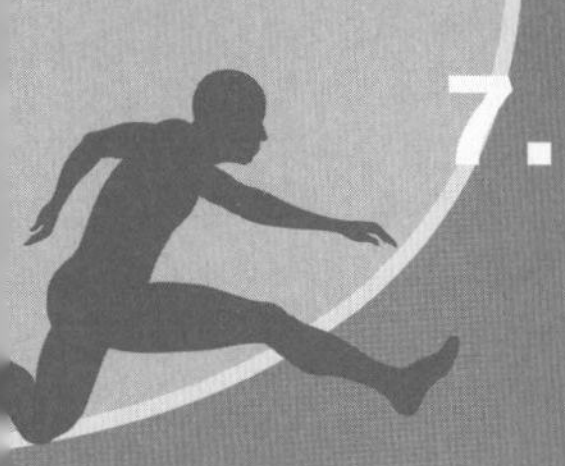

7. Pathology of the Gastrointestinal System

Disorders of the upper gastrointestinal tract

The mouth and oropharynx

Congenital abnormalities

Cleft palate and cleft (hare) lip

These are the most common major congenital malformations of the mouth, and they frequently occur together as a result of the same process, namely a failure of fusion of during the embryonic period.

Etiology—A few cases are associated with a chromosomal abnormality (e.g., trisomy 13 or 18) but, in the majority of cases, no teratogenic factor can be identified.

Morphology:

- Cleft lip—may be unilateral or bilateral, involving the lip only or extending upwards and backwards to include the floor of the nose and the alveolar ridge (Fig. 7.1).
- Cleft palate—considerable variation, from a small defect in the soft palate (bifid uvula) which causes little disability to a complete separation of the hard palate combined with a cleft lip (Fig. 7.2).

The effects are an abnormal facial appearance, defective speech, and feeding difficulty with extensive lesions (child is unable to suck).

Management is by artificial feeding, with plastic surgery recommended between 1 and 2 years of age.

Infections and inflammation

Noninfective stomatitis

Aphthous ulcers These are tiny, painful, shallow ulcers on a background of red mucosa typically occurring on the lips, tongue, or buccal mucosa. The ulcer crater is covered by a creamy exudate composed of fibrin and inflammatory cells, mainly neutrophils.

Etiology and pathogenesis are unknown. These ulcers may be associated with Crohn's disease, celiac disease, and Behçet's syndrome, but they also occur in 20% of the normal population.

Aphthous ulcers are extremely common (most common oral ulcers), recurrent (but usually of short duration), and occur singly or in groups.

Rarely, large ulcers (up to 3cm across) occur, sometimes persisting for several weeks before healing with fibrosis.

Infective stomatitis The majority of infections of the lips and buccal cavity are due to either viruses or fungi. The most common conditions are described below.

Herpes simplex virus Viral infections of the lips and mouth usually manifest as large blisters or crops of small painful vesicles, which eventually erode to form shallow tender ulcers.

Infection of the mouth with herpes simplex virus (HSV) is known as herpetic stomatitis.

Blisters develop on the gingiva and palate, which eventually rupture leaving shallow ulcers. Severe herpetic stomatitis is important in immunosuppressed patients, particularly those with acquired immune deficiency syndrome (AIDS).

Oral candidiasis This is an infection of the mouth with *Candida albicans* (also known as oral thrush). It is common in infants but less common in adults unless there are predisposing factors such as diabetes mellitus, or an immunosuppressed state (e.g., immunosuppressive therapy, advanced malignancy, or human immunodeficiency virus (HIV) infection).

The condition develops as white patches on palatal, buccal, and tongue surfaces. Lesions are composed of tangled fungal hyphae mixed with acute inflammatory cells and some desquamated epithelium. Underlying epithelium is acutely inflamed and red.

Glossitis This inflammation of the tongue either arises as a result of infective stomatitis (see above), or else it is due to a deficiency of nutritional factors, especially niacin, riboflavin, folic acid, and vitamin B_{12}:

- Acute deficiency: tongue is red, raw, and painful because of atrophy of papillae.
- Chronic deficiency: tongue appears moist and unduly clean.

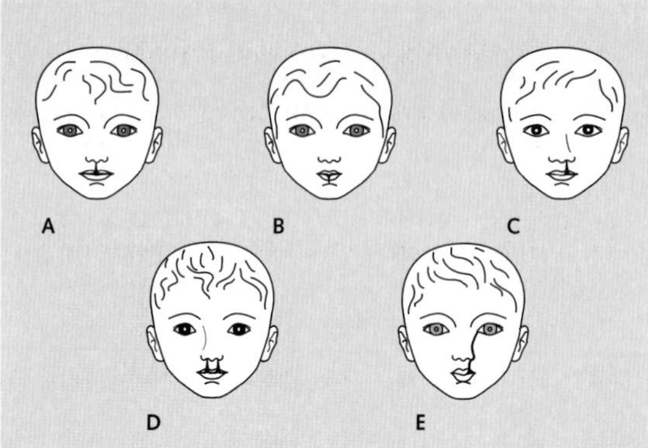

Fig. 7.1 Different types of cleft lip. (A) Median cleft upper lip. (B) Median cleft lower lip. (C) Unilateral cleft lip. (D) Bilateral cleft lip. (E) Oblique facial cleft.

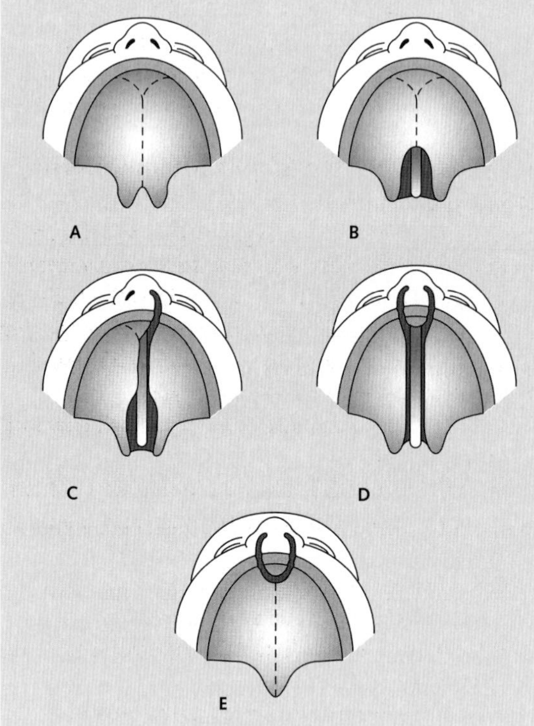

Fig. 7.2 Different types of cleft palate. (A) Cleft uvula. (B) Cleft soft and hard palate. (C) Total unilateral cleft palate and cleft lip. (D) Total bilateral cleft palate and cleft lip. (E) Bilateral cleft lip and jaw.

Oral manifestation of systemic disease Many oral pathologies are manifestations of systemic diseases. Examples include aphthous ulcers occurring in Crohn's and celiac disease, and angular cheilitis/glossitis in iron-deficiency anemia.

Neoplastic disease

Precancerous and benign

Leukoplakia (keratosis) This condition is characterized by white, firm, smooth patches (hyperkeratosis) beginning at the side of the tongue and later spreading over the dorsum. In the early stages, the tongue is not painful but later, the patches are split by tender fissures.

This condition can also affect the oral mucosa, but this is less typical. Biopsy is required to rule out carcinoma, since leukoplakia is not a diagnostic but merely a descriptive term.

Erythroplakia (erythroplasia) Less common than leukoplakia, this is characterized by the presence of red velvety patches of epithelial atrophy and pronounced dysplasia. It is seen mainly in elderly males on the buccal mucosa or the palate.

Malignant

Squamous cell carcinoma This is the most common tumor of the mouth, and it is derived from lining epithelium. It may arise in pre-existing dysplasia. It affects 2 per 100,000 in the U.S., affecting men more than women by about 2:1. The risk factors are:

- Smoking: direct relationship between number of cigarettes smoked per day and the risk of developing oral cancer.
- Alcohol: moderate intake = decreased risk; excessive intake = increased risk.
- Nutritional deficiencies.
- Candidal infection.
- Viral infections.

Macroscopically, there are raised nodular lesions and central ulceration with hard raised edges.

Microscopically, the tumor is typically well-differentiated and keratinizing.

The sites are:

- Lips (most common)—usually recognized early and amenable to surgery.
- Tongue—typically occurring on the lateral border of the anterior two-thirds.
- Cheek or floor of the mouth—generally asymptomatic, resulting in extensive local invasion and making surgical removal difficult.

Prognosis—May infiltrate locally and metastasize to regional lymph nodes in the neck. Five-year survival is about 50%.

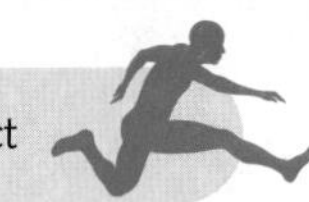

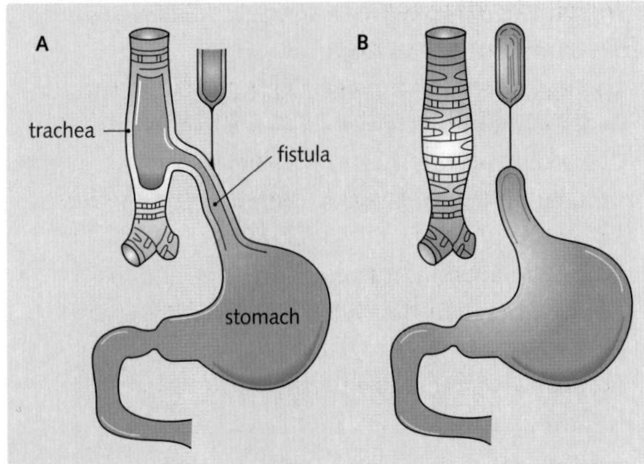

Fig. 7.3 Esophageal atresia. (A) Blind ending of esophagus with fistula formed between lower part and trachea. (B) Esophageal atresia with no fistulous communication—very rare.

The esophagus

Congenital abnormalities

Esophageal atresia

In esophageal atresia, the upper end of the esophagus is intact, but it ends in a blind pouch. Esophageal atresia affects 1 per 4000 live births, and more than 85% of cases are associated with the tracheo-esophageal fistula (Fig. 7.3).

Esophageal atresia with the tracheo-esophageal fistula

The lower esophagus is normal at the gastro-esophageal junction, but it tapers proximally and communicates with the trachea. The cause is a deviation of the tracheo-esophageal septum in a posterior direction.

The effects are:

- Fetus: inability to swallow amniotic fluid results in polyhydramnios, the accumulation of an excessive amount of amniotic fluid.
- Neonate: initially appears healthy, but swallowed fluid returns through the nose and mouth and respiratory distress occurs.

Esophageal stenosis

There is a narrowing of the lumen of the esophagus, usually occurring in the distal third either as a web or as a long segment of esophagus with a threadlike lumen. The causes are:

- Incomplete recanalization of the esophagus during development.
- Failure of blood vessels to develop in affected area → atrophy of a segment.

Predisposing factors of reflux esophagitis	
Factors that increase intra-abdominal pressure	Over-eating Pregnancy Poor posture
Factors that render the lower esophageal sphincter lax or incompetent	Hiatus hernia Smoking Alcohol ingestion

Fig. 7.4 Predisposing factors of reflux esophagitis.

Webs and rings

These localized constrictions of the esophagus are caused by mucosal folds or muscular contractions.

In Plummer–Vinson or Paterson–Brown–Kelly syndrome, upper esophageal webs are associated with dysphagia in patients with iron-deficiency anemia, cheilosis, and glossitis. This is a rare but important condition because of an association with the development of postcricoid and oral carcinoma.

Inflammation of the esophagus (esophagitis)

Reflux esophagitis

Inflammation of the esophagus caused by reflux of gastric acid into its lower part is the most common esophageal abnormality. The condition affects 3–4% of the general population; it can occur at any age (but with increased incidence over the age of 55 years), and it affects males more than females.

See Fig. 7.4 for a table of the predisposing factors of reflux esophagitis.

Symptoms are a burning pain in the centre of the lower chest or hypochondrium commonly known as "heartburn."

The complications are:

- Peptic ulceration of lower esophagus: development of small ulcers which become chronic with fibrosis.
- Lower esophageal stricture: chronic peptic ulceration causes progressive fibrous thickening of the lower esophagus wall producing difficulty in swallowing.
- Barrett's esophagus (also termed columnar epithelial-line esophagus): persistent esophageal reflux causes metaplasia of lower esophageal mucosa, the squamous epithelium being replaced by glandular columnar epithelium composed of tall columnar cells. Metaplasia of the esophagus predisposes to the development of adenocarcinoma.

Relevant investigations include endoscopy and 24-hour intraluminal pH monitoring.

Management is by:

- Life-style alterations: stop smoking, decrease alcohol intake.
- Drug therapy: antacids, alginates, mucosal-protective agents, H_2 receptor antagonists, proton pump inhibitors.
- Surgery: vagotomy, repair of hiatal defect, or fundal plication.

Other less common causes of esophagitis are:

- Infective agents: *Candida albicans*, herpes simplex and cytomegalovirus are important causes of acute esophagitis in the immunosuppressed.
- Physical agents: irradiation or ingestion of caustic agents.
- Skin diseases (e.g., pemphigus, epidermolysis bullosa, and Behçet's syndrome) may cause esophageal ulceration with extensive separation of epithelium from submucosa, producing blistering followed by erosion.

Lesions associated with motor dysfunction

Achalasia

Achalasia is a condition in which muscular contraction of the esophagus and relaxation at its lower end are not coordinated, leading to retention of the food bolus. This may occur at any age, but it is mainly seen in middle-aged individuals. The cause is unknown, but reduced numbers of ganglion cells in the muscle plexus have been noted in long-standing cases.

The consequences are:

- Difficulty in swallowing (dysphagia): increasing slowly over years.
- Regurgitation of undigested food.
- Occasional severe chest pain caused by esophageal spasm.
- Megaesophagus: esophageal distension occurs over a period of time.
- Increased predisposition to development of carcinoma of the esophagus.

Chagas' disease

Infection by *Trypanosoma cruzi* causes a condition similar to achalasia with destruction of the myenteric plexus. It is common in South America.

Others

Hiatus hernia This is a common condition in which the upper part of the stomach herniates through the diaphragmatic esophageal opening (hiatus) into the thoracic cavity.

The incidence is 5 per 1000 in the U.S., but it is 50–100 times less common in Asia and Africa.

The causes are:

- Congenital (rare)—short esophagus.
- Acquired (majority)—a consequence of increased intra-abdominal pressure and loss of diaphragmatic muscular tone with ageing.

There are two types (Fig. 7.5):

- Sliding hiatus hernia (90%)—stomach herniates through esophageal diaphragmatic hiatus.
- Rolling (paraesophageal) hiatus hernia (10%)—stomach protrudes through a separate defect alongside the esophagus.

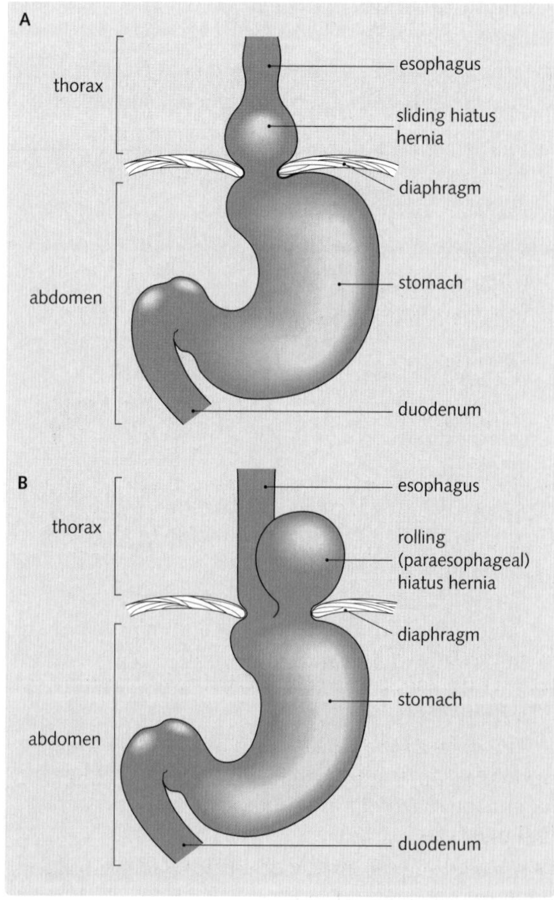

Fig. 7.5 Types of hiatus hernia. (A) Sliding hiatus hernia. (B) Rolling hiatus hernia.

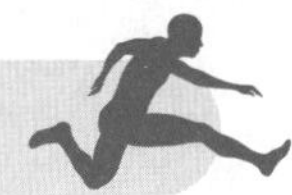

The complications are reflux esophagitis and peptic ulceration in the intrathoracic part of the stomach and the lower esophagus.

Diverticula Esophageal diverticula are outpouchings of one or more layers of the esophageal wall. They can develop by either:

Pulsion: pressure from within the esophagus creates a diverticulum. This is common immediately above sphincters.

Traction: external forces pull on the wall, usually from adherent inflammatory lesions—classically tuberculous lymph nodes. This is common near the midpoint of the esophagus.

The site may be:

- Immediately above the upper esophageal sphincter (Zenker's diverticulum).
- Near the midpoint of the esophagus (traction diverticulum).
- Immediately above the lower esophageal sphincter (epiphrenic diverticulum).

The complications are dysphagia (where the diverticula frequently become permanently distended with retained food and cause difficulties in swallowing) and an increased risk of esophageal perforation on endoscopy.

Lacerations Esophageal perforation is rare, but it may be caused by:

- Traumatic rupture: usually associated with vomiting.
- Impaction of a sharp foreign body.
- Intubation of strictures.

Mallory–Weiss tear is an esophageal laceration as a result of vomiting. A classical symptom is vomiting of clear fluid (pre-tearing), followed by vomiting of blood (post-tearing).

Esophageal varices

Esophageal varices are varicosed, dilated submucosal veins in the esophagus.

The condition is caused by portal hypertension (most commonly associated with cirrhosis of the liver).

Pathogenesis

Esophageal veins normally drain into both systemic and portal venous systems.

Increased pressure in the portal venous system (e.g., as a result of severe diffuse long-standing liver disease) causes dilatation of the esophageal veins to form esophageal varices, which often protrude into the lumen.

Rupture of the varices, or ulceration of overlying mucosa, can produce a torrential hemorrhage into the esophagus and stomach, often precipitating vomiting of blood.

Management

There are three stages:

1. Local measures to control bleeding: sclerotherapy, ballon tamponade, and transjugular intrahepatic portosystemic stent shunting (TIPSS).
2. Reduction of portal venous pressure: drug therapy with vasopressin and somatostatin.
3. Prevention of recurrent bleeding: sclerotherapy, banding, and TIPSS.

Neoplastic disease

Barrett's esophagus

Definition—Metaplastic replacement of normal squamous esophageal epithelium with glandular columnar epithelium. There are three types of mucosa seen: junctional type, atrophic type, and specialized mucosa.

The condition is caused by persistent esophageal reflux; approximately 10% of these patients will develop Barrett's esophagus.

Barrett's esophagus predisposes to the development of adenocarcinoma. Metaplastic glandular epithelium can progress to epithelial dysplasia and then to frank adenocarcinoma.

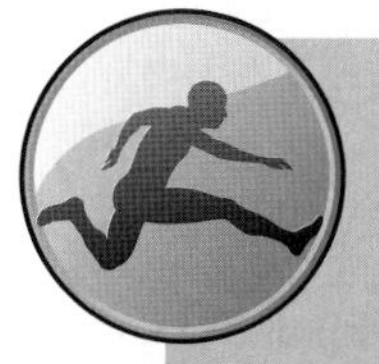

Barrett's esophagus is a classic example of metaplasia, and it is a good example to quote in an examination.

Benign neoplastic disease

Benign tumors of the esophagus are rare. The majority are leiomyomas derived from the smooth muscle of muscularis propria, the minority being derived from nerves (i.e., schwannomas and neurofibromas).

Malignant neoplastic disease

The most common malignant tumors of the esophagus are squamous carcinomas and adenocarcinomas. Risk factors are:

- Smoking/alcohol.
- Diet (tannic acid, food colorings).
- Barrett's esophagus.
- Corrosives.
- Achalasia.
- Iron-deficiency anemia.
- Infection: viruses (HPV). Interestingly some esophageal cancers contain HPV. Current research is trying to determine whether the virus is involved in the process of carcinogenesis (oncogene activation).

Squamous cell carcinomas These mostly develop in men who are heavy alcohol drinkers or heavy smokers and may be preceded by an epithelial dysplastic change. They usually present late when the tumor is large enough to compromise the esophageal lumen and cause dysphagia. They are most common in the middle and lower esophagus.

Adenocarcinomas These mainly occur in the lower esophagus and are increasing in prevalence, representing about 50% of all esophageal cancers. The majority arise in areas of epithelial metaplasia (Barrett's esophagus), but some are primary carcinomas of the stomach that have infiltrated the lower esophagus.

Clinical features of esophageal tumors

- Common: dysphagia, anorexia, weight loss, anemia (acute or chronic).
- Rare: hoarse voice (involvement of larynx or left recurrent laryngeal nerve palsy), supraclavicular lymphadenopathy, tracheo-esophageal fistula, aorto-esophageal fistula.

Investigations are:

- Chest x-ray: mediastinal mass, pulmonary metastases, pleural effusion.
- Barium swallow.
- Upper gastrointestinal (GI) endoscopy: proximal extent of tumor, biopsy, dilatation.
- CT/MRI: check other organs for metastases.
- Endoscopic ultrasound: good for staging disease.
- Respiratory function tests: prognostic for resection.

Management:

- Palliative: usually for treatment of dysphagia (intubation, dilatation, bypass, laser treatment).
- Curative: surgery or radiotherapy.

The prognosis is poor for both types of malignant esophageal tumors. However, the prognosis for squamous carcinoma is slightly better because it is more responsive to radiotherapy.

Survival post treatment—30% at 1 year, 20% at 2 years, 5% at 5 years.

Disorders of the stomach

Congenital abnormalities

Diaphragmatic hernias

These are described in the previous section (p. 106).

Pyloric stenosis

Marked narrowing of the pylorus (gastric outflow tract) causes obstruction to the passage of food such that the stomach becomes markedly distended and the stomach's contents are expelled with considerable force. This disorder can be congenital or acquired.

Congenitally, it is a common anomaly, affecting 4 per 1000 live births, males more than females by 5:1. Hypertrophy of pyloric circular and longitudinal muscle layers causes projectile vomiting.

Acquired causes are:

- Fibrous stricture from a duodenal ulcer.
- Edema from a pyloric channel or duodenal ulcer.
- Carcinoma of stomach antrum.
- Adult hypertrophic pyloric stenosis.

Symptoms are mainly nausea and vomiting. Signs include wasting, dehydration, and a succussion splash, which may be elicited 4 hours or more after the last meal or drink.

Inflammation

Acute gastritis

This superficial acute inflammation of the gastric mucosa is typically caused by ingested chemicals, the most common being alcohol, aspirin, and other nonsteroidal anti-inflammatory drugs (NSAIDs).

Acute erosive gastritis

Focal loss of the superficial gastric epithelium causes dyspepsia with vomiting and occasionally, if the erosions are numerous, hematemesis may occur.

Causes are:

- NSAIDs.
- Heavy acute alcohol ingestion.

- Severe stress or shock (e.g., after major trauma or burns).
- Hypotension: acute hypoxia of surface epithelium.

Chronic gastritis

Chronic inflammation of the gastric mucosa is a common condition. It increases with age, and it is more common in developed countries.

The condition is present in over 90% of patients with duodenal ulceration, in about 70% of those with gastric ulceration, and it is also common in those with gastric cancer.

There are three etiological types of classification:

- Infectious—*Helicobacter pylori*-associated gastritis.
- Immune—pernicious anemia and atrophic gastritis without pernicious anemia.
- Reactive—post gastrectomy or adjacent to erosions/ulcers.

Helicobacter-associated gastritis

This is the most common form of chronic gastritis, accounting for more than 90% of cases, and it may arise at any age. The pyloric antrum is the most severely affected area, but damage is also seen in the fundus.

Pathogenesis is as follows:

- Colonization: *Helicobacter pylori* colonizes epithelial surface beneath thin layer of mucus. This causes an initial acute neutrophilic gastritis, which gives way to chronic (lymphocytic) gastritis.
- Urease production: the bacterium produces the enzyme urease, which breaks down urea to give CO_2 and NH_3, the latter providing protection from the acid secretions of the stomach.
- Immune response: the presence of the organism results in an immune response → epithelial damage.
- Persistence of infection: once established infection may persist for years.

The morphological features are:

- Mucin depletion leading to damage to the underlying epithelium.
- Atrophy of gastric glands.
- Mixed acute and chronic inflammatory cell reaction in lamina propria and superficial epithelium.
- Intestinal metaplasia: normal gastric epithelium is replaced by a type similar to that of small intestine.

The tests available for diagnosis of *H. pylori* infection are listed in Fig. 7.6.

Autoimmune chronic gastritis

This organ-specific autoimmune disease associated with pernicious anemia is generally seen in elderly patients with the development of severe atrophy of the mucosa (atrophic gastritis). It particularly affects the body of the stomach.

Antibodies are of two types:

- Antibodies against gastric parietal cells (90%): associated with decreased hydrochloric acid production (hypochlorhydria).
- Antibodies against intrinsic factor (60%) → failure of absorption of dietary vitamin B_{12} → interference with normal erythropoiesis in bone

Test for diagnosis of *Helicobacter pylori* infection

Type	Test	Diagnosis
Non-invasive	Urea breath test	Radiolabelled urea is administered; urease produced by *H. pylori* → radioactive CO_2, which can be detected on the breath
	Serology	Antibodies to *H. pylori* can be detected in serum
Invasive	Histology	Organisms can be seen in biopsy material
	Culture	Can be cultured from biopsy material
	CLO (*Campylobacter*-like organism) test	Biopsy added to test kit containing urea. If urease present, NH_3 produced causes change in color of indicator

Fig. 7.6 Diagnosis of *Helicobacter pylori* infection.

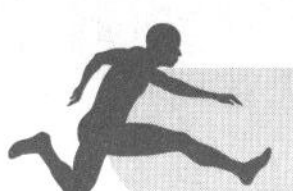

marrow → megaloblastic, macrocytic anemia (pernicious anemia).

The most common form is atrophic gastritis with achlorhydria but without pernicious anemia. In this condition, antibodies of both types are often present, but there is a residual ability to absorb vitamin B_{12}. However, patients may develop pernicious anemia with time.

The morphological features are:

- Loss of specialized cells.
- Fibrosis.
- Infiltrate of plasma cells and lymphocytes.
- Intestinal metaplasia.

Reactive gastritis (reflux gastritis)

In this pattern of mucosal injury the dominant feature is epithelial change with minimal inflammatory cell infiltrates. The causes are threefold:

- Idiopathic: majority of cases.
- Reflux of alkaline bile-containing duodenal fluid into the lower part of the stomach. This may be caused by motility disturbances (e.g., due to gallstones or cholecystectomy) or pyloric incompetence (as a result of previous surgery to the pyloric area).
- Drugs: NSAIDs may cause direct damage to the mucus layer.

Morphological features are:

- Epithelial desquamation.
- Foveolar hyperplasia.
- Vasodilatation.
- Mucosal edema.

Complications of chronic gastritis

Regardless of cause, all forms of chronic gastritis can cause intestinal metaplasia (producing an increased predisposition to undergo dysplastic change with eventual transformation into carcinoma), and peptic ulcerations caused by damage to the gastric lining by acidic gastric secretions.

Gastric ulceration

Peptic ulcers

Peptic ulcers are ulcers of the esophagus, stomach, or duodenum caused by damage to the epithelial lining by gastric secretions, particularly acid.

It is estimated that about 10% of the Western population experience peptic ulceration at some time. Ulcers usually develop in adulthood, and they have a natural history of repeated healing and relapse over many years.

Sites are:

- Lower esophagus (due to gastric reflux).
- Stomach: most common on distal lesser curve.
- Duodenum: most common site of peptic ulceration.
- Gastroenterostomy sites.

Etiology is probably multifactorial. Ulcers are commonly associated with *H. pylori*, NSAIDs, and stress. Less commonly, they may be associated with acid hypersecretion (e.g., gastrinoma), infection, duodenal obstruction/disruption, vascular insufficiency, or radiation.

Other factors, such as chronic gastritis, smoking, and genetic predisposition, are also believed to play a role in the pathogenesis, although the mechanisms are poorly understood.

Pathogenesis

Upper GI mucosa is normally protected by either squamous epithelium (esophagus) or an acid-resisting mucus barrier containing neutralizing bicarbonate ions. Peptic ulceration occurs when the aggressive action of acid and pepsin is not opposed by adequate mucosal protective mechanisms:

- Esophageal ulceration: the most important cause is reflux of acid gastric secretion on to the unprotected esophageal mucosa.
- Duodenal ulceration: the most important factor is hypersecretion of acid by the stomach.
- Gastric ulceration: predisposing factors include regurgitated bile in pyloric incompetence and surface epithelial damage by *H. pylori* infection or by NSAIDs.

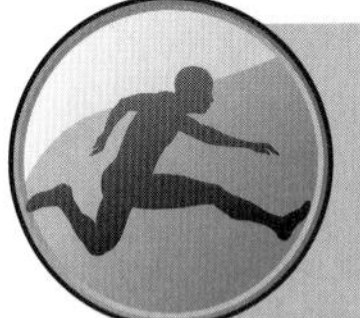

Peptic ulceration represents the adverse result of a conflict between erosive forces and defense mechanisms of the stomach and duodenum.

Macroscopically, peptic ulcers are typically 1–2 cm in diameter (but they can be much larger) with sharply defined borders surrounding the ulcer crater.

Microscopically, the ulcer crater usually penetrates into the muscularis propria of the stomach and it has four histological zones, namely:

1. Superficial layer of fibrin and inflammatory exudate.
2. Fibrinoid necrosis.
3. Granulation tissue.
4. Fibrosis.

Complete healing of the ulcer leads to fibrous replacement of muscle with regrowth of epithelium over the scar. Clinical features include epigastric pain (alleviated by antacids), nausea, and heartburn (esophageal ulcers).

Sequelae

Complications and sequelae are as follows:

- Healing: usually occurs slowly but can be hastened by acid-inhibiting agents or mucosal protectants.
- Hemorrhage: a common cause of upper GI bleeding.
- Adherence and erosion: ulcer penetrates full thickness of the stomach or duodenal wall, adhering and eroding into underlying tissue, particularly the pancreas or liver.
- Perforation: ulcer perforates, leading to peritonitis.
- Fibrous strictures: seen in peptic ulcers of the esophagus; fibrous thickening caused by healing leads to scarring of the esophagus and obstruction. In the stomach, ulcers may cause pyloric stenosis.
- Malignant change (very rare).

Management

Management is by:

- Life-style alterations: stop smoking, decrease alcohol intake, stress reduction.
- Medical: eradication of *H. pylori* (antibiotics), acid suppression, e.g., antacids, proton pump inhibitors, H_2 receptor antagonists).
- Surgery: partial gastrectomy, vagotomy.

Acute gastric ulcer

Acute peptic ulcers usually develop from areas of erosive gastritis, and they are predisposed by the same conditions as erosive gastritis. In contrast to chronic ulcers, they are generally multiple and shallow with minimal surrounding inflammation or fibrosis.

Acute ulcers may heal without scarring, or they may progress to chronicity.

Hypertrophic gastropathy

Ménétrier's disease

This rare disease of unknown cause is characterized by gross hyperplasia of gastric pits, atrophy of glands, and a marked overall increase in mucosal thickness. It is associated with hypoalbuminemia as a result of gastric protein loss via superficial ulcerations.

Hypertrophic hypersecretory gastropathy

An extremely rare condition, this is characterized by acid hypersecretion and gastric protein loss.

Zollinger–Ellison syndrome

This syndrome of gastric hypersecretion, multiple peptic ulcers, and diarrhea is caused by the gastrin secreting tumor (gastrinoma) of the pancreatic G cells (see Chapter 9).

Neoplastic disease

Benign

Benign gastric polyps are rare compared with the incidence of malignant tumors of the stomach. The types are:

- Hyperplastic polyps—most common polyp of the stomach, formed by regeneration of mucosa, often at the edge of an ulcer.
- Adenomatous polyps—true benign tumors of the surface epithelium ranging up to 5 cm in size. Very rare, but may carry a risk of malignant change.
- Fundal polyps—cystic glandular lesions seen mainly in women.
- Hamartomatous polyps—occur in Peutz–Jeghers syndrome (hereditary condition of multiple polyps in the small intestine associated with pigmented areas around the lips, inside mouth, and on palms and soles).

Other benign tumors of the stomach are derived from mesenchymal tissues, the most common being leiomyomas. These appear as mucosal or intramural nodules and are usually asymptomatic.

Malignant

Gastric adenocarcinomas

The vast majority of gastric carcinomas are adenocarcinomas derived from mucus-secreting epithelial cells. They affect 20–40 people per 100,000 per year, and they are typically seen in patients after the age of 30 years, the incidence rising greatly after the age of 50 years. Males are affected more than females by 3:2.

They are common in the Far East and certain parts of South America and Scandinavia, but less so in Western Europe and North America.

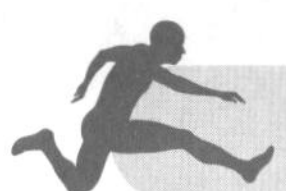

The sites are:

- Pylorus (60%): often produce symptoms of obstruction to the gastric outlet.
- Fundus (20–30%): typically a fungating, ulcerating mass.
- Cardia (5–20%): may produce dysphagia.

Unlike chronic peptic ulcers of the stomach, they are not confined to the lesser curvature.

Etiology is unknown but dietary factors are suggested to account for geographical variation (e.g., ingestion of smoked and salted preserved foods). Other risk factors include:

- Chronic gastritis and intestinal metaplasia.
- Gastric adenomatous polyps.
- Postgastrectomy patients with persisting gastric inflammation.
- Gastric cancer families (rare).
- *H. pylori* infection: prevalence of *H. pylori* infection frequently runs parallel with the incidence of gastric cancer, and patients with antibodies to the bacterium have a higher risk of gastric cancer.

Mechanisms linking *H. pylori* to gastric cancer include:

- Proliferating *H. pylori* are capable of converting compounds in the diet into potentially carcinogenic compounds.
- Reactive oxygen species produced by activated macrophages and polymorphs may cause DNA damage.
- *H. pylori* infection promotes a high cell turnover (increased proliferation), which compromises DNA repair.

The sequence of events in the development of gastric carcinomas is as follows:

normal mucosa → chronic gastritis → intestinal metaplasia → dysplasia → intramucosal carcinoma (early gastric cancer) → invasive carcinoma

Several genetic changes have been reported in gastric cancer, including alterations of p53, K-*ras*, and the APC gene. Overexpression of oncogenes such as c-*myc* has also been demonstrated.

Gastric cancers are classified as either early or advanced according to the extent of their spread through the stomach wall.

Early gastric cancer This is confined to the mucosa and/or submucosa regardless of whether spread has occurred to regional lymph nodes. It is associated with a good prognosis.

The cancer is further divided into three types according to macroscopic appearance (Fig. 7.7).

Advanced gastric tumors These extend into or beyond the main muscle coats, and they are associated with a poor prognosis. They are further divided into three types macroscopically (Fig. 7.8):

- Polypoid: protrudes into stomach lumen and presents early due to a feeling of gastric discomfort and bleeding of protrusion when traumatized. Usually amenable to surgical excision, and it has the best prognosis.

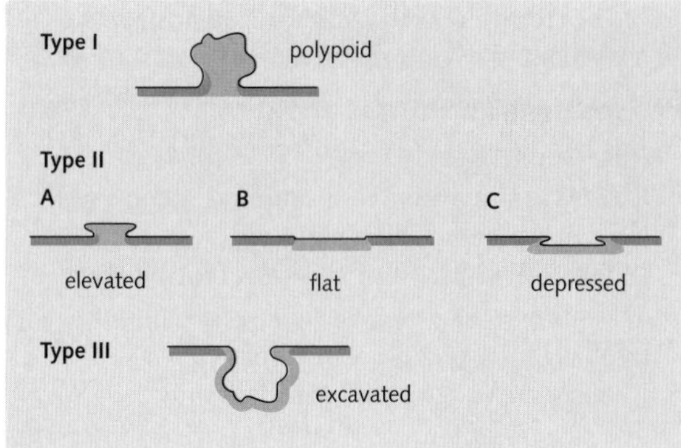

Fig. 7.7 Macroscopic classification of early gastric cancers: type I polypoid; type II is further divided into (A) elevated, (B) flat, and (C) depressed; type III excavated.

Comparison of the types of advanced gastric carcinomas

	Polypoid	Ulcerative	Diffuse infiltrative
Incidence	Common	Very common	Rare
Hemorrhage	Yes	Yes	Not until late stage
Prognosis	Good	Intermediate	Poor
Involvement	Focal	Focal	Diffuse

Fig. 7.8 Comparison of the types of advanced gastric carcinomas.

- Ulcerating (most common type): similar in appearance to benign peptic ulcers but with a raised edge, necrotic shaggy base, and an absence of the radiating folds seen in benign peptic ulcers. Nonhealing ulcers after adequate medical therapy, must always be biopsied to rule out carcinoma.
- Diffuse infiltrative pattern (linitis plastica): presents late, and has the worst prognosis. Tumor spreads extensively within mucosa and submucosa producing a shrunken, inexpansible, rigid stomach. Symptoms are usually non-specific; loss of appetite and vomiting due to small capacity of the stomach and its inability to distend under a food load. Surface ulceration is not a prominent feature and so hematemesis is not common until the later stages. Metastatic spread to lymph nodes and the liver is usually present at time of clinical presentation.

Other gastric tumors

Other forms of malignancy are rare in the stomach, but include lymphomas (see Chapter 12), carcinoid tumors (p. 149), lymphomas, and stromal tumors.

General aspects of hepatic damage

Patterns of hepatic injury

Following hepatic injury, the liver has a limited set of responses:

- Necrosis.
- Inflammation.
- Regeneration.
- Fibrosis.

All pathological processes of the liver result in one or more of the above reactions.

Necrosis

Acute hepatocellular injury can result in variable forms of necrosis. The underlying type of necrosis depends on etiology.

Coagulative necrosis

This is typically a result of ischemia (see Chapter 3).

Councilman bodies

During the death of individual liver cells (by apoptosis), single, dead hepatocytes form brightly eosinophilic, shrunken structures known as Councilman bodies.

Hydropic degeneration

This is the ballooning of individual hepatocytes, generally as a result of viral hepatitis. It is a mild, often reversible change, but it may progress to necrosis.

Focal necrosis

Necrosis of small groups of hepatocytes, which occurs in acute viral- or drug-induced hepatitis.

Zonal necrosis

Necrosis confined to certain zones is seen with certain diseases; for example, the centrilobular area (zone 3) is affected in paracetamol toxicity (Fig. 7.9).

Massive necrosis

Necrosis of the majority of hepatocytes. Occurs with fulminant hepatic damage and is seen in some cases of viral- and toxin-induced damage.

Piecemeal necrosis

Liver cells at the interface between parenchyma and fibrous tissue are destroyed, together with lymphocytic or plasma cell infiltrate.

Inflammation

Inflammation of the liver is known as hepatitis, and it is a common response to a wide array of damage (e.g., viral infection, autoimmune disorders, drugs, and toxins).

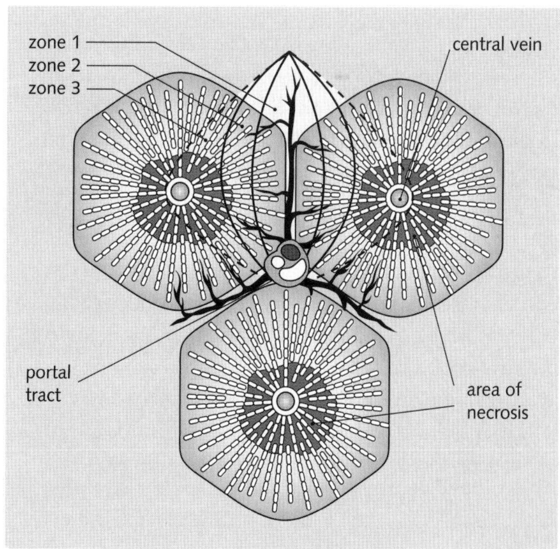

Fig. 7.9 Centrilobular (zone 3) zonal necrosis.

Regeneration

Under normal circumstances there is very little liver cell proliferation. However, following hepatic injury, liver cell regeneration occurs to restore liver function; this is a crucial phenomenon for recovery for patients with fulminant or subfulminant liver failure.

Fibrosis

Repeated chronic damage to the liver can result in fibrosis. Growth factors produced as part of a inflammatory response are thought to stimulate proliferation and differentiation of mesenchymal cells (the normally inconspicuous fat-storing cells of Ito located in the space of Disse) into collagen-secreting fibroblasts.

Development of fibrosis is an important complication of several liver diseases, and it is one of the characteristic features of cirrhosis.

Cirrhosis

Cirrhosis is an irreversible condition in which the liver's normal architecture is diffusely replaced by nodules of regenerated liver cells separated by bands of collagenous fibrosis. Cirrhosis represents the end-stage of many processes: it is not a specific disease in itself. It involves:

- Long-standing destruction of liver cells.
- Chronic inflammation that stimulates fibrosis.
- Regeneration of hepatocytes to cause nodules.

Macroscopically, the liver is tawny and characteristically knobbly (due to nodules). On a cut surface, parenchyma is replaced by nodules of regenerated hepatocytes separated by fine fibrosis.

Microscopically, the nodules of hepatocytes are separated by bands of collagenous tissue. Bile ducts and portal vessels run in the fibrous septa.

Cirrhosis can be classified either according to the size of regenerative nodules (Fig. 7.10) or according to its etiology (Fig. 7.11). However, an etiological classification is most useful in determining prognosis and treatment. The clinical features of cirrhosis are illustrated in Fig. 7.12.

Consequences are:

- Liver failure: reduced hepatocyte function (decreased synthesis of proteins, failure of detoxification).
- Portal hypertension and its complications (see below): a result of impeded blood flow through liver.

Classification according to nodular size	
Type	**Nodule size**
Micronodular	≤3mm
Macronodular	3mm–2cm
Mixed micro- and macronodular	Mixture of small and large

Fig. 7.10 Classification of cirrhosis according to nodular size.

Classification according to incidence in the Western world	
Common	Alcoholic liver disease Cryptogenic (no cause found) Chronic hepatitis caused by hepatitis B and C viruses
Uncommon	Autoimmune chronic hepatitis Primary biliary cirrhosis Chronic biliary obstruction (biliary cirrhosis) Cystic fibrosis
Treatable but rare	Hemochromatosis Wilson's disease
Rare	α_1-antitrypsin deficiency Galactosemia Glycogenosis type IV Tyrosinemia

Fig. 7.11 Classification of cirrhosis according to incidence in the Western world.

- Reduced immune competence → increased susceptibility to infection.
- Increased risk of development of hepatocellular carcinoma.
- Increased risk of development of portal vein thrombosis.

Portal hypertension, ascites, and splenomegaly

Portal hypertension

This is a continued elevation in portal venous pressure, normal portal venous pressure being less than 7mm Hg. Causes of portal hypertension can be classified according to whether the site of obstruction to flow is:

- Prehepatic—blockage of vessels before the hepatic sinusoids.

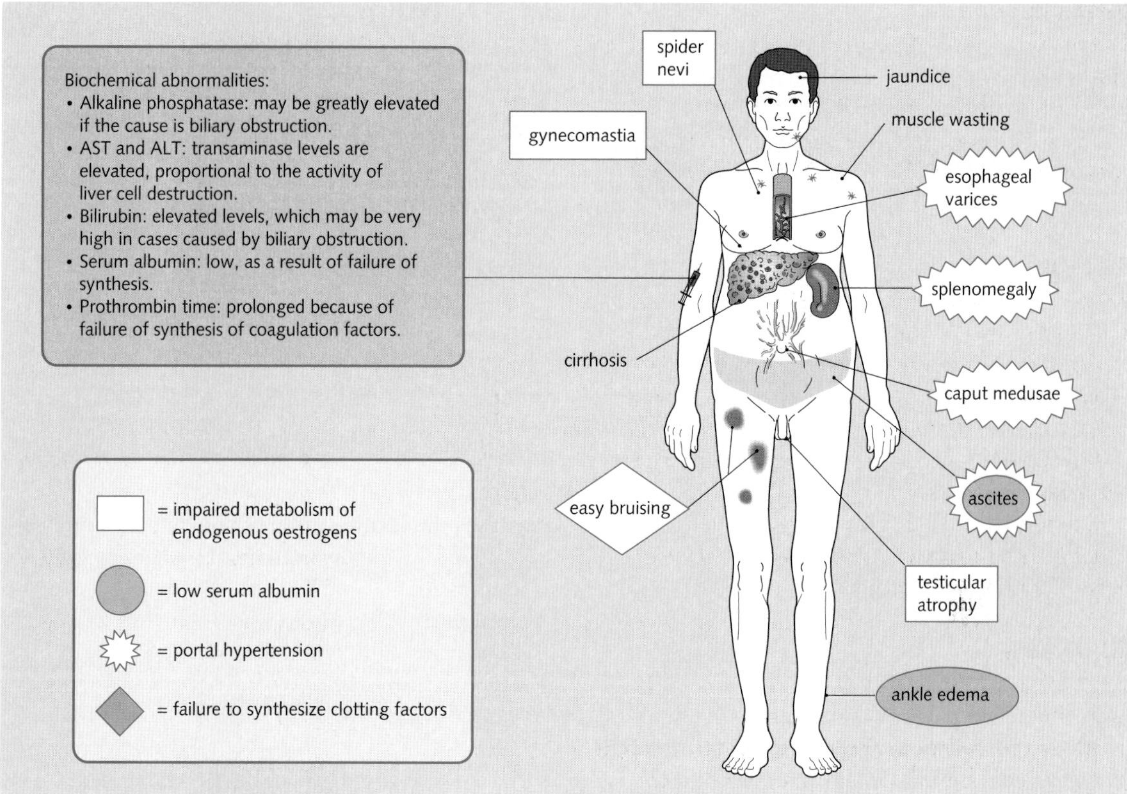

Fig. 7.12 Clinical signs of cirrhosis.

Classification of portal hypertension	
Prehepatic	**Portal vein thrombosis**
Hepatic	Cirrhosis Idiopathic portal hypertension Hepatic fibrosis: caused by schistosomiasis (important cause in endemic areas) Polycystic disease of the liver
Posthepatic	Disease of hepatic veins and branches

Fig. 7.13 Classification of portal hypertension.

- Hepatic—blockage in the hepatic sinusoids.
- Posthepatic—blockage in the central veins, hepatic veins, or vena cava.

See Fig. 7.13 for a table of the causes of portal hypertension.

Complications—Portal hypertension causes back-pressure in the portal vascular bed leading to splenomegaly, ascites, and varicose venous channels.

New varicose venous channels open up between the portal venous system and systemic venous system. Main sites are the lower esophagus (esophageal varices (see p. 107), which may cause catastrophic bleeding), the umbilicus (channels are called caput medusae), and the anus (rectal varices).

The causes and effects of portal hypertension are shown in Fig. 7.14.

Main causes of portal hypertension are:

- Cirrhosis of the liver (most common).
- Portal vein thrombosis.
- Hepatic vein thrombosis (Budd–Chiari syndrome).

Portosystemic shunts

Venous communications that link portal and systemic venous systems become enlarged in portal hypertension. The four sites of portal–systemic anastomosis are:

- Lower third of the esophagus: left gastric vein (portal tributary) anastomoses with esophageal veins (systemic tributary).

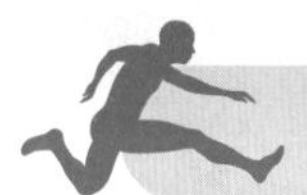

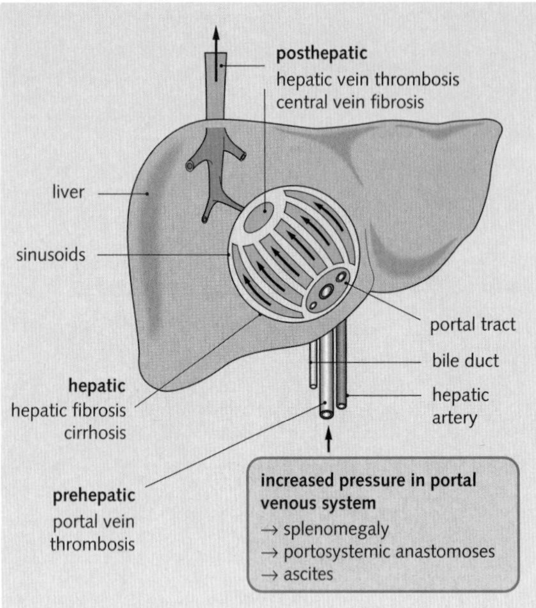

Fig. 7.14 Causes and effects of portal hypertension.

- Halfway down the anal canal: superior rectal veins (portal tributary) draining upper half of anal canal anastomose with middle and inferior rectal veins (systemic tributaries).
- Paraumbilical veins: connect left branch of the portal vein with superficial veins of anterior abdominal wall (systemic tributaries).
- Veins of ascending colon, descending colon, duodenum, pancreas, and liver (portal tributaries) anastomose with renal, lumbar, and phrenic veins (systemic tributaries).

Pathogenesis—Under normal conditions, portal venous blood traverses the liver and drains into the inferior vena cava of systemic venous circulation by way of the hepatic veins. In portal hypertension, this direct route is blocked and the portal venous blood is forced through smaller communications that exist between the portal and systemic systems.

Anastomotic channels become dilated resulting in the development of varicose venous channels, namely:

- Esophageal varices (see p. 107): may cause severe bleeding.
- Caput medusae: distention of paraumbilical veins.
- Hemorrhoids.

Types of ascites	
Transudate **low protein fluid (<30 g/L)**	**Exudate** **high protein fluid (>30 g/L)**
Cirrhosis Constrictive pericarditis Cardiac failure Hypoalbuminemia, e.g., nephrotic syndrome	Malignancy Peritonitis Pancreatitis Budd-Chiari syndrome Hypothyroidism Lymphatic obstruction (chylous ascites)

Fig. 7.15 Types of ascites.

Ascites

Ascites is the accumulation of fluid in the peritoneal cavity.

Causes are:

- Peritonitis.
- Malignancy in the peritoneal cavity.
- Hypoproteinemia.
- Portal hypertension.

Pathogenesis of ascites in cirrhosis—Increased transudation of fluid in ascites occurs as a result of:

- ↑ Hydrostatic pressure in portal veins.
- ↓ Plasma oncotic pressure (due to lowered albumin synthesis by damaged liver cells).

Fig. 7.15 is a table describing the types of ascites.

Clinical features are abdominal distention with fullness in the flanks, shifting dullness on percussion, and fluid thrill.

Management is by:

- Restricted Na^+ intake.
- Diuretic drugs (e.g., spironolactone).
- Paracentesis: drainage of 3–5 liters over 1–2 hours is used for immediate relief. Drainage to dryness must be supported by giving colloid (e.g., plasma) as required.
- LeVeen shunt: a long tube with a one-way valve running subcutaneously from the peritoneum to the internal jugular vein in the neck. This allows ascitic fluid to pass directly into the systemic circulation. Complications of infection, thrombosis, and pulmonary edema limit its use.
- TIPSS (see p. 107): relieves portal hypertension.

Prognosis—Only 10–20% of patients survive 5 years from its appearance.

Splenomegaly

Increased pressure in the portal vein is transmitted to the splenic vein resulting in splenomegaly (see Chapter 13).

Jaundice and cholestasis

Jaundice

This presents as a yellowing of the skin or sclerae, indicating excess bilirubin in the blood.

The biochemical definition of jaundice is an increase in the plasma bilirubin level above the normal level of about 18–24μmol/L (i.e., 1.2mg/dL).

Clinical jaundice is when levels of bilirubin are above 50μmol/L (i.e., 2.5mg/dL), manifesting as a yellow discoloration of the sclerae and skin.

The metabolism of bilirubin is illustrated in Fig. 7.16.

Cholestasis

Failure of bile flow caused by the obstruction of either small (intrahepatic) or large (extrahepatic) bile ducts results in jaundice due to conjugated hyperbilirubinemia.

Jaundice can be classified according to etiology (Fig. 7.17) or according to chemical analysis of the bilirubin in the blood (Fig. 7.18).

Unconjugated versus conjugated hyperbilirubinemia

Unconjugated

Excess bilirubin is not water soluble and it cannot be excreted in urine. Urine is, therefore, of normal color but feces may be slightly darker because of increased excretion of fat-soluble bilirubin into the bile.

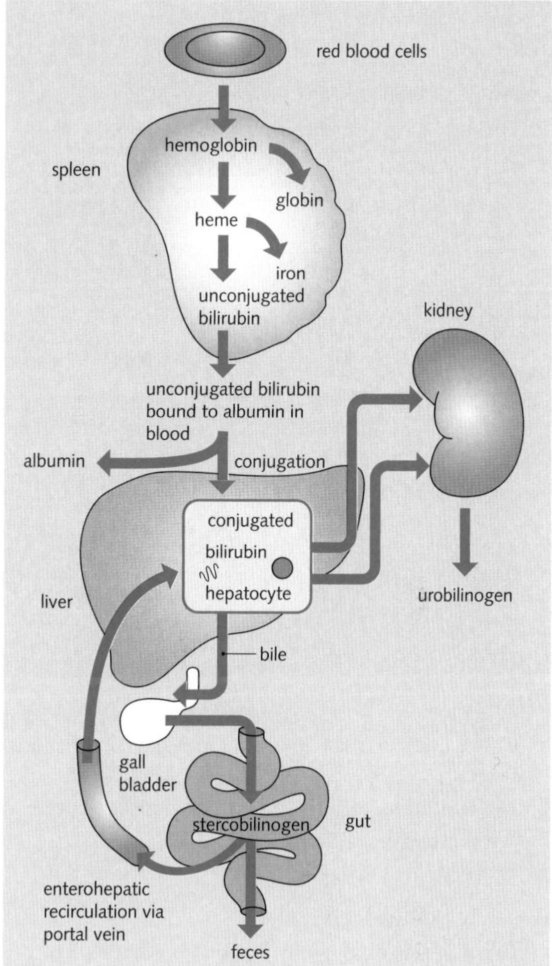

Fig. 7.16 Bilirubin metabolism.

Causes of jaundice	
Cause	**Clinical consequence**
Prehepatic causes	Hemolysis (most common cause)
Intrahepatic causes	Hereditary enzyme defects, e.g., Dubin-Johnson, Rotor's, Gilbert's, and Crigler-Najjar syndromes Drugs causing intrahepatic cholestasis Pregnancy-associated cholestasis Hepatocellular damage, e.g., alcohol, virus hepatitis
Posthepatic (obstructive) causes	Large duct obstruction as a result of: • gallstones • strictures caused by inflammation or fibrosis • extrahepatic biliary atresia • compression by extrinsic masses, e.g., carcinoma of the pancreas, enlarged lymph nodes

Fig. 7.17 Causes of jaundice.

Classification of jaundice according to chemical composition of bilirubin			
Type	**Cause**	**Example**	**Features**
Unconjugated hyperbilirubinemia	Prehepatic	Hemolysis	Urine: normal Feces: dark
	Intrahepatic	Impaired bilirubin uptake (Gilbert's syndrome) Impaired bilirubin conjugation Crigler–Najjar syndrome Drugs, e.g., rifampicin	Increased risk of pigment gallstones No itching (excess urobilinogen with hemolysis)
Conjugated hyperbilirubinemia	Intrahepatic non-cholestatic	Impaired bilirubin excretion into bile: • Dubin–Johnson syndrome • Rotor's syndrome	Urine: dark Feces: pale Itching
	Intrahepatic cholestatic	Small bile duct obstruction: • acute/chronic hepatitis • cirrhosis • intrahepatic tumors • pregnancy-associated cholestasis • sclerosing cholangitis • intrahepatic biliary atresia	Urine: dark Feces: pale Itching
	Posthepatic	Large bile duct obstruction	Urine: dark Feces: pale Itching

Fig. 7.18 Classification of jaundice according to chemical composition of bilirubin.

Unconjugated hyperbilirubinemia is not associated with itching.

Conjugated

Excess bilirubin is conjugated to form bilirubin–glucuronate, which is water soluble. The features of conjugated hyperbilirubinemia are:

Pale stools: bilirubin conjugate is not excreted into the intestine, but it accumulates in the liver either as a result of biliary obstruction (cholestasis) or as a result of its impaired excretion into the bile (rare).

Dark urine: conjugated bilirubin (water soluble) accumulates in the liver, and it is excreted in the urine.

Pruritus: conjugated bilirubin is deposited in the skin, causing severe itching.

> Two important points to note about jaundice:
> - Liver disease is not the only cause of jaundice; there are other causes (e.g., hemolysis).
> - Many patients with significant liver disease are not jaundiced.

Hepatic failure

Hepatic encephalopathy

A neuropsychiatric syndrome caused by liver disease, this occurs most often in patients with cirrhosis but it is also seen in more acute form in fulminant hepatic failure.

Pathogenesis is:

- Liver failure: the liver is unable to remove exogenous/endogenous compounds from the circulation. Neurotoxins accumulate and mimic the action of endogenous neurotransmitters.
- Shunting: in portal hypertension, there is shunting of portal blood past the liver directly into the systemic circulation.

The overall effect is a biochemical disturbance of brain function. The condition is reversible and rarely shows marked pathological changes in the brain.

Hepatorenal syndrome

Renal failure secondary to liver failure occurs in advanced cirrhosis, and almost always in conjunction with ascites.

The kidneys themselves are normal. Renal failure is thought to result from altered systemic blood flow including diminished renal flow.

Prognosis—Recovery depends on improvement of liver function but in chronic liver disease this seldom occurs.

Liver transplantation

Liver transplantation is, necessarily, a treatment for liver failure for which there is no other medical therapy.

Conditions for which liver transplantation is most commonly performed

These are shown below in decreasing order of frequency.

Chronic liver disease (end-stage)

The conditions are:

- Primary biliary cirrhosis.
- Primary sclerosing cholangitis.
- Alcoholic liver disease.
- Metabolic liver disease.

Fulminant hepatic failure

Examples of this include disease due to viral hepatitis or idiosyncratic drug reactions.

Hepatic tumors

Transplantation is only considered in the absence of extrahepatic malignancy.

Indications

Signs of end-stage liver disease:

- Sustained or increased jaundice (bilirubin more than 100μmol/L).
- Ascites not responding readily to medical therapy.
- Malnutrition.
- Hypoalbuminemia (<30g/L).
- Prothrombin time increased.

Risks and prognosis

Risks involved are:

- Rejection: immunosuppressives used to lower risk.
- Sepsis: prophylactic antibiotic therapy.
- Poor biliary drainage due to biliary strictures of leaks.

Prognosis is very good and improving. One year survival is 75–85%.

Disorders of the liver and biliary tract

Congenital errors of metabolism

Hemochromatosis

This condition is caused by excessive deposition of iron in the tissues. There are two types: primary hemochromatosis, which is an autosomal recessive trait that leads to excessive absorption of iron from the gut (also known as hereditary hemochromatosis); and secondary hemochromatosis, which results from excessive iron accumulation caused by other primary diseases (also called hemosiderosis).

Effects of iron accumulation

Iron accumulates as haemosiderin in many tissues including the liver, pancreas, pituitary, heart, and skin. Affected tissues appear rusty brown due to hemosiderin in cells, as follows:

- In the liver: hepatocyte necrosis (possibly from generation of free radicals), ultimately resulting in cirrhosis often with hepatomegaly.
- In the heart: infiltration of cardiac muscle can cause cardiomyopathy with heart failure.
- In the pancreas: damage to pancreatic islets may result in diabetes mellitus.
- In the skin: leaden grey pigmentation of skin due to excess melanin, especially in exposed parts—axillae, groins, and genitalia.

Diagnosis—In the blood there is a high saturation of transferrin, and high serum iron and ferritin levels; in the liver, biopsy shows heavy iron deposition and hepatic fibrosis, which may have progressed to cirrhosis.

Management:

- Reduction of dietary ferritin.
- Weekly venesection (bleedings) of 500mL until serum iron is normal.
- Therapy for cirrhosis and diabetes mellitus.

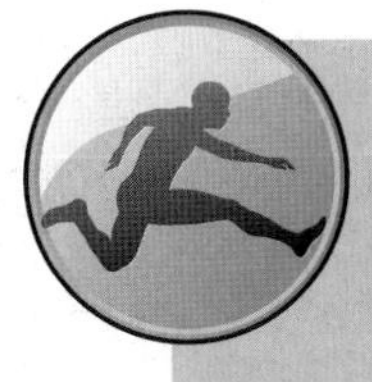

The term "bronzed diabetes" is often used to describe hemochromatosis due to the combination of diabetes and hyperpigmentation.

Wilson's disease

This autosomal recessive disorder of copper metabolism results in chronic destructive liver disease.

Normally, dietary copper is taken up by the liver, complexed to ceruloplasmin (a copper-binding protein), and then the whole complex is secreted into the plasma. Circulating ceruloplasmin is subsequently recycled by the liver, with any remaining associated copper being re-excreted into the bile.

In Wilson's disease, a mutation in a copper transport ATPase gene results in failure of the liver to secrete the copper–ceruloplasmin complex into the plasma. The copper complex accumulates within the hepatocytes, and, on saturation of ceruloplasmin, free copper overspills into the blood and is deposited in the brain and cornea.

The effects are:

- Liver: chronic hepatitis, which progresses to cirrhosis.
- Brain: psychiatric disorders, abnormal eye movements, and movement disorders resembling Parkinson's disease.
- Eye: development of greenish-brown discoloration around cornea (Kayser–Fleischer rings).

Diagnosis—Low levels of serum ceruloplasmin in the blood; confirm by liver biopsy.

Management is by copper chelators (e.g,. penicillamine).

Alpha$_1$-antitrypsin deficiency

Affected individuals with this inherited condition fail to produce the normal active extracellular protease inhibitor α_1-antitrypsin.

Pathogenesis—α_1-antitrypsin is normally produced and secreted by the liver to inhibit the activity of protease enzymes. Mutations in the genes encoding the inhibitor prevent their secretion such that protease enzymes are not inhibited.

In heterozygotes, there is an increased risk of lung damage, especially emphysema in smokers. Homozygotes develop emphysema and liver disease (cholestatic jaundice in the neonate, and chronic hepatitis, and cirrhoses).

Others

Reye's syndrome

This rare syndrome is characterized by acute encephalopathy with cerebral edema as a result of sudden severe impairment of hepatic function (fulminant hepatic failure). It occurs primarily in children and adolescents following an infectious illness such as influenza or chickenpox, which has often been treated with aspirin.

Neonatal hepatitis

This clinical condition with many causes presents as neonatal jaundice.

Main causes are:

- Idiopathic (50% of cases).
- α_1-antitrypsin deficiency (30% of cases).
- Viral hepatitis.
- Hepatitis due to toxoplasma, rubella, cytomegalovirus or herpes simplex (i.e., TORCH group).
- Metabolic causes (e.g., galactosemia or hereditary fructose intolerance).
- Extrahepatic biliary atresia.
- Congenital hepatic fibrosis.

Prognosis—Children with neonatal hepatitis generally recover. However, cases associated with biliary atresia require a surgical bile drainage operation.

Infectious and inflammatory disease

Viral hepatitis

This viral infection is a common cause of acute hepatitis. The main so-called hepatitis viruses are a group of hepatotrophic viruses. Although all cause a primary hepatitis, they are unrelated and they belong to different viral types.

Clinical features are similar in all forms of acute hepatitis regardless of etiology.

Symptoms are nausea, anorexia, low-grade pyrexia, and general malaise. Signs are hepatomegaly with tenderness, and jaundice 1 week after onset of symptoms, peaking at about 10 days.

Investigations—Raised serum levels of conjugated bilirubin and liver enzymes (aspartate transaminase and alanine transaminase, normal <40IU/L).

Hepatitis A

This RNA virus of the picorna group is prevalent in tropical countries, but less common in developed countries.

Transmission is via the fecal–oral route; for example, from:

- Nurseries or institutions where hygiene levels are inadequate (person to person via hand-to-hand contact).

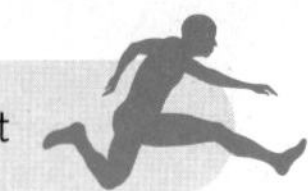

- Recreational activities in waters contaminated by sewage outfalls.
- Ingestion of sewage-contaminated shellfish.
- (Sexual) oral–anal contact (rare).

Its time course is illustrated in Fig. 7.19.

Prognosis—The majority of patients recover fully with restoration of normal liver function tests. However, a small minority (1–3 per 1000) develop fulminant hepatic failure with a mortality rate of 85%.

The disease never causes chronic hepatitis and infection confers subsequent immunity. A vaccine is available for long-term immunity.

Hepatitis B

This is a DNA virus of the Hepadna group. It can integrate into host DNA.

Transmission can be:

- Bloodborne—blood transfusions, IV drug abusers, tattooing, acupuncture.
- Sexual—sexual intercourse.
- Vertical—transmission from mother to child; perinatal (transplacental), postnatal (breast milk).

There are five clinical patterns of infection (Fig. 7.20):

- Asymptomatic infection (65%): subclinical infection but may progress to chronic hepatitis or the patient may become a carrier.
- Acute self-limiting hepatitis (25%): patients develop jaundice, malaise, and anorexia, but the majority recover (about 1% mortality) and they have lifelong immunity.
- Fulminant acute hepatitis (rare) causing massive necrosis of liver cells.
- Chronic hepatitis (5–10% of cases): may progress to cirrhosis, or the patient may recover to become asymptomatic carrier.
- Asymptomatic carrier state: may later develop chronic hepatitis.

The time course for hepatitis B is illustrated in Fig. 7.21.

Complications are cirrhosis (as a result of chronic hepatitis) and hepatocellular carcinoma, as carriers of hepatitis B are 200 times more likely to get liver cancer (typically 20–30 years post infection) than non-carriers.

Treatment is with large doses of interferon-α/β for carriers. Vaccination is available, but up to 10% of normal individuals fail to produce protective antihepatitis B antibodies.

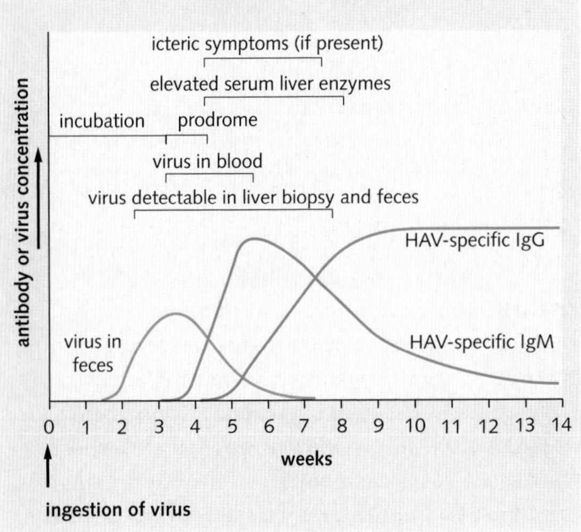

Fig. 7.19 Course of infection in hepatitis A.

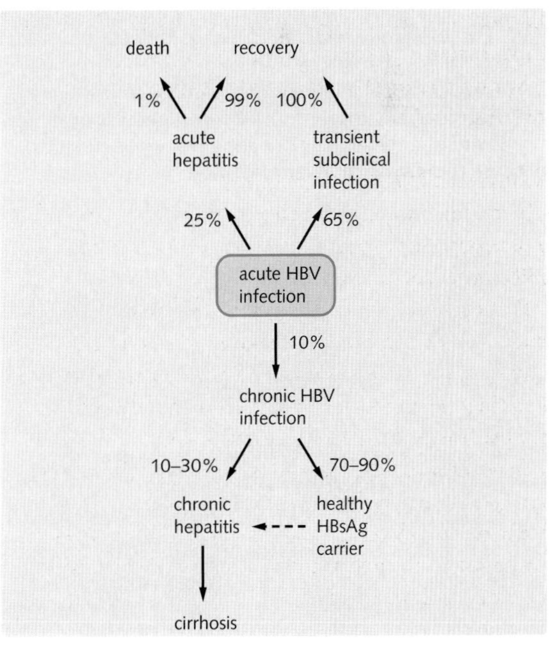

Fig. 7.20 Diagram summarizing possible courses of infection. (Adapted with permission from *Clinical Medicine*, 3rd edn, by P. Kumar and M. Clarke, Baillière Tindall, 1994.)

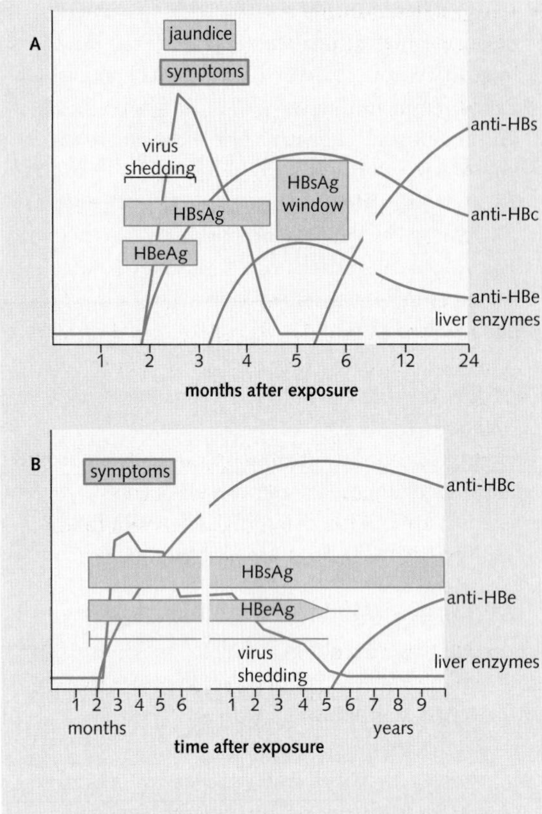

Fig. 7.21 Course of infection in hepatitis B. (A) Acute hepatitis. (B) Chronic hepatitis. (HBsAg, hepatitis B surface antigen; HBeAg, hepatitis B e antigen; anti-HBs, antibody to HBsAg; anti-HBc, antibody to hepatitis B core antigen; anti-HBe, antibody to HBeAg.) HBsAg window is time point where neither HBsAg nor anti-HBs can be detected because of immune complex formation.

Hepatitis C, D, and E

Hepatitis C This RNA viral infection was formerly known as non-A non-B hepatitis.

Transmission is as for hepatitis B.

Infection is asymptomatic in 10–35% of cases although it may progress to the carrier state. However, the majority of patients develop acute hepatitis (in 65–90% of cases).

Chronic hepatitis develops in 50–75% of those infected, following a relapsing and remitting course.

Treatment is with interferon-α and ribavirin.

Hepatitis D This RNA virus can only cause infection in the presence of hepatitis B virus; transmission is as for hepatitis B virus. Both viruses may be acquired simultaneously or hepatitis D may be acquired later as a superinfection.

The virus increases the severity of chronic hepatitis, and it may predispose to the development of fulminant hepatitis.

Hepatitis E This is an RNA virus with a transmission as for hepatitis A. Infection by hepatitis E is clinically similar to hepatitis A infection.

Other viruses

Other viruses may also cause hepatitis. Examples include group B arbovirus (yellow fever), Epstein–Barr virus, and cytomegalovirus.

Autoimmune hepatitis

This chronic form of hepatitis is also known as lupoid hepatitis. It has a prevalence of about 4 per 10,000, and it typically occurs in women (70%) between the ages of 20 and 40 years.

Etiology is unknown, and, despite the name, no immune mechanism has been proven. However, the condition is associated with hyperglobulinemia, autoantibodies (antismooth muscle antibodies and antinuclear antibodies) in the serum, and with other autoimmune disorders such as thyroiditis, arthritis, and Sjögren's syndrome (dry eyes and mouth).

Clinically, there is insidious onset of anorexia, malaise, and fatigue accompanied by abdominal distention and mild jaundice (with dark urine and itching).

Complications are cirrhosis, liver cell failure, and hepatocellular carcinoma.

Investigations:

- Liver function tests: hyperbilirubinemia, moderately raised transaminase levels, slight elevation of alkaline phosphatase.
- Full blood count: erythrocyte sedimentation ratio (ESR) is typically elevated, and there may be normochromic anemia.
- Serology: presence of antinuclear antibodies and antismooth muscle antibodies.

The disease may run a relapsing and remitting course, but it progresses inexorably to cirrhosis.

Treatment is with corticosteroids, and azathioprine can slow the progression of the disease.

Prognosis—Patients who do not respond to treatment will almost always progress to cirrhosis. Also, many patients develop cirrhosis despite having a response to treatment. If end-stage liver disease develops, liver transplantation is an effective procedure.

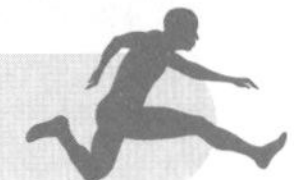

Fulminant hepatitis

This rare syndrome of hepatic encephalopathy results from sudden severe impairment of hepatic function.

Etiology—Any cause of acute liver damage if sufficiently severe such as:

- Viral infections (most common cause; e.g., hepatitis B).
- Postviral infections (e.g., Reye's syndrome).
- Drugs (e.g., acetaminophen overdose).
- Poisons (e.g., carbon tetrachloride).
- Nonviral infections (e.g., *Leptospira*, *Toxoplasma gondii*, *Coxiella burnetii*).
- Metabolic: Wilson's disease, pregnancy.
- Ischemic: shock, severe cardiac failure, Budd–Chiari syndrome.

> Fulminant hepatitis is distinguished from hepatic encephalopathy as a result of deterioration in chronic liver disease by its occurrence within 8 weeks of onset of the precipitating illness, in the absence of evidence of pre-existing liver disease.

The pathogenesis of hepatic encephalopathy has already been described (see p. 118)

Clinical features are:

- Cerebral disturbance (mental changes progressing from confusion to stupor and coma).
- Weakness, vomiting, and nausea.
- Rapidly developing jaundice.
- Asterixis: flapping tremor.
- Ascites and edema.

The liver may enlarge initially, but later it becomes impalpable; disappearance of hepatic dullness on percussion indicates shrinkage and a bad prognosis.

Complications:

- Cerebral edema: may cause intracranial hypertension.
- Respiratory failure: as a result of both cerebral edema and pulmonary edema.
- General vasodilatation: hypotension and hypothermia.
- Infection.
- Coagulation disorders.
- Necrotic cirrhosis.
- Pancreatitis.
- Renal failure: deterioration parallels that of liver failure.
- Metabolic: hypoglycemia, hypokalemia, hypocalcemia, hypomagnesemia, acid–base disturbance.

There is no specific treatment. Management is by close observation in a high dependency or intensive care unit so that complications can be corrected promptly.

Prognosis:

- 66% of patients with minor signs survive.
- Only 10% of patients with coma survive.
- Those who recover from fulminant hepatic failure usually regain normal hepatic structure and function.

Postnecrotic cirrhosis

This rapidly developing cirrhosis follows extensive necrosis (e.g., postfulminant hepatitis).

Liver abscess

This localized collection of pus within the liver is walled off and surrounded by damaged and inflamed liver tissue. Liver abscesses are rare but important as they are inevitably fatal if untreated.

Pyogenic abscesses

The most common causative organisms are *Escherichia coli*, various streptococci, and other enterobacteria.

Mode of infection:

- Bloodborne: via portal vein (mesenteric infections) or hepatic artery (bacteremia).
- Ascending spread from colonization of biliary tract (most common): almost always predisposed by biliary obstruction.
- Penetrating trauma.

Clinical features:

- Symptoms: fever, malaise, rigors and weight loss, pain in right upper quadrant sometimes with radiation to right shoulder (may be pleuritic).
- Signs: hepatomegaly in 50% of patients, mild jaundice.

Investigations include liver imaging, and needle aspiration at ultrasound examination to confirm diagnosis and provide pus for culture.

Management is by antibiotics and drainage of the abscess.

Prognosis—The mortality of liver abscesses is 20–40%, usually through failure to make the diagnosis.

Amoebic abscess

The most common causative organism is *Entamoeba histolytica*, which is transmitted from the bowel to the liver via the blood. The disease is rare in the U.S. but common worldwide, and it must be considered in patients travelling from endemic areas such as Africa, Asia, and South America.

Alcohol, drugs, and toxins

Alcoholic liver disease

Alcohol abuse is the most common cause of liver disease in Western countries, and women are more prone to alcohol-induced liver damage than men.

Alcohol is metabolized almost exclusively in the liver, and liver damage is related to daily alcohol intake. Toxicity of ethanol is probably caused by the generation of its metabolic breakdown product, acetaldehyde, which binds to liver proteins and damages hepatocytes. Alcohol also stimulates collagen synthesis in the liver leading to fibrosis.

Its effects are fatty liver, acute hepatitis, and cirrhosis.

Fatty liver (hepatic steatosis)

This is the most common lesion of alcoholic liver disease. The condition is characterized by the accumulation of fat globules within the cytoplasm of hepatocytes, and it is reversible on cessation of alcohol ingestion.

Metabolism of ethanol takes precedence over metabolism of fat, so that fat accumulates in the liver cells. The condition reflects severe metabolic derangement, and it may affect a few or almost all hepatocytes.

Alcoholic hepatitis

This is acute hepatitis with focal necrosis of liver cells. At high concentrations, alcohol causes toxic injury to hepatocytes, evoking an inflammatory reaction, which is reversible on abstinence. However, continued alcohol consumption causes the development of fibrosis around central veins. The result is hepatic fibrosis that may progress to cirrhosis.

The illness resembles acute viral hepatitis (see p. 120) and liver function tests show raised levels of transaminases and γ-glutamyl transpeptidase.

Alcoholic cirrhosis

Irreversible architectural disturbance occurs as a result of sustained alcoholic liver injury.

Normal liver architecture is diffusely replaced by nodules of regenerated liver cells separated by bands of collagenous fibrosis. This may develop after episodes of acute alcoholic hepatitis or may be insidious in its onset presenting only as end-stage liver disease.

It affects fewer than 10% of patients suffering from chronic alcoholism.

Drugs and toxins

The liver is the main organ of drug metabolism and, consequently, drugs are a common cause of liver disease. Hepatotoxic drugs may be divided into two main groups: intrinsic hepatotoxins and idiosyncratic hepatotoxins.

Intrinsic hepatotoxins

These have dose-dependent, predictable toxic effects. They are responsible for a high incidence of toxic damage to the liver via either direct toxicity of an unmetabolized drug or normal hepatic conversion to a toxic metabolite.

Idiosyncratic hepatotoxins

These have non-dose-dependent, unpredictable toxic effects. They cause liver disease in a small percentage of exposed individuals as a result of hypersensitivity (drug-mediated autoimmunity) or abnormal drug metabolism.

Circulatory disorders of the liver

Overview

Vascular disorders of the liver (Fig. 7.22) can be classified into one of three categories depending on their pathogenetic mechanisms:

- Obstruction to outflow: hepatic vein obstruction.
- Lobular compromise.
- Obstruction to inflow: obstruction of portal vein or hepatic artery occlusion.

Diseases causing obstruction to outflow (hepatic vein obstruction)

- Veno-occlusive disease: widespread occlusion of central hepatic veins.
- Budd–Chiari syndrome: obstruction occurs in the larger hepatic veins.
- Cardiac disease: right-sided cardiac failure causes congestion of the inferior vena cava.

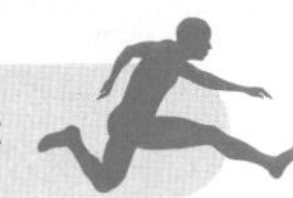

Vascular disorders of the liver	
Cause	**Example**
Outflow (hepatic vein) obstruction	Veno-occlusive disease Budd-Chiari syndrome Right-sided cardiac failure
Lobular compromise	Cirrhosis Non-cirrhotic fibrosis: • infective, e.g., schistosomiasis • drugs, e.g., alcohol, hypervitaminosis A, vinyl chloride, arsenic • congenital, e.g., congenital hepatic fibrosis, infantile polycystic disease • nodular regenerative hyperplasia Systemic circulatory disturbances, e.g., shock
Inflow obstruction	Extrahepatic • portal vein obstruction: portal vein thrombosis extrinsic compression of portal vein congenital stenosis • hepatic artery occlusion: hepatic artery thrombosis embolism, e.g., infective endocarditis accidental ligation Intrahepatic • occlusion of intrahepatic portal vein branches

Fig. 7.22 Vascular disorders of the liver.

Clinical manifestations depend on the cause and speed with which obstruction develops, but congestive hepatomegaly and ascites are features in all patients.

Diseases resulting in lobular compromise

- Cirrhosis: distortion and destruction of the hepatic vascular architecture causes sinusoid occlusion.
- Noncirrhosis fibrosis: fibrotic damage to the liver does not amount to a true cirrhosis, e.g., schistosomiasis infection.
- Systemic circulatory disturbances: shock from any source causes severe hypoperfusion, resulting in zonal necrosis.

Diseases resulting in obstruction to inflow

- Extrahepatic: portal vein obstruction (thrombosis, extrinsic compression) hepatic artery occlusion (thrombosis, embolism).
- Intrahepatic: occlusion of intrahepatic portal vein branches causes areas of venous infarction.

Liver infarction

True infarction of the liver is rare because of its dual blood supply and rich anastomosis of blood flow through the sinusoids. However, hepatic blood flow may be compromised in the following conditions:

- Surgical trauma or accidental ligation of hepatic artery.
- Therapeutic arterial embolization of the liver or therapeutic hepatic arterial ligation (performed to treat isolated neoplastic masses).
- Bacterial endocarditis: embolism.
- Eclampsia.
- Polyarteritis nodosa.

Portal vein obstruction

Obstruction of the portal vein results in portal hypertension and its associated complications (see p. 107). The causes may be thrombotic or non-thrombotic.

Thrombotic conditions (those that predispose to portal vein thrombosis) are:

- Inflammatory: thrombophlebitis and intra-abdominal sepsis (e.g., appendicitis, cholecystitis, pancreatitis).
- Neoplastic: hepatocellular carcinoma, metastatic liver tumors, and hematological malignancies (e.g., polycythemia rubra vera, essential thrombocytosis, myelofibrosis).
- Cirrhosis: leads to portal hypertension and stasis.
- Splenic vein thrombosis by propagation.

Nonthrombotic conditions are external compression (e.g., by tumor masses) and cirrhosis.

Passive congestion

Congestive cardiac failure causes venous outflow obstruction in the liver due to back pressure transmitted as described below:

inferior vena cava → hepatic vein → central veins → centrilobular congestion

Centrilobular sinusoids are dilated by blood, and the centrilobular hepatocytes undergo atrophy and necrosis (centrilobular necrosis), giving rise to the appearance of what is described as a "nutmeg liver" (chronic passive venous congestion).

The condition is common in tricuspid valve incompetence when the liver is pulsatile.

Arterial hypotension may complicate right-sided cardiac failure, causing necrosis of the centrilobular hepatocytes with elevation of serum transaminase levels.

Budd–Chiari syndrome

This rare condition is caused by occlusion of the main hepatic vein or (more rarely) the intrahepatic vena cava (Fig. 7.23).

Obstruction of the hepatic vein causes severe hepatic congestion with atrophy and/or necrosis of liver cells in the affected areas. Fibrous scarring eventually occurs in areas of hepatocyte necrosis. True cirrhosis supervenes in a minority of cases.

Clinical manifestations—Patients develop severe acute disease with:

- Painful hepatomegaly.
- Acute portal hypertension.
- Rapid development of ascites.
- Jaundice.

Death results, unless therapeutic portosystemic vascular anastomosis is performed.

Veno-occlusive disease

This condition is caused by widespread occlusion of central hepatic veins leading to clinical features similar to those of Budd–Chiari syndrome (see above).

Causes are hepatic irradiation, cytotoxic drugs, and the ingestion of plants containing toxic alkaloids (common in Jamaica and certain areas of Africa in those who drink herbal teas).

Etiology of Budd-Chiari syndrome	
Idiopathic	Underlying cause cannot be found in more than half of cases
Thrombotic causes	Hematological diseases, e.g. • primary proliferative polycythemia • paroxysmal nocturnal hemoglobinuria • deficiencies of antithrombin III, proteins C and S Pregnancy/oral contraceptives
Local compression of hepatic vein (rare)	Obstruction due to tumors, e.g., liver, kidneys, or adrenals Congenital venous webs Inferior vena caval stenosis

Fig. 7.23 Etiology of Budd–Chiari syndrome.

Pathogenesis is unclear, but it involves fibrosis around central veins ultimately resulting in obliteration of the vein lumen.

Clinical features, investigations, and management of veno-occlusive disease are similar to those of Budd–Chiari syndrome.

Hepatic disease in pregnancy

Pre-eclampsia and eclampsia

Pre-eclampsia

This is high blood pressure (more than 140/90mmHg) developing during pregnancy in a woman whose blood pressure was previously normal. It occurs in about 10% of pregnancies.

HELLP syndrome

This syndrome of hemolysis, elevated liver tests, and low platelets in the blood occurs in approximately 10% of all women with pre-eclampsia. The liver may be destroyed by the development of disseminated intravascular coagulation (see Chapter 12). Irregular areas of necrosis occur as a result of fibrin thrombi deposition in adjacent portal vessels.

- Mild cases: liver function remains normal, although liver blood tests may be abnormal.
- Severe cases: large parts of the liver may be damaged or destroyed leading to symptoms similar to severe viral hepatitis.
- Extremely severe cases: life-threatening hemorrhage into parts of the liver or abdomen may occur.

This disease resolves immediately after delivery, and the liver generally heals itself within days to weeks. However, whilst the disease is ongoing, the mother is at risk of complications of liver damage and bleeding, and the baby is at risk of premature delivery or stillbirth.

Eclampsia

This is the occurrence of one or more convulsions not caused by other conditions such as epilepsy or cerebral hemorrhage in a woman with pre-eclampsia. It is associated with severe epigastric pain, nausea and vomiting, and severe hepatic damage. Fetal and maternal death may occur.

Liver histology shows fibrin deposition and ischemic necrosis.

Acute fatty liver of pregnancy

This serious but rare condition presents in the third trimester with symptoms of fulminant hepatitis

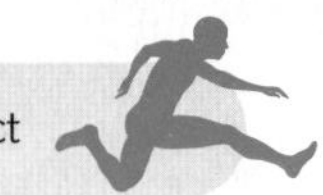

(jaundice, vomiting, abdominal pain, and possibly coma), affecting 1 in 4000 pregnancies.

Pathogenesis is unknown, but it is characterized by widespread centrilobular microvesicular fatty change in hepatocytes.

Untreated cases are associated with a high maternal and fetal mortality. Early recognition of the condition and treatment by Caesarean section have greatly improved the outlook.

Intrahepatic cholestasis of pregnancy

Cholestasis occurring as a result of intrahepatic causes appears in the second or third trimester, lasts for the duration of the pregnancy, and resolves within 2–4 weeks of delivery.

Etiology of the syndrome is uncertain but it is probably caused by an inherited susceptibility of a patient's liver cells to oestrogens. The condition is sometimes precipitated by oral contraceptives.

Symptoms are pruritus (almost always starts in third trimester and remits within about 2 weeks of delivery) and jaundice (occurs in about half of the patients).

The fetus remains unharmed but the condition tends to recur in subsequent pregnancies.

Neoplasia of the liver

Benign tumors

Hepatic adenomas

These typically affect premenopausal women, and they are predisposed by estrogen-containing oral contraceptives.

The macroscopic appearance is of well-circumscribed nodules up to 20cm in size.

The microscopic appearance closely resembles that of a normal liver, except that no portal structures are seen.

Complications—The majority of lesions are asymptomatic, but they may cause problems if they rupture, leading to intra-abdominal bleeding.

Bile duct adenomas

These are very common lesions composed of abnormal bile ducts in a collagenous stroma that appear as small white nodules, often beneath the liver capsule. They may be mistaken for metastatic tumor deposits at laparotomy.

Hemangioma

These are common hamartomas composed of abnormal vascular channels in a collagenous stroma. They are found at autopsy in 2–5% of the population, typically seen beneath the capsule as a dark lesion (usually 2–3cm in size).

Malignant

Primary

Hepatocellular carcinoma (liver cell carcinoma)
Carcinoma of hepatocytes is the most common primary tumor of the liver. Uncommon in the U.S. (affects about 1 per 100,000) it is up to 100 times more common in parts of Africa and the Far East, probably because of the higher incidence of hepatitis B and contaminating mycotoxins. Males are affected more than females by 8:1.

Predisposing factors are cirrhosis (independent of cause), hepatitis B infection with chronic carrier state, and mycotoxins-contaminated food (e.g., aflatoxins produced by the fungus *Aspergillus flavus*, which frequently contaminates stored nuts and grains in tropical countries).

Hepatocellular carcinomas often produce α-fetoprotein. This protein is secreted into the blood, where its presence is a useful diagnostic marker. Prognosis is very poor with median survival of less than 6 months from diagnosis.

Cholangiocarcinoma This is an adenocarcinoma arising from the intrahepatic bile duct epithelium. It accounts for 5–10% of all cases of primary liver tumors.

Predisposing factors:

- Chronic inflammatory disease of intrahepatic biliary tree, particularly sclerosing cholangitis.
- Disease caused by Chinese liver flukes (*Clonorchis sinensis*) (rare).

Lesions are associated with a very poor prognosis; most patients do not survive more than 6 months from diagnosis.

Angiosarcomas These highly malignant tumors are derived from vascular endothelium, and characterized by multifocal hemorrhagic nodules within the liver. The tumors are rare unless there has been exposure to:

- Thorotrast (a radiological contrast agent used until the 1950s).
- Vinyl chloride monomer (used in plastics industry to make PVC).
- Arsenic (administered in the past in certain tonics).
- Anabolic steroids.

Secondary tumors

The majority of malignant liver tumors are metastatic. The most common primary carcinomas, which metastasize to the liver, are of the lung, breast, colon, and stomach.

Many other tumors also spread to the liver (e.g., lymphomas, melanomas, leukemias), but they are numerically less frequent.

Mode of spread is via the bloodstream, through the portal vein (tumors of the GI tract) and the systemic circulation (other tumors). There are usually multiple metastatic deposits with a central area of necrosis.

Clinically, the liver is enlarged, hard, and craggy on palpation.

Small deposits of tumor have little clinical effect. However, extensive metastases cause compression of the intrahepatic bile ducts leading to obstructive jaundice.

Disorders of the biliary tree

Disorders associated with biliary cirrhosis

Biliary cirrhosis is the result of the long-standing obstruction of bile ducts leading to the development of obstructive jaundice, liver cell necrosis, and fibrosis with regenerative nodules. The main causes:

- Primary biliary cirrhosis: intrahepatic bile duct destruction of unknown etiology.
- Secondary biliary cirrhosis: unrelieved obstruction of the main extrahepatic bile ducts.
- Sclerosing cholangitis: inflammation and fibrosis of bile ducts.

Biliary obstruction causes edema and expansion of intrahepatic portal tracts with portal tract fibrosis. Bile droplets develop in biliary canaliculi, which may rupture and cause death of adjacent hepatocytes (so-called "bile infarct"). Over a long period of time, liver cell death, regeneration, and fibrosis result in cirrhosis.

Primary biliary cirrhosis

This cirrhosis occurs as a result of a chronic destruction of intrahepatic bile ducts. (Also known as chronic destructive non-suppurative cholangitis.) It affects 5 per 100,000, typically among the middle-aged population. Females are affected more than males by 10:1.

Etiology is unknown, but it is thought to involve immune phenomena (antimitochondrial antibodies in more than 90% of cases).

It is often associated with other autoimmune diseases (e.g., rheumatoid arthritis (RA), thyroiditis, systemic lupus erythematosus (SLE), scleroderma, and Sjögren's syndrome (dry eyes and mouth)).

Pathogenesis is progressive, chronic, granulomatous, and inflammatory. Inflammatory damage with fibrosis may spread from portal tracts to the liver parenchyma. The condition eventually leads to cirrhosis and its complications over a period of about 10 years.

There are four stages:

1. Florid bile-duct inflammation with granulomata.
2. Ductular proliferation (periportal).
3. Scarring (bridging fibrosis).
4. Cirrhosis.

Clinical features in the early stages are tiredness, fatigue, and arthralgia, with pruritus and mild jaundice. In the late stages, patients develop true cirrhosis with features of:

- Jaundice.
- Pruritus with excoriation.
- Hepatosplenomegaly.
- Malabsorption (weight loss, osteomalacia, osteoporosis).
- Xanthelasma and possible xanthomata.
- Other complications of liver failure.

Investigations are:

- Blood: liver function tests show features of cholestasis (raised alkaline phosphatase, cholesterol, and bile acids); demonstration of antimitochondrial antibodies.
- Liver biopsy showing compatible histology.
- ERCP (endoscopic retrograde cholangiopancreatography) shows patent and nondilated biliary tree (rules out obstructive causes of cirrhosis).

Management—No specific therapy is available. Treatment with drugs is ineffective and liver transplantation is often necessary.

Secondary biliary cirrhosis

This occurs as a result of prolonged mechanical obstruction to bile flow in large ducts outside the liver or within the porta hepatis. Causes are:

- Gallstones: impacted in common bile duct.
- Tumors (e.g., carcinoma of bile duct, carcinoma of the pancreas).
- Strictures: usually following surgery.

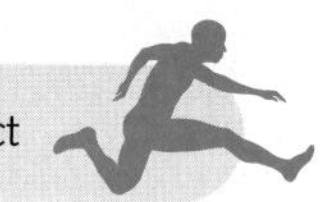

- Congenital diseases: choledochal cyst, extrahepatic biliary atresia.
- Parasitic obstruction (rare).

Histological features—Bile pigment accumulates in hepatocytes, in dilated biliary canaliculi and in Kupffer cells. Prolonged obstruction causes:

- Extravasation of bile from dilated canaliculi with development of characteristic "bile infarcts."
- Extravasation of bile from small intrahepatic bile ducts with development of characteristic portal tract lesions—"bile lakes."
- Eventual development of cirrhosis.

Complications are cholangitis (inflammation of the bile ducts, usually as a result of superimposed infection) and those of cirrhosis (p. 114).

Primary sclerosing cholangitis

Chronic inflammation and fibrosis of bile ducts with stricture formation causes progressive obstructive jaundice. The condition affects 1 per 100,000 with peak incidence between 25 and 40 years, males more so than females. Etiology is unknown.

There is a strong association with ulcerative colitis as 60% of patients with primary sclerosing cholangitis also have ulcerative colitis.

This disease is not associated with immunological features of primary biliary cirrhosis.

The effects are:

- Large intrahepatic and extrahepatic bile ducts: development of fibrous strictures with segmental dilatation causing the "beaded" appearance on ERCP.
- Medium-sized ducts, and ducts in portal tracts: inflammation with concentric fibrosis around ducts.
- Small bile ducts in portal tracts: replaced by collagenous scarring (vanishing bile ducts).

Clinical features—Patients develop cholestatic jaundice (pale stools, dark urine, and itching of the skin) with progression to cirrhosis over a period of about 10 years. There is an increased risk of developing cholangiocarcinomas.

Fig. 7.24 shows a summary of disorders associated with biliary cirrhosis.

Summary of disorders associated with biliary cirrhosis

	Primary biliary cirrhosis	Secondary biliary cirrhosis	Primary sclerosing cholangitis
Prevalence	5 per 100,000	?	1 per 100,000
Sex association	Females > males by 10:1; typically affecting middle-aged population	?	Males > females with peak incidence between 25 and 40 years
Etiology	Unknown, probably autoimmune	Gallstones Tumors Strictures Congenital diseases Parasitic obstruction (rare)	Unknown
Bile duct changes	Progressive chronic granulomatous inflammatory damage with fibrosis Eventual cirrhosis	Development of bile infarcts and bile lakes Bile duct hyperplasia Eventual cirrhosis	Narrowing and obliteration of intra- and extrahepatic bile ducts Eventual cirrhosis
Lab findings			
Liver function tests	Features of cholestasis (increased alkaline phosphatase, cholesterol and bile acids)	Same	Same
Serology	Antimitochondrial antibodies	—	—
ERCP	Patent and non-dilated biliary tree	Dilation of large ducts	Fibrous strictures with segmental dilatation → "beaded" appearance

Fig. 7.24 Summary of disorders associated with biliary cirrhosis.

Risk factors for cholesterol stones	
Age	↑ Cholesterol secretion
Female	↑ Cholesterol secretion
Pregnancy	↑ Cholesterol secretion ↓ Bile secretion Impaired gallbladder motility
Obesity	↑ Cholesterol secretion
Rapid weight loss	↑ Cholesterol secretion
Racial	↑ Cholesterol secretion
Gallbladder stasis Brief fast Parenteral therapy Spinal cord injury	Impaired gallbladder motility

Fig. 7.25 Risk factors for cholesterol stones.

Diseases of the gallbladder

Gallstones (cholelithiasis)

Gallstones (stones formed in the gallbladder) are the most common cause of disease affecting the biliary tree. They occur in 10% of all adults in the U.S., females more often than males by 2.5:1. The number of stones per patient has varied from one to 26,000.

However, despite the high incidence of gallstones, only about 1% of total patients with gallstones develop complications.

There are two types of gallstone: cholesterol stones (80% of all stones) and pigment stones (20% of all stones). Both types also contain calcium salts (e.g., bilirubinate, carbonate, phosphate, and palmitate).

Cholesterol stones

Here, the major constituent of the stone is cholesterol.

Pathogenesis:

- Hypersecretion of cholesterol (most common mechanism).
- Decreased secretion of bile salts, due to either defective bile synthesis or excessive intestinal loss of bile salts.
- Abnormal gallbladder function.

Risk factors for cholesterol stones are shown in Fig. 7.25.

Bile pigment stones

Here, the major constituent of the stones is bile pigment (calcium bilirubinate). They are typically found in patients with chronic hemolysis due to increased bilirubin production, hence pigment stones are typically black.

Complications, investigations, and management

Gallstones may be asymptomatic (80% have no symptoms), symptomatic (pain and other symptoms), or complicated.

Complications include:

- Cholecystitis: inflammation of gallbladder caused by impaction of stone in neck of gallbladder or cystic duct.
- Jaundice: impaction of stone in common bile duct (choledolithiasis), leading to biliary obstruction.
- Cholangitis: inflammation of bile duct usually as a result of biliary obstruction complicated with bacterial infection.
- Pancreatitis: impaction of stone distal to opening of pancreatic duct.
- Predisposition to carcinoma of the gallbladder.

Investigations are:

- Abdominal X-ray: stones are calcified in 10–20%.
- ERCP.
- Percutaneous transhepatic angiogram.
- Ultrasound (most useful).

Management is by:

- Surgery (cholecystectomy).
- Bile acids (chenodeoxycholic or ursodeoxycholic): prevents formation of new stones but cannot dissolve pre-existing ones.
- Lithotripsy: useful for those patients unsuitable for surgery.

Cholecystitis

This is inflammation of the gallbladder. Etiology is almost always associated with gallstones. There are two types, acute and chronic.

Acute cholecystitis

This acute inflammation of the gallbladder is precipitated by the chemical effects of concentrated static bile. It is typically due to obstruction of gallbladder outflow by gall stones, and it may be exacerbated by secondary infection with enteric organisms such as *E. coli*.

In severe cases, the lumen distends with pus causing increased risk of perforation and peritonitis.

Empyema is an inflamed gallbladder greatly distended with pus.

Chronic cholecystitis

Invariably associated with gallstones, in chronic cholecystitis the gallbladder wall is thickened and rigid from fibrosis, with variable chronic inflammatory infiltration of the mucosa and submucosa. The thickened wall may contain sinuses (Aschoff–Rokitansky sinuses).

Hartmann's pouch is a pathological dilatation in the neck of the gallbladder formed by increased intraluminal pressure or stone.

Mucocoele

This is sterile obstruction of the neck by a gallstone. A lack of inflammation permits the gallbladder to distend.

Carcinoma of the gallbladder

This is usually an adenocarcinoma, invariably associated with gallstones and chronic cholecystitis. Most cases are seen in women over the age of 70 years. There is a poor prognosis due to liver invasion.

Disorders of the exocrine pancreas

Pancreatitis

Acute pancreatitis

This acute inflammation of the pancreas is caused by the destructive effect of enzymes released from pancreatic acini. It affects 5–10 per 100,000 per year in Western communities. By far the most common causes of acute pancreatitis are gallstones (50% of cases) and alcohol ingestion (20%). These and other causes are classified in Fig. 7.26.

Causes of acute pancreatitis

Cause	Example
Mechanical obstruction of pancreatic ducts	Gallstones Trauma Postoperative
Metabolic/toxic causes	Alcohol Drugs, e.g., corticosteroids, thiazide diuretics, azathioprine Hypercalcemia Hyperlipidemia
Vascular/poor perfusion	Shock Atherosclerosis Hypothermia Polyarteritis nodosa (PAN)
Infections	Mumps

Fig. 7.26 Causes of acute pancreatitis.

A useful mnemonic for memorizing the causes of pancreatitis is GET SMASHED: **G**allstones, **E**thanol, **T**rauma, **S**hock, **M**umps, **A**utoimmune (PAN), **S**corpion bites (rare in the U.S.!), **H**yperlipidemia (also hypercalcemia and hypothermia), **E**RCP, and **D**rugs.

Pathogenesis

Duct obstruction Impaction of a gallstone distal to the site of union of a common bile duct and pancreatic duct results in:

- Reflux of bile up pancreatic duct → toxic injury to pancreatic acini.
- Increased intraductal pressure → enzymatic leakage from pancreatic ducts.

Note: chronic alcohol ingestion may also produce increased intraductal pressure due to production of a protein-rich pancreatic fluid, which can form solid plugs in smaller pancreatic ducts.

Direct acinar injury Less common causes of pancreatitis (e.g., viruses, drugs, and trauma) may produce direct acinar damage. The three patterns of pancreatic necrosis are:

- Periductal necrosis: necrosis of acinar cells adjacent to ducts. Typically caused by duct obstruction, particularly associated with gallstones and alcohol.
- Perilobular necrosis: necrosis of the periphery of lobules. Caused by poor vascular perfusion of their zone as a result of shock and hypothermia.
- Panlobular necrosis: necrosis affects all portions of the pancreatic lobule. This may be due to spread from initial periductal perilobular necrosis or it may be panlobular from the start.

Regardless of the cause of pancreatitis, acinar damage leads to the liberation of lytic enzymes (proteases and lipases), causing necrosis of normal tissue. A vicious circle of events is begun in which enzymatic release results in further acinar damage, etc.:

- Lipases → fat necrosis. Causes discoloration of skin around abdominal wall (Cullen's or Grey Turner's sign).
- Proteases → destruction of pancreatic parenchyma. Endocrine destruction results in hyperglycemia.
- Elastase and other enzymes → vascular damage with hemorrhage into pancreas or peritoneum.
- Extensive hemorrhage is known as acute hemorrhagic pancreatitis.

Clinical features

Clinical features are:

- Symptoms: severe central abdominal pain of sudden onset, often radiating into back. Nausea and vomiting.
- Signs: tachycardia, fever, jaundice, shock, ileus, rigid abdomen, discoloration around the umbilicus (Cullen's sign) or in the flanks (Grey Turner's sign).

Complications, investigations, and management

Complications may be local affecting the pancreas (pancreatic pseudocyst, abscess formation) and GI (gastric and duodenal erosions, intestinal ileus) or systemic (shock, diabetes mellitus, ARDS, renal failure, peritonitis).

Investigations are:

- Full blood count: neutrophil leucocytosis.
- Blood sugar: hyperglycemia in severe disease.
- Liver function tests: ↑ bilirubin, ↑ alkaline phosphatase, ↓ albumin.
- Serum amylase: greatly elevated.

Management is by physiological support and treatment of shock, respiratory failure, and pain.

Prognosis

Mortality is about 20% (negligible in mild cases, but up to 50% in cases with a severe hemorrhagic pancreatitis).

Death may be from shock, renal failure, sepsis, or respiratory failure with contributory factors being protease-induced activation of complement, kinin, and the fibrinolytic and coagulation cascades.

Chronic pancreatitis

This is chronic inflammation and fibrosis of the pancreas with a relapsing and remitting course.

It is a relatively rare disease but with increasing incidence due to a rise in the incidence of alcoholism. Typically, it occurs between the ages of 35 and 45 years; males more so than females.

Etiology—The main causes of chronic pancreatitis are outlined in Fig. 7.27.

Pathogenesis is thought to be similar to the mechanisms involved in acute pancreatitis. However, there is permanent impairment of function.

Morphological features:

- Chronic inflammation.
- Fibrous scarring.
- Loss of pancreatic parenchymal elements.
- Duct strictures with formation of intrapancreatic calculi (stones).

Clinical features are:

- Recurrent bouts of severe abdominal pain.
- Malabsorption (due to reduced lipase and protease secretion): steatorrhea (fat in feces); creatorrhea (undigested meat in feces).
- Diabetes mellitus (destruction of pancreatic parenchyma).

Episodes of acute pancreatitis may complicate chronic pancreatitis.

Relevant investigations include imaging and function tests.

Imaging is by plain radiograph (for calcification of the pancreas), ultrasound and CT, and ERCP.

Main causes of chronic pancreatitis		
	Cause	**Pathogenesis**
Common	Chronic alcoholism (majority of cases)	Protein plugs form in ducts and become calculi; ducts are obstructed, inflamed and scarred
	Biliary tract disease	Gallstones or anatomical abnormalities of pancreatic ducts
	Idiopathic chronic pancreatitis	Pathogenesis uncertain
Rare	Cystic fibrosis	Protein plugs in ducts
	Familial pancreatitis	Autosomal dominant
	Tropical pancreatitis	Uncertain cause; prevalent in India and Africa

Fig. 7.27 Main causes of chronic pancreatitis.

Function tests are:
- Secretin/CCK/stimulation test.
- Glucose tolerance test.
- 5-day stool collection for fat excretion (steatorrhea).
- Liver function tests.

Management is by:
- Abstinence from alcohol.
- Pancrax: pancreatic extract with or without antacids to prevent inactivation by gastric acid.
- Supplementation of fat-soluble vitamins A, D, E, and K.
- Diet and insulin for diabetics.
- Surgery for pseudocysts and biliary obstruction.

Pseudocysts

A collection of fluid and necrotic inflammatory debris is localized either within the pancreas itself or more commonly in the adjacent tissue, particularly the lesser sac. They are not "true" cysts (as they have no epithelial lining), but they are surrounded by a zone of inflammatory granulation tissue, and they communicate into the pancreatic duct system. They occur in both acute and chronic forms of pancreatitis.

Neoplasms of the pancreas

Cystic tumors

These benign, well-circumscribed masses are composed of multiple cystic cavities lined by either serous or mucin-secreting epithelium.

Carcinoma of the pancreas

This common tumor accounts for 3–5% of cancer deaths in the U.S. It is typically seen in patients over 60 years of age, but occasionally in younger people, and more often in males than females.

Associations include cigarette smoking, alcohol, a high fat and carbohydrate diet, and diabetes in women.

Macroscopic appearance—gritty, gray, hard nodules invading adjacent gland and local structures.

The tumor arises with different frequencies in different parts of the pancreas: 60% in the head, 10% in the body, 10% in the tail; and 20% of pancreatic cancers exhibit a diffuse pattern.

Carcinoma in the head of the pancreas tends to present early with obstructive jaundice. As a result, tumors are on average smaller at diagnosis than in other sites.

Microscopic appearance—Lesions are typically moderately differentiated adenocarcinomas composed of glandular spaces in a fibrous stroma.

Routes of spread:
- Local: causes obstructive jaundice, or invasion of the duodenum.
- Lymphatic: spread to adjacent lymph nodes.
- Blood: spread to the liver.

Clinical features are:
- Weight loss, anorexia and chronic persistent pain in epigastrium radiating to the back.
- Obstructive jaundice with painless palpable dilatation of gallbladder (Courvoisier's sign).
- Migratory thrombophlebitis: development of multiple thromboses in superficial and deep leg veins (Trousseau's syndrome).
- Diabetes mellitus: extensive replacement of the gland with carcinoma and destruction of the islets of Langerhans.

Management is by:
- Curative resection (Whipple's procedure): rarely possible due to extensive disease.
- Palliative surgery: often performed to bypass obstruction of the bile duct (relieving jaundice) and obstruction of the duodenum.

Prognosis is extremely poor: 90% of patients die within 6 months of diagnosis. This is largely due to the critical location of the tumor in proximity to critical structures.

Disorders of the intestine

Congenital abnormalities

Meckel's diverticulum

Diverticulum (outpouching) of the ileum is caused by persistence of part of the yolk stalk. This arises as a result of incomplete regression of the yolk stalk (vitello-intestinal duct) during the embryonic period, such that a tubular diverticulum is present in the ileum.

Meckel's diverticulum occurs in 2% of the population, and in males more than females by about 3:1.

Macroscopically, it is 5 cm long and located 61 cm from the ileocecal junction.

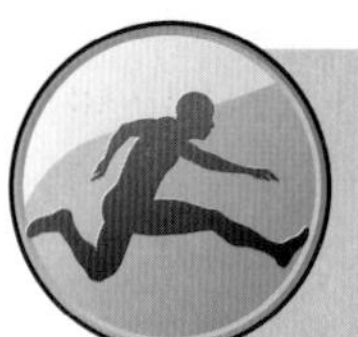

Rule of 2s for Meckel's diverticulum:
- Prevalence: 2% of the population.
- Site: 2 feet (60cm) from the ileocecal junction.
- Length: 2 inches (5cm)

Microscopically, there is a muscular wall and a lining similar in nature to small bowel epithelium, often mixed with gastric acid-secreting epithelium or heterotopic pancreatic tissue.

Complications—The majority of these diverticula are asymptomatic; however, the complications include volvulus, inflammation, peptic ulceration, and intussusception.

Congenital aganglionic megacolon (Hirschsprung's disease)

This congenital condition is characterized by dilatation of the colon due to the absence of the normal myenteric plexus distal to dilatation. It results from the failure of neuroblast cells to migrate from the vagus into the developing gut. It occurs in 1 per 5000 live births.

This condition always involves the rectum, and it may be present in continuity for a variable distance along the bowel. Some cases involve only short segments of rectum, others the rectosigmoid segment, and in rare cases there may be total colonic or total intestinal aganglionosis.

Macroscopically, there is a narrowing of an abnormally innervated bowel segment, and dilatation and muscular hypertrophy of a proximal bowel segment.

Microscopically, there is an absence of normal myenteric and submucosal plexus ganglion cells, and hypertrophy of nerve fibres within submucosa and muscularis mucosae, with extension of abnormal axons up into lamina propria.

Clinical features—The disease usually presents in early childhood with symptoms of colonic obstruction (i.e., constipation, abdominal distension, and vomiting).

Diagnosis—Radiological examination with small amounts of barium demonstrates a small, empty rectum, a narrowed segment above, and wide dilatation of the colon full of retained feces. A biopsy of the rectal mucosa will confirm the diagnosis.

Treatment is by excision of the abnormal segments of colon and rectum.

Note that megacolon can also be a result of acquired disease. However, acquired megacolon differs macroscopically from Hirschsprung's disease in that there is no narrowed segment, dilatation extends down to the anus, and the rectum is full of feces.

Causes of acquired megacolon:

- Psychogenic megacolon: disregard for the urge to defecate.
- Prolonged laxative abuse: degeneration of myenteric plexus.
- Smooth muscle disorders: degeneration of colonic smooth muscle (e.g., scleroderma).
- Chagas' disease: infection by *Trypanosoma cruzi* with destruction of myenteric plexus. Common in South America.
- Obstruction (e.g., in the case of a polypoid colorectal carcinoma).
- Toxic megacolon: complication of ulcerative colitis (see below).

Atresia and stenosis

Atresia results in complete intestinal obstruction (failure in recanalization), whereas stenosis (narrowing) results in incomplete obstruction. These defects are most common in the duodenum and small intestine; they are rare in the colon. Thirty per cent of children with Down syndrome have duodenal atresia.

They are probably caused by infarction of fetal bowel as a result of impaired blood supply due to fetal vascular accident; for example, an excessively mobile loop of intestine may become twisted, thereby interrupting its blood supply and leading to necrosis of the section of bowel involved.

In turn, infarction leads to failure of the gut to canalize and failure of a segment to develop during fetal growth.

Anorectal anomalies

Numerous anorectal anomalies exist, the most common of which are imperforate anus and anorectal agenesis.

Imperforate anus

This common anomaly affects 1 per 5000 live births, males more so than females. The anus is in the normal position but a thin layer of tissue separates the anal canal from the exterior. The membrane is thin enough to bulge on straining, and it appears blue from the presence of meconium above it.

Its cause is the failure of the anal membrane to perforate at the end of the eighth week.

Anorectal agenesis

The rectum ends superior to the puborectalis muscle, accounting for about two thirds of anorectal defects. There are two types:

- With fistula (most common): in males—rectovesical fistula (to bladder) or rectourethral fistula (to urethra). Meconium may be observed in the urine. In females—rectovaginal fistula (to vagina) or rectovestibular fistula (to vestibule of vagina). Meconium may be present in the vestibule of the vagina.
- Without fistula (rectal agenesis): anal canal and rectum are present, but they are separated.

Infections and enterocolitis

Diarrhea and dysentery

Definitions

Diarrhea means frequent bowel evacuation or the passage of abnormally soft or liquid feces. Dysentery is an inflammatory disorder of the intestinal tract causing severe diarrhea with blood and mucus.

Classification

Diarrhea can be classified as:

- Secretory: diarrhea caused by a combined effect of excessive intestinal secretions and decreased absorption. Stool volumes may be very high, and diarrhea persists even when there is total fasting.
- Osmotic: diarrhea caused by the presence of unabsorbed solute in the colon, which prevents the absorption of fluid. Ceases on fasting long enough to empty the small bowel.
- Exudative: diarrhea due to inflammatory exudate consisting of extracellular fluid and pus mixed with blood.
- Deranged motility: diarrhea as a result of either increased or decreased motility of the small intestine.
- Malabsorption: diarrhea occurring as a result of malabsorption (see below).

The classification and causes of diarrhea are described in Fig. 7.28.

Infectious enterocolitis

Enterocolitis (inflammation of the colon and small intestine) is common and is often a result of infection.

Viral gastroenteritis

Viruses are the most common cause of gastroenteritis in infants and young children, and they account for 10% of all food poisoning outbreaks in the U.S. Transmission is typically by a fecal–oral route. Symptoms are cramps, vomiting, and fever, but no blood in stools.

In children most cases are caused by three viruses:

- Rotavirus: causes 50% of infantile diarrhea and accounts for some adult cases.
- Adenovirus (especially types 40, 41): second to rotavirus as cause of acute diarrhea in young children.
- Astrovirus: most infections occur in childhood and are mild.

In adults, the Norwalk virus accounts for 30% of cases of gastroenteritis, and it is responsible for the "winter vomiting disease." Recently there have been numerous outbreaks on cruise ships.

Bacterial enterocolitis

The types of pathogenic mechanisms are as follows:

- Preformed toxin: ingestion of food contaminated with bacterial toxins (e.g., from *S. aureus*, *Bacillus cereus*, *Clostridium botulinum*). Incubation period is very short (1–7 hours).
- Toxigenic organism: ingestion of bacteria that produce toxins in the gut (e.g., *Vibrio cholerae*, enterotoxigenic *E. coli* (ETEC), and *C. perfringens*).
- Enteroinvasive organism: ingestion of bacteria that invade the intestinal mucosa and may cause dysentery as a result of severe inflammation (e.g., *Salmonella typhi*, *Campylobacter jejuni*, *Shigella*, enterohemorrhagic *E. coli* (EHEC)).
- Antibiotic-associated diarrhea: occurs as a result of overgrowth of one type of bacteria because of disruption of normal gut flora following antibiotic treatment. Main culprit is *C. difficile*, which causes a condition known as pseudomembranous colitis (forms a false membrane in the colon). Other pathogens are *C. perfringens* and *S. aureus*.
- Necrotizing enterocolitis: rare condition arising through a combination of ischemia and infection. Ischemia progresses to intestinal infarction and necrosis of the intestines. Infection of infarcted

Classification and causes of diarrhea	
Type	**Causes**
Secretory	Infections: bacteria producing enterotoxins, viral diarrhoea, *Giardia* Irritants: laxatives, bile acids, hydroxy fatty acids Hormonal: VIP, glucagon, medullary carcinoma of the thyroid, Addison's disease Mucosal infiltration: villous adenoma, lymphoma, collagen diseases Congenital: chloridorrhea
Osmotic	Osmotic laxatives, e.g., lactulose, magnesium sulphate Disaccharidase deficiency Malabsorption syndromes Congenital, e.g., chloridorrhea (secretory and osmotic), hexose malabsorption
Exudative	Inflammatory diseases, e.g., ulcerative colitis, Crohn's disease Infections: bacteria causing invasion of the mucosa, i.e., enteroinvasive bacteria such as *Shigella*, *Campylobacter*, enterohemorrhagic *Escherichia coli*; and *Entamoeba histolytica*
Deranged motility	Decreased motility: • systemic sclerosis and other collagen disorders • intestinal pseudo-obstruction • diabetic autonomic neuropathy Increased motility: • carcinoid syndrome • postvagotomy state • thyrotoxicosis • unabsorbed bile salts entering colon
Malabsorption	May be a mixture of secretory, osmotic, and exudative diarrhea (see Fig. 7.33)

Fig. 7.28 Classification and causes of diarrhea.

tissue results in gas gangrene (see Chapter 3), sepsis, and shock with paralytic ileus. Most cases are seen in neonates. Adult cases are related to C. *perfringens* infection.

See Fig. 7.29 for a summary of common bacterial GI infections.

Pseudomembranous colitis

Caused by overgrowth with C. *difficile*, this is almost invariably associated with antibiotic therapy.

Clostridial toxin produced by bacteria causes necrosis of colonic mucosa. Patients develop fever, abdominal pain, and diarrhea.

Other diseases of the colon that allow clostridial overgrowth (gastrointestinal surgery, ischemia, shock, and burns) also predispose to its development.

Protozoa

Chagas' disease Infection by *Trypanosoma cruzi* results in the destruction of the myenteric plexus over a period of years with resulting dilatation of various parts of the alimentary canal, especially the colon and esophagus. Common in South America.

Amoebic dysentery This infection by *Entamoeba histolytica* is common throughout the tropics and occasionally seen in Britain. Cysts are ingested in water or uncooked food. The condition follows a chronic course with abdominal pains and two or more unformed stools a day. Periods of diarrhea alternating with constipation are common.

Other protozoal infections include giardiasis (*Giardia lamblia*), balantidiasis (*Balantidium coli*), cryptosporidiosis (*Cryptosporidium*), and schistosomiasis (*Schistosoma mansoni*).

Inflammatory disorders of the bowel

The idiopathic inflammatory bowel diseases

This group of disorders are characterized by primary inflammation of the intestinal wall.

Crohn's disease

A granulomatous inflammation of unknown cause that affects the full thickness of the bowel wall anywhere in the GI tract from mouth to anus, this disease is characterized by a relapsing and remitting course. Its prevalence is about 30–50 per 100,000 in the U.S.

Summary of common bacterial GI infections							
Mechanism	**Bacterium**	**Incubation period**	**Duration (days)**	**V**	**C**	**F**	**B**
Preformed toxin	*Staphylococcus aureus*	2–7 hours	1	+	+	±	–
	B. cereus	1–6 hours	1	+	+	–	–
Toxigenic organisms	*Vibrio cholerae*	2–3 days	Up to 7	+	–	–	–
	Escherichia coli (ETEC)	12 hours–3 days	2–4	+	–	–	–
	Clostridium perfringens	8 hours–1 day	0.5–1	–	+	–	–
Enteroinvasive bacteria	Non-typhoidal *Salmonella*	8–48 hours	4–7	+	±	+	±
	Campylobacter jejuni	2–11 days	3–21	–	+	+	+
	Shigella	1–4 days	2–3	–	+	+	+
	E. coli (EHEC)	1–5 days	1–4	+	+	+	+
Antibiotic-associated bacteria	*C. difficile*	–	–	–	+	+	±

Fig. 7.29 Summary of common bacterial GI infections. (V, vomiting; C, abdominal cramps; F, fever; B, blood in the stools; ETEC, enterotoxigenic *Escherichia coli*; EHEC, enterohemorrhagic *E. coli*.)

It usually presents in early adult life, with 90% of patients aged between 10 and 40 years, although a secondary peak occurs in the elderly. Females are affected more than males. There is a higher incidence in northern Europe and the U.S. than elsewhere.

Pathogenesis Cause and pathogenesis are unknown, but several hypotheses have been suggested:

- Infectious (e.g., mycobacteria, *Chlamydia*, and viruses), but no direct evidence.
- Immune: abnormal immune response to gut antigens.
- Dietary: increased carbohydrate, decreased fiber.
- Genetic: often associated with family history.
- Vascular: focal small vessel narrowing claimed to precede development of inflammation.
- Smoking: increased incidence in smokers. (Note: this is different from ulcerative colitis.)
- Miscellaneous: food antigens, psychosomatic, and other factors have been proposed.

Macroscopic appearance Site—Most commonly affects the terminal ileum, but it may affect any part of the GI tract from the mouth to the anus in a discontinuous pattern. Two thirds of cases affect only the terminal ileum, one sixth affect only the colon, and one sixth are in the terminal ileum and colon.

Pattern:

- "Skip" lesions: disease is characterized by a discontinuous distribution with normal bowel areas present between diseased segments.
- Edema of submucosa and mucosa.
- Hemorrhagic ulcers: initially small and discrete, those progress to form deep, linear, fissured ulcers ("rose thorn" ulcers).
- Cobblestone pattern of bowel mucosa due to submucosal edema and interconnecting deep fissured ulcers.
- Thickened bowel wall due to edema and fibrosis.
- Fibrous strictures may cause partial obstruction.
- Dilatation of normal bowel proximal to diseased segment due to partial obstruction.
- Enlargement of mesenteric lymph nodes.

Microscopic appearance

- Transmural inflammation: all layers of bowel wall may be affected. Forms basis of fissures, adhesions, fistulae, and sinuses.
- Lymphoid aggregates develop deep in bowel wall.
- Submucosal edema.
- Ulceration.
- Noncaseating granulomas present in inflamed bowel wall and in mesenteric lymph nodes in about 60% of cases.
- Evidence of persistent and inappropriate T cell and macrophage activation with increased

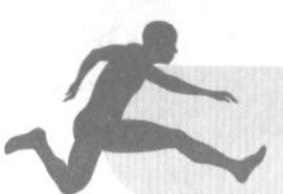

production of inflammatory cytokines (interleukins—IL-1, IL-2, IL-6, IL-8—interferon-γ and TNF-α).

Clinical features Clinical features are symptoms of abdominal pain, diarrhea, and weight loss, with signs of anemia, clubbing, fever, mouth ulcers, and abdominal mass (inflamed bowel loops, abscesses).

Complications The natural history of Crohn's disease is one of remissions and relapses of inflammation punctuated by complications.

Local complications are:

- Fistulae and sinuses: inflammation of serosal layer leads to the formation of adhesions to other bowel loops, to parietal peritoneum of anterior abdominal wall, or to the bladder.
- Stricture formations lead to intestinal obstruction.
- Fibrous adhesions lead to intestinal obstruction.
- Perforation of the bowel by deep fissured ulcers leads to intra-abdominal abscesses.
- Carcinoma of bowel: increased incidence after many years.
- Hemorrhage: significant bleeding from areas of ulceration (rare).

Systemic complications, which develop in a minority of patients with Crohn's, are:

- Malabsorption due to diseased bowel or surgical resections.
- Skin disease: pyoderma gangrenosum, erythema nodosum.
- Eye disease: uveitis.
- Joint disease: polyarthropathy, sacroiliitis, ankylosing spondylitis.
- Chronic liver disease: pericholangitis, gallstones.
- Finger clubbing.
- Systemic amyloidosis (rare).

Ulcerative colitis

This diffuse superficial inflammation of the colorectum is of unknown cause, and characterized by relapses and remissions. It affects about 80 per 100,000 in the U.S., with much lower rates in developing countries with warmer climates. (Ulcerative colitis has a similar age distribution to Crohn's, but the sex incidence is equal.)

Pathogenesis This is unknown, but the same hypotheses as for Crohn's have been proposed with the exception of smoking, which unusually is associated with a decreased risk. Again, inappropriate and persistent T cell activation may play an important role in the pathogenesis.

Macroscopic appearance The site and pattern are important to note as described below.

Site—Ulcerative colitis usually begins distally as proctitis and then spreads proximally to affect the whole of the large bowel, and may affect the terminal ileum ("backwash" ileitis).

The pattern is one of shallow ulceration (which may become confluent), with "pseudopolyps," hyperemia, and hemorrhage.

Microscopic appearance Inflammation is diffuse and is limited to mucosa, with infiltration of both acute and chronic inflammatory cells. Other features are crypt abscesses with ulceration, crypt atrophy, and Paneth's cell metaplasia.

Clinical features Clinical features are symptoms of bloody diarrhea, mucus, cramping discomfort, and weight loss, signs of fever, tachycardia, pallor, and abdominal tenderness.

Complications Acute local complications include perforation, dilatation, hemorrhage, and dehydration (blood and fluid loss from extensive ulceration).

Chronic local complications include strictures, dysplasia, and carcinoma.

Systemic complications are:

- Anemia.
- Malabsorption due to diseased bowel or surgical resections.
- Skin disease: pyoderma gangrenosum, erythema nodosum.
- Eye disease: uveitis, hypopyon.
- Joint disease: polyarthropathy, sacroiliitis, ankylosing spondylitis.
- Chronic liver disease: primary sclerosing cholangitis.
- Finger clubbing.
- Systemic amyloidosis (rare).

A comparison of Crohn's and ulcerative colitis

Both Crohn's and ulcerative colitis are examples of inflammatory bowel disease, and they have many features in common. However, in the majority of cases (about 90%), it is possible to distinguish between these two conditions (Figs 7.30–7.32).

Diagnosis Diagnosis is by colonoscopy, barium and small bowel enema. With colonoscopy, biopsy specimens can be taken for histological examination (see Fig. 7.32 for differences in microscopical

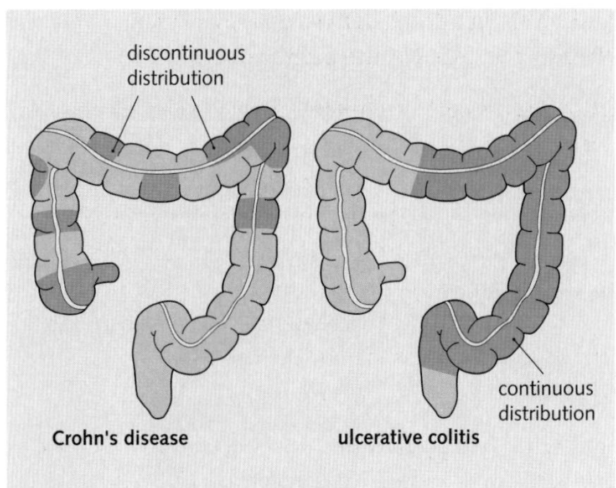

Fig. 7.30 Comparisons of distribution along the bowel.

appearance). This investigation is also important in the surveillance of patients with long-standing colitis as it allows severe dysplasia and early invasive cancer to be detected.

Barium and small bowel enema:

- Crohn's is characterized by a discontinuous distribution, often with rectal sparing. Diseased segments have a "cobblestone" appearance caused by deep longitudinal and transverse ulcers. "Rose thorn" ulcers may be present, which sometimes perforate to produce fistulous tracks.
- Mild ulcerative colitis is characterized by a disturbed mucosal pattern with small ulcers. Long-standing severe disease may show loss of haustral markings with a featureless, shortened hosepipe colon.

Management Management can be medical or surgical.

Medical:

- Corticosteroids: effective in inducing remission (local—topical steroid enemas used for exacerbations of distal proctocolitis; systemic—oral prednisolone).
- Sulfasalazine: can be used to maintain remission once remission has been induced by corticosteroids.
- Azathioprine: helpful in patients with chronic disease for whom surgery is inappropriate.

Surgical:

- Minimal resections for strictures, fistulae, or perforations.
- Colectomy: indicated in cases of chronic disease, side effects from long-term high dosages of steroids, premalignant change on colonoscopic surveillance, and in patients at high risk of developing chronic cancer (early onset disease, extensive colonic involvement, and continuous rather than episodic symptoms).
- Colectomy and pouch formation: younger patients with ulcerative colitis can have a sphincter-preserving operation in which a pouch is constructed from a duplicated (J pouch) or triplicated (Park's pouch) loop of ileum. The pouch is anastomosed to the dentate line following excision of the rectum. Crohn's patients are not suitable for pouch formation as recurrent disease may affect the ileum used in constructing the pouch.

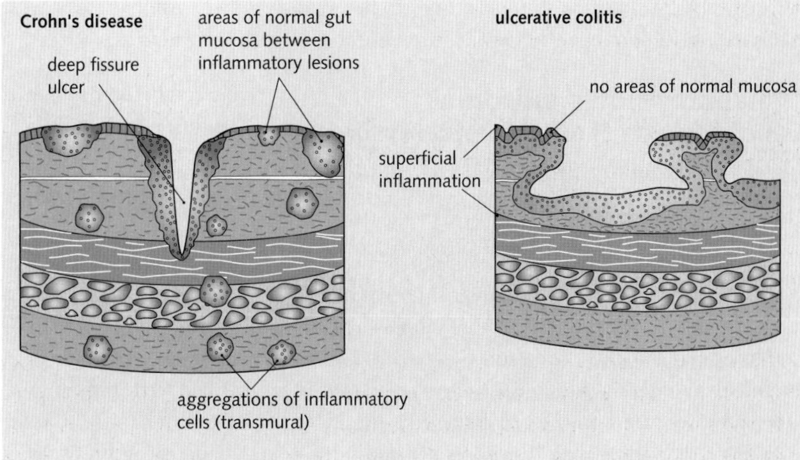

Fig. 7.31 Depth and distribution of lesions in the bowel wall.

Comparison of the basic features of Crohn's disease and ulcerative colitis		
	Crohn's disease	**Ulcerative colitis**
Prevalence in U.S.	~30–50 per 100,000 in U.S.	~80 per 100,000
Site	Any part of GI system but typically terminal ileum	Colon and rectum only
Macroscopic: • disease continuity • bowel wall • ulcers	 Discontinuous Thickened with strictures and adhesions Deep fissures form basis of fistulae	 Continuous Not thickened Flat based; do not extend to submucosa
Microscopic: • pattern of inflammation • crypt pattern	 Transmural Focal Granulomas (in 60% of cases) Little distortion	 Mucosal and submucosal Diffuse No granulomas Distorted in long-standing disease; crypt abscesses
Anal lesions	Present in 75%; anal fistulae; ulceration or chronic fissure	Present in <25%
Frequency of fistula	10–20% of cases	Uncommon
Risk of developing cancer	Slightly increased	Significantly increased

Fig. 7.32 Comparison of the basic features of Crohn's disease and ulcerative colitis.

Miscellaneous intestinal inflammatory disorders

Gastrointestinal manifestations of HIV disease

AIDS is associated with fulminant bowel infection which often causes severe diarrhea.

Malabsorptive or colitic syndromes

These are described below.

Diarrhea in bone marrow transplantation graft vs. host disease

Bone marrow transplants contain competent T lymphocytes, which can react against HLA antigens of the recipient, causing skin rash, liver toxicity, and diarrhea—which may be torrential in severe forms.

Malabsorption syndromes

General aspects of malabsorption syndromes

Malabsorption may be caused by disorders of:

- Intraluminal digestion: pancreas secretes digestive enzymes into the gut lumen (these are necessary for breakdown of macromolecules).
- Intraluminal solubilization: liver secretes bile acids required for solubilization and absorption of fats.
- Terminal digestion: mucosa is the site of a set of enzymes located on the brush border which hydrolyse large molecules for absorption, especially complex sugars (e.g., sucrase for sucrose and lactase for lactose).
- Transepithelial transport: mucosa is specialized for absorption—transverse mucosal folds and finger-like villi provide a vast surface area.

Systemic effects of the malabsorption syndromes:

- Weight loss.
- Abdominal distention.
- Diarrhea (loose, bulky stools).
- Steatorrhea: malabsorption of fat, producing pale, foul-smelling stools that characteristically float in water.
- Anemia.

Classification of malabsorption syndromes This is described in Fig. 7.33.

Specific malabsorption syndromes

Celiac disease

There is atrophy of small intestinal villi and crypt hyperplasia caused by an abnormal sensitivity to gluten, which is a protein in wheat flour. It affects about 1 per 2000 in most populations in western Europe (but 1 per 300 in western Ireland).

It can present at any age, but it is an important cause of failure to thrive in infants and children.

Causes of malabsorption	
Defective intraluminal digestion or solubilization	Pancreatic insufficiency: • chronic pancreatitis • cystic fibrosis • carcinoma of the pancreas Liver disease: failure of bile secretion into gut
Primary mucosal cell abnormalities	Lactase deficiency
Reduced surface area of small intestine	Conditions that cause villus atrophy: • celiac disease • tropical sprue • Crohn's disease • malnutrition Iatrogenic: • extensive small intestine resection • jejunal ileal bypass procedures • postradiotherapy
Infection	Parasitic infestation of gut Bacterial overgrowth in blind loops of diverticulae Postinfective malabsorption Giardiasis Whipple's disease
Lymphatic obstruction	Primary lymphangiectasia Lymphoma
Drug-induced	Cytotoxic drugs Drugs that bind bile salts, e.g., cholestyramine and some antibiotics such as neomycin (which cause steatorrhea)
Miscellaneous	Thyrotoxicosis → increased gastric emptying and motility Zollinger-Ellison syndrome Diabetes mellitus → bacterial overgrowth Hypogammaglobulinemia → infection

Fig. 7.33 Causes of malabsorption.

It is caused by an immune response to the protein gliadin, a component of gluten. Anti-gliadin antibodies are present in the majority of cases. There is an increased incidence of disease in first-degree relatives of those affected, and linkage with certain HLA-B8 groups has been shown. It often occurs concurrently with dermatitis herpetiformis (itchy, blistering skin disease).

Macroscopically, the lumenal surface becomes flattened developing a mosaic-like pattern of crypt openings (Fig. 7.34).

Microscopically there is:

- Mucosal inflammation with lymphocytic infiltration.
- Loss of villous architecture ranging from blunting (partial villous atrophy) to complete flattening (total villous atrophy) due to a high rate of cell loss.
- Increase in the depth of crypts with epithelial cell hyperplasia to compensate for those lost through damage.

Long-term complications are:

- Chronic ulceration of the small intestine: may lead to strictures.
- Development of primary T-cell lymphoma of the small intestine.
- Development of adenocarcinoma (rare).

Diagnosis is by biopsy of the small bowel mucosa; and by the gluten-challenge, in which gluten is withdrawn from the diet. Improvement should result, followed by relapse of the disease on the subsequent reintroduction of gluten.

Management is by the complete withdrawal of gliadin from the diet (i.e., a gluten-free diet), which

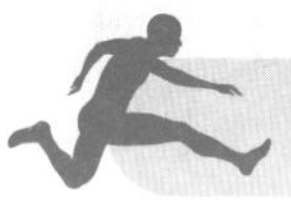

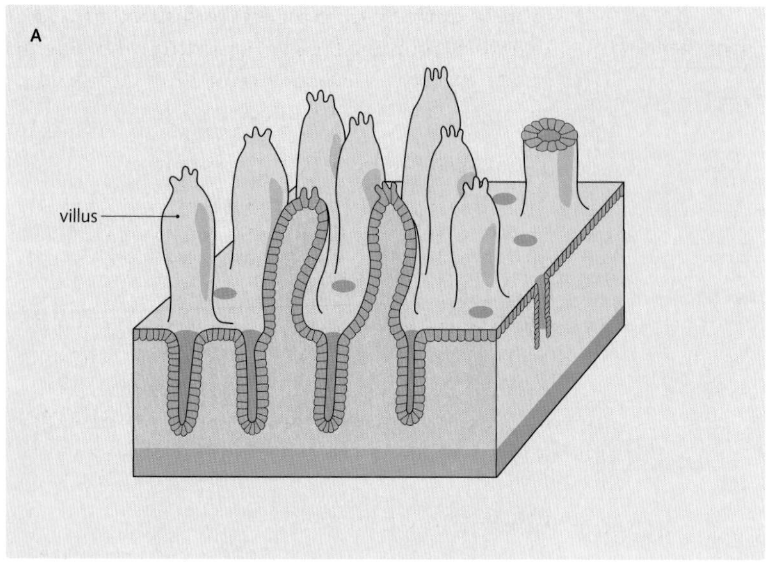

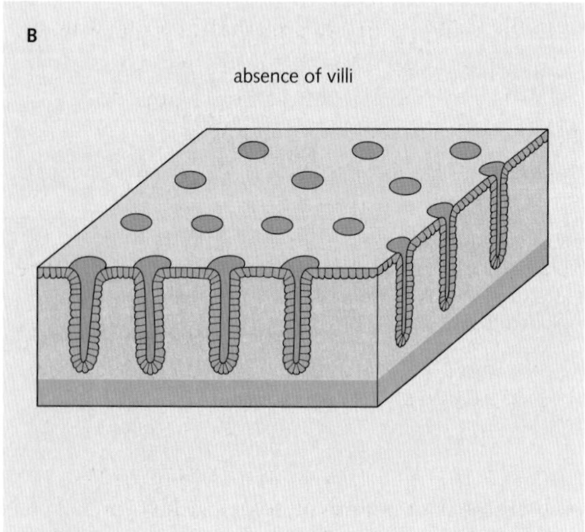

Fig. 7.34 Comparison of normal jejunal mucosa (A) and jejunal mucosa in celiac disease with total villous atrophy (B).

leads to gradual recovery of the villous structure that may be partial or complete.

Tropical sprue

This persistent malabsorption syndrome without a definable cause is seen in patients who live or have lived in the tropics, and in the absence of other intestinal disease or parasites. The disease occurs mainly in the West Indies including Sri Lanka, southern India, Malaysia, and Indonesia.

Etiology is unclear; however, the condition is thought to be infective, probably toxigenic *E. coli*.

Clinical features and histological appearances resemble those of celiac disease. However, a gluten-free diet has little beneficial effect.

Whipple's disease

Whipple's disease is a multisystem disorder involving malabsorption, weight loss, lymphadenopathy, and joint pain. The causative agent has recently been identified as *Tropheryma whippelii*. This rare condition is characterized by tissue infiltration with foamy macrophages containing intracellular bacilli.

Bacterial overgrowth syndrome

In this syndrome, there is malabsorption secondary to excessive bacteria in the small intestine, usually the jejunum. (It is also known as contaminated bowel syndrome, blind loop syndrome, and small intestine stasis syndrome.)

Causes of small intestinal bacterial overgrowth	
Cause	**Example**
Excessive entry of bacteria	Achlorhydria Infected bile ducts Gastrocolic fistula Gastric surgery Resection of ileocecal valve
Defective immune mechanisms	Immune deficiencies Malnutrition Old age
Stagnant region	Blind loops Enterocolic fistulae Jejunal diverticula Strictures or other obstruction Continent ileostomy
Disturbed motility	Systemic sclerosis Intestinal pseudo-obstruction Diabetes autonomic neuropathy

Fig. 7.35 Causes of small intestinal bacterial overgrowth.

Causes of small intestinal bacterial overgrowth are outlined in Fig. 7.35.

Malabsorption is as a result of:

- Deconjugation of bile salts by the bacteria, hence steatorrhea.
- Damage to the small intestinal mucosa, probably by bacterial products.
- Binding of vitamin B_{12} by bacteria, hence vitamin B_{12} deficiency.

Diarrhea is both secretory (due to bacterial products affecting mucosa) and osmotic (due to unabsorbed products and deficiency of disaccharidases because of mucosal damage).

Clinical features are weight loss, diarrhea, and anemia (due to vitamin B_{12} deficiency).

Diagnosis is by the reversal of symptoms with broad-spectrum antibiotics and by the demonstration of the causative lesion.

Management is by antibiotic therapy and surgical resection for a localized abnormality, e.g., stricture, fistula.

Giardiasis

This disease is caused by the parasitic protozoan *Giardia lamblia* in the small intestine. Infection occurs by eating food or water contaminated with parasitic cysts. Symptoms include diarrhea, nausea, abdominal pain, and flatulence, as well as the passage of pale fatty stools. The disease occurs worldwide, and it is particularly common in children.

Disaccharidase deficiency (alactasia)

This is the absence or deficiency of the enzyme lactase, which is essential for the digestion of milk sugar (lactose). All babies have lactase in their intestines but the enzyme disappears during childhood in about 10% of northern Europeans, 40% of Greeks and Italians, and 80% of Africans and Asians. The presence of undigested lactose in the small intestine (following consumption of raw milk) causes diarrhea and abdominal pain.

Abetalipoproteinemia

This rare condition is characterized by the absence of plasma β-lipoproteins resulting in:

- Abnormally-shaped red blood cells with spikes on the surface (acanthocytosis).
- Retinitis pigmentosa leading to blindness.
- Progressive ataxia.
- Fatty infiltration of enterocytes.
- Steatorrhea.

Beta-lipoproteins are thought to be necessary for the transport of lipids from the enterocyte into lacteals, and for the transport of nutrients into the CNS and red blood cells. Plasma vitamin E levels are very low since vitamin E is carried primarily on the β-lipoproteins.

Early intensive and continued repletion with vitamin E prevents neurological deterioration. Steatorrhea is managed by a low fat diet and nutritional supplements.

Obstruction of the bowel

Major causes of bowel obstruction

Obstruction and pseudo-obstruction can be classified as follows:

- Simple mechanical obstruction: the bowel above the obstructing lesion becomes distended with fluid and gas.
- Strangulation obstruction: occlusion of the blood supply by constricting agents.
- Paralytic ileus: may arise as a consequence of peritonitis, pancreatitis, or retroperitoneal bleeding.
- Pseudo-obstruction: abnormal gut motility rather than an organic obstructive lesion.

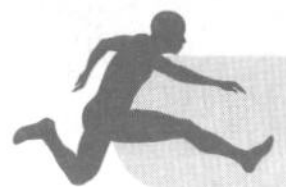

Major causes of bowel obstruction	
Cause	**Example**
Simple mechanical obstruction	Intraluminal: • foreign bodies • gallstone ileus • fecaliths • meconium in cystic fibrosis Bowel wall: • adhesions • carcinoma • strictures • atresia • imperforate anus
Strangulation obstruction	Intussusception Infarction Volvulus Internal/external hernias Bands
Adynamic obstruction (paralytic ileus)	Abdominal causes: postoperative, peritonitis, vascular occlusion Systemic causes: electrolyte disorders, uremia, hypothyroidism Drugs: anticholinergics, opiates

Fig. 7.36 Major causes of bowel obstruction.

Examples of simple mechanical obstruction, strangulation obstruction, and paralytic ileus types of obstructions are listed in Fig. 7.36.

Hernias

Definition This is the protrusion of the whole or part of a viscus from its normal position through a defect in the cavity wall in which it is contained. About 1 per 100 people have a hernia at some time. Hernias can be congenital or acquired.

Acquired:

- Secondary to increased intra-abdominal pressure: resulting from cough, straining at the stool, cysts, carcinoma, pregnancy.

Iatrogenic: incisional hernias.
Classification:

- Reducible: contents of sac can be completely returned to abdominal cavity.
- Irreducible/incarcerated: content of sac cannot be completely returned to the abdominal cavity.

Common sites of abdominal hernias are inguinal (70%), femoral (20%), and umbilical (10%). Others are supraumbilical or linea alba, incisional hernias, and hiatus hernia (see p. 106).

Complications:

- Obstruction: constriction at the neck of hernial sac causes obstruction of bowel loops within it.
- Strangulation: constriction at the neck of sac prevents venous return leading to venous congestion, arterial occlusion, and gangrene. This may result in perforation leading to peritonitis/groin abscess.

Note that strangulation can occur without obstruction if only one wall of the viscus pouches into the sac (Richter's hernia).

Hernias must be repaired because of potential complications. The principles of surgical repair are identification of the sac and contents, mobilization of the sac, reduction of the contents, ligation of the sac, and repairing the fascial defect.

Inguinal hernia The most common type of hernia, this is much more prevalent in men than in women. There are two types: indirect inguinal (85%) and direct inguinal (15%).

Indirect inguinal hernia

The hernial sac enters the inguinal canal through the deep ring (lateral to the inferior epigastric artery) and then traverses through the canal to the superficial ring, where it may eventually reach the scrotum or labium major.

Its origin is congenital (due to patency of processus vaginalis), and it is most common in children and young adults. Males are more affected than females by 20:1!

Strangulation is a common complication due to the narrow neck of the hernial sac.

Direct inguinal hernia

The hernial sac protrudes through a weakness in fascia transversalis (medial to inferior epigastric artery) and it does not normally descend into the scrotum or labium major.

It originates as a result of weakened abdominal muscles. It is most common in the elderly, and it affects males more than females. The neck of the sac is wide so strangulation is rare.

Clinically, it is difficult (often impossible) to distinguish between direct and indirect inguinal hernias. Often, differentiation can only be made at operation from the position of the neck of the hernial sac relative to the inferior epigastric artery.

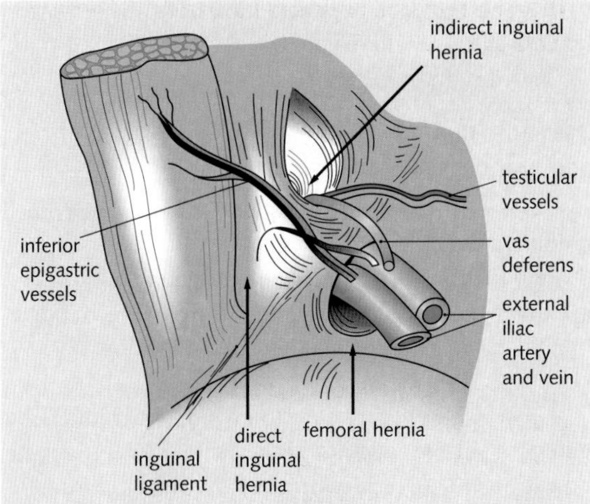

Fig. 7.37 Sites of direct inguinal, indirect inguinal and femoral herniations. (Adapted with permission from *Principles and Practice of Surgery*, 3rd edn, by A.P.M. Forrest, P.C. Carter and I.B. Macleod, Churchill Livingstone, 1995.)

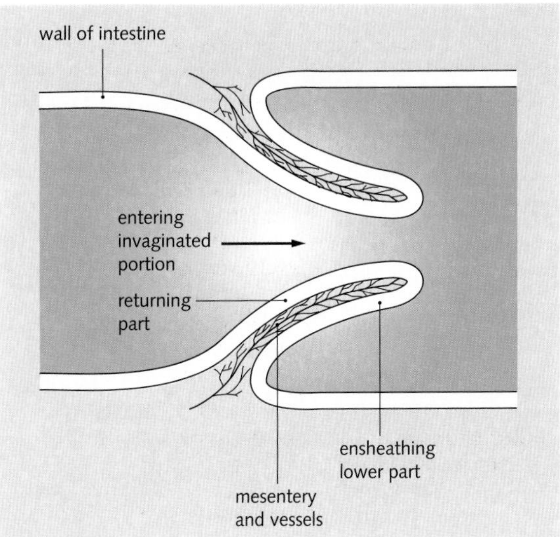

Fig. 7.38 Intussusception.

Femoral hernia The hernial sac protrudes through the femoral canal inferior to the inguinal ligament (Fig. 7.37). There is an increasing incidence with age, and females are affected more than males by 2:1 (but inguinal hernia is still more common in both males and females). The most common complication is strangulation.

Adhesions

Adhesions are by far the most common cause of mechanical obstruction in the small bowel, and they are defined as areas of fibrosis between adjacent membranes or organs resulting in their fusion. The causes can be congenital (e.g., bands in small children) or acquired.

Acquired causes are as follows:

- Inflammation (e.g., Crohn's disease, sclerosing peritonitis).
- Infection (e.g,. appendicitis, diverticulitis, tuberculosis, peritonitis).
- Trauma (e.g., stab wounds).
- Iatrogenic: post-surgery introduction of foreign bodies (starch granules, talc, nonabsorbable sutures), irradiation.
- Vascular: infarction/gangrene.
- Malignancies.

Intussusception

This is invagination of one part of the bowel into the adjoining segment (Fig. 7.38). The ileocecal valve is the most common site with the ileum invaginating into the cecum. It typically affects children under the age of 4 years.

Adult cases are extremely rare, and they are almost invariably precipitated by structural abnormalities of the small intestinal wall, e.g., benign tumors (leiomyoma or lipoma) or Meckel's diverticulum.

As the contents of the intestine are pushed onwards by muscular contraction, more and more intestine is dragged into the adjoining bowel. The net effect is venous congestion of the invaginated portion causing bleeding from the mucosa as well as intestinal obstruction.

Symptoms are intermittent colic or pain, vomiting, and the passing of "red currant jelly" with the stools.

Complications—If the bowel remains invaginated, infarction and shock from gangrene may result.

Management is by barium reduction in children or by resection in adults because of the high incidence of organic causes.

Volvulus

This is a twisting of part of the GI tract, usually leading to partial, or complete obstruction (Fig. 7.39). Sites:

- Gastric volvulus: twisting of the stomach, usually in a hiatus hernia.
- Small intestinal volvulus: twisting of part of the bowel around an adhesion.

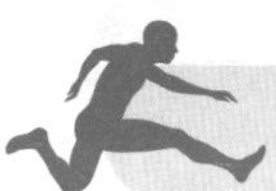

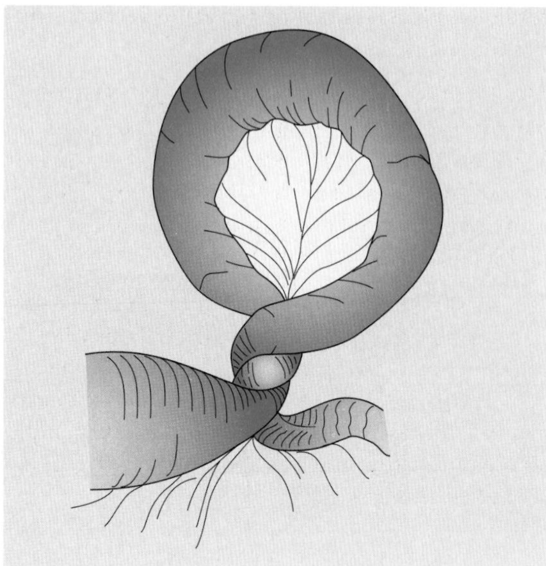
Fig. 7.39 Intestinal volvulus.

- Sigmoid volvulus: twist of the sigmoid colon, usually when this loop is particularly long.

The most common complication is strangulation (reduction of blood supply causing infarction and possibly gangrene).

Management—May untwist spontaneously but surgical manipulation is usually performed.

Colonic diverticulosis

Definitions

Diverticulum means a sac or pouch formed at weak points in the wall of the alimentary tract, and diverticulosis means a condition in which diverticula exist in a segment of the intestine without evidence of inflammation. Diverticulitis is inflammation of a diverticulum, most commonly of one or more colonic diverticula.

Pathogenesis of diverticula

Congenital diverticula are true diverticula containing all three coats of the bowel wall, e.g., Meckel's diverticulum (see p. 133).

Acquired diverticula may contain some (false diverticula) or all (true diverticula) coats of the bowel wall.

Pathogenesis of acquired diverticula—Typically develop during adult life as a result of:

- Pulsion from increased intraluminal pressure causing protrusion at points of focal weakness (e.g., at the sites of penetration of blood vessels).
- Traction due to extrinsic disease.

Colonic diverticulosis

This acquired diverticulosis of the colon is caused by a chronic lack of dietary fiber. It is also known as colonic diverticular disease.

Though rare before 35 years of age, by 65 years of age at least one third of the population of developed countries are affected—but it is rare in countries with high fiber diets.

Diverticula are most common in the sigmoid colon emerging between mesenteric and antimesenteric teniae.

Pathogenesis—Increased intraluminal pressure (e.g., as a result of straining at the stool) causes herniation of intestinal mucosa through the circular muscle at points of weakness, notably sites of penetration of the blood vessels.

The clinical course may be either asymptomatic or symptomatic, with left-sided colicky abdominal pain and alteration of bowel habit (usually constipation) or rectal bleeding.

Complications are:

- Inflammation (peridiverticulitis): may cause pain and tenderness in left iliac fossa, alteration of bowel habit, fever, leukocytosis. There may be a palpable mass.
- Perforation: results in peritonitis.
- Obstruction: due to edema or fibrosis in the inflamed segment of colon or to adherence of small bowel loops.
- Stricture formation: long-standing diverticular disease may cause stricture formation and subacute intestinal obstruction.
- Fistula: most common cause of colovesical fistula.
- Bleeding: common complication.

Diagnosis is by barium enema and colonoscopy.

Treatment:

- Conservative: high-fiber diet results in improvement in most patients.
- Surgery: sigmoid colectomy with end-to-end anastomosis if there are persistent symptoms or when carcinoma cannot be excluded by radiology or colonoscopy.

Vascular disorders of the bowel

Ischemic bowel disease

Ischemic bowel disease may affect the small or large bowel, and it is most commonly seen in elderly patients with severe atherosclerosis.

Causes of bowel ischemia

Vessel disease These are:

- Vascular occlusion: emboli lodge in the superior mesenteric artery, which supplies all the small intestine except for the first part of duodenum. The extent of the bowel infarction depends on whether occlusion is in proximal or distal branch. Emboli are derived from mural thrombus (myocardial infarct, thrombotic vegetations on mitral or aortic valves, left atrial thrombosis).
- Vascular stenosis (less common): occurs with thrombosis in severely atherosclerotic mesenteric artery. Typically located in its proximal part shortly after its origin from aorta. Resultant small bowel infarction is extensive and usually fatal.
- Vasculitic syndromes (p. 67), e.g., polyarteritis nodosa, Henoch–Schönlein purpura, SLE.

Strangulation Thin-walled veins which drain blood from the small bowel become occluded by extrinsic pressure; for example, from:

- Loop of bowel in a narrow hernial sac.
- Intussusception.
- Volvulus.
- Adhesions.

Venous occlusion causes congestion and edema of the bowel wall. Increased pressure prevents entry of oxygenated arterial blood leading to ischemic necrosis.

Hypoperfusion In severe hypotension, blood is shunted preferentially away from the superficial mucosa, which is the layer of the wall most susceptible to injury because of its high metabolic requirements.

In infants, poor perfusion of the mucosa followed by infection produces a rapidly fatal condition known as neonatal necrotizing enterocolitis. The bowel wall is thickened from congestion, and there is extensive superficial mucosal ulceration. Predisposing factors are prematurity, ARDS, Hirschsprung's disease and cystic fibrosis with meconium ileus.

Classification of severity

Ischemic infarcts are classified according to the depth of involvement, either mucosal infarction, mural infarction, or transmural infarction.

Mucosal infarction This transient or reversible infarction may be followed by complete regeneration. However, increased permeability to toxic substances can bring about further cardiovascular deterioration and gradual progression to a transmural infarct.

Mural infarction Here, there is infarction of mucosa and submucosa up to muscularis propria. The mucosa is ulcerated, edematous, and hemorrhagic. Healing occurs by granulation tissue formation. Mural infarction may lead to the development of fibrous strictures.

Transmural infarction Necrosis extends through the muscularis propria, and it is synonymous with gangrene. The bowel is flaccid, dilated, and liable to perforation. Surgical resection is an option, but many patients already have peritonitis, endotoxemia, and severe circulatory problems at the time of diagnosis, so the prognosis is poor.

Watersheds of ischemic bowel disease

Progression of mural infarction to stricture formation occurs in about 50% of patients with ischemic bowel disease. The splenic flexure and left colon are the common sites affected. Most patients ultimately require resection but a minority of patients will improve spontaneously.

Angiodysplasia

In this condition, abnormal venous dilatations develop in the submucosa of the large intestine (typically the right side) often causing occult or massive intestinal bleeding. It occurs in the elderly and is associated with hypertension and left-sided valvular heart disease.

It is thought to be a degenerative process resulting in increasing obstruction of the mucosal veins. Obstruction results in repeated episodes of transient elevated pressure causing dilatation and tortuosity of the submucosal veins and subsequently of the venules and capillaries of the mucosal units draining into the veins.

Hemorrhoids (piles)

These are dilated varicose veins forming in the anal canal. The most common of all anal conditions, they affect as much as 40% of the population at some time.

Etiology:

- Increased intra-abdominal pressure: constipation and straining at the stool, pregnancy.
- Portal hypertension (rare).

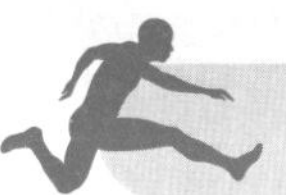

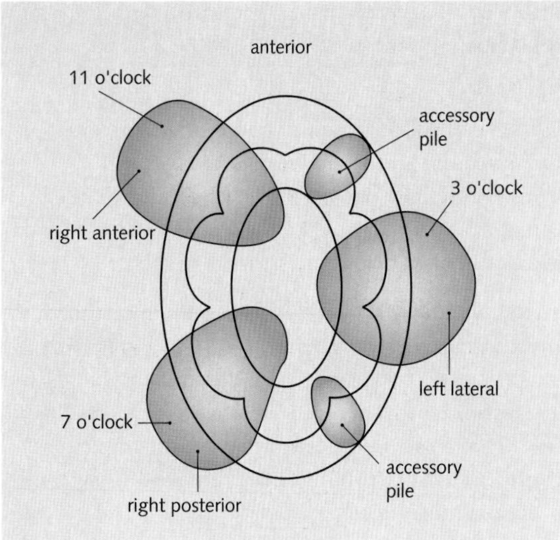

Fig. 7.40 Diagram to illustrate the 3, 7, 11 distribution of hemorrhoids around the anus. (Adapted with permission from *Surgery of the Anus, Rectum and Colon*, 5th edn, by J. Goligher, Baillière Tindall, 1984.)

Classification:

- Internal hemorrhoids: proximal to superior hemorrhoidal plexus, above anorectal margin.
- External hemorrhoids: below the anorectal margin.

Internal hemorrhoids

These are caused by the enlargement of the normal, spongy, blood-filled cushions found in the wall of the anus. They most commonly occur at three main points equidistant to the circumference of the anus (Fig. 7.40). There are four types of internal hemorrhoids:

First degree: present in the lumen but does not prolapse.

Second degree: prolapse on defecation but return spontaneously.

Third degree: remains prolapsed but can be digitally replaced.

Fourth degree: long-standing prolapsed hemorrhoids, which cannot be replaced in the anal canal.

Diagnosis is by proctoscopy (to visualize the hemorrhoids) or by sigmoidoscopy (to exclude coexisting rectal pathology).

Treatment:

- Sclerotherapy: injection with 5% phenol in almond oil induces submucosal fibrosis.
- Rubber-band ligation: hemorrhoid is pulled down through proctoscope and a rubber band is applied around the mucosa-covered part.
- Infrared photocoagulation: causes coagulation within hemorrhoid with reduction in size.
- Hemorrhoidectomy.

External hemorrhoids

There are two types: prolapsed internal hemorrhoids, and perianal hematomas or residual skin tags remaining after a perianal hematoma has healed.

Complications

Both internal and external hemorrhoids have the following complications:

- Prolapse.
- Bleeding.
- Ulceration.
- Thrombosis.
- Strangulation.

Neoplastic disease of the intestine

Primary tumors of the small intestine are rare; those that do arise are outlined in Fig. 7.41. In contrast, tumors of the large bowel are extremely common. The colon and rectum are frequently affected by both benign and malignant tumors.

Classification of intestinal tumors

Intestinal tumors can be classified according to Fig. 7.41.

Neoplastic epithelial lesions

Adenomas

These premalignant tumors are derived from the glandular epithelium of the large bowel. Common in older subjects, they are present in up to 50% of persons aged over 60, males more than females by 2:1.

Etiology is probably multifactorial. Both genetic and environmental (dietary) factors have been implicated.

There are three types:

- Tubular—rounded lesions (0.5–2cm in size). Often pedunculated (i.e., have a stalk of normal mucosa). Microscopically composed of tube-shaped glands.
- Villous—frond-like lesions about 0.6cm thick, which occupy a broad area of mucosa (about 1–5cm in diameter). Microscopically composed of finger-like epithelial projections.

Types of intestinal tumors		
	Small intestine	**Large bowel**
Non-neoplastic polyps	Hamartomas Juvenile polyps Adenomatous polyps (in familial adenomatous polyposis and Gardner's syndrome) Inflammatory fibroid polyps	Hyperplastic polyps: small, flat, pale lesions typically 5mm in size, which occur most commonly in the rectum and sigmoid colon Hamartomatous polyps: typically occur in childhood and in adolescence: • Peutz–Jeghers syndrome • juvenile polyps (autosomal dominant) • sporadic Inflammatory "pseudopolyps" (of ulcerative colitis)
Neoplastic epithelial lesions	Adenocarcinomas	Pre-malignant: • adenomas (dysplastic): tubular adenoma villus adenoma tubulovillus adenoma • familial adenomatous polyposis Malignant: • colorectal carcinoma
Mesenchymal lesions	Benign: lipoma, neurogenic tumors, leiomyoma and hemangioma Malignant: some smooth muscle tumors (leiomyosarcomas)	Rare; usually incidental findings or at post mortem: seldom responsible for symptoms; lipomas, leiomyomas, hemangiomas, neurofibromas
Lymphoma	Common site for primary lymphoma of the GI tract: celiac disease is a major predisposing factor	Very uncommon in large bowel
Carcinoid tumors (neuroendocrine tumors)	Most common site for carcinoid tumors (especially appendix); lesions typically scattered singly throughout GI tract; may secrete gut hormones, e.g., somatostatin, cholecystokinin, pancreatic polypeptide and vasoactive intestinal polypeptide (VIP)	Rare; do not usually produce functioning hormones

Fig. 7.41 Types of intestinal tumors.

- Tubulovillous—raised lesions (1–4cm in size). Pedunculated but composed of both tube-shaped glands and finger-like epithelial projections.

Epithelium of all three types shows dysplastic features, which can be subjectively graded as mild, moderate, or severe.

Progression from adenoma to carcinoma

Most carcinomas of the colon develop from previous adenomas. Progression from adenoma to carcinoma is the well-established basis of the polyp–cancer sequence for development of carcinoma of the colon (see Fig. 2.6).

Risk of malignant change is greatest where adenomas show the following features:

- Large: less than 1cm (1% malignant); 1–2cm (12% malignant); more than 2cm (30% malignant).
- Villous: villous adenomas are more likely to undergo malignant transformation.
- Severe dysplasia.

Familial adenomatous polyposis

Familial adenomatous polyposis (FAP) is an autosomal dominant condition caused by a mutation in the FAP gene located on the long arm of chromosome 5. It is characterized by the presence of innumerable adenomata of the large bowel from about the age of 25. There is a 100% risk of developing a carcinoma of the colon by the age of 45.

Hereditary nonpolyposis colon cancer

This is an inherited form of colon cancer, without adenomas, which is due to mutation in DNA mismatch repair genes. This is associated with microsatellite instability.

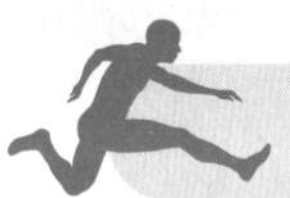

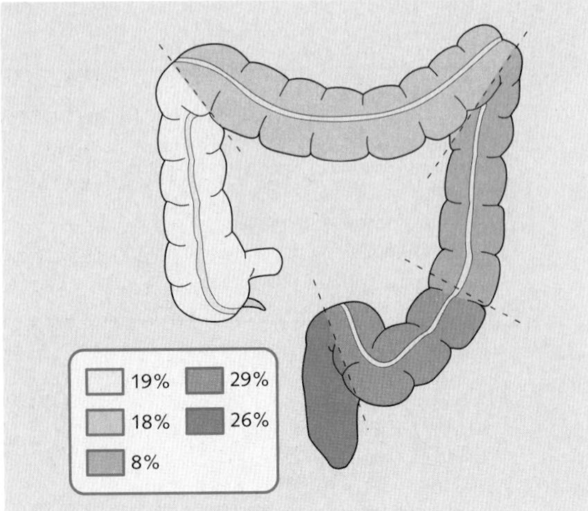

Fig. 7.42 Site and incidence of carcinomas of the large intestine.

Colorectal carcinoma

This adenocarcinoma is derived from the glandular epithelium of the large bowel mucosa.

It is the second most common cause of death from neoplasia, with a peak incidence between 60 and 70 years of age; it is rare under the age of 40.

It is rare in Africa but there is a high incidence in developed countries. Environmental factors are thought to play a large role in the etiology of colorectal cancer. Risk factors are:

- High-fat, high-protein, low-fiber diets (effects on bowel transit time, bacterial flora, and levels of cellulose, amino acids, and bile acids in the bowel contents).
- Presence of multiple sporadic adenomatous polyps.
- Ulcerative colitis.
- Familial adenomatous polyposis.

Macroscopically, the most common sites for colorectal carcinomas are illustrated in Fig. 7.42.

Types of colorectal carcinomas are:

- Polypoid—cauliflower-like growth.
- Annular—small, circumferential carcinomas which may cause stenosis.
- Ulcerated—tumors that present mainly with bleeding.
- Diffusely infiltrative—rare, but virtually identical to that seen in stomach. Often associated with carcinoma that develops in association with inflammatory bowel disease.

Right-sided carcinomas (ascending colon):

- Type of growth: polypoid.
- Pathogenesis: fecal material is soft in ascending colon, and so lesions grow to large size before causing obstruction.
- Presentation: later than for left-sided carcinomas.

Left-sided carcinomas (descending colon):

- Type of growth: annular, ulcerating.
- Pathogenesis: lesions develop where fecal material is more solid.
- Presentation: earlier due to mechanical obstruction to passage of feces.

Microscopical features—The majority of colorectal carcinomas are moderately or well-differentiated adenocarcinomas forming recognizable glandular structures. Poorly differentiated carcinomas have a poorer prognosis.

Spread:

- Local: into adjacent bowel wall and adherent structures (e.g., bladder).
- Lymphatic: to draining nodes.
- Blood: to liver and then elsewhere.
- Transcoelomic: along peritoneal cavity.

Prognosis of carcinoma of the colon is related to the stage of the disease, which is assessed using a modification of a staging system originally proposed for carcinoma of the rectum by Dukes (Fig. 7.43).

Disorders of the peritoneum

Inflammation—peritonitis

Peritoneal infection

This can either be of primary or secondary infection. Primary infection (less common) is seen in patients with nephrotic syndrome (peritoneal dialysis), cirrhosis with ascites, or abdominal trauma.

Secondary infection (most common) is typically an extension of inflammatory processes from the abdominal cavity. For example:

- Appendicitis.
- Ruptured ulcers: peptic, ulcerative colitis, typhoid ulcers, ulcerated neoplasms.
- Cholecystitis, pancreatitis, salpingitis.
- Diverticulitis.
- Strangulated bowel.

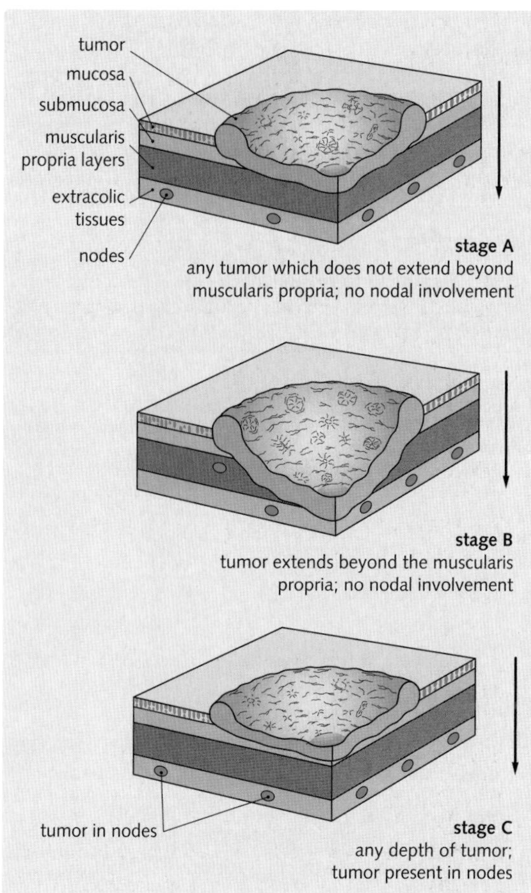

Fig. 7.43 Staging of carcinoma of the colon using the Dukes system.

Organisms involved are typically a mixture of normal gut commensals with a predominance of anaerobic bacteria and coliforms.

Irritation of the peritoneum by leaking bile, gastric juice, pancreatic enzymes, or urine produces an exudate that is initially sterile but which usually becomes infected within 6–12 hours.

As peritonitis develops, inflammation of visceral and parietal peritoneum produces a purulent exudate; the intestine becomes flaccid, dilated, and covered with fibrinous plaques that form adhesions between bowel loops.

Clinical features are:

- Tenderness, guarding, and rebound tenderness.
- Board-like abdominal rigidity.
- Absent bowel sounds (paralytic ileus).
- Increased pulse and temperature.

Complications are:

- Hypovolemic shock.
- Severe toxemia from absorbed bacterial products.
- Paralytic ileus: paralysis of gut motility as a result of inflammation of the serosa of the small bowel.
- Fibrous adhesions as a result of organization of fibrinous adhesion by granulation tissue.
- Abscesses, particularly in the paracolic gutters and beneath the diaphragm (subphrenic recesses).
- Portal pyophlebitis: spread via the portal vein to the liver.

Diagnosis is by clinical examination and erect abdominal X-ray, which may show air under the diaphragm from perforated viscus.

Management is by:

- Treatment of shock.
- Antibiotic therapy.
- Surgery: removal of contaminating source, e.g., appendicitis or perforated bowel.
- Peritoneal toilet and lavage.

See Fig. 7.44 for a summary of peritoneal infection.

Sclerosis retroperitonitis

This dense progressive fibrosis of the peritoneum particularly affects the visceral peritoneum of the small intestine. It is thought to be a side effect of practolol (β-blocker), now withdrawn from use. It is also seen in patients undergoing long-term continuous ambulatory peritoneal dialysis.

Mesenteric cysts

Sequestered lymphatic channels (cystic lymphangiomas)

These cystic developmental abnormalities of lymphoid type are typically asymptomatic and discovered incidentally at laparotomy or autopsy.

Punched-off enteric diverticula (enterogenous cysts)

These common lesions are found either incorporated in the bowel wall or in mesentery detached and separated from the tract. They are usually surrounded by smooth muscle, and they have a mucosal lining of alimentary type epithelium.

Urogenital ridge derivations

These developmental cysts are of urogenital origin.

"Walled-off" infections

This localized peritonitis is due to the capacity of omentum to wall off infection.

Summary of peritoneal infection	
Etiology	Primary infection (less common): nephrotic syndrome, peritoneal dialysis, cirrhosis with ascites, abdominal trauma Secondary infection (most common): typically an extension of inflammatory processes from abdominal cavity, e.g., appendicitis, ruptured ulcers (peptic, ulcerative colitis, typhoid ulcers, ulcerated neoplasms), cholecystitis, pancreatitis, salpingitis, diverticulitis, strangulated bowel
Organisms involved	Normal gut commensals with anaerobic bacteria and coliforms predominating
Pathogenesis	Leaking bile, gastric juice, pancreatic enzymes or urine cause irritation and inflammation of peritoneum producing an exudate that typically becomes infected; intestine becomes flaccid, dilated, and covered with fibrinous plaques forming adhesions between bowel loops
Clinical features	Guarding and rebound tenderness Board-like abdominal rigidity Absent bowel sounds (paralytic ileus) Increased pulse and temperature
Complications	Local: ileus, fibrinous adhesions, abscesses, portal pyophlebitis Systemic: hypovolemic shock, severe toxemia

Fig. 7.44 Summary of peritoneal infection.

Neoplasms

Primary mesothelioma

A rare condition, this is associated with exposure to asbestos. It corresponds to the much more common pleural mesothelioma (see Chapter 6).

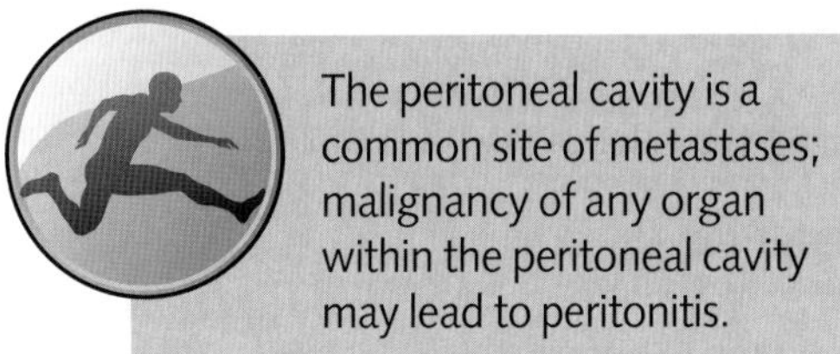
The peritoneal cavity is a common site of metastases; malignancy of any organ within the peritoneal cavity may lead to peritonitis.

Secondary

The most common tumors to metastasize to the peritoneal cavity are of the stomach, ovary, pancreas, and colon.

Metastases result in the effusion of protein-rich fluid into the cavity (i.e., an exudate) containing neoplastic cells, which also grow as tiny white nodules on the mesothelial surface of the cavity. Nodules eventually coalesce to form tumor sheets over the surface of the viscera.

- Name the common developmental abnormalities of the mouth, and state their prevalence.
- What are aphthous ulcers? Describe neoplastic lesions of the mouth.
- Describe the features of reflux esophagitis.
- What is Barrett's esophagus?
- Describe the three main patterns of chronic gastritis.
- Name the sites affected and the pathogenesis of peptic ulcers.
- Describe the pathologies associated with *Helicobacter pylori* infection.
- Define cirrhosis and list the most common causes.
- State the causes of portal hypertension and ascites.
- Compare the pathologies of hepatitis A, B, and C.
- Describe the pathogenesis of alcoholic liver disease.
- Describe the etiology and pathogenesis of acute pancreatitis.
- List the complications of acute pancreatitis.
- Name the risk factors associated with development of carcinoma of the pancreas.
- Compare and contrast the features of Crohn's disease with those of ulcerative colitis.
- Describe the pathology of celiac disease.
- State the major causes of bowel obstruction.
- What are the causes of ischemic bowel disease?
- Summarize the features of colorectal carcinomas.
- What are the complications of peritonitis?

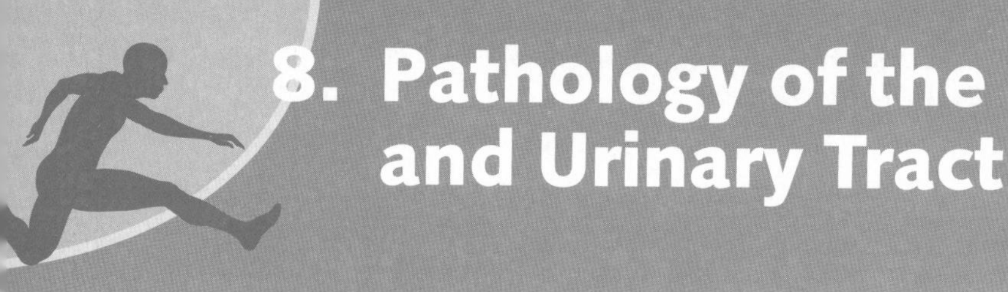

8. Pathology of the Kidney and Urinary Tract

Abnormalities of kidney structure

Congenital abnormalities of the kidney

Congenital anomalies of kidneys are common, affecting 3–4% of newborn infants.

Agenesis of the kidney

Unilateral

Unilateral agenesis occurs in 1 in 1000 births, and it may occur along side other congenital disease such as spina bifida. The remaining kidney undergoes marked hypertrophy, and it is susceptible to infections and trauma. It affects males more than females by 2:1; the left kidney is usually the absent one.

Bilateral

Occurrence of bilateral agenesis is 1 in 3000 births, as part of Potter's syndrome. Affected infants have abnormal facies, and they often have abnormalities of the lower urinary tract, lungs, and nervous system.

Characteristically, there is oligohydramnios in pregnancy, as the kidneys are not present to contribute to amniotic fluid (absence of fetal urine). The disorder is not compatible with postnatal life.

Hypoplasia

Kidneys fail to reach the normal adult size either as a result of a congenital maldevelopment or due to shrinkage, which may have occurred as a result of chronic infection in early life.

Ectopic kidneys

One or both kidneys may be in an abnormal position: most commonly the pelvis, but some lie in the inferior part of the abdomen.

Pancake kidney

Here, there is fusion of the pelvic kidneys to form a round discoid mass.

Unilateral fused kidney

The kidneys fuse together in the pelvis, then, as one kidney ascends to the "normal" position, the other is carried with it so that both kidneys end up on the same side.

Horseshoe kidney

The poles of the kidneys are fused, usually inferiorly, to form a large U-shaped (horseshoe) kidney. This affects about 1 in 500 people, but it is typically asymptomatic as the collecting system develops normally. However, Wilms' tumors are 2 to 8 times more frequent in children with horseshoe kidneys than in the general population (p. 171).

Cystic diseases of the kidney

Overview of cystic kidney disease

This heterogeneous group of diseases comprises:

- Hereditary disorders.
- Developmental (but not hereditary) disorders.
- Acquired disorders.

Each disease is distinguished by a characteristic distribution of cysts, illustrated in Fig. 8.1. Fig. 8.2 provides a summary of cystic diseases of the kidney.

Accurate diagnosis of cystic diseases is important for two reasons:

- Appropriate patient management to delay onset of renal failure.
- Appropriate genetic counseling to patients/relatives in the case of hereditary cystic diseases.

Cystic renal dysplasia

Here, the failure of differentiation of metanephric tissues affects the whole or just one segment of a kidney, either unilaterally or bilaterally. Affected areas are replaced by solid or cystic masses, in which cartilage is usually prominent.

The condition often presents in childhood as an abdominal mass and it requires surgical excision to exclude a malignant tumor (e.g., nephroblastoma). Prognosis is good for unilateral lesions.

Adult polycystic kidney disease

Adult polycystic kidney disease (APKD) is a hereditary disease. Both kidneys are progressively

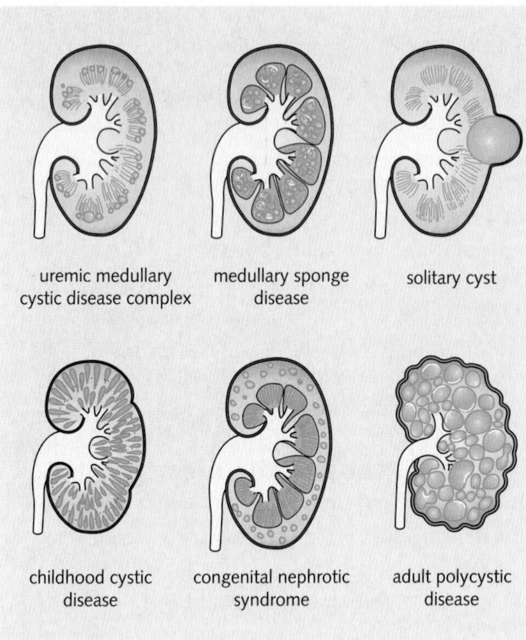

Fig. 8.1 Macroscopic features of cystic diseases of the kidney.

Summary of cystic diseases of the kidney	
Type of cystic disease	**Clinical features**
Hereditary:	
• adult polycystic disease (autosomal dominant) • infantile polycystic disease (autosomal recessive)	Chronic renal failure and hypertension
• medullary cystic disease (autosomal dominant) • juvenile nephronophthisis (autosomal recessive)	Early-onset chronic renal failure
• medullary sponge kidney (occasionally familial)	Renal stones predispose to renal colic and infection
Developmental:	
• cystic renal dysplasia	Typically asymptomatic
Acquired:	
• simple renal cysts • dialysis-associated cystic disease	Typically asymptomatic Increased risk of renal carcinoma

Fig. 8.2 Summary of cystic diseases of the kidney.

replaced by cysts, which develop and enlarge over a period of years.

Incidence is 1 per 1250 live births, accounting for 10% of all end-stage renal disease, with the sexes equally affected.

It is inherited as an autosomal dominant disorder (but about 50% are new mutations); 90% of cases are linked to the α-globin cluster located on the small arm of chromosome 16 (autosomal dominant polycystic kidney disease-1, ADPKD-1). Associations are berry aneurysms of the cerebral arteries, and cysts of the liver, pancreas, and lung.

The condition is asymptomatic at first, but eventually replacement and compression of the functioning renal parenchyma by the enlarging cysts leads to slowly progressive impairment of renal function.

Macroscopically, in fully developed APKD, the kidneys are asymmetrically enlarged, and they are composed of a mass of large cysts (which may be up to 5cm in diameter). Hemorrhage into the cysts is common, leading to bloodstained contents.

Microscopically, the cysts are lined by flattened cuboidal epithelium and communicate both with calyces and with each other. Surrounding parenchyma often shows extensive fibrosis and arteriosclerosis.

Clinical features—This presents in adult life (typically the fourth decade or later) usually with a large lobulated abdominal mass, pain, or hematuria. There is progressive renal insufficiency and hypertension.

Complications are as follows:

- Uremia.
- Hypertension: often preceding development of cardiac failure.
- Intracranial hemorrhage (10% of cases): combination of berry aneurysms and hypertension predisposes to cerebral hemorrhage.

Diagnosis is by:

- Intravenous urography: reveals irregular renal enlargement with calyceal distortion.
- Ultrasound: shows multiple cysts of variable sizes.

Management is by:

Control of blood pressure: uncontrolled hypertension accelerates the development of renal failure.

- Treatment of urinary infections.
- Relief of cardiac failure.
- Eventual dialysis or transplantation.

Infantile (childhood) polycystic disease

This is a less common autosomal recessive disorder, in which there is cystic replacement of both kidneys present at birth. Cysts are composed of dilated tubules and collecting ducts.

This is a rare condition (at 1 per 10,000 live births), with associations of cysts of the liver, pancreas, and lungs.

It presents in stillborn or neonates with enlarged kidneys (12–16 times normal size) containing a radiating cystic pattern in the medulla and cortex ("sunburst" pattern; Fig. 8.1). Rarely, it may present in childhood with renal insufficiency.

Prognosis—Affected infants usually die within the first 2 months of life.

Cystic diseases of the renal medulla

Medullary sponge kidney (tubular ectasia)

In this condition, multiple cysts develop in renal papillae, with an incidence of 1 in 20,000. Renal function is not impaired and the main clinical problem is the development of renal stones that predispose to renal colic and infection.

Acquired dialysis-associated cystic disease

This is seen in kidneys left *in situ* while patients are treated by dialysis or transplantation for chronic renal failure. There is an increased risk of renal cell carcinoma.

Simple cysts

These common lesions occur as solitary or occasionally multiple cystic spaces in otherwise normal kidneys, and are extremely common, incidence increasing with age.

The abnormality is widely believed to be acquired, but the cause is unknown.

Macroscopically, cysts are of variable size (generally being no larger than 5–6cm), and they contain clear watery fluid.

Microscopically, they are lined by flattened cuboidal epithelium and surrounded by a thin fibrous capsule. Clinically, cysts may cause renal enlargement, but they have no effect on renal function. However, they require clinical differentiation from tumors and other cystic disorders.

Diseases of the glomerulus

Overview of glomerular disease

Glomerular diseases are typically caused by disturbances of structure. There are four significant components of the glomerulus that may be damaged:

- Endothelial cells lining the capillary.
- Glomerular basement membrane.
- Mesangium: supporting mesentery to the capillary comprised of mesangial cells (phagocytic support cells) and associated extracellular material (mesangial matrix).
- Epithelial cells or podocytes, which form an outer coating to the capillary. These cells are in contact with the outer surface of the basement membrane via a series of foot processes.

Patterns of glomerular disease

Although a small number of diseases affect all glomeruli in a uniform manner, most glomerular diseases affect different glomeruli to varying degrees. A nomenclature has been agreed for the various patterns of disease:

- Global: affecting the whole glomerulus uniformly.
- Segmental: affecting one glomerular segment while sparing the others within that glomerulus.
- Diffuse: affecting all glomeruli in both kidneys.
- Focal: affecting a proportion of glomeruli, sparing others.

Thus a glomerular disease may be described as one of "diffuse global," "diffuse segmental," "focal global," or "focal segmental." The vast majority are either "diffuse global" or "focal segmental."

This explains how some glomerular diseases cause sudden acute renal failure (diffuse global diseases), whereas others cause a selective partial renal failure (focal segmental diseases).

Etiology of glomerular diseases

Glomerular diseases may be classified as (Fig. 8.3):

- Primary (majority): disease process appears to start within the glomerulus. These are further classified into four main histological types—proliferative (majority), membranous, glomerulosclerotic, and minimal change lesions.
- Secondary: disease process is secondary to systemic disease, either immune complex-mediated, metabolic, or vascular conditions. These are covered on p. 164.

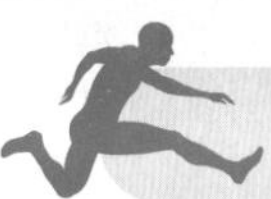

Etiology of glomerular disorders		
Type	**Etiology**	**Example**
Primary	Antiglomerular basement membrane disease: • proliferative	Goodpasture's syndrome
	Immune complex-mediated lesions: • proliferative	Diffuse proliferative glomerulonephritis Focal proliferative glomerulonephritis Membranoproliferative glomerulonephritis Crescentic glomerulonephritis
	• membranous	Membranous glomerulopathy
	• glomerulosclerosis	Focal glomerulosclerosis
	• minimal change	Minimal change disease
Secondary	Immune complex-mediated conditions	Systemic lupus erythematosus Henoch-Schönlein purpura Infective endocarditis
	Metabolic conditions	Diabetes mellitus Renal amyloidosis Multiple myeloma
	Vascular conditions	Polyarteritis nodosa Wegener's granulomatosis Hemolytic uremic syndrome Idiopathic thrombocytopenic purpura Disseminated intravascular coagulation
Hereditary	—	Alport's and Fabry's syndromes

Fig. 8.3 Etiology of glomerular disorders.

- Hereditary: Alport's syndrome, Fabry's disease, and congenital nephrotic syndrome.

Steps in diagnoses of glomerular lesions

Clinical presentation

This is to identify the type of urinary abnormality (see below).

Histological identification

Identification of the pattern of glomerular response to injury. Percutaneous needle biopsy of the kidney allows histological examination of the glomeruli and tubules to identify structural abnormalities and to characterize patterns of damage.

Immunological investigation

This is for the detection of immune complex deposition and serological changes (see below).

Clinical manifestations of glomerular disease

Patients with glomerular disease usually present with one of five possible syndromes (described below).

Asymptomatic hematuria

This is a hematuria without significant proteinemia, which may be continuous or intermittent, and it varies in severity from macroscopic to microscopic. The condition does not cause renal failure.

Asymptomatic proteinuria

This proteinuria (>0.3g every 24 hours) without hematuria may be continuous, orthostatic (postural), or transient. It is typically detected at a routine medical examination.

Acute nephritic syndrome

This presents with a sudden onset of hematuria, proteinuria (often with urinary casts), and hypertension. Loin pain and headache may be present and the patient will often feel unwell. In children there is often generalized oedema, especially around the eyes.

Nephrotic syndrome

Here, there is proteinuria (usually >3.5g every 24 hours) with hypoproteinemia and edema. There is also hypercholesterolemia. It may be due to primary or secondary glomerular disease.

Chronic renal failure

This is an irreversible deterioration in renal function caused by the destruction of more and more individual nephrons over a long period of time. Impairment of excretory, metabolic, and endocrine functions of the kidney leads to the clinical syndrome of uremia.

Fig. 8.4 gives the symptoms and signs of renal failure.

Management—Excretory function of the kidney can be partially replaced by dialysis. However, replacement of the endocrine and metabolic functions can only be achieved by successful renal transplantation.

Unless some form of supportive therapy, such as dialysis or transplantation, is available, chronic renal failure is eventually fatal.

Summary

Many of the diseases causing the above clinical syndromes are listed in Fig. 8.5.

However, there is considerable overlap—several diseases may give rise to the same clinical picture, and conversely many conditions fall into more than one clinical group.

The mechanism of glomerular injury

Many glomerular diseases are caused by immune-mediated damage with five main mechanisms (listed below). Different patterns of immune-mediated damage point to different diagnoses. Therefore, it is important to identify the site, type, and pattern of

Symptoms and signs of renal failure

Symptoms	Signs
General malaise Breathlessness on exertion Nausea and vomiting Disordered GI motility Headaches Pruritus Pigmentation	Uremia Anemia Metabolic bone disease (renal osteodystrophy) Hypertension Acidosis Neuropathy Generalized myopathy endocrine abnormalities

Fig. 8.4 Symptoms and signs of renal failure.

Clinical manifestations of glomerular disease and the conditions that cause them

Clinical manifestations	Causative renal disease
Asymptomatic hematuria	Exercise hematuria IgA nephropathy Henoch–Schönlein purpura Bacterial endocarditis Systemic lupus erythematosus (SLE) Polyarteritis nodosa (PAN)
Asymptomatic proteinuria	Primary: • focal segmental glomerulosclerosis • membranoproliferative glomerulonephritis Secondary: • Henoch–Schönlein purpura • SLE • PAN • bacterial endocarditis
Acute nephritic syndrome	Primary: • poststreptococcal glomerulonephritis • rapidly progressive glomerulonephritis • Goodpasture's syndrome Secondary: • SLE • PAN • Wegener's granulomatosis • Henoch–Schönlein purpura • essential cryoglobulinemia
Nephrotic syndrome	Primary: • minimal change disease • membranous glomerulopathy • membranoproliferative glomerulonephritis • focal proliferative glomerulonephritis • focal glomerulosclerosis Secondary: • immune complex-mediated conditions SLE Henoch–Schönlein purpura infective endocarditis • metabolic conditions diabetes mellitus renal amyloidosis • vascular conditions PAN Wegener's granulomatosis hemolytic uremic syndrome • infections malaria, syphilis, hepatitis B
Chronic renal failure	All of above except minimal change disease

Fig. 8.5 Clinical manifestations of glomerular disease and the conditions that cause them.

immune complexes and complement within the glomerulus by immunohistochemistry and electron microscopy.

Circulating immune complex nephritis

This is the most common pattern of immunological disease.

Mechanism

Antigen–antibody complexes circulating in the blood are trapped at the basement membrane, the mesangium, or both. Complexes activate the complement cascade via the classical pathway (see Fig. 3.6). Activated components of complement bring about the characteristic acute inflammation of glomerulonephritis by attracting neutrophil polymorphs, increasing vascular permeability, and causing membrane damage (see Fig. 3.7). Damage to the basement membrane results in alteration of its properties leading to some of the urinary abnormalities observed clinically.

Example

Poststreptococcal glomerulonephritis.

In-situ immune complex formation

Mechanism

Circulating antigens become trapped in the glomerulus, where they are targeted by circulating antibodies such that immune complexes are formed within the glomerulus. This in-situ formation explains why, in contrast to circulating immune complex nephritis described above, there is little complement and no inflammatory or proliferative responses.

Example

This is believed to occur in certain cases of systemic lupus erythematosus (SLE) when free DNA in the blood is trapped in the glomerular basement membrane, subsequently binding to anti-DNA antibodies.

Cytotoxic antibodies

Mechanism

Autoantibodies are directed to a component of the glomerular basement membrane (anti-GBM antibodies). This is an uncommon form of immune-mediated damage.

Example

This is the basis of Goodpasture's syndrome, in which autoantibodies cause direct damage to the glomerular basement membrane. The Goodpasture antigen (which is the target of the anti-GBM antibodies) has been identified as a domain on the α_3 type IV collagen chain.

Activation of the alternate complement pathway

Mechanism

The alternative complement pathway is normally activated by the presence of bacterial cell walls, and it is independent of immune complex formation (see Fig. 3.6). However, in certain disease conditions, the alternative pathway can be activated by different mechanisms.

Example

In type II membranoproliferative glomerulonephritis, a circulating autoantibody (termed "C3 nephritic factor") activates complement via the alternate pathway by stabilizing the enzyme, C3-convertase. This enzyme normally activates C3, but it has a very short half-life. Thus, stabilization of C3-convertase prolongs the activation of C3.

Cell-mediated immunity

Cell-mediated immunological mechanisms are uncommon in the initiation of acute glomerular diseases, but they are thought to play a role in the progression of acute glomerulonephritis to a chronic phase.

Proliferative glomerulonephritis

This group of disorders is characterized histologically by varying degrees of proliferation of mesangial and epithelial (and sometimes endothelial) cells within the glomerulus.

The majority of cases of glomerulonephritis (over 70%) belong to this group.

Proliferative glomerulonephritis can be divided according to certain histological appearances into:

- Diffuse proliferative.
- Rapidly progressive.
- Focal proliferative.
- Membranoproliferative.

However, it must be emphasized that these subdivisions are not diagnoses, but rather describe a pattern of reaction caused by glomerular insult.

Diffuse proliferative glomerulonephritis

Diffuse, global, acute inflammation of glomeruli is caused by the deposition of immune complexes in the glomeruli, stimulated by a preceding infection.

Etiology is as follows:

- Poststreptococcal (most common): onset is 1–2 weeks after a primary pharyngeal infection with β-hemolytic streptococci of Lancefield group A.
- Nonstreptococcal (less common): a range of bacterial, viral and protozoal infections can also stimulate this pattern of disease.

Those antibodies produced to combat initial infection cross-react with cellular antigens producing immune complexes. These complexes circulate in the blood, and they are filtered out in the glomerulus producing four main histological changes:

- Immune complex deposition: in lumps on the epithelial side of glomerular basement membrane.
- Neutrophil infiltration: activation of complement attracts neutrophils into the glomerulus.
- Endothelial cell proliferation: degranulation of neutrophils damages endothelial cells, stimulating their proliferation.
- Mild mesangial cell proliferation: mediated by factors derived from complement and platelets.

Rapidly progressive glomerulonephritis (crescentic glomerulonephritis)

Rapidly progressive glomerulonephritis (RPGN) is a manifestation of severe glomerular injury characterized by the formation of cellular crescent-shaped masses within the Bowman's space. It occurs in a small percentage of patients with poststreptococcal glomerulonephritis (see above), but it can also be associated with many other forms of glomerular damage.

If damage to the glomerular capillaries is severe, fibrin and blood leak into Bowman's space stimulating epithelial cell proliferation, and infiltration of macrophages and neutrophils. Crescent-shaped cellular masses composed of epithelial cells and macrophages are formed within the Bowman's space. These crescents are associated with glomerular ischemia and ultimately they result in permanent glomerular damage.

Focal proliferative glomerulonephritis

Here, there is an acute inflammation with cellular proliferation occurring in only a proportion of all glomeruli (focal) and usually affecting only one segment of the glomerular tufts (segmental). Therefore, the condition is more accurately described as focal segmental proliferative glomerulonephritis.

Several diseases can cause this pattern of response. These can be classified into two groups:

- Primary: mainly mesangial IgA disease and Goodpasture's syndrome (Fig. 8.6).
- Secondary: associated with other systemic diseases including infective endocarditis, vasculitis and connective tissue diseases.

Immunohistochemistry and electron microscopy are required to distinguish them.

Proliferative glomerulonephritis

Condition	Features
Mesangial IgA disease (Berger's disease)	A focal proliferative glomerulonephritis. Serum IgA levels are raised and IgA is deposited in the mesangium and basement membrane
Goodpasture's syndrome	A focal proliferative glomerulonephritis. The Goodpasture antigen is a domain of type IV collagen in the basement membrane; this is a target for the autoantibodies
Type I MPGN	An immune complex disease thought to involve a disorder of complement, characterized by subendothelial deposits. There is a persistently low serum C3
Type II MPGN	An autoimmune-mediated abnormality of complement. There is marked thickening of the capillary walls due to deposition of C3 (dense deposit disease)

Fig. 8.6 Examples of proliferative glomerulonephritic disease (MPGN, membranoproliferative glomerulonephritis).

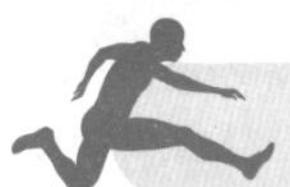

Membranoproliferative glomerulonephritis

Membranoproliferative glomerulonephritis (MPGN) is a diffuse, global pattern of glomerulonephritis with features of both proliferation and membrane thickening (hence the name). It is also known as mesangiocapillary glomerulonephritis.

Diseases causing MPGN can be classified into two groups:

- Primary (majority): idiopathic. Subdivided according to clinical and pathological features into type I (90% of cases) and type II (10% of cases) (Fig. 8.6).
- Secondary: a few are secondary to systemic disorders such as SLE, infective endocarditis, malaria, and infected ventricular cerebrospinal fluid (CSF) shunts.

Membranous nephropathy

In membranous nephropathy there is a pattern of reaction in which the glomerular capillary basement membrane is uniformly thickened. Unlike the proliferative types of glomerulonephritis, there is no associated inflammation or endothelial/epithelial proliferation, although the mesangial cell population may be slightly increased.

It affects all age groups, but the highest incidence is between fifth and seventh decades. Males are affected more than females.

Etiology is as follows:

- Primary: 80–90% of cases have no apparent reason for development of immune complexes, and are classed as primary or idiopathic membranous nephropathy.
- Secondary: membranous nephropathy is found in association with a number of conditions, which are listed in Fig. 8.7.

There are four pathological stages:

- In-situ formation of immune complexes on the epithelial side of the basement membrane (diffuse, global pattern).
- Mild mesangial increase.
- New basement membrane is deposited around immune complex deposits.
- Immune complex deposits disappear, leaving thickened "lacy" basement membrane.

Over many years, the abnormal glomeruli develop increased mesangial matrix produced by the mesangial cells. This, together with membrane thickening, causes gradual hyalinization of the glomeruli (glomerulosclerosis) and death of individual nephrons.

Conditions associated with membranous nephropathy

Type	Example
Infection	Malaria Syphilis Hepatitis B
Malignancy	Carcinoma (lung, breast, GI) Lymphoma
Drugs	Gold, mercury, penicillamine, captopril
Systemic disease	SLE (10% of renal involvement is of the membranous pattern)

Fig. 8.7 Conditions associated with membranous nephropathy.

Abnormality of the basement membrane renders it unusually permeable resulting in heavy proteinuria. This may cause nephrotic syndrome. Indeed, membranous nephropathy is one of the most important causes of nephrotic syndrome.

Prognosis is variable and related to cause, but, in crude figures, 25% of patients undergo remission and 25% develop stable persisting proteinuria; 50% develop chronic renal failure over a period of about 10 years.

Minimal change disease (lipoid nephrosis)

The characteristic feature in this neuropathy (and the reason for the name) is that no significant abnormalities can be detected by light microscopy.

It mainly affects children under the age of 6 years, and it is less common in adults, but still accounts for 10–25% of cases of nephrotic syndrome. Males are affected more than females.

Etiology is unknown.

Pathogenesis is postulated to be immunologically related (cell-mediated damage to be basement membrane) because of the universal satisfactory response to corticosteroid therapy. Ultimately, polyanionic charges of the glomerular basement membrane are depleted, leading to failure of protein retention.

Morphological features—With electron microscopy, there is a diagnostic loss of epithelial foot processes. Tubules may show accumulation of lipid in lining cells, giving rise to the alternative name of "lipoid nephrosis."

Prognosis in children is good, with no permanent renal damage. In adults, the outlook is variable.

Focal segmental glomerulosclerosis

The glomerulus is partially replaced by hyaline material, which, in most cases, is excess mesangial matrix.

Etiology is variable and related to age:

- Primary (most common): idiopathic disease affecting children and young adults.
- Secondary: in later adult life the condition is usually secondary to other disorders, especially previous focal proliferative glomerulonephritis.

Pathogenesis is unknown, but it is probably immune-mediated.

Focal glomerulosclerosis initially affects the juxtamedullary glomeruli, causing an increase in mesangial matrix, which gradually expands to destroy the surrounding lobule, until global sclerosis occurs. In time, similar lesions appear in glomeruli throughout the cortex.

The patient presents with nephrotic syndrome. Later, hematuria, hypertension, and renal failure are common.

Prognosis is poor with progression of disease over many years leading to chronic renal failure.

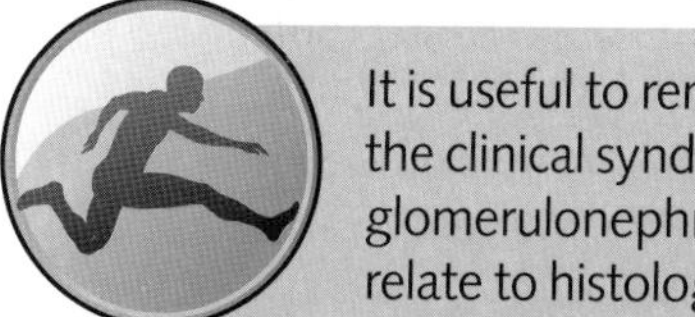

It is useful to remember that the clinical syndromes of glomerulonephritis broadly relate to histological findings:

- Asymptomatic proteinuria and nephrotic syndrome are associated with basement membrane thickening as a result of either structural change or deposition of excessive mesangial matrix (e.g., membranous nephropathy, glomerulosclerosis).
- Asymptomatic hematuria and nephritic syndrome are associated with proliferation of the endothelial or mesangial cells (e.g., diffuse, global glomerulonephritis).
- Mixed nephritic/nephrotic syndrome is associated with combined damage to the basement membrane and cell proliferation (e.g., membranoproliferative glomerulonephritis).

Hereditary glomerulonephritis

Alport's syndrome

This syndrome is characterized by the clinical triad of deafness, glomerulonephritis, and ocular lesions. Inheritance is complex, and it is X-linked in 50% of families (mutation of COLIVα5 gene).

The clinical features are:

- Glomerulonephritis: usually presents as microscopic hematuria and proteinuria in childhood. There is subsequent development of nephrotic syndrome with progression to renal failure, occurring by the second decade in males, but often not until the fifth decade in females.
- Ocular disease: occurs in only severely affected patients.
- Deafness: only for high-pitched sounds, and it may be difficult to demonstrate.

Fabry's syndrome

A rare, X-linked recessive syndrome of glycosphingolipid metabolism resulting in painful extremities, red hyperkeratotic papules on skin, proteinuria, and renal failure.

Congenital nephrotic syndrome

A rare disorder characterized by nephrotic syndrome occurring at or shortly after birth. It is often associated with a bulky placenta, congenital heart disease, and raised α-fetoprotein levels in maternal amniotic fluid. Etiology is an autosomal recessive pattern of inheritance.

There are two types:

- Finnish type: shows slight glomerular mesangial proliferation and progressive glomerulosclerosis.
- Non-Finnish type: shows focal and segmental glomerulosclerosis.

Both types ultimately progress to renal failure.

Chronic glomerulonephritis

Chronic renal failure associated with small, contracted kidneys, in which all the glomeruli are hyalinized (end-stage kidneys).

This may be caused by many diseases, particularly proliferative types of acute glomerulonephritis.

In patients who present for the first time with chronic glomerulonephritis, it is often not possible to ascertain the cause because of diffuse global glomerular destruction. However, it is likely that many patients presenting for the first time have had IgA mesangial disease.

Macroscopically, affected kidneys are small and there is granularity of the external surface, reflecting fine scarring due to nephron hyalinization. However, the pelvicalyceal system is normal, an important distinction from cases of end-stage kidney due to chronic pyelonephritis.

Microscopically, there is hyalinization of the glomeruli, tubular atrophy and interstitial fibrosis.

It is helpful to remember that the patterns of glomerular damage that occur secondary to systemic disease mimic the various patterns of primary glomerulonephritis.

Glomerular lesions in systemic disease

Systemic lupus erythematosus

Glomerular lesions are the main abnormalities of renal involvement in SLE. These vary in severity from minor abnormalities such as asymptomatic proteinuria to severe glomerular disease leading to renal failure.

The basis of glomerular damage is immune complex deposition in the basement membrane (leading to basement membrane thickening), or in the mesangium (leading to mesangial expansion).

Patterns of glomerular damage that may occur include:

- Diffuse MPGN: associated with a mixed nephritic/nephrotic syndrome and rapid progression to renal failure.
- Focal segmental proliferative glomerulonephritis: associated with hematuria, proteinuria, and slow progression.
- Diffuse membranous nephropathy: associated with nephrotic syndrome and slow progression to chronic renal failure.

Immune complexes

The immune complexes of SLE are characterized by the presence of IgG, IgA, IgM, C3, and C1q (known as a "full-house" of deposits). The detection of this pattern of immunoglobulins and complement factors, together with the particular location of the immune complexes in relation to the glomerular basement membrane, is an important factor in distinguishing lupus glomerulonephritis from non-lupus patterns.

Note that although glomerular lesions are the main abnormalities of renal involvement in SLE, there may also be extraglomerular vascular abnormalities and tubular damage, particularly interstitial nephritis.

Henoch–Schönlein purpura

This immune complex-mediated systemic vasculitis affects small arteries in the skin, joints, intestine, and kidneys (see Chapters 5 and 12).

Significant renal damage occurs in over one third of cases, ranging from proteinuria, possibly with nephrotic syndrome, to RPGN.

Bacterial endocarditis

Renal lesions in infective endocarditis are caused by two mechanisms:

- Immune complex deposition—immune complexes (formed with antigens of infecting organisms) are deposited in the glomerulus causing a focal segmental proliferative glomerulonephritis or a diffuse proliferative glomerulonephritis.
- Embolism-mediated infarction—embolic vegetations from heart valves cause multiple renal infarcts.

Renal lesions typically subside when the bacterial source of the antigen is removed by intensive antibiotic therapy.

Diabetic glomerulosclerosis

Diabetic glomerular damage causes an increase in the permeability of the glomerular capillary basement membrane, leading to proteinuria and occasionally nephrotic syndrome.

The pathogenesis of basement membrane changes is not fully understood, but it includes deficiency of proteoglycans that are responsible for the polyanionic nature of the membrane, glomerular hypertrophy, basement membrane thickening, ECM expansion, and mesangial cell hypertrophy. Factors which mediated these changes are hyperglycemia, hyperfiltration (increased glomerular blood flow in diabetes), and nonenzymic glycosylation of proteins.

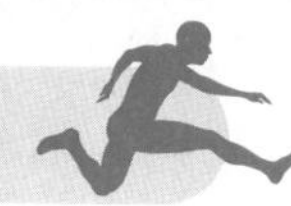

Histologically there are three types of glomerular lesions that occur, representing a continuous spectrum of increasing severity:

- Capillary wall thickening—mild proteinuria.
- Diffuse glomerulosclerosis—excess mesangial matrix formation in an even pattern throughout the glomerulus combined with capillary thickening eventually encroaches on the capillaries.
- Nodular glomerulosclerosis (Kimmelstiel–Wilson nodules)—nodular expansion of the mesangium at the tips of the glomerular lobules is very characteristic of diabetes.

Diabetic sclerosis causes progressive hyalinization of glomeruli with obliteration of capillary loops and death of individual nephrons. Over a period of years this leads to chronic renal failure.

Prognosis—Approximately 10% of all diabetics die in renal failure. This rises to 50% if patients developing diabetes in childhood are considered separately.

Amyloidosis

This is a condition in which amyloid, an extracellular fibrillar protein, is deposited in a variety of tissues (see Chapter 12). Amyloidosis is an important cause of the nephrotic syndrome in adults.

Amyloid is deposited as fibrils in the glomerular basement membrane and in the mesangium of the kidney, resulting in membrane thickening and increased mesangial matrix formation. The net result is the development of:

- Proteinuria—membrane thickening leads to an increase in membrane permeability so that the first manifestation of amyloidosis is often proteinuria.
- Nephrotic syndrome—increased deposition of amyloid causes increased protein loss until the patient develops features of the nephrotic syndrome.
- Chronic renal failure—combined effect of amyloid deposition and increased mesangial matrix formation eventually leads to expansion of the mesangium causing compression of the glomerular capillary system and transition into chronic renal failure.

Amyloid is also deposited in the walls of intrarenal vessels, particularly the afferent arterioles.

Polyarteritis nodosa

Polyarteritis nodosa is a systemic disease characterized by inflammatory necrosis of the walls of small and medium-sized arteries (see Chapter 5). Necrosis of medium-sized arteries causes small infarcts in the kidney; necrosis of arterioles and the glomerular tuft produces infarction of entire glomeruli or segments. This is visible as fibrinoid necrosis.

Wegener's granulomatosis

This immune complex-mediated systemic necrotizing vasculitis primarily affects the nose, upper respiratory tract, and kidneys. Renal involvement is of variable severity causing one of the following:

- Focal segmental glomerulonephritis (asymptomatic hematuria or nephritic syndrome).
- Rapidly progressive glomerulonephritis (rapidly progressive acute renal failure).

This condition usually responds to immunosuppressive therapy.

Diseases of the tubules and interstitium

Acute tubular necrosis

This acute, but usually reversible, renal failure is caused by necrosis of renal tubular epithelial cells resulting from metabolic or toxic disturbances. The causes of acute tubular necrosis (ATN) are shown in Fig. 8.8.

The etiology is:

- Ischemic (most common): caused by failure of renal perfusion, typically the result of hypotension and hypervolemia in shock.
- Toxic: uncommon (heavy metals, organic solvents).

There are three phases to ATN (oliguric, polyuric, and recovery) as follows:

- Oliguric phase—necrosis of renal tubular cells causes tubule blockage and reduced glomerular blood flow and filtration.
- Polyuric phase—tubules slowly open as phagocytic cells begin to remove necrotic material. Regenerated renal tubule cells are undifferentiated.

Causes of acute tubular necrosis	
Type of ATN	**Causes**
Ischemic	Major surgery Extensive acute blood loss Severe burns Hemorrhage
Toxic	Endogenous products: hemoglobinuria and myoglobinuria Heavy metals: lead, mercury Organic solvents: chloroform, carbon tetrachloride Drugs: antibiotics, NSAIDs, ciclosporin Others: paraquat, phenol, ethylene glycol, poisonous fungi

Fig. 8.8 Causes of acute tubular necrosis.

- Recovery phase—differentiated tubular cells restore renal function.

The morphological features are:
- Ischemic ATN: kidneys are pale and swollen. Histology reveals flattened, vacuolated epithelial cells along the entire length of the tubules.
- Necrotic ATN: kidneys are red and swollen. Histology reveals flattened, vacuolated epithelial cells restricted to proximal tubular cells, those of the distal tubule being spared.

Clinical features are oliguria (50–500mL daily) with features of renal failure (Fig. 8.4) and polyuria.

A knowledge of the etiology (ischemic vs. toxic) and an understanding of the pathogenesis (oliguric and polyuric phases) of ATN make the morphological and clinical features easy to remember.

Treatment:
- Oliguric phase: supportive measures to prevent hyperkalemia and fluid overload.
- Polyuric phase: replacement of fluid and electrolytes to compensate for excessive loss from urine.

The prognosis depends on the speed and efficiency with which corrective measures are put into operation, on the prompt recognition and effective treatment of complications, and on the nature and severity of the causal disorder.

Tubulointerstitial nephritis

Urinary tract infection and pyelonephritis

Acute pyelonephritis

Inflammation of the tubules and interstitium is caused by bacterial infection. There are three age peaks—childhood, pregnancy, and in the elderly.

Most cases of infection are caused by enterobacteria from the patient's fecal flora (e.g., *E. coli*, *Proteus*, and *Klebsiella*) or by staphylococci from skin (perineal) flora. The organism may enter the kidney by one of two routes: ascending infection from the lower urinary tract (in pregnancy, DM, stasis of urine) or via the blood in bacteremia/septicemia.

Macroscopically, the condition is characterized by numerous abscesses throughout the kidney:
- Cortical abscesses—small, yellowish-white abscesses, usually spherical, under 2mm in diameter, and sometimes surrounded by a zone of hyperemia. Most prominent on subcapsular surface.
- Medullary abscesses—yellowish-white linear streaks which converge on the papilla. Pelvicalyceal mucosa is hyperemic or covered with a fibrinopurulent exudate.

Microscopically, there is focal inflammation with infiltration of tubules by neutrophils and interstitial edema.

Clinical features are fever, rigors, and pain in the back.

This condition is often associated with dysuria and urgency of micturition—signs of a lower urinary tract infection.

Complications and sequelae include resolution, healing with scarring, chronicity, pyonephrosis, renal papillary necrosis, perinephric abscess, or death.

Diagnosis is by examination of midstream urine, especially cultured to demonstrate responsible organisms:
- Significant bacteriuria is defined as $> 10^5$ culture-forming units per mL (to eliminate cases of extraneous bacterial contamination).
- Significant pyuria is defined as > 10 neutrophil polymorphs per high power field.

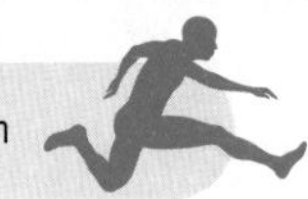

Treatment is by oral antibiotic therapy (e.g., trimethoprim, ampicillin, amoxycillin, or ciprofloxacin: all are generally active against *E. coli*). Intravenous antibiotic therapy is used for more severe or septicemic cases.

Untreated, infection may spread to cause Gram-negative septicemia with shock.

Chronic pyelonephritis

Chronic inflammation of the tubules and interstitium is associated with nephron destruction and coarse scarring of the kidneys. There are two forms (obstructive and reflux-associated) as described below.

Obstructive chronic pyelonephritis

Obstruction of pelvicalyceal drainage causes recurrent episodes of infection (discussed in more detail on p. 173).

Reflux-associated chronic pyelonephritis

Reflux of urine from the bladder into the ureter predisposes to recurrent bouts of inflammation. It is most common in childhood and early adult life, with males affected more than females.

Normally, the ureter enters the bladder obliquely so that contraction of the bladder wall during micturition closes the ureteric orifice. In patients with vesicourethral reflux, the terminal portion of the ureter is short and orientated at approximately 90° to the mucosal surface. Contraction of the bladder tends to hold the ureteric orifice open, thus facilitating reflux of urine, enabling organisms to gain access to the kidney from the bladder.

Macroscopically, the kidneys have irregular areas of scarring seen as depressed areas, 1–2cm in size, most commonly sited in the renal calyces at the poles of the kidney, but often associated with fibrous scarring of the renal papilla. Involvement may be either bilateral or unilateral.

Microscopically, kidneys have irregular areas of interstitial fibrosis with chronic inflammatory cell infiltration. Tubules are atrophic, or they may be dilated and contain proteinaceous casts. Glomeruli show periglomerular fibrosis and many demonstrate complete hyalinization.

Clinical features are symptoms of urinary tract infection and of uremia.

Diagnosis is by:

- Intravenous urography: reveals reduction in kidney size and localized contraction of renal substance associated with clubbing of the adjacent calyces.
- Urine culture: for identification of infecting organism.

Treatment is by antibiotic therapy, control of hypertension, and removal of the source of obstruction.

Prognosis—The course is usually long and punctuated by acute exacerbations.

Other diseases of the tubules and interstitium are illustrated in Fig. 8.9.

Diseases of the tubules and interstitium

Condition	Features
Toxic and drug induced	Inflammation of the renal interstitium and tubules (tubulointerstitial nephritis) due to exposure to toxic agents. Two types: acute and chronic
Urate nephropathy	Affects a small group of patients with hyperuricemia
Hypercalcemia and nephrocalcinosis	Hypercalcemia causes calcification of the renal parenchyma and tubular damage
Multiple myeloma	Some types of myeloma are characterized by proliferating plasma cells, which produce monoclonal free light chains. These cause physical obstruction and damage to the tubules

Fig. 8.9 Diseases of the tubules and interstitium.

Diseases of the renal blood vessels

Benign nephrosclerosis

This hyaline arteriosclerosis of the kidney is associated with benign hypertension.

The condition is an important complication of long-standing benign hypertension (p. 49), chronic renal failure being one of its major sequelae.

This is the most common form of nephropathy, found in approximately 75% of autopsies over the age of 60 years.

(The causes of hypertension are listed in Fig. 5.11.)

In long-standing benign hypertension, there is reduced flow of blood to the glomeruli caused by vascular changes that affect:

- Branches of the renal artery: thickening of arterial walls due to fibroelastic intimal proliferation, elastic lamina reduplication, and muscular hypertrophy of the media. Results in focal areas of ischemia with scarring.
- Afferent arterioles: undergo hyalinization (arteriolosclerosis), their muscular walls being replaced by a rigid and inelastic amorphous material.

A progressive reduction in blood flow to the nephrons leads to chronic ischemia with slow conversion of individual glomeruli into a mass of hyaline tissue devoid of capillary lumina (Fig. 8.10).

Blood supply to the tubules is also derived from glomerular blood flow, therefore there is eventual ischemic destruction of the associated tubule.

The process gradually destroys individual nephrons over a period of many years.

Clinical features—Initially, there are no clinical symptoms, although a gradual increase in blood levels of urea and a reduction in creatinine clearance occur.

Eventually, critical numbers of nephrons become dysfunctional and the patient develops manifestations of chronic renal failure.

Prognosis—Less than 5% of patients with well-developed benign nephrosclerosis die from renal failure. Death in the great majority of cases of benign hypertension occurs from congestive heart failure, coronary insufficiency, and cerebral vascular accidents.

Malignant nephrosclerosis

Renal disease is associated with malignant, accelerated hypertension.

renal muscular artery | glomerulus

normal

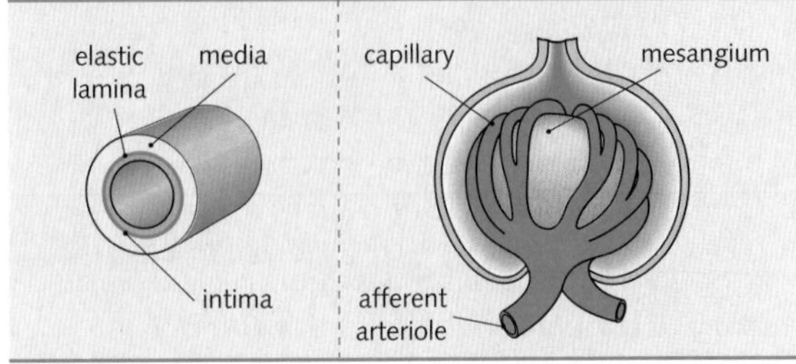

benign hypertension

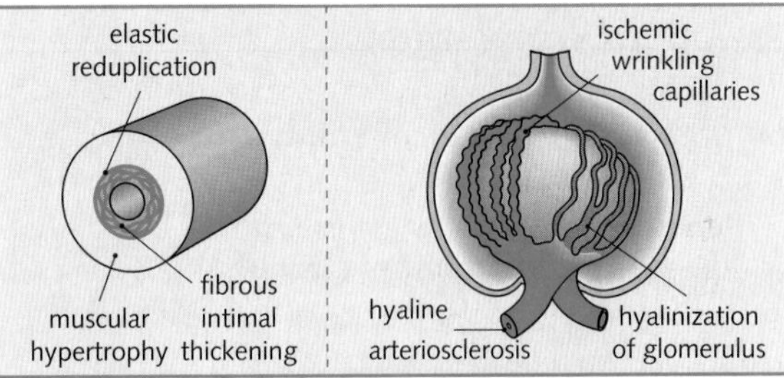

malignant hypertension

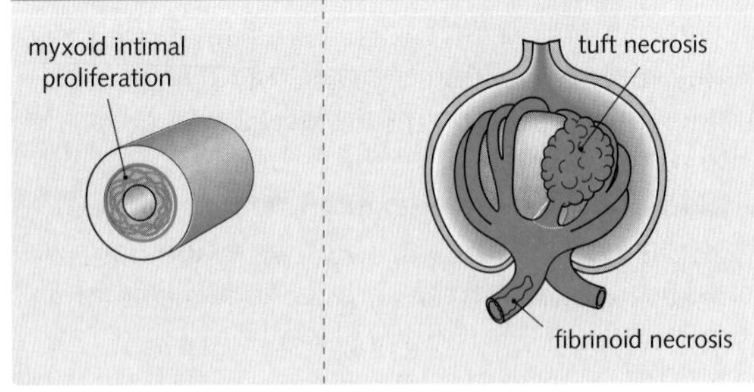

Fig. 8.10 Vascular changes associated with hypertensive renal disease.

Pathogenesis—In accelerated hypertension, the rise in blood pressure is very rapid, causing a pattern of renal damage that differs from that seen in benign hypertension:

- Larger muscular vessels undergo fibroelastic proliferation of the intima, but no muscular hypertrophy.
- Afferent arterioles frequently undergo necrosis, often with fibrin in their damaged walls (fibrinoid necrosis) following exposure to the sudden high pressures.
- Glomerular capillary network: segmental fibrinoid necrosis of glomerular tuft.

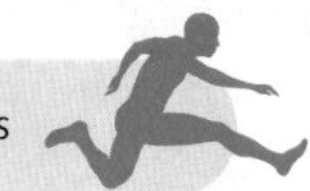

The patient develops acute renal failure when sufficient nephrons are rendered nonfunctional because of damage to glomerular tufts and afferent arterioles.

The renal changes seen in benign and accelerated hypertensive nephrosclerosis are summarized in Fig. 8.10.

Untreated accelerated hypertension causes death from renal failure in 90% of cases, usually with marked rapidity. However, if hypertension is treated adequately, before there is evidence of impairment of renal function by a raised blood urea, then prognosis is good and subsequent renal failure unusual.

Renal artery stenosis

This is a narrowing of renal arteries, typically caused by generalized atherosclerosis, but it may rarely be caused by arterial fibromuscular dysplasia.

Atherosclerotic occlusion of the renal artery is usually most severe at its origin from the aorta. Renal artery stenosis at this point can lead to two main pathological processes:

- Chronic ischemia of the affected kidney—reduction in function of all nephrons on that side produces an end-stage shrunken kidney. However, the contralateral kidney undergoes compensatory hypertrophy, so that renal function is largely unaffected.
- Renovascular hypertension—inadequate perfusion of the kidney caused by renal artery stenosis may lead to hyper-reninism, and subsequent abnormal activation of the renin–angiotensin system. This condition is important in that it is one of the recognized causes of hypertension that is amenable to surgical correction.

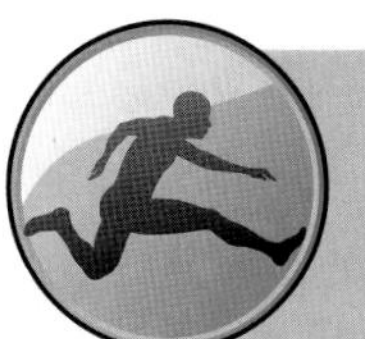

A useful diagnostic pointer for renal artery stenosis is to look for associated features of:

- Vascular disease elsewhere.
- Severe or drug-resistant hypertension.
- Abdominal bruits.

Thrombotic microangiopathies

Hemolytic uremic syndrome

Hemolytic uremic syndrome (HUS) is a complex syndrome of disordered platelet function that is characterized by the triad of thrombocytopenia, hemolysis, and acute renal failure.

Classification

There are three subtypes of HUS—childhood, adult, and secondary.

Childhood HUS

This usually affects children under 4 years of age. The etiology is unknown, but the prognosis is better than for adult and secondary types.

Adult HUS

This is more frequently fatal than childhood HUS, and it is associated with the following conditions:

- Pregnancy: occurring postpartum even several months after delivery.
- Estrogen therapy: contraceptive pills or estrogen therapy for men with prostatic carcinoma.
- Infections (e.g., typhoid, viruses, and shigellosis).

Secondary HUS

This occurs as a complication of:

- Malignant hypertension.
- Progressive systemic sclerosis.
- SLE.
- Transplant rejection.

Pathogenesis

Platelets adhere to the endothelium of small vessels, including the glomerular capillaries, where they undergo aggregation and trigger fibrin deposition. Fibrin strands form a tight mesh which deforms the erythrocytes as they are forced through the obstruction (microangiopathic hemolysis).

Morphological features are:

- Endocapillary proliferation: in response to fibrin and platelet deposition in glomerular tufts.
- Luminal narrowing: arterioles and small arteries show fibrin and erythrocytes in the walls, often with thrombosis which, when extensive, can result in cortical necrosis.

Clinical features and prognosis

Clinical features are:

- Sudden onset of oliguria with hematuria and occasionally melena.
- Jaundice.
- Anemia with schistocytes (fragmented erythrocytes) and thrombocytopenia.
- Hypertension in 50% of cases.

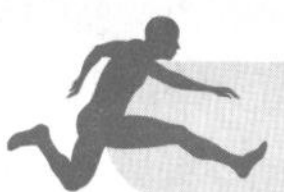

In childhood HUS, symptoms are often preceded by a prodromal episode of diarrhea or flu-like illness lasting for 5–15 days.

Prognosis depends on the severity of attack but mortality may be as high as 40%.

Thrombotic thrombocytopenic purpura

Thrombotic thrombocytopenic purpura (TTP) and HUS are thought to represent the same disease process but with a different distribution of thrombotic lesions. In TTP, occlusive plugs lead to widespread ischemic organ damage, especially of the brain and kidney, resulting in neurological abnormalities and progressive renal impairment.

Renal infarcts

There are two mechanisms of renal infarction: embolic infarction and diffuse cortical necrosis.

Embolic renal disease Renal infarcts are usually due to the passage of emboli down renal arterial branches. The most common causes are:

- Embolization of atheromatous material.
- Thrombotic material arising from the left side of the heart.
- Bacterial vegetation from infective endocarditis.

Resultant infarcts may be clinically silent or may result in hematuria and loin pain. Macroscopically, infarcts are pale or white and have a characteristic wedge shape with the apex directed toward the hilum.

Diffuse cortical necrosis This rare pattern of renal infarction is associated with conditions resulting in severe hypotension, the most common of which are hypovolemic shock, severe sepsis, and eclampsia of pregnancy.

The pathogenesis is uncertain, but diffuse spasm of renal blood vessels is thought to play a major part in precipitating ischemic damage.

Macroscopically, necrosis is confined to the outer part of the renal cortex, which in the acute stages is pale and focally hemorrhagic.

This condition results in acute renal failure, and prognosis depends on the extent of the damage.

Sickle cell disease nephropathy

Vascular occlusion of vasae rectae in sickle cell disease (p. 277) causes papillary necrosis, leading to the development of hematuria and polyuria.

Neoplastic disease of the kidney

Benign tumors of the kidney

These are common incidental findings at post mortem examination in about 20% of all patients; however, they rarely cause clinical problems.

Cortical adenoma

These are benign epithelial tumors derived from renal tubular epithelium.

Macroscopically, they are discrete nodules usually less than 20mm in diameter, situated in the cortex of the kidney.

Microscopically, appearances are similar to those of well-dfferentiated renal cell carcinomas, both being composed of well-differentiated large clear cells with small nuclei.

Difficulty in differentiating between these tumors has prompted the adoption of an arbitrary cut-off of 3cm in size to distinguish between the smaller adenomas and the typically larger carcinomas. However, the distinction is unreliable since some small lesions suspected of being adenomas may in fact be carcinomas capable of metastasis.

Renal fibroma or hamartoma (renomedullary interstitial cell tumor)

This is the most common benign tumor of the kidney. It is composed of spindle cells.

Macroscopically, there are firm white nodules situated in the medulla, typically 3–10mm in size.

Microscopically, it is composed of spindle cells that surround the adjacent tubules.

They are of no functional or clinical significance.

Angiomyolipoma

This hamartoma is composed of a mixture of smooth muscle, blood vessels, and fat, and it is situated either in the cortex or in the medulla. It is mainly seen in association with tuberous sclerosis.

Oncocytoma

This benign epithelial tumor is composed of large cells with granular, eosinophilic cytoplasm filled with mitochondria. It is a variant of the renal adenomas, and it can attain a considerable size leading to clinical confusion with renal cell carcinoma.

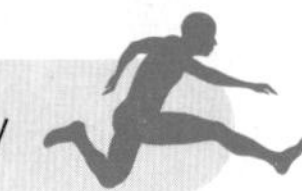

Malignant tumors of the kidney

Renal cell carcinoma (renal adenocarcinoma; hypernephroma)

An adenocarcinoma derived from the renal tubular epithelium in adults, this tumor accounts for about 3% of all carcinomas, and about 90% of primary malignant renal tumors. It is usually seen after the age of 50 years. Males are more often affected than females by 3:1.

There is an increased incidence in those who smoke tobacco and also in patients with von Hippel–Lindau syndrome, a rare hereditary condition (suggesting a genetic predisposition).

Associations—Paraneoplastic syndromes of hypercalcemia, hypertension, and polycythemia.

Macroscopically, tumors occur most commonly at the upper pole of a kidney. They are usually rounded masses, with a yellowish cut surface marked with areas of hemorrhage and necrosis.

Microscopically, they are composed of either clear or granular cell types. The most common is the "clear cell pattern," in which tumor cells have clear cytoplasm because of the high content of glycogen and lipid. Granular cell types are derived from tubular and papillary carcinomas.

Route of spread is:

- Local: eroding through renal capsule into perinephric fat.
- Lymphatic: to para-aortic and other nodes.
- Bloodborne metastasis: involving the lungs, bone, brain, and other sites as a result of tumor invasion of the renal vein. A characteristic feature is that large tumors may grow as a solid core along the main renal vein even entering the inferior vena cava.

Clinical features are:

- Common presenting symptoms: hematuria, loin pain, loin mass.

Occasional presenting symptoms: bone metastasis, brain metastasis, or polycythemia.

Prognosis depends on the stage at presentation. If the tumor is confined within a renal capsule there is a 70% chance of 10 years' survival. However, prognosis is very poor if metastases are present at diagnosis.

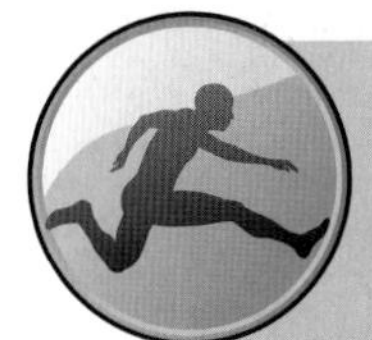

Differential diagnosis of unilateral enlargement of the kidney is:

- Hydronephrosis.
- Tumor.
- Renal vein thrombosis.
- Postcontralateral nephrectomy.
- Contralateral kidney failure.

Urothelial carcinoma of the renal pelvis

This malignant tumor of the renal pelvis is derived from the transitional cells of the urothelium, and it is mainly caused by environmental agents. It is associated with analgesic abuse and exposure to aniline dyes used in the dye, rubber, and plastics industries. Some cases have also been reported to develop many years after the use of Thorotrast, an α-particle-emitting contrast agent used in retrograde pyelography.

Tumors generally present early with hematuria or obstruction.

Histologically, tumors are similar in nature to those seen in the bladder (p. 175).

Wilms' tumor (nephroblastoma)

This malignant embryonal tumor is derived from the primitive metanephros. A common malignant tumor of childhood, its peak incidence is between the ages of 1 and 4 years. Males and females are equally affected.

At least three different types of genes are important in the formation of Wilm's tumor. The most characterized one being the tumor suppressor gene WT1, located on chromosome 11.

Macroscopically, large amounts of kidney are replaced by rounded masses of solid, fleshy, white lesions with frequent areas of necrosis. The tumor is aggressive and rapidly growing; extension beyond the capsule into perinephric fat and even into the root of mesentery is frequent. Spread to lungs is identified in a high proportion of cases at the time of diagnosis.

Microscopically, it is composed of up to four elements:

- Primitive, small-cell, blastematous tissue: resembles developing metanephric blastema.
- Immature-looking, glomerular structures.
- Epithelial tubules.

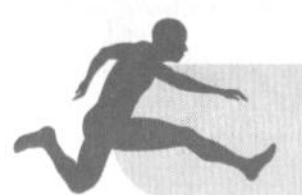

- Stroma composed of spindle cells and striated muscle.

Clinical presentation—Abdominal mass or hematuria.

Prognosis is related to the spread of the tumor at diagnosis (stage). Treatment is by a combination of radiotherapy and intensive chemotherapy, achieving a high cure rate.

Disorders of the urinary tract

Congenital abnormalities of the urinary tract

Ureteric abnormalities

Double and bifid ureters

The most common ureteric abnormality, these often occur in association with the duplication of the renal pelvis. They may be associated with vesicoureteric reflux, and they are predisposed to recurrent infections.

Ureteropelvic junction obstruction

This is most commonly caused by a stricture that may be either intrinsic (within the wall of the ureter) or extrinsic (associated with external factors such as an aberrant vessel). The condition causes an increase in the relative amount of fibrous tissue at the site of the stricture. This appears to provide a barrier to the conduction of a wave of contraction of the ureter.

Diverticulum

This is a rare outpouching of the ureter.

Megaloureter

In this common congenital anomaly, retention of urine within the enlarged ureter results in hydroureter. The condition predisposes to reflux and recurrent infections.

Bladder abnormalities

Diverticula

Congenital diverticula are rare and are more often acquired as a result of bladder outlet obstruction. Symptoms are due to stasis and the resultant infection.

Urethral abnormalities

Hypospadias

The urethra opens on to the underside of the penis, either on the glans (glandular hypospadias), at the junction of the glans with the shaft (coronal hypospadias), or on the shaft itself (penile hypospadias).

Epispadias

The urethra opens on to the dorsal (upper) surface of the penis.

All varieties can be corrected surgically.

Urinary tract obstruction and urolithiasis

Urinary tract obstruction

This is obstruction of urine drainage from the kidney occurring at any level within the urinary tract. Obstruction may be caused by either a structural lesion (majority) or congenital neuromuscular defects that prevent contraction waves, and thus the flow of urine.

Structural lesions can be classified into:

- Intrinsic lesions: within ureteric wall or lumen (e.g., urinary calculus (most common), caseous or necrotic debris, fibrosis following trauma or infection, tumor).
- Extrinsic lesions: cause pressure from without (e.g., tumors of the rectum, prostate, and bladder, aberrant renal arteries, retroperitoneal fibrosis, pregnancy).

Causes vary according to the site of the obstruction (Fig. 8.11), where * indicates the most common sites of obstruction:

- Renal pelvis: calculi, tumors.
- Pelviureteric junction*: stricture, calculi, extrinsic compression.
- Ureter: calculi, extrinsic compression (pregnancy, tumor, fibrosis).
- Bladder neck*: tumor, calculi.
- Urethra*: prostatic hyperplasia or carcinoma, urethral valves, urethral stricture.

Pathogenesis—Obstruction at any point in the urinary tract causes increased pressure superior to the blockage, with dilatation of the renal pelvis and calyces (hydronephrosis):

- Obstruction at the pelviureteric junction → hydronephrosis.
- Obstruction of the ureter → hydroureter with subsequent development of hydronephrosis.
- Obstruction of the bladder neck or urethra → bladder distension with hypertrophy of its muscle (seen on cystoscopic examination as

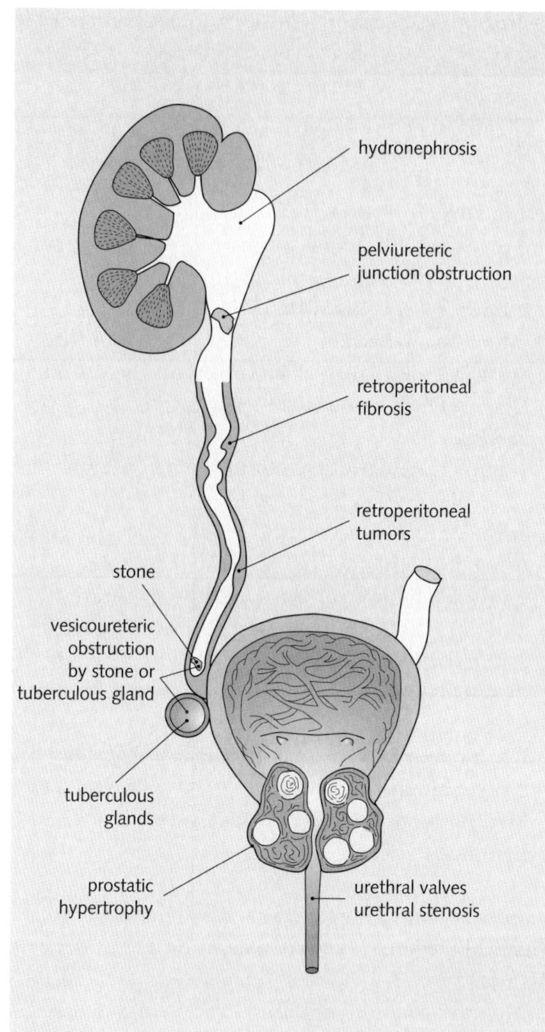

Fig. 8.11 Urinary tract showing common sites of obstruction.

trabeculation). Subsequently leads to hydroureter and hydronephrosis.

Hydronephrosis

Hydronephrosis may be:

- Unilateral: caused by obstruction at the level of the ureter, pelviureteric junction, or renal pelvis. Obstruction is typically detected late, because renal function is maintained by the non-obstructed kidney. Renal parenchyma becomes severely atrophic and renal function is permanently impaired (end-stage hydronephrosis).
- Bilateral: caused by obstruction at the level of the bladder or urethra. Obstruction is typically detected at an earlier stage, as renal failure develops before severe atrophy of both kidneys.

In both forms, urinary tract obstruction predisposes to infection of the bladder (cystitis) and kidney (pyelonephritis or pyonephrosis) as well as stone formation.

Effects of hydronephrosis The net result of hydronephrosis is that fluid entering the collecting ducts cannot empty into renal pelvis, and intrarenal resorption of fluid occurs.

If the obstruction is removed at this stage, then renal function returns to normal. However, persistence of obstruction leads to atrophy of the renal tubules with glomerular hyalinization and fibrosis.

Clinical features depend on the cause and site of the lesion.

Obstruction above the bladder will cause either an acute onset of renal colic or a gradual onset of aching pain in the loins, sometimes aggravated by drinking.

The clinical feature of obstruction below the bladder is difficulty in micturition, occasionally with distension of the bladder; it may progress to a bilateral ache in the loins.

Superimposed infection causes malaise, fever, dysuria, and sometimes septicemia.

Management is by removal of the obstruction and treatment of the infection.

Urolithiasis (urinary calculi)

This is the formation of stones in the urinary tract. It affects 1–5% of the population in the U.S. and onset is typically after 30 years of age, with males affected more than females.

Stones can form anywhere in the urinary tract but the most common site is within the renal pelvis.

Composition of stones:

- Calcium oxalate (75–80%).
- Triple phosphates (15%): magnesium ammonium phosphate stones.
- Uric acid (5%).
- Calculi in cystinuria and oxalosis.

Etiology is:

- Acquired: as a result of urinary tract obstruction, persistent urinary tract infection, reduced urine volume (low fluid intake or excessive sweating).

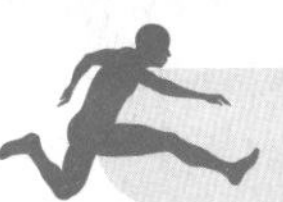

- Inherited: primary metabolic disturbances (e.g., cystinuria, xanthinuria)

The mechanism of stone formation is not well understood, but it is thought to involve an excess of solute in the urine (due to either a primary increase in metabolite, or stasis) or reduced solubility of solute in the urine (due to persistently abnormal urinary pH).

Calculi vary greatly in size, from sand-like particles to large round stones. "Staghorn calculi" fill the whole renal pelvis and branch into calyces. Deposits of calcium may be present throughout renal parenchyma giving rise to nephrocalcinosis.

The condition may present with:

- Renal colic often with nausea and vomiting: caused by the passage of small stones along the ureter.
- Dull ache in the loins: due to the presence of stones in the kidney.
- Strangury (the desire to pass something that will not pass): caused by stones in the bladder.
- Recurrent and intractable urinary tract infection, hematuria, or renal failure.

Occasionally, the condition is asymptomatic, discovered only during radiological examination for another disease.

Management is by bed rest, application of warmth to the site of pain, and administration of analgesia.

Small stones (<0.5cm) in diameter are usually passed naturally. Larger stones may require surgical intervention.

Inflammation of the urinary tract

Cystitis

This is inflammation of the bladder and it is extremely common—most women will have one or more episodes of cystitis. Females are affected more often than males because they have a short urethra (i.e., less travelling distance for bacteria).

Etiology

The condition is most commonly due to infection, but it is occasionally caused by physical agents (e.g., radiation or mechanical irritants).

Infective causes:

- Bacterial infection (most common): usually gram-negative coliform bacilli (e.g., *E. coli* and *Proteus*), but *Streptococcus faecalis*, *Pseudomonas aeruginosa*, and staphylococci are also common.
- Viral infection: adenovirus may cause hemorrhagic cystitis in children.
- Parasites: *Schistosoma haematobium*, which is common in Africa.
- Fungi: *Candida*.

Risk factors are:

- Urinary retention: due to obstruction, bladder paralysis, diverticula, calculi, foreign bodies, tumors, uterine prolapse.
- Infection of adjacent structures (e.g., prostatitis, urethritis, and diverticular disease of the colon).
- Diabetes mellitus.
- Pregnancy.
- Trauma (e.g., catheterization).

Routes of infection are:

- Ascending infection (most common): from urethral infection, or introduction of bacteria directly into the bladder via the urethra (e.g., on catheterization).
- Descending infection: from the kidney (e.g., renal tuberculosis).
- Direct spread: from adjacent organs (e.g., diverticulitis).
- Hematogenous: rare.
- Lymphatic: extremely rare.

Macroscopically, there is acute inflammation with edema, erythema, and later ulceration of bladder mucosa.

Microscopically, there is infiltration of mucosa with acute inflammatory cells.

Clinical features—Urinary tract infections may present with any of the following features:

- Disorders of micturition: increases in frequency, urgency, dysuria, hematuria, and incontinence.
- Pain in the right iliac fossa, loin, and suprapubic area.
- Pyrexia.

Investigation, treatment, and sequelae

Investigations—Examination of midstream urine (see p. 166 for definitions of significant bacteruria and pyuria).

Treatment is by:

- Increased fluid intake to flush out organisms.
- Antibiotic therapy (e.g., trimethoprim).
- Treatment of any underlying causes (e.g., obstruction).

Sequelae:

- Resolution (which is common).
- Chronicity if the underlying cause is untreatable.
- Development of pyelonephritis and associated complications.

Interstitial cystitis (Hunner's ulcer)

This is a condition of unknown etiology, in which the bladder is inflamed, fibrotic and of small capacity, but the urine is sterile. It is characterized clinically by suprapubic pain and increased frequency.

Macroscopically, there is linear ulceration and erythema.

Microscopically, there is fibrosis and lymphocytic infiltration through the full thickness of the bladder wall.

Malakoplakia

A rare variant of cystitis, the bladder mucosa develops yellow plaques composed of a mixture of chronic inflammatory cells including characteristic granule-containing macrophages. Granules (known as Michaelis–Gutmann bodies) are composed of calcified bacterial debris, and they are thought to reflect defective macrophage functions.

Plaques may subsequently undergo ulceration thus mimicking a bladder tumor.

Ureteritis

This inflammation of the ureter is usually due to an ascending urinary tract infection.

Causative organisms are the same as for cystitis.

Pathogenesis—In most cases, lower urinary tract infection remains localized to the urethra and bladder. Occasionally, organisms may ascend the ureter and enter the pelvicalyceal system, particularly when there is an obstructive lesion. Thus, an acute bacterial cystitis may lead to an ascending ureteritis and pyelitis (inflammation of the renal pelvis and calyces).

Complications—Organisms may gain access to the renal parenchyma to produce acute pyelonephritis, with the formation of abscesses in the renal medulla and cortex.

Ureteritis follicularis

This ureteritis presents with large aggregates of lymphoid cells.

Ureteritis cystica

This is a complication of chronic ureteritis in which epithelial nests become trapped by fibrosis and subsequently develop into thin-walled cysts.

Neoplastic disease of the urinary tract

Tumors of the ureter

Tumors of the ureter are extremely rare and almost always epithelial.

Fibroepithelial polyps

These are benign papillary tumors.

Malignant urothelial tumors

These tumors arise from the transitional cell epithelium of the ureter. They are mainly caused by environmental agents (see below), and they are identical to those seen in the bladder.

Bladder metaplasia

Metaplasia

Glandular metaplasia (cystitis glandularis)

These small, rounded collections of urothelial cells are found just below the urothelial surface (Brunn's nests). They develop a central lumen surrounded by cuboidal or columnar cells. These are quite common and often seen in the normal bladder.

Occasionally, there is metaplasia to an intestinal variant of cystitis glandularis, lined by colonic, mucin-secreting epithelium.

Adenomatous metaplasia (nephrogenic adenoma)

This benign condition is characterized by metaplasia of the urothelium to cuboidal epithelium. Metaplastic areas resemble collecting tubules of the kidney. It is associated with chronic infections (e.g., tuberculosis).

Squamous metaplasia There are two types:

- Keratinizing squamous metaplasia (leukoplakia): the bladder mucosa develops white plaques, which are often secondary to chronic irritation (e.g., calcul). This occurs in both males and females, and a significant proportion progress to squamous carcinoma of the bladder.
- Nonkeratinizing squamous metaplasia (vaginal metaplasia): white plaques are seen on the trigone. This only occurs in women and it has no pathological significance.

Tumors of the bladder

Transitional cell papilloma

These are rare benign tumors of the bladder that may represent the first stage of transitional cell carcinoma. A fibrovascular stalk attaches their branched structure to the mucosa.

Transitional cell carcinoma

These are tumors of the urothelium, affecting 1 in 5000 in the U.S. and accounting for 3% of all cancer deaths. They are found in those aged 60–70 years, with males affected more than females by 3:1.

Etiology is as follows:

- Chemicals: exposure to environmental agents excreted in high concentrations in the urine. Known carcinogens are associated with cigarette smoking, aniline dyes, and the rubber industry.
- Leukoplakia (see above): associated with bladder stones.
- Bladder diverticula: about 3% are complicated with tumor.

Most tumors are at the base of trigone and around the ureteric orifices.

Morphological types:

- Papillary (most common): warty masses projecting into the lumen with little or no invasion of the bladder wall. Only a small percentage evolve into invasive carcinoma.
- Solid: tumors grow directly into the bladder wall and are often ulcerated or encrusted. Most are invasive from the outset.
- Mixed papillary and solid.
- Flat in-situ carcinoma: reddened mucosal surface due to underlying telangiectatic blood vessels. May become invasive.

The majority of urothelial cancers are caused by exposure to environmental agents. Therefore, bladder tumors are usually multiple, and they are often found in conjunction with urothelial tumors at other sites of the lower urinary tract (e.g., renal pelvis, ureters, or urethra).

Other tumors of the bladder

Only a small proportion of bladder cancers are of squamous origin (squamous cell carcinoma). They are most often associated with calculi and schistosomiasis. Adenocarcinomas and mesenchymal tumors are rare. Secondary tumors usually occur following direct invasion from the cervix, prostate, or rectum.

Grading and staging of bladder carcinomas

The degree of differentiation (grade) and extent of spread (stage) are important indicators for prognosis.

Grading

Transitional cell carcinomas are graded I–III:

- Grade I (well differentiated): vast majority are papillary growths with no evidence of invasion.
- Grade II (moderately well differentiated): usually papillary, but many are either invasive at presentation or become so. Cells show significant atypicality and an increase in mitotic figures.
- Grade III (poorly differentiated): mainly solid lesions which are extensively invasive. Cells are pleomorphic with numerous mitoses.

TNM (tumor–node–metastasis) staging

The TNM staging is as follows:

- T1: tumor confined to mucosa or submucosa.
- T2: superficial muscle involved.
- T3: deep muscle involved.
- T4: invasion beyond the bladder.

Spread is as follows:

- Local: to pelvic structures.
- Lymphatic: to iliac and para-aortic lymph nodes.
- Hematogenous: to liver and lung.

Clinically, the disease commonly presents with painless (or painful) hematuria or recurrent urinary tract infections. Rarely, it may present with hydronephrosis (from ureteric obstruction), pneumaturia from vesicocolic fistula, or incontinence from vesicovaginal fistula.

Treatment depends on the stage at diagnosis:

- Diathermy via cystoscope: for T1 and T2 stages (± chemo- or radiotherapy).
- Radical radiotherapy, cystectomy, or a combination of the two for T3 stage.
- Palliative radiotherapy for T4 stage.

Prognosis depends on the histological type of the tumor and extent of spread. Papillary, noninvasive tumors have an excellent prognosis, whereas solid, invasive, urothelial tumors only have an overall 35% 5-year survival rate.

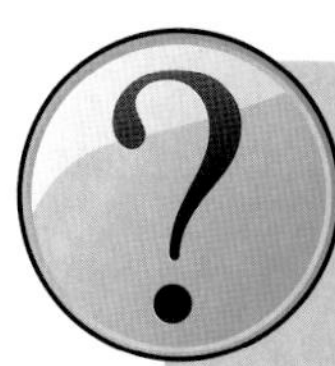

- List the types of cystic diseases of the kidney.
- Describe the pathology of adult polycystic kidney disease (autosomal dominant). Compare with infantile polycystic disease (autosomal recessive).
- List the distribution patterns of glomerular disease.
- Explain the differences between nephritic and nephrotic syndrome.
- State the mechanisms of immune-mediated glomerulonephritic injury.
- Describe the two types of membranoproliferative glomerulonephritis.
- Describe the patterns of glomerulonephritis that may occur in SLE.
- Name the vasculitic diseases that cause glomerulonephritis.
- Describe the glomerular lesions that occur in diabetic glomerulosclerosis.
- State the causes of acute tubular necrosis.
- Describe the pathogenesis of acute tubular necrosis.
- List the complications of acute pyelonephritis.
- What is nephrocalcinosis?
- How does multiple myeloma cause tubular interstitial nephritis?
- Describe the effects of renal artery stenosis and the mechanism of renal infarcts.
- Describe the pathology of renal cell carcinoma and Wilms' tumor.
- What are the common congenital abnormalities of the ureter, bladder, and urethra?
- List the causes of urinary tract obstruction. What are the types of kidney stones?
- State the risk factors for development of cystitis.
- Name the metaplastic tumors of the bladder.

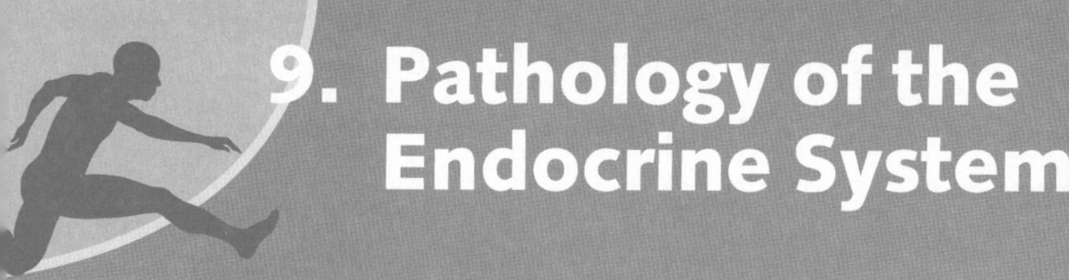

9. Pathology of the Endocrine System

Disorders of the pituitary

The pituitary (hypophysis) is a small gland (500–1000mg) lying in the sella turcica in the base of the skull. It is composed of two parts:

- Anterior lobe (adenohypophysis): synthesizes and secretes a number of hormones (Fig. 9.1), most of which act on other endocrine glands.
- Posterior lobe (neurohypophysis): stores and secretes two hormones synthesized in the hypothalamus, namely antidiuretic hormone (ADH; vasopressin) and oxytocin. This lobe is in direct continuity with the hypothalamus.

Secretion of the pituitary hormones is regulated by neural and chemical stimuli from the hypothalamus, diseases of which cause secondary abnormalities in pituitary function.

The anterior pituitary: hyperpituitarism

Hyperpituitarism is defined as excessive secretion of one or more of the pituitary hormones. Its most common causes are functioning (hormone-secreting) adenomas of the anterior lobe.

Anterior lobe adenomas

Anterior lobe adenomas comprise about 10% of all intracranial tumors (posterior lobe adenomas do not occur). These tumors do not usually metastasize, but they are often life-threatening because of their position and ability to secrete excess hormone.

Effects of pituitary adenomas

Pituitary adenomas cause problems because of a combination of endocrine effects (excessive secretion of a particular hormone) and compressive effects, caused by an increase in local pressure of the following:

- Remainder of the pituitary → hypopituitarism.
- Optic chiasm → visual field defects, notably bitemporal hemianopia.
- Brain (large tumors) → distortion of the midbrain with internal hydrocephalus.
- Dura → headaches.
- Cavernous sinus → CN III, IV, or VI nerve palsies.

The endocrine effects depend on which hormone is being excessively secreted (see below).

Investigations:

- Imaging: plain X-ray (can detect enlargement of sella turcica and erosion of the clinoid processes), computed tomography (CT) scans, magnetic resonance imaging (MRI), cisternography.
- Hormone assays (e.g., growth hormone, prolactin).
- Functional testing of the pituitary–adrenal axis.
- Visual field assessment.

Types of functioning adenomas

Functioning adenomas may produce any of the adenophyseal (anterior lobe) hormones, but the majority produce either prolactin (produced by prolactinomas—lactotroph adenomas), growth hormone (produced by somatotroph adenomas), or adrenocorticotrophic hormone (ACTH; produced by corticotroph adenomas).

Prolactinomas

Abnormally increased prolactin secretion is associated in women with menstrual irregularity and infertility, and in men with ejaculatory failure or impotence.

Galactorrhea is present in about 30% of affected women, but it is rare in men since estrogen priming is required for lactation.

Somatotroph adenoma

This results in hypersecretion of growth hormone, the effects of which depend on the developmental stage of the affected individual:

- Pre-epiphyseal union (prepubertal) leads to gigantism (syn. giantism), i.e., excessive growth in a regular and initially well-proportioned manner. Most giants also show some features of acromegaly with disproportionate enlargement (e.g., of the hands and jaw).
- Postepiphyseal union (adults) leads to acromegaly, which is characterized by enlargement of the hands, feet, and head. They may also present with

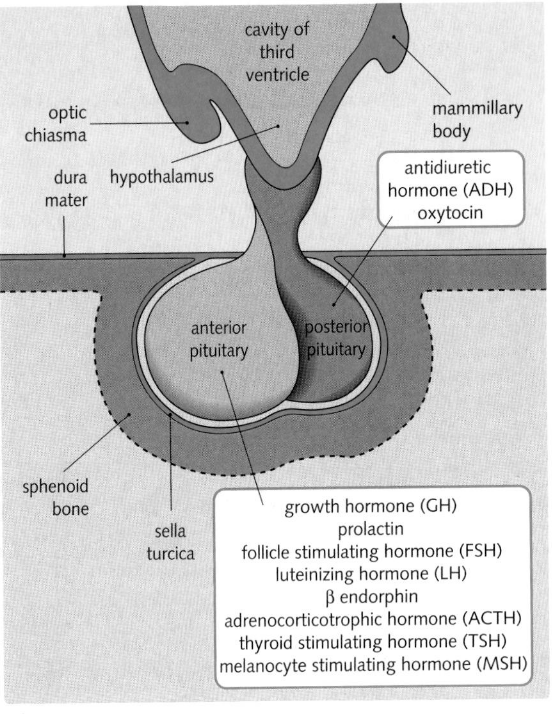

Fig. 9.1 Pituitary and hypothalamus and their hormones.

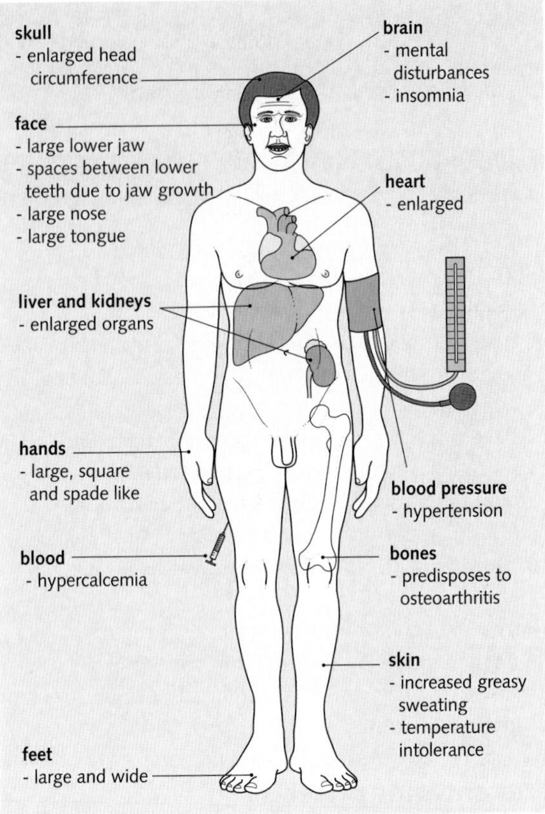

Fig. 9.2 Features of acromegaly.

secondary diabetes (growth hormone is an insulin antagonist) or cardiovascular effects (Fig. 9.2).

There are three types of treatment:

- Surgery—hypophysectomy (transfrontal or transphenoidal), especially where there are signs of compression of adjacent structures.
- Radiotherapy—fewer complications than surgery, but less successful.
- Drug therapy—bromocriptine lowers growth hormone levels in uncomplicated acromegaly.

Corticotroph adenoma

Overproduction of ACTH by the pituitary gland (Cushing's disease) causes adrenal hyperplasia, resulting in the excessive secretion of glucocorticoids causing Cushing's syndrome, the effects of which are described in "Disorders of the Adrenal Gland" (p. 192).

Other functioning adenomas

Other endocrine secreting adenomas (e.g., of thyroid-stimulating hormone (TSH), luteinizing hormone (LH), and follicle-stimulating hormone (FSH)), are extremely rare.

The anterior pituitary—hypopituitarism

Hypopituitarism is defined as insufficient secretion of the pituitary hormones. The clinical features are dependent on the patient's age, and the type and severity of the hormone deficiencies (Fig. 9.3).

Hypopituitarism can be caused by either hypothalamic lesions or pituitary lesions.

Hypothalamic lesions are:

- Idiopathic deficiency of one or more of the releasing factors, such as GnRH (gonadotrophin-releasing factor) (Kallmann's syndrome), GHRH (growth-hormone releasing factor), or more rarely TRH (thyrotrophin-releasing factor) or CRF (corticotrophin-releasing factor).
- Infarction.
- Inflammation.
- Suprasellar tumors (e.g., craniopharyngioma) or more rarely pinealoma, teratoma, or a secondary tumor from another site.

Clinical features associated with specific forms of hypopituitarism		
Hormone deficiency	**Clinical features**	**Tests to exclude hypofunction of anterior pituitary**
Gonadotrophin deficiency	Prepubertal: • failure to enter puberty • undescended testes • obesity • eunuchoidism Postpubertal: • infertility • amenorrhea • oligospermia • progressive loss of secondary sex characteristics (hypogonadism) • osteoporotic collapse of spine → loss of stature	LH reserves adequate if: • males have a normal testosterone • females are ovulating FSH reserves adequate if: • males have normal spermatogenesis • females are ovulating
GH deficiency	Children: failure of longitudinal growth Adults: tendency to hypoglycemia	GH reserves adequate if: • random plasma level >20mU/L • stress or otherwise elevated GH peak >20mU/L
TSH deficiency	Fetus or newborn: cretinism Adults: hypothyroidism	TSH reserves adequate if serum thyroxine within normal range
ACTH deficiency	Features of primary hypoadrenalism but with decreased pigmentation (rather than an increase)	ACTH reserves adequate if: • random plasma cortisol >550nmol/L • stress-induced cortisol rise >550nmol/L

Fig. 9.3 Clinical features associated with specific forms of hypopituitarism.

Pituitary lesions are:
- Idiopathic deficiency of one or more of the pituitary hormones.
- Nonfunctioning chromophobe pituitary adenomas: adenomas of the anterior pituitary (usually derived from non-hormone-secreting chromophobe cells), which may cause hypopituitarism by compression or obliteration of normal pituitary tissue.
- Sheehan's syndrome: ischemic necrosis of the adenohypophysis due to hypotensive shock occurring as a result of intrapartum or postpartum hemorrhage.
- Empty sella syndrome: occupation of the sella by a CSF-containing arachnoid space. This may be a primary anatomical variant or it may follow spontaneous infarction, surgery, or radiotherapy of a tumor.
- Trauma, including surgery and radiotherapy.
- Granulomatous lesions: sarcoidosis, tuberculosis, histiocytosis.

Management
Management is by substitution therapy according to the deficiencies demonstrated, such as cortisol replacement for ACTH deficiency, thyroid hormone replacement for TSH deficiency.

The posterior pituitary
Diseases of the posterior pituitary are much less common than those of the anterior pituitary, and they are usually the result of damage to the hypothalamus by tumor invasion or infarction. Posterior pituitary diseases typically cause disorders of abnormal ADH secretion. There are no known effects of abnormal oxytocin secretion.

Diabetes insipidus
Diabetes insipidus (DI) is a rare condition characterized by the persistent excretion of excessive quantities of dilute urine and by constant thirst.

There are two types:
- Cranial DI: caused by the failure of ADH production.
- Nephrogenic DI: distal tubules are refractory to the water reabsorptive action of ADH (Fig. 9.4).

Clinical features—Regardless of etiology, reabsorption of water from the glomerular filtrate in the renal collecting ducts does not occur, resulting in

Causes of cranial and nephrogenic diabetes insipidus (DI)		
	Cause	**Features**
Cranial DI	Hypothalamic or pituitary stalk damage	Surgical damage, usually in the course of tumor removal Head injury, usually transient Hypothalamic tumor (either primary or secondary) Hypothalamic inflammatory lesions, e.g., sarcoidosis, encephalitis, meningitis
	Genetic defects	Dominant Recessive: DIDMOAD syndrome–association of DI with diabetes mellitus (DM), optic atrophy (OA), and deafness (D)
	Idiopathic	About 30% of cases have no known cause
Nephrogenic DI	Hereditary	Abnormality of ADH receptors
	Metabolic abnormalities	Hypokalemia Hypercalcemia
	Drug therapy	Lithium Demethylchlortetracycline
	Poisoning	Heavy metals

Fig. 9.4 Causes of cranial and nephrogenic diabetes insipidus (DI).

the excretion of large quantities of dilute urine (polyuria) with a high risk of body water depletion. DI is potentially lethal without appropriate therapy.

Investigations—Water deprivation test for 8 hours or until 3% of the body weight is lost. Demonstration of continued polyuria and increased hemoconcentration indicates DI. This test serves to differentiate DI from psychogenic polydipsia. The test is then followed by ADH administration to differentiate between cranial DI (kidneys are responsive to ADH) or nephrogenic DI (kidneys are unresponsive to ADH).

Treatment of mild DI—The effects of dehydration can be counteracted by greatly increasing water intake (polydipsia).

Treatment of moderate to severe DI:

- Cranial DI: treatment with desmopressin (ADH analog but without vasoactive effects).
- Nephrogenic DI: treatment with thiazide diuretics, producing a decrease in urine volume by approximately 50%.

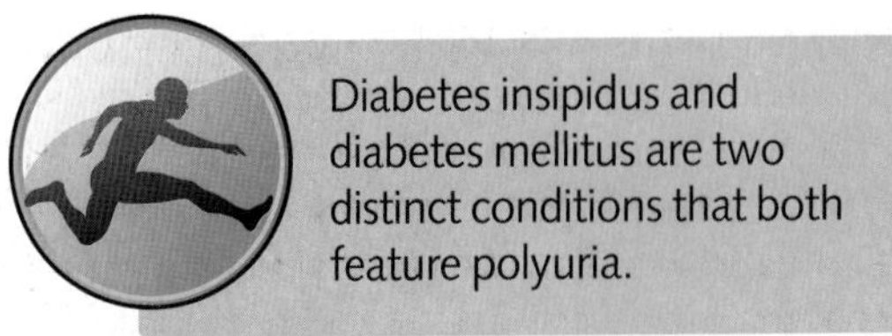

Syndrome of inappropriate antidiuretic hormone secretion

Increased secretion of ADH occurs as a complication of other diseases. (Primary hypersecretion of ADH is not recognized.) The condition is characterized by water retention with hemodilution, and, in severe cases, cerebral edema supervenes with impaired consciousness.

The causes are:

- Idiopathic.
- Tumors: ectopic secretion of ADH, especially by oat cell carcinomas of the lung and some neuroendocrine tumors.
- Trauma: skull fracture, head injury, or surgery may produce transiently increased secretion of ADH.
- Intracranial inflammation: meningitis, tuberculosis, syphilis.
- Thoracic diseases (e.g., pneumonia, pulmonary embolus), probably due to involvement of intrathoracic baroreceptors.

Fig. 9.5 shows a comparison table of features of DI with those of inappropriate ADH secretion.

Disorders of the pineal gland

The pineal gland is located above the third ventricle and secretes the hormone melatonin. Melatonin is

Comparison of features of diabetes insipidus with those of inappropriate ADH secretion			
Condition	**Imbalance**	**Urinary and plasma osmolality**	**Symptoms**
Diabetes insipidus	↓ ADH	Low urinary osmolality High plasma osmolality	Polyuria (5–20L/day) Thirst Polydipsia (may lead to severe dehydration, exhaustion, coma)
Syndrome of inappropriate ADH secretion	↑ ADH	High urinary osmolality Low plasma osmolality (dilutional hyponatremia)	Oliguria Water intoxication (may lead to confusion, neurological disturbances, coma)

Fig. 9.5 Comparison of features of diabetes insipidus with those of inappropriate ADH secretion.

thought to function in circadian rhythm control and gonadal maturation.

Pinealomas (germinomas)

These common tumors of young adults and children are often called germinomas. They are thought to originate from primitive germ cells, and histologically they resemble testicular seminomas and/or teratomas:

- Pressure on the midbrain may produce Parinaud's syndrome (paralysis of the conjugate upward gaze without paralysis of convergence).
- Pressure on the hypothalamus can produce symptoms of DI, emaciation, or precocious puberty.

Thyroid disorders

Thyrotoxicosis (hyperthyroidism)

This syndrome is caused by the excessive secretion of thyroid hormones (typically both thyroxine, T_4, and tri-iodothyronine, T_3) in the bloodstream. Symptoms include tachycardia, sweating, tremor, anxiety, increased appetite, loss of weight, and intolerance of heat.

Hyperthyroidism can be classified on the basis of etiology into:

- Primary hyperthyroidism (↑ thyroid hormones, ↓ TSH): hypersecretion of thyroid hormones, which is not secondary to increased levels of TSH.
- Secondary hyperthyroidism (↑ thyroid hormones, ↑ TSH): overstimulation of the thyroid gland caused by excess TSH produced by a tumor in the pituitary or elsewhere (rare).

The causes of primary hyperthyroidism:

- Graves' disease (exophthalmic goiter): most common cause of thyrotoxicosis, characterized by a diffusely enlarged thyroid gland, which is stimulated to produce excess hormone by an IgG autoantibody.
- Toxic multinodular goiter (Plummer's disease): second most common cause of hyperthyroidism.
- Toxic adenoma: solitary thyroid nodule producing excess hormone with remainder of the thyroid gland being suppressed.
- Ingestion of large doses of thyroid hormone (thyrotoxicosis factitia).

Effects of thyrotoxicosis

Signs and symptoms of thyrotoxicosis are a consequence of an increase in the body's metabolism, which occurs as a direct result of increased concentrations of the thyroid hormones. The most important symptoms diagnostically are:

- Heat intolerance and excessive sweating (hyperhidrosis).
- Nervousness and irritability.
- Weight loss with normal or increased appetite.
- Goiter (an enlargement of the thyroid gland).

Other symptoms are summarized in Fig. 9.6.

Investigations—Hyperthyroidism is confirmed by raised serum thyroxine and/or lowered serum TSH.

Management is by:

- Surgery: reduces the amount of functioning thyroid tissue.
- Radioactive iodine to destroy part of the gland.
- Drugs (such as carbimazole or propylthiouracil) that interfere with the production of thyroid hormones.

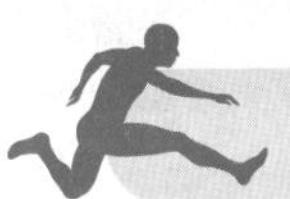

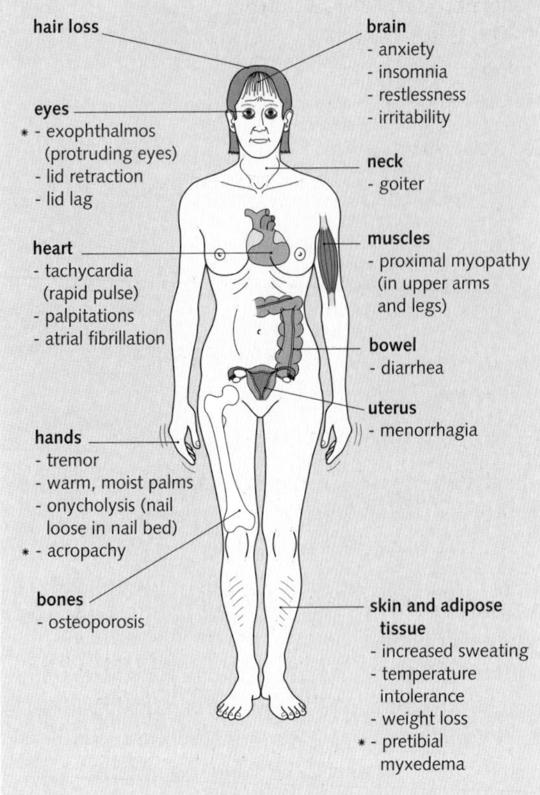

Fig. 9.6 Summary diagram illustrating features of thyrotoxicosis. (* = additional features seen only in Graves' disease.)

Hypothyroidism

Decreased activity of the thyroid gland results in decreased production of thyroid hormones. There are two forms:

Hypothyroidism present at birth → cretinism or congenital hypothyroidism.

Hypothyroidism in adults → myxedema.

Cretinism (congenital hypothyroidism)

This condition occurs as a result of extreme hypothyroidism during fetal life, infancy, or childhood. It has the following types and etiology:

- Endemic cretinism, which occurs in iodine-deficient countries where goiter is common. The mother almost always has a goiter, and the thyroid of the affected infant is usually enlarged and nodular.
- Sporadic cretinism, which is caused by congenital hypoplasia or absence of the thyroid gland and often associated with deaf mutism.
- Dyshormonogenesis, which is a congenital familial recessive enzyme defect leading to inability to complete the formation of thyroid hormones. TSH is increased, and the thyroid gland is enlarged and shows epithelial hyperplasia.

The clinical features of cretinism are:

- Mental retardation.
- Retarded growth: skeletal growth is inhibited more than soft tissue growth, hence the cretinism appearance of the obese, stocky, short child.
- Coarse, dry skin.
- Lack of hair and teeth.
- Pot belly (often with umbilical hernia).
- Protruding tongue.

Management is by early detection and treatment with thyroxine, which can prevent an irreversible mental defect and cerebellar damage. Many countries now have screening programs measuring serum TSH and/or thyroxine levels on heel-prick blood samples taken on the fourth or fifth day of life.

Hypothyroidism in adults (myxedema)

This common clinical condition is associated with decreased function of the thyroid gland and a decrease in the circulating level of thyroid hormones. It affects 8 per 10,000 people in the U.S., with females more than males by 4 to 1, and it can present at any age but most commonly between 30 and 50 years of age.

Note that, strictly speaking, myxedema describes a nonpitting, edematous reaction characteristic of hypothyroidism caused by the deposition of a mucoid substance ("myxo–" is a prefix denoting mucus) in the skin and elsewhere in the body. However, the terms "myxedema" and "hypothyroidism of adults" are now frequently used interchangeably.

Hypothyroidism can be classified according to etiology:

Primary (↓ thyroid hormones, ↑ TSH): failure of the thyroid gland itself. (This is much more common than secondary hypothyroidism.)

Secondary (↓ thyroid hormones, ↓ TSH): failure of TSH production due to pituitary disease.

The causes of primary hypothyroidism are:

- Autoimmune thyroiditis: atrophic form (e.g., primary atrophic thyroiditis) and goitrous form (such as Hashimoto's thyroiditis).

- Graves' disease: approximately 5% of patients with thyrotoxicosis develop hypothyroidism in later years, unrelated to treatment. Probably caused by a spectrum of antithyroid antibodies, some of which stimulate TSH receptor and some of which are destructive.
- Treatment of hyperthyroidism: surgical ablation, radioiodine, or drug treatment.
- Severe iodine deficiency (rare in the U.S.): iodine must be virtually absent from the diet before myxedema develops.

The effects of hypothyroidism are shown in Fig. 9.7.

Signs and symptoms of hypothyroidism are a consequence of widespread effects (which decrease the body's metabolism due to reduced concentrations of thyroid hormones) and of localized effects (myxedema due to the accumulation of mucoproteins). The most important symptoms diagnostically are:

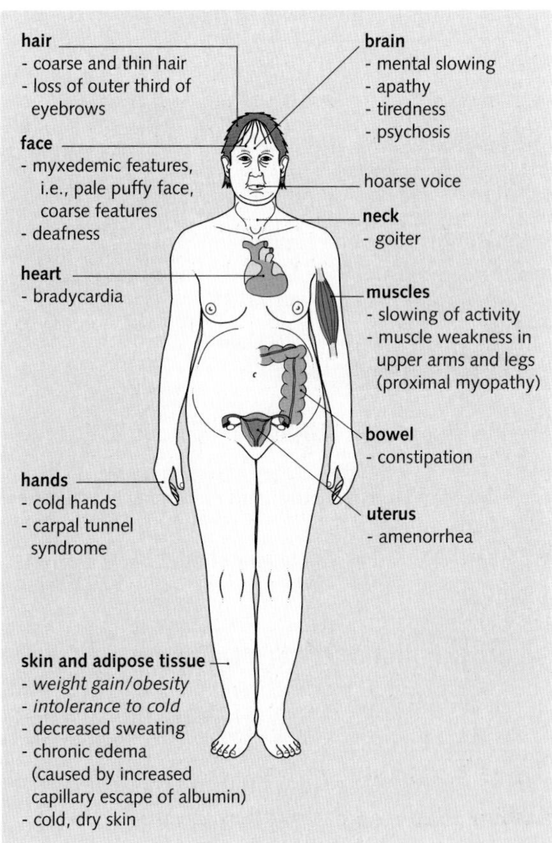

Fig. 9.7 Summary diagram illustrating features of hypothyroidism in the adult (myxedema).

- Mental and physical slowness.
- Tiredness.
- Cold intolerance.
- Dryness of skin and hair.

Investigations are:
- Serum thyroxine concentration (decreased in hypothyroidism).
- Serum TSH concentration (reduced in secondary hypothyroidism but increased in primary hypothyroidism).

The treatment is oral thyroxine daily for life.

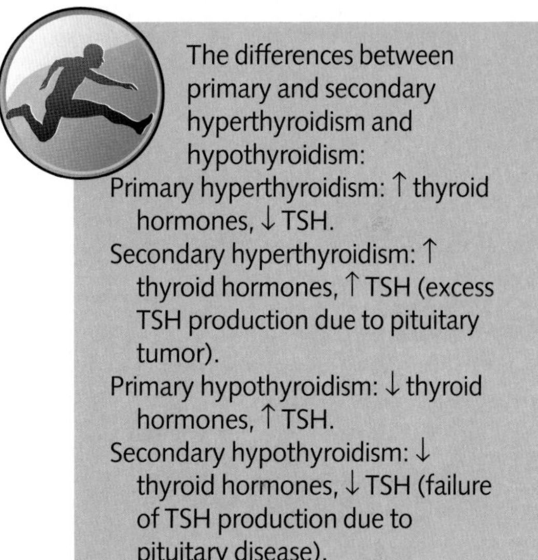

The differences between primary and secondary hyperthyroidism and hypothyroidism:

Primary hyperthyroidism: ↑ thyroid hormones, ↓ TSH.

Secondary hyperthyroidism: ↑ thyroid hormones, ↑ TSH (excess TSH production due to pituitary tumor).

Primary hypothyroidism: ↓ thyroid hormones, ↑ TSH.

Secondary hypothyroidism: ↓ thyroid hormones, ↓ TSH (failure of TSH production due to pituitary disease).

Congenital disorders of the thyroid

Development of the thyroid

The thyroid gland develops from an endodermal thickening in the floor of the primitive pharynx at a point later indicated by the foramen caecum of tongue (Fig. 9.8). As the embryo grows, the thyroid

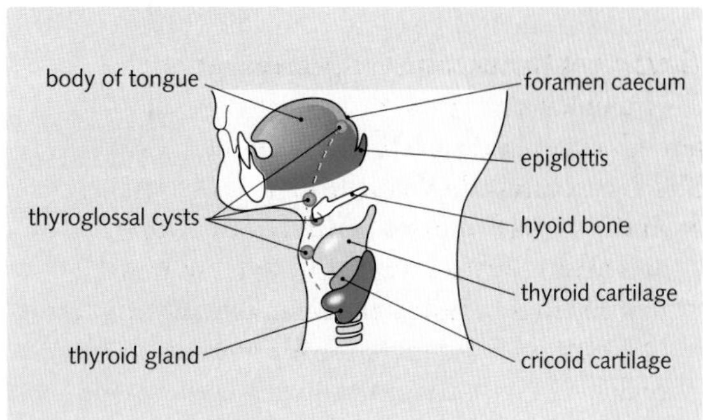

Fig. 9.8 Path of descent of thyroid gland (broken line) and localization of thyroglossal cysts.

descends into the neck, passing anterior to the hyoid and laryngeal cartilages. During migration, the gland remains connected to the tongue by a narrow canal, the thyroglossal duct, which later becomes solid and finally disappears.

Thyroglossal cysts

Cystic remnants of parts of the thyroglossal duct are known as thyroglossal cysts (Fig. 9.8). These cysts may form anywhere along the course of descent, but they are always located near or in the midline of the neck, most commonly just inferior to the hyoid bone. Cysts usually develop as painless, progressively enlarging, and movable masses. Infection of cysts may result in the formation of sinuses that open through the skin.

Thyroiditis

This is inflammation of the thyroid gland, which may have a viral or autoimmune etiology.

Hashimoto's thyroiditis (most common cause of hypothyroidism)

This organ-specific autoimmune disease results in destructive thyroiditis. It can occur at any age, but it typically affects the middle-aged, and females more than males by 12:1.

The most common autoantibodies are antimicrosomal antibody and antithyroglobulin. The disease is associated with the HLA-DR5 and HLA-B8 haplotypes, and patients with Hashimoto's disease (and Graves' disease) show a high incidence of other autoimmune diseases.

Macroscopically, the thyroid gland is usually:

- Diffusely enlarged (typically 2–5 times normal size).
- Firm in consistency.
- White or gray on a cut surface as a result of the disappearance of brown (iodine-rich) colloid (thyroglobulin), and its replacement by lymphocytes.

Microscopically, the thyroid gland shows:

- Small thyroid follicles infiltrated by lymphocytes and plasma cells.
- Lymphoid follicle formation and increased fibrous tissue stroma.
- Acini lined with abnormal, highly eosinophilic epithelial cells (mitochondria proliferation) termed Askanazy cells, Hürthle cells, or oncocytes.
- Reduced colloid content of disrupted acini.

The condition may present with a goiter or with hypothyroidism. However, damage to thyroid follicles may lead to the release of thyroglobulin into the circulation causing a transient phase of thyrotoxicosis. Some cases proceed to primary atrophic thyroiditis. Furthermore there is an increased incidence of non-Hodgkin's lymphoma originating in the thyroid of patients with Hashimoto's thyroiditis.

Treatment is by oral thyroxine, which overcomes hypothyroidism and reduces the size of the goiter.

De Quervain's thyroiditis

A rare, viral thyroiditis seen in young and middle-aged women as a slightly diffuse tender swelling of the thyroid, this is also known as subacute, giant cell, or granulomatous thyroiditis. The condition usually occurs in association with a transient febrile illness, often during various viral epidemics.

Characteristic features are:

- Painful enlargement of the thyroid (about twice normal size; normal weight is 20–30g).
- History of usually short duration.
- Preceded by general malaise, pyrexia, or upper respiratory infection.

Histological examination shows:

- Inflammation with a giant cell granulomatous reaction engulfing leaked colloid (hence the synonyms giant cell or granulomatous thyroiditis).
- Degeneration of follicles with inflammatory cell infiltration (neutrophils, plasma cells, lymphocytes, and histiocytes).
- Fibrous scarring.

The illness is usually self-limiting and settles in a few weeks. Transient hyperthyroidism can result from the release of thyroglobulin and excessive amounts of thyroid hormone.

Severe thyroiditis may be fatal in the elderly and debilitated.

Subacute lymphocytic thyroiditis

This form of autoimmune thyroiditis is characterized by focal lymphocytic infiltration of the thyroid (also known as focal lymphocytic thyroiditis).

Histological changes are similar to those in Hashimoto's thyroiditis but they are focal rather than diffuse. The disease is less severe than Hashimoto's thyroiditis, and it is often asymptomatic (Fig. 9.9).

Summary of features of thyroiditis			
	Hashimoto's thyroiditis	De Quervain's thyroiditis	Subacute lymphocytic thyroiditis
Etiology	Autoimmune	Viral	Autoimmune
Histological features	Diffuse lymphocytic infiltration of thyroid	Giant cell granulomatous inflammatory reaction	Focal lymphocytic infiltration of thyroid
Hypothyroidism	Common	Rare	Rare

Fig. 9.9 Summary of features of thyroiditis.

Note that some degree of progressive lymphocytic infiltration of the thyroid is seen in 5–10% of thyroid autopsies, and these are thought to be a normal ageing change. However, in subacute lymphocytic thyroiditis, lymphocytic infiltration is in excess of what would normally be expected for age-related change.

Graves' disease

Graves' disease is an organ-specific autoimmune disorder that results in thyrotoxicosis due to overstimulation of the thyroid gland by autoantibodies. It is the most common form of thyrotoxicosis, females being affected more than males by 8:1, and it is usually associated with a diffuse enlargement of the thyroid.

Pathogenesis—IgG-type immunoglobulins bind to TSH membrane receptors, and they cause prolonged stimulation of the thyroid, lasting for as long as 12 hours (cf. 1 hour for TSH). The autoantibody binds at a site different to the hormone-binding locus, and it is termed long-acting thyroid stimulator (LATS) or thyroid-stimulating immunoglobulin (TSI).

Histologically, the gland shows hyperplasia of acinar epithelium, reduction of stored colloid, and local accumulations of lymphocytes with lymphoid follicle formation.

The clinical features of Graves' disease are similar to those of general thyrotoxicosis but with some additional features, namely:

- Exophthalmos (protrusion of the eyeballs in their sockets) due to the infiltration of orbital tissues by fat, mucopolysaccharides, and lymphocytes. May cause compression of the optic nerve, hence blindness. However, only about 5% of Graves' patients show signs of exophthalmos.
- Thyroid acropachy: enlargement of fingernails.
- Pretibial myxedema: accumulation of mucoproteins in the deep dermis of the skin.
- Clubbing of the fingers.

Treatment is as for thyrotoxicosis.

Thyroid goiters

Definitions

A goiter is any enlargement of part or whole of the thyroid gland. There are two types:

- Toxic goiter, i.e., goiter associated with thyrotoxicosis.
- Nontoxic goiter, i.e., goiter associated with normal or reduced levels of thyroid hormones.

Toxic goiter

Graves' disease

This is the most common cause of toxic goiter (described above).

Toxic multinodular goiter

This results from the development of hyperthyroidism in a multinodular goiter (see below).

Nontoxic goiters

Diffuse nontoxic goiter (simple goiter)

This diffuse enlargement of the thyroid gland is classified into:

- Endemic goiter—due to iodine deficiency. Rare in the U.S., but may occur in certain geographical areas remote from the sea.
- Sporadic goiter—caused by goitrogenic agents (substances that induce goiter formation) or may be familial in origin. Examples of goitrogenic agents include certain cabbage species because of their thiourea content, and specific drugs or

chemicals, such as iodide, paraminosalicylic acid, and drugs used in the treatment of thyrotoxicosis. Familial cases show inherited autosomal recessive traits, which interfere with hormone synthesis at various enzyme pathways (these are dyshormonogenic goiters).
- Physiological goiter—enlargement of the thyroid gland in females during puberty or pregnancy; the reason is unclear.

Multinodular goiter

This is the most common cause of thyroid enlargement, and seen particularly in the elderly. The etiology is uncertain but it may represent an uneven responsiveness of various parts of the thyroid to fluctuating TSH levels over a period of many years.

Morphological features are:

- Irregular hyperplastic enlargement of the entire thyroid gland due to the development of well-circumscribed nodules of varying size.
- Larger nodules filled with brown, gelatinous colloid, consequently, it is often termed multinodular colloid goiters.

Most patients have normal thyroid function, and they generally seek treatment for cosmetic reasons (an unsightly swelling in the neck) or compression symptoms, such as pressure on the trachea producing stridor or pressure on the recurrent laryngeal nerve producing hoarseness.

However, toxic changes occasionally occur in a multinodular goiter resulting in hyperthyroidism, and the goiter is then termed a toxic multinodular goiter.

Neoplasms of the thyroid

Tumors of the thyroid are generally benign. Carcinomas are rare, and lymphomas are rarer still.

Benign tumors

Thyroid adenomas

These are solitary, or multiple, encapsulated solid nodules. Compression of the adjacent gland is a common feature, and the center may show areas of hemorrhage and cystic changes. The most common type is follicular adenoma, which consists of colloid-containing microfollicles and columns of larger cells of alveolar arrangement.

Rarely, follicular adenomas may synthesize excess thyroid hormones, causing thyrotoxicosis.

Malignant tumors

These rare tumors account for less than 1% of total cancer deaths in the U.S., with females affected more than males by 3:1. Types of malignant thyroid tumors and their basic features are outlined in Fig. 9.10.

Papillary adenocarcinoma

This is a well-differentiated tumor most commonly found in younger patients. It presents as a non-encapsulated infiltrative mass, but it is a slow growing tumor with an excellent prognosis.

Histologically, it consists of epithelial papillary projections between which calcified spherules may

Types and features of malignant thyroid tumors						
	Tumor type	Origin of tumor	Frequency (%)	Typical age range (years)	Spread	Prognosis (% for 10-year survival)
Differentiated carcinoma	Papillary	Follicular cells	70	20–40	Lymph nodes	90
	Follicular	Follicular cells	10	40–60	Bloodstream	60
Undifferentiated carcinoma	Anaplastic	Follicular cells	5	>60	Aggressive local invasion; bloodstream	1
Medullary carcinoma	—	Parafollicular C cells	5–10	>40	Local, lymphatic, and blood	50 (but very variable)
Lymphoma	—	Lymphocytes	5–10	>60	Lymphatic	10

Fig. 9.10 Types and features of malignant thyroid tumors.

be present. Epithelial cell nuclei are characteristically large with optically clear areas centrally (described as "Orphan Annie nuclei").

Follicular adenocarcinoma

This well-differentiated, single, encapsulated lesion is histologically similar to follicular adenoma, but it can be differentiated by its invasion of the capsule and/or blood vessels. Spread is usually to bones and the lungs via the bloodstream.

Many of these tumors retain the ability to take up radioactive iodine (^{131}I), which may be used as a highly effective targeted form of radiotherapy. The prognosis is, therefore, good.

Anaplastic carcinoma

This highly malignant, poorly differentiated adenocarcinoma usually presents in the elderly as a diffusely infiltrative mass.

Histologically, the dominant features are those of a spindle cell tumor with or without giant cell areas, or a small cell pattern.

The prognosis is very poor due to the rapid local invasion of structures such as the trachea, producing respiratory obstruction.

Medullary carcinoma

This rare tumor arises from parafollicular C cells, which commonly synthesize and secrete calcitonin but which may also secrete 5-hydroxytryptamine (serotonin), various peptides of the tachykinin family, ACTH, and prostaglandins. As a consequence, carcinoid syndrome and Cushing's syndrome have been described in association with medullary carcinoma.

High levels of serum calcitonin are useful diagnostically, but they produce no clinical effects.

Although medullary carcinoma is most common in the elderly, it also occurs in younger individuals, where it is commonly associated with other endocrine tumors—multiple endocrine neoplasia (MEN) syndromes IIa and IIb (p. 192).

Lymphomas

Most thyroid lymphomas are regarded as tumors of mucosa-associated lymphoma tissue. Interestingly non-Hodgkin's B cell lymphomas occasionally arise in long-standing, autoimmune thyroiditis, especially Hashimoto's disease.

Parathyroid disorders

Parathyroid hormone

Parathyroid hormone (PTH) is a polypeptide (84 amino acid residues) secreted by the chief cells of the parathyroid glands (four glands: two in each of the superior and inferior lobes of the thyroid; total weight 120 mg).

The main action of PTH is to increase serum calcium and decrease serum phosphate. Its actions are mediated by the bones and kidneys as described below.

In bone, PTH stimulates osteoclastic bone resorption and inhibits osteoblastic bone deposition. The net effect is the release of calcium from bone.

In the kidney, PTH has the following effects:

- Increases calcium reabsorption.
- Decreases phosphate reabsorption.
- Increases 1-hydroxylation of 25-hydroxyvitamin D (i.e., activates vitamin D).

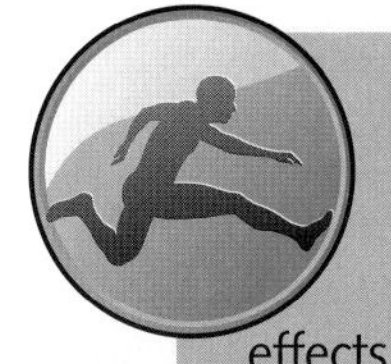

Understanding the physiological functions of PTH is essential to an understanding of the clinical effects produced by its hypo- or hypersecretion.

Hyperparathyroidism

Hyperparathyroidism is defined as an elevated secretion of PTH, of which there are three main types:

- Primary: hypersecretion of PTH by adenoma or hyperplasia of the gland.
- Secondary: physiological increase in PTH secretions in response to hypocalcemia of any cause.
- Tertiary: supervention of an autonomous hypersecreting adenoma in long-standing secondary hyperparathyroidism.

Primary hyperparathyroidism

This is the most common of the parathyroid disorders, with a prevalence of about 1 per 800 in the U.S. More than 90% of patients are over 50 years of age, and the condition affects females more than males by about 2:1. The etiology of primary hyperparathyroidism is outlined in Fig. 9.11.

Etiology of primary hyperparathyroidism		
Type	**Frequency**	**Features**
Adenoma	75%	Orange–brown, well-encapsulated tumor of variable size but seldom >1 cm diameter Tumors are usually solitary, affecting only one of the parathyroids, the others often showing atrophy; they are deep seated and rarely palpable
Primary hyperplasia	20%	Diffuse enlargement of all the parathyroid glands
Parathyroid carcinoma	5%	Usually resembles adenoma but is poorly encapsulated and invasive locally

Fig. 9.11 Etiology of primary hyperparathyroidism.

Effects of hyperparathyroidism

The clinical effects are the result of hypercalcemia and bone resorption (as described below).

Effects of hypercalcemia:

- Renal stones due to hypercalcuria.
- Excessive calcification of blood vessels.
- Corneal calcification.
- General muscle weakness.
- Tiredness.
- Thirst and polyuria.
- Anorexia and constipation.
- Peptic ulceration (rare) due to enhanced gastrin secretion.

Effects of bone resorption:

- Osteitis fibrosa: increased bone resorption with fibrous replacement in the lacunae.
- "Brown tumors": hemorrhagic and cystic tumor-like areas in the bone, containing large masses of giant osteoclastic cells.
- Osteitis fibrosa cystica (von Recklinghausen's disease of bone): multiple brown tumors combined with osteitis fibrosa.
- Changes may present clinically as bone pain, fracture, or deformity.

However, about 50% of patients with biochemical evidence of primary hyperparathyroidism are asymptomatic.

Investigations are:

- Biochemical: increased PTH and Ca^{2+}, and decreased PO_4^{3-}.
- Radiological: 90% normal; 10% show evidence of bone resorption, particularly phalangeal erosions.

Management is by the surgical removal of abnormal parathyroid and by conservative treatment with oral phosphate to reduce plasma calcium.

Secondary hyperparathyroidism

This is compensatory hyperplasia of the parathyroid glands, occurring in response to diseases of low serum calcium or increased serum phosphate.

Its causes are:

- Chronic renal failure and some renal tubular disorders.
- Steatorrhea and other malabsorption syndromes.
- Osteomalacia and rickets.
- Pregnancy and lactation.

Morphological changes of the parathyroid glands are:

- Enlargement of all parathyroid glands, but to a lesser degree than in primary hyperplasia.
- Increase in "water clear" cells and chief cells of the parathyroid glands, with loss of stromal fat cells.

Clinical manifestations—Symptoms of bone resorption are dominant.

Renal osteodystrophy

Skeletal abnormalities, arising as a result of raised PTH secondary to chronic renal disease, are known as renal osteodystrophy.

The pathogenesis of renal osteodystrophy is shown in Fig. 9.12.

Abnormalities vary widely according to the nature of the renal lesion, its duration and the age of the patient, but include:

- Osteitis fibrosa (see above).
- Rickets or osteomalacia due to reduced activation of vitamin D.
- Osteosclerosis: increased radiodensity of certain bones, particularly the parts of vertebrae adjacent to the intervertebral discs.

Note that the symptoms of hypercalcemia are not a feature of secondary hyperparathyroidism as calcium

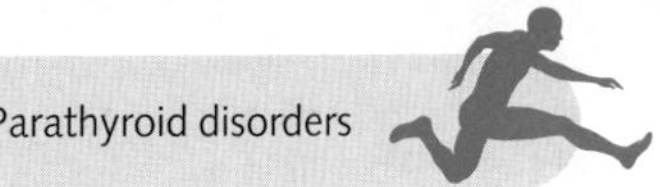

Fig. 9.12 Pathogenesis of renal osteodystrophy.

renal disease → ↓ vit. D activation + ↓ Ca^{2+} reabsorption → ↓ serum Ca^{2+} → ↑ PTH → ↑ bone resorption

Comparison of primary, secondary, and tertiary hyperparathyroidism

	Primary	**Secondary**	**Tertiary**
Serum PTH and Ca^{2+}	↑ PTH; ↑ Ca^{2+}	↑ PTH; normal or ↓ Ca^{2+}	↑ PTH; ↑ Ca^{2+}
Etiology	Adenoma Hyperplasia Carcinoma	Chronic renal failure Malabsorption Osteomalacia and rickets Pregnancy and lactation	Adenoma resulting from overstimulation of glands in secondary hyperthyroidism
Predominant effects	Hypercalcemia	Increased bone resorption	Hypercalcemia and increased bone resorption

Fig. 9.13 Comparison of primary, secondary, and tertiary hyperparathyroidism.

levels are usually normal or reduced (PTH is secreted as a compensatory response to reduced calcium levels).

The investigations are both biochemical (raised PTH and normal or lowered Ca^{2+}) and radiological (higher incidence of bone resorption than in primary hyperparathyroidism).

Management is by treatment of the underlying disease, and oral calcium supplements to correct hypocalcemia.

Tertiary hyperparathyroidism

This condition, resulting from chronic overstimulation of the parathyroid glands in renal failure, causes one or more of the glands to become an autonomous hypersecreting adenoma with resultant hypercalcemia.

Fig. 9.13 gives a comparison of primary, secondary, and tertiary hyperparathyroidism.

Hypoparathyroidism

Hypoparathyroidism is a condition of reduced or absent PTH secretion, resulting in hypocalcemia and hyperphosphatemia.

The causes of hypoparathyroidism are:

- Removal or damage of the parathyroid glands during thyroidectomy: most common cause of hypothyroidism resulting from inadvertent damage (e.g., by interference with their blood supply) or deliberate removal during surgery of the thyroid gland.
- Autoimmune parathyroid disease: usually occurs in patients who have another autoimmune endocrine disease (e.g., Hashimoto's disease or Addison's disease).
- Congenital deficiency (DiGeorge syndrome): rare, congenital disorder caused by arrested development of the third and fourth branchial arches, resulting in an almost complete absence of the thymus (see Chapter 12) and parathyroid gland.

The effects of hypoparathyroidism are:

- ↓ Release of Ca^{2+} from bones.
- ↓ Ca^{2+} reabsorption but ↑ PO_4^{3-} reabsorption by kidney.
- ↓ 1-Hydroxylation of 25-hydroxyvitamin D by kidney.

Most symptoms of hypoparathyroidism are those of hypocalcemia:

- Tetany: muscular spasm provoked by lowered plasma Ca^{2+}.
- Convulsions.
- Paresthesias.
- Psychiatric disturbances (e.g., depression and irritability).
- Rarely: cataracts, alopecia, brittle nails.

Management is by treatment with large doses of oral vitamin D; the acute phase requires intravenous calcium and calcitriol (1,25-dihydroxycholecalciferol, i.e., activated vitamin D).

Multiple endocrine neoplasia syndromes

These are syndromes in which patients develop tumors in a number of different endocrine organs. Patients are younger than those who develop single sporadic tumors and usually have a strong family history of multiple endocrine tumors with autosomal dominant inheritance.

There are three main types of MEN syndrome:

- MEN I (Werner's) syndrome.
- MEN IIa (Sipple's) syndrome.
- MEN IIb (sometimes called MEN III) syndrome.

MEN I (Werner's) syndrome

Patients usually show a combination of hyperparathyroidism (usually chief cell hyperplasia), pituitary adenomas, and pancreatic tumors (gastrin and insulin producing). Rarely, there may also be thyroid tumors and adrenal cortical adenomas.

MEN IIa (Sipple's) syndrome

Patients have a combination of pheochromocytoma (50% bilateral) and medullary carcinoma of the thyroid (often bilateral and multinodular). Rarely, there may also be hyperparathyroidism due to parathyroid hyperplasia.

MEN IIb (MEN III) syndrome

Patients have all of the features of MEN IIa with additional features of:

- Neuromas and ganglioneuromas in the dermis and submucosal regions throughout the body.
- Marfanoid body habitus with poor muscle development.
- Skeletal abnormalities (e.g., kyphosis, pes cavus, and high arch palate).

The facial appearance is characteristic with thick, bumpy lips, broad-based nose, everted eyelids, and grossly abnormal dental enamel.

Disorders of the adrenal gland

Hormones of the adrenal gland

The adrenal gland has two distinct endocrine components derived from different embryonic tissue: the cortex and the medulla.

Cortex

This is the outer part of the gland, which is derived from the mesoderm. It synthesizes, stores, and secretes various cholesterol-derived hormones, namely:

- Glucocorticoid hormones (e.g., hydrocortisone).
- Mineralocorticoid hormones (e.g., aldosterone).
- Sex steroids.

Medulla

This is the inner part of the gland, which is derived from the neuroectoderm, forming part of the sympathetic nervous system. It synthesizes and secretes the vasoactive amines adrenaline (epinephrine) and noradrenaline (norepinephrine).

Hyperfunction of the adrenal cortex

Cushing's syndrome

The symptoms and signs of Cushing's syndrome are associated with prolonged inappropriate elevation of free corticosteroid levels (Fig. 9.14).

Clinical features—The main effects of sustained elevation of glucocorticoid secretion are:

- Central obesity and moon face.
- Plethora and acne.
- Menstrual irregularity.
- Hirsutism and hair thinning.
- Hypertension.
- Diabetes.
- Osteoporosis: may cause collapse of vertebrae, rib fractures.
- Muscle wasting and weakness.
- Atrophy of skin and dermis: paper thin skin with bruising tendency, purple striae.

Pathogenesis—Patients with Cushing's syndrome can be classified into two groups on the basis of whether the etiology of the condition is ACTH-dependent or ACTH-independent (Fig. 9.15).

ACTH-dependent etiology:

- Pituitary hypersecretion of ACTH (Cushing's disease): bilateral adrenal hyperplasia secondary

Fig. 9.14 Systemic effects of Cushing's syndrome.

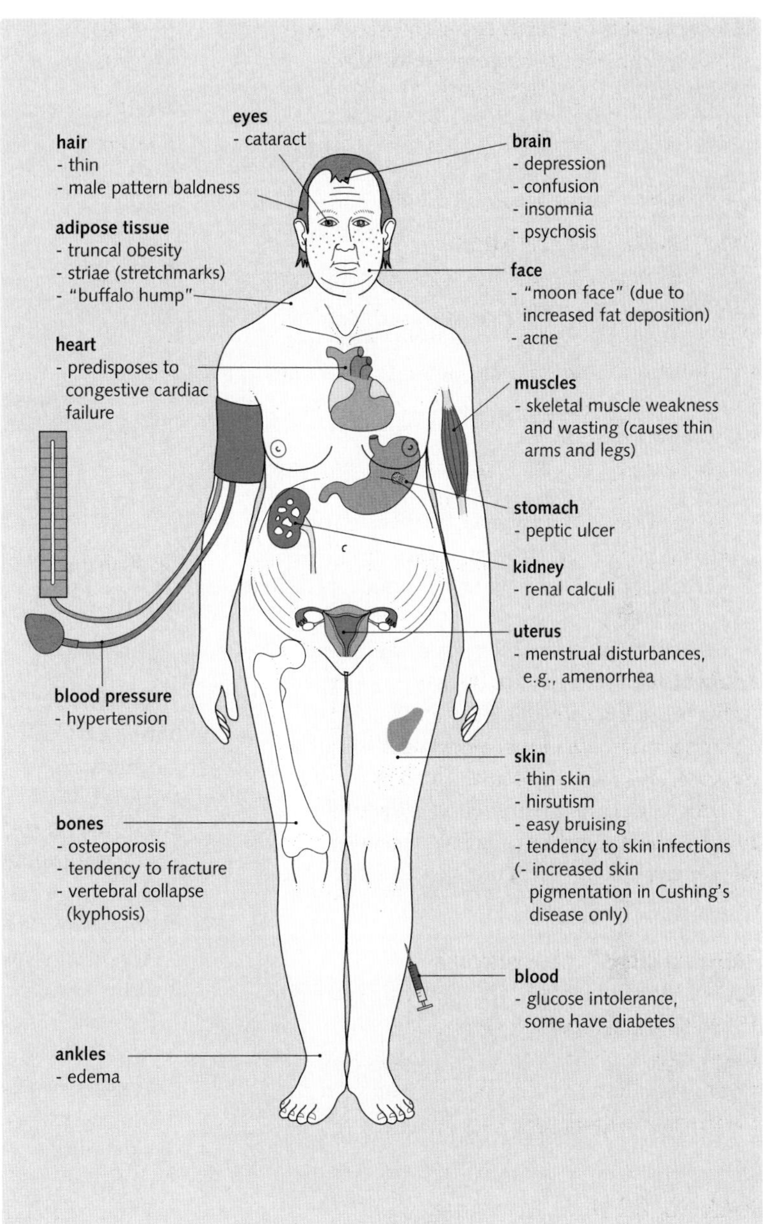

to excessive secretion of ACTH by the pituitary gland (p. 180).

- Ectopic ACTH or CRH (corticotrophin-releasing hormone) production by nonendocrine neoplasm (e.g., oat cell carcinoma of bronchus and some carcinoid tumors). In cases of malignant bronchial tumor, the patient rarely survives long enough to develop any physical features of Cushing's syndrome.

Non-ACTH-dependent etiology:

- Iatrogenic steroid therapy: most common cause of Cushing's syndrome.
- Adrenal cortical adenoma: well-circumscribed yellow tumor usually 2–5 cm in diameter. Extremely common as an incidental finding in up to 30% of all post mortem examinations. The yellow color is due to stored lipid (mainly cholesterol) from which the hormones are

Classification of Cushing's syndrome	
Type	**Cause**
ACTH-dependent	Iatrogenic (ACTH therapy) Pituitary hypersecretion of ACTH Ectopic ACTH syndrome (benign or malignant non-endocrine tumor)
Non-ACTH-dependent	Iatrogenic, e.g., prednisolone Adrenal cortical adenoma Adrenal cortical carcinoma

Fig. 9.15 Classification of Cushing's syndrome.

synthesized. The vast majority have no clinical effects (i.e., they are nonfunctioning adenomas), with only a small percentage producing Cushing's syndrome.

- Adrenal cortical carcinoma: rare and almost always associated with the overproduction of hormones, usually glucocorticoids and sex steroids. Patients usually have features of Cushing's syndrome mixed with androgenic effects which are particularly noticeable in women. Tumors are usually large and yellowish-white in colour. Local invasion and metastatic spread are common.

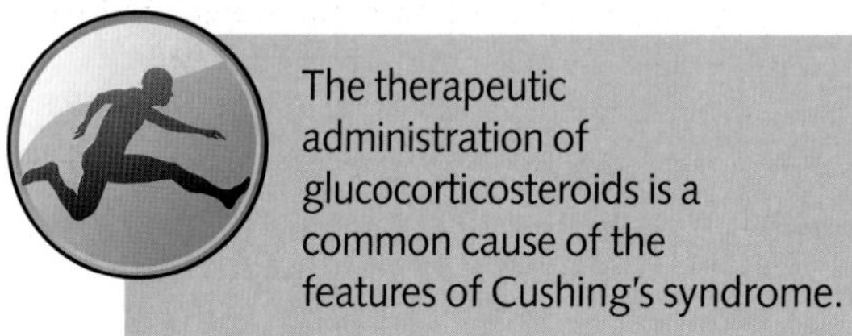

Regardless of the etiology, the diagnosis is based on clinical features and the demonstration of a raised plasma cortisol level.

The etiology of the disorder is elucidated through:

- Dexamethasone suppression test (suppression of cortisol levels in Cushing's disease due to suppression of pituitary ACTH secretion).
- MRI and CT scan visualization of pituitary and adrenal glands.
- Analysis of blood ACTH (high = pituitary adenoma or ectopic ACTH source; low = primary adrenal tumor).

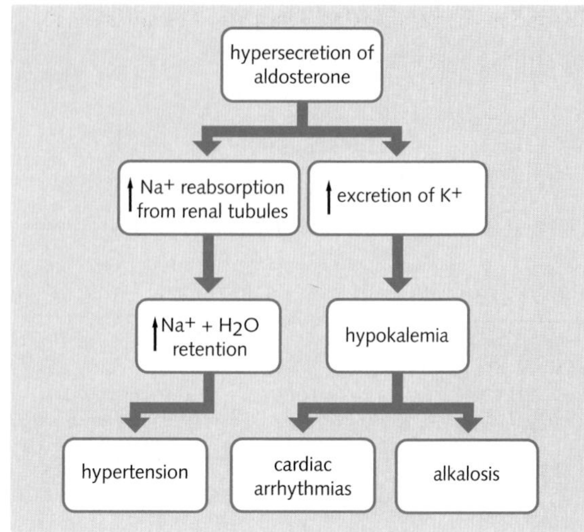

Fig. 9.16 Effects of hyperaldosteronism.

Treatment of the underlying cause is essential as untreated Cushing's syndrome has a 50% 5-year mortality rate.

Hyperaldosteronism

Excessive production of aldosterone by the zona glomerulosa of the adrenal cortex results in increased Na^+ retention and increased K^+ loss.

The etiology is as follows:

- Primary hyperaldosteronism: autonomous hypersecretion of aldosterone, which is almost invariably caused by adrenal cortical adenoma (Conn's syndrome).
- Secondary hyperaldosteronism: hypersecretion of aldosterone secondary to an increased production of angiotensin II following activation of the renin–angiotensin system. May be precipitated by congestive cardiac failure, cirrhosis, nephrotic syndrome, hypertension. This is more common than primary form of disorder.

The effects of hyperaldosteronism are shown in Fig. 9.16.

Clinical features are:

- Hypertension: often the only presenting feature. Commonly occurs in the younger age group.
- Hypokalemia: usually accompanies hypertension and may give rise to polyuria, nocturia, polydipsia, paraesthesia, cardiac arrhythmias, muscle weakness, or paralysis.

Secondary hyperaldosteronism also has additional features of underlying disease.

Biochemical diagnosis:

- ↑ Na^+, ↓ K^+.
- ↑ Aldosterone.
- Plasma renin: ↓ in Conn's syndrome but ↑ in secondary hyperaldosteronism.

Radiological diagnosis is by visualization of adrenal cortical adenoma by CT scan or MRI.

Management:

- Primary hyperaldosteronism: surgical removal of the affected adrenal.
- Secondary hyperaldosteronism: treatment of the underlying cause.

Congenital adrenal hyperplasia

This rare, autosomal recessive disorder is caused by a deficiency of the enzyme 21-hydroxylase, required for the synthesis of both cortisol and aldosterone. Failure of cortisol production produces an increase in ACTH secretion by the pituitary and hyperplasia of the adrenal cortex.

Production of androgens by the adrenal cortex does not require 21-hydroxylase, consequently, adrenal hyperplasia causes excessive secretion of androgens resulting in masculinization of females and precocious puberty in males. Also, aldosterone deficiency is serious, causing a life-threatening salt loss unless replacement therapy is given.

Hypofunction of the adrenal cortex

Addison's disease

This rare condition of chronic adrenal insufficiency is due to a lack of glucocorticoids and mineralocorticoids. Its estimated prevalence in the developed world is 0.8 cases per 100,000 population.

The clinical features outlined in Fig. 9.17 are a result of glucocorticoid deficiency together with mineralocorticoid insufficiency, loss of adrenal androgen production, and increased ACTH secretion.

Etiology—Autoimmune destruction of the cortex of both adrenals is the most common cause of Addison's disease. It is often associated with autoimmune thyroid disease, autoimmune gastritis, and other endocrine organ autoimmune diseases. Adrenal insufficiency is also a well-recognized complication of patients with acquired immune deficiency syndrome (AIDS) and may result from a variety of causes, including bilateral adrenal tuberculosis (caseous necrosis) and fungal infections.

Clinical features of Addison's disease

Hormonal abnormality	Clinical features
Glucocorticoid insufficiency	Vomiting and loss of appetite Weight loss Lethargy and weakness Postural hypotension Hypoglycemia
Mineralocorticoid insufficiency	↓ serum Na^+, ↑ serum K^+ Chronic dehydration Hypotension
Increased ACTH secretion	Brownish pigmentation of skin and buccal mucosa
Loss of adrenal androgen	Decreased body hair, especially in females

Fig. 9.17 Clinical features of Addison's disease.

Other rarer causes of Addison's disease are adrenal destruction by tumor, hemochromatosis, and amyloidosis.

Biochemical diagnosis:

- Measurement of plasma ACTH and cortisol: ↑ ACTH, ↓ cortisol.
- ACTH stimulation test: ACTH is administered and plasma cortisol levels are monitored. Failure of cortisol levels to rise indicates Addison's disease.
- Plasma electrolytes: ↓ Na^+, normal or ↑ K^+, ↑ urea
- Blood glucose: usually low.
- ↑ Plasma renin activity and normal or ↓ aldosterone.

Management is by glucocorticoid replacement therapy and usually mineralocorticoid therapy.

Primary acute adrenocortical insufficiency (adrenal crisis)

This may occur as a result of:

- Iatrogenic: abrupt cessation of prolonged high-dose therapeutic corticosteroids (prolonged corticosteroid therapy produces lowered endogenous steroid production, leading to atrophy of the adrenal cortex).
- Bilateral adrenal hemorrhage: caused by Gram-negative (usually meningococcal) septicemia (Waterhouse–Friderichsen syndrome) and adrenal

vein thrombosis secondary to retroperitoneal hemorrhage.
- Complication of chronic adrenal failure: Addisonian crisis.

Clinical features are:
- Profound hypotension.
- Vomiting.
- Diarrhea.
- Abdominal pain.
- Pyrexia.

An adrenal crisis is a medical emergency and requires intravenous hydrocortisone and fluid replacement. The precipitating cause should be sought and if possible treated.

Secondary adrenocortical insufficiency

This adrenocortical insufficiency is caused by adrenal atrophy secondary to:
- Hypothalamic or pituitary disease (tumors or surgical destruction), which produces lowered ACTH, hence lowered endogenous glucocorticoids and aldosterone.
- Glucocorticoid therapy, which produces lowered ACTH (suppression), hence lowered endogenous glucocorticoids and aldosterone.

The adrenal medulla

Pheochromocytoma

This is a rare tumor of the adrenaline- and noradrenaline-secreting cells (chromaffin cells) of the adrenal medulla (see Chapter 14).

Tumors of extra-adrenal paraganglia

Neuroblastomas

These rare tumors are derived from neuroblasts. Affected sites are the adrenal medulla, the mediastinum (usually in association with the sympathetic chain), and the celiac plexus.

They are almost exclusively tumors of children, but they may occur very rarely above 5 years of age. The tumor is highly malignant and usually inoperable.

Ganglioneuroma

A benign tumor derived from sympathetic nerves, this is most commonly found in the posterior mediastinum, but 10% of cases arise in the adrenal medulla.

Disorders of the endocrine pancreas

Diabetes mellitus

Diabetes mellitus (DM) is a multisystem disease of an abnormal metabolic state characterized by hyperglycemia due to inadequate insulin action/production. It can be classified into primary and secondary.

Primary DM is a primary disorder of insulin production/action, and this accounts for 95% of diabetic cases.

In 5% of cases, diabetes may be secondary to:
- Pancreatic diseases (e.g., chronic pancreatitis or hemochromatosis).
- Hypersecretion of hormones which antagonize the effects of insulin (e.g., glucocorticoids in Cushing's syndrome, growth hormone in acromegaly, adrenaline in pheochromocytomas).

Primary DM is by far the most important cause of diabetes, and it is further classified into:
- Type 1, also known as insulin-dependent DM (IDDM) or juvenile-onset diabetes.
- Type 2, also known as non-insulin-dependent DM (NIDDM) or mature-onset diabetes.

The basic features of these two types of diabetes are described in Fig. 9.18.

Type 1 diabetes mellitus

Etiology and pathogenesis—Type 1 diabetes mellitus is an organ-specific, autoimmune-induced disorder characterized by antibody-mediated destruction of the endocrine cell population of the islet of Langerhans.

Two main factors are thought to predispose to autoimmunity:
- Genetic predisposition: patients with type 1 diabetes are usually HLA-DR3 or HLA-DR4 positive, a feature that is also seen in other organ-specific autoimmune diseases. However, identical twins show a 40% concordance in the development of the disease indicating the additional importance of environmental factors.
- Viral infection: viral infection may trigger the autoimmune reaction; viruses implicated include mumps, measles, and coxsackie B.

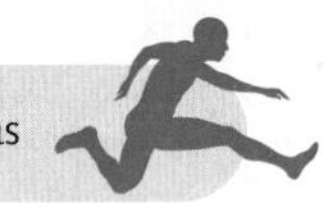

Table comparing type I and type II diabetes mellitus (DM)	
Type I	**Type II**
Childhood/adolescent onset	Middle-aged/elderly onset
1/3 of primary diabetes	2/3 of primary diabetes
Females = males	Females > males (by 4:1)
Acute/subacute onset	Gradual onset
Thin	Obese
Ketoacidosis common	Ketoacidosis rare
Plasma insulin absent or low	Plasma insulin normal or raised
Insulin sensitive	Insulin insensitive (end-organ resistance)
Autoimmune mechanism (islet cell antibodies present)	Non-autoimmune mechanism (no islet cell antibodies)
Genetic predisposition associated with HLA-DR genotype	Polygenic inheritance

Fig. 9.18 Table comparing type 1 and type 2 diabetes mellitus (DM).

One postulated mechanism is that viruses induce mild structural damage to the islet cells, thereby altering their antigenicity, and that certain individuals with the genetic predisposition to organ specific autoimmune disease then mount an autoimmune response against the damaged insulin-secreting cells.

Histologically, the pancreas shows lymphocytic infiltration and destruction of insulin-secreting cells of islets of Langerhans (β-cells). Destruction of insulin-secreting cells results in insulin deficiency with hyperglycemia and other secondary metabolic complications.

Type 2 diabetes mellitus

Etiology and pathogenesis—The precise etiopathogenesis of type 2 diabetes is unclear, but the following factors are thought to be involved:

- Genetic factors: familial tendency with >90% concordance rate among identical twins. However, there are no HLA associations, and inheritance is considered to be polygenic.
- Relative insulin deficiency: reduced secretion compared with the amounts required, possibly related to islet cell ageing.
- Insulin resistance: tissues are unable to respond to insulin because of an impairment in the function of insulin receptors on the surface of target cells.

Diagnosis of diabetes mellitus

Regardless of etiology, the diagnosis of DM depends on the finding of hyperglycemia. However, the distribution curve of blood glucose concentration for whole populations is unimodal with no clear division between normal and abnormal values.

Diagnostic criteria (Fig. 9.19) are, therefore, arbitrary, and in general diabetes mellitus is indicated by either:

- Fasting venous blood glucose level of >7.8 mmol/L.
- Random venous blood glucose level of >11.1 mmol/L on two occasions.

A distinction is made between diabetes mellitus and impaired glucose tolerance in cases where fasting or random blood sugar level is borderline; in this case, the response to an oral load of glucose can be assessed via a glucose tolerance test.

> The complications of DM are important. Eighty percent of adult diabetics die from cardiovascular disease and patients frequently develop serious renal and retinal disease.

Complications of diabetes mellitus

Acute complications

Diabetics are particularly prone to several types of coma. These result from (in decreasing order of frequency):

- Hypoglycemia: complication of overtreatment with insulin.
- Ketoacidosis: common in type 1 diabetes due to ↑ breakdown of triglycerides → ↑ production of ketone bodies → ketoacidosis → impaired consciousness.
- Hyperosmolarity (aketotic or nonketotic coma): ↑ plasma glucose concentration → ↑ plasma osmolarity → cerebral dehydration → coma. More common in type 2 diabetes.

Diagnostic criteria for diabetes mellitus using an oral glucose tolerance test		
Diagnosis	Venous whole blood glucose	
	Fasting sample	2 hours after 75g glucose load
Normal	<5.6mmol/L	<6.7mmol/L
Impaired glucose tolerance	<6.7mmol/L	6.7–10mmol/L
Diabetes mellitus	>6.7mmol/L	>10.0mmol/L

Fig. 9.19 Diagnostic criteria for diabetes mellitus using an oral glucose tolerance test.

- Lactic acidosis: increased concentrations of lactic acid (produced as an end product of glycolysis instead of pyruvate) may cause coma.

Chronic complications

In recent years, with the advent of insulin therapy and various oral hypoglycemic agents, morbidity and mortality associated with DM are more commonly the result of the chronic rather than the acute complications of the disorder (Fig. 9.20).

The most important chronic complications of diabetes are:

- Vascular disease: atherosclerosis and diabetic microangiopathy.
- Renal disease: diabetic nephropathy.
- Eye disease: diabetic retinopathy.
- Predisposition to infections.
- Peripheral nerve damage: diabetic neuropathy.

Vascular disease Atherosclerosis—Diabetics suffer from an increased severity of atherosclerosis than nondiabetics of the same age and gender, probably due to the increased plasma levels of cholesterol and triglycerides.

The main clinical sequelae of this are seen in:

Heart → ischemic heart disease.

Brain → cerebral ischemia.

Legs and feet → gangrene: ischemia of toes and areas on the heel is a characteristic feature of diabetic gangrene.

Kidney → chronic nephron ischemia, an important component of the multiple renal lesions in diabetes.

Diabetic microangiopathy—Small arterioles and capillaries show a characteristic pattern of wall thickening, which is due to a marked expansion of the basement membrane termed hyaline arteriolosclerosis.

The abnormality is widespread and contributes to ischemic changes that are symptomatic in the kidney, the retina, the brain, and peripheral nerves.

Diabetic nephropathy Diabetes is now one of the most common causes of end-stage renal failure. Associated renal disease can be divided into three forms:

- Complications of diabetic vascular disease: atherosclerosis (atheroma affecting aorta and renal arteries → ischemia); diabetic microangiopathy (glomerular capillary basement membrane thickening (hyaline arteriolosclerosis) → ischemic glomerular damage).
- Diabetic glomerulosclerosis (diffuse and nodular types): ↑ leakage of plasma proteins through capillary wall into glomerular filtrate → proteinuria and progressive glomerular hyalinization with eventual chronic renal failure.
- Increased susceptibility to infections → papillary necrosis. Acute pyelonephritis is a common complication of diabetes mellitus and it occurs as a result of the relative immune suppression seen in diabetics together with reduced neutrophil function.

Eye disease Diabetes is the commonest cause of acquired blindness in the Western world, and it can affect the eyes in five main ways:

- Background retinopathy: small vessel abnormalities in the retina leading to hard exudates, hemorrhages, and microaneurysms. Does not usually affect acuity.
- Proliferative retinopathy: extensive proliferation of new capillaries in the retina. Sudden deterioration in vision may result from vitreous hemorrhage as a consequence of proliferating new vessels or from the development of retinal detachment.

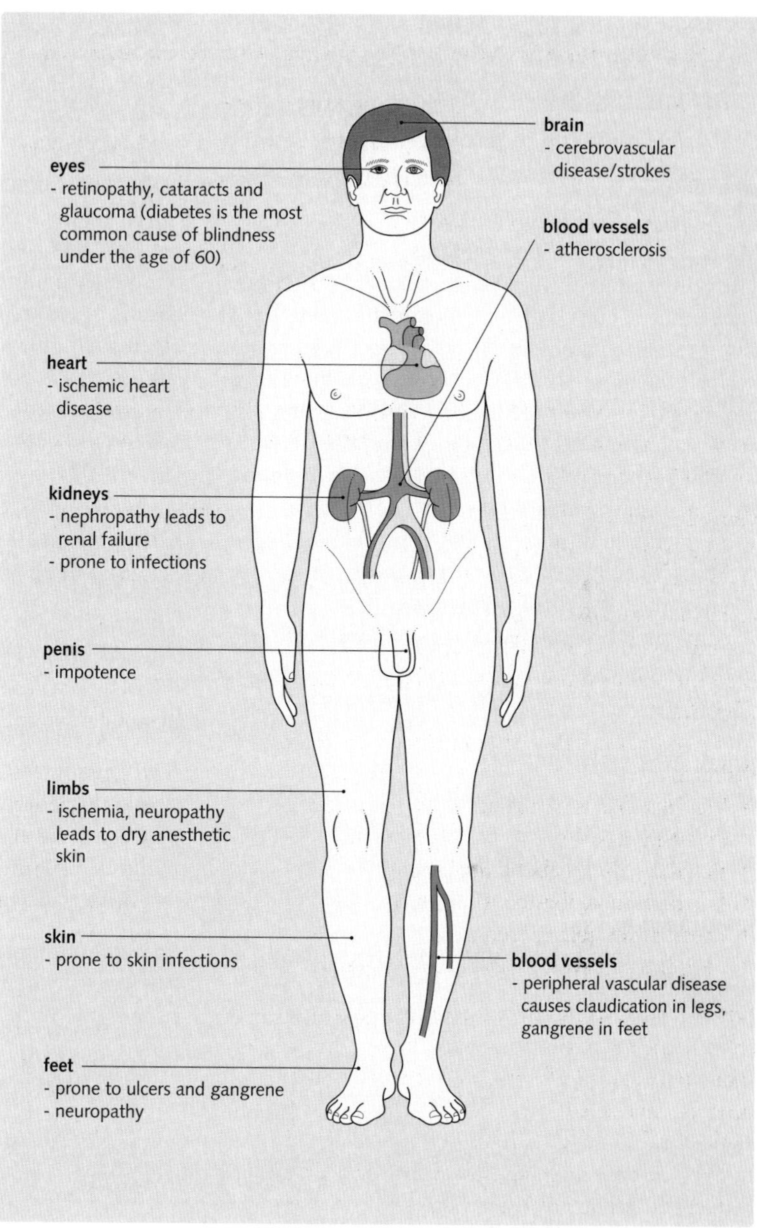

Fig. 9.20 Chronic complications of diabetes mellitus.

- Maculopathy: caused by edema, hard exudates, or retinal ischemia and results in a marked reduction of acuity.
- Cataract formation: greatly increased incidence in diabetics.
- Glaucoma: increased incidence in diabetics due to neovascularization of the iris (rubeosis iridis).

Predisposition to infections Patients with diabetes have an increased tendency to develop infections, usually of a bacterial or fungal nature. The main target organs are:

- Skin—folliculitis, erysipelas, cellulitis, and superficial fungal infections.
- Oral and genital mucosae—especially with *Candida*.

- Urinary tract—increased predisposition to acute pyelonephritis, often associated with recurrent lower urinary tract infections.

Diabetic neuropathy This is possibly due to a disease of the small vessels supplying the nerves (see Chapter 5, p. 52).

Management of diabetes mellitus

The primary aim of treatment is to maintain a normal or near normal blood glucose level at all times. The closer the blood glucose concentration is kept to normal, the more normal the body's total metabolic profile and the lower the incidence of vascular disease. Regardless of the etiology, the type of treatment required is determined by the circulating plasma insulin concentration.

Three methods of treatment are:

- Diet alone: 50% of diabetic patients.
- Diet and oral hypoglycemic drugs (e.g., sulphonylureas and biguanides): 20–30% of diabetic patients.
- Diet and insulin: 20–30% of diabetic patients.

Islet cell tumors

These tumors are rare compared with those of the exocrine pancreas, and they occur most commonly in the 30–50-year age group.

Insulinomas

The most common islet cell tumors, these are derived from pancreatic β-cells:

- Produce hypoglycemia through hypersecretion of insulin.
- May produce permanent brain damage.
- Majority are solitary, nonmetastasizing lesions (10% are multiple and 10% are malignant).

Zollinger–Ellison syndrome

This syndrome of gastric hypersecretion, multiple peptic ulcers, and diarrhea is caused by the gastrin-secreting tumor (gastrinoma) of the pancreatic G-cells. Tumors are multiple in 50% of cases, and are often malignant, with 10–20% occurring in other sites (e.g., the duodenum).

It may also be part of the MEN I syndrome, with adenomas also present in other endocrine glands (see p. 192).

Other islet cell tumors

For a summary of islet cell tumors see Fig. 9.21.

VIPomas

These produce vasoactive intestinal polypeptide (VIP), resulting in a syndrome of watery diarrhea, hypokalemia, and achlorhydria (WDHA).

Glucagonomas

These glucagon-secreting tumors are derived from pancreatic α-cells, and they cause secondary diabetes mellitus (usually mild), necrolytic migratory erythema (skin rash), and uremia.

Somatostatinomas

These somatostatin-producing tumors derived from pancreatic δ-cells are associated with diabetes mellitus, cholelithiasis and steatorrhea.

Summary of islet cell tumors

Islet cell tumor	Occurrence	Clinical features
Insulinoma	70–75%	Hypoglycemia
Gastrinoma	20–25%	Zollinger-Ellison syndrome: gastric hypersecretion, multiple peptic ulcers, and diarrhea
VIPoma	Rare	Watery diarrhea, hypokalemia, and achlorhydria
Glucagonoma	Rare	Secondary diabetes mellitus, necrolytic migratory erythema, and uremia
Somatostatinoma	Rare	Diabetes mellitus, cholelithiasis, and steatorrhea

Fig. 9.21 Summary of islet cell tumors.

- What are the most common adenomas of the anterior lobe? Describe their effects.
- State the causes of hypopituitarism.
- Describe the individual forms of hypopituitarism.
- What are the causes of diabetes insipidus?
- State the causes and effects of hyperthyroidism.
- State the causes of hypothyroidism.
- Name three types of thyroiditis, and outline their basic features.
- Describe the pathogenesis of Graves' disease and its clinical features.
- What are the types and features of malignant thyroid tumors?
- Define primary, secondary, and tertiary hyperparathyroidism.
- Describe the etiology and clinical effects of primary and secondary hyperparathyroidism.
- Describe the etiology and clinical effects of hypoparathyroidism.
- Define the multiple endocrine neoplasia syndromes, and name the organs involved in each type.
- Describe the etiology and features of Cushing's disease.
- Describe the etiology and features of hyperaldosteronism.
- What are the clinical effects of congenital adrenal hyperplasia?
- Name the diseases associated with hypofunction of the adrenal cortex.
- What clinical effects are associated with Addison's disease?
- Compare the pathogenesis and features of type 1 and type 2 diabetes mellitus.
- List the acute and the chronic complications of diabetes mellitus.

10. Pathology of the Reproductive Systems

Disorders of the vulva, vagina, and cervix

Infections of the lower genital tract

Bartholin's cyst

This common, benign, mucus-secreting cyst on the vulva is derived from Bartholin's glands (mucus-secreting glands in the posterior part of the labia majora). Frequently there is superimposed infection—Bartholin's abscess.

Viral infection

Viral infections of the vulval skin are typically due to either herpes simplex virus (HSV) or human papillomavirus (HPV).

Herpes simplex virus

HSV type 2 infection of the vulva (herpes vulvitis) produces initially painless blisters, which subsequently break down to form a painful, sore, eroded area. Infection is acquired through sexual contact and the disease is more common in young women.

Human papillomavirus

This sexually transmitted disease may present with a thickening of the vulval skin and mucosa (flat condyloma) in the labia minora, or as multiple protuberant warts (condylomata acuminata) that may be either sessile or pedunculated. There is a strong link between HPV infections of the vulva and intra-epithelial neoplastic change in both the vulva (see below) and cervix.

Bacterial and protozoal infections

Gardnerella vaginalis

This Gram-negative coccobacillus is often associated with other sexually-spread infections. The patient complains of a foul-smelling discharge, which is thin, greyish, and sometimes shows bubbles. Examination confirms both the discharge and the odor.

Chlamydia trachomatis

The main feature of this disease is the production of painful superficial groin nodes (lymphogranuloma venereum), which may rupture through the skin. It is preceded by a painless vulval ulceration that is often overlooked. Later, chronic lymphatic obstruction leads to nonpitting edema of the external genitalia.

Trichomonas vaginalis

This sexually transmitted flagellated protozoan organism is typically asymptomatic in men, but in women it often produces an intensely irritating vaginal discharge with inflammation of the vulva, vagina, and cervix. The discharge is often frothy and offensive in odor.

Treponema pallidum

A rare sexually transmitted spirochetal bacterium responsible for syphilis, this disease typically involves three stages (primary, secondary, and tertiary):

- Primary: small indurated lesions (chancres) develop at the site of entry of the organism (vulva, vagina, or perianal area).
- Secondary: characterized by multiple, moist, warty, vulvovaginal, and perineal lesions (condylomata lata). There is often a papular eruption on the trunk, limbs, palms, and soles with generalized lymphadenopathy.
- Tertiary: involves the CNS (see Chapter 14).

Fungal and yeast infection

Fungal infections are usually caused by either superficial dermatophytes or *Candida albicans*. There is usually associated fungal vaginitis presenting with a copious vaginal discharge and vulval reddening and soreness.

Candida albicans

This is a normal commensal of the vagina, but its proliferation is usually suppressed by commensal vaginal flora. (*Candida* was formerly known as *Monilia*.)

Conditions that predispose to candidial overgrowth are:

- Pregnancy/estrogen contraceptives: high concentration of estrogens in the blood.
- Immunosuppressive therapy (e.g., cytotoxic drugs and corticosteroids).
- Glycosuria (e.g., diabetes, pregnancy (due to lowering of the renal threshold for sugar)).
- Antibiotic therapy: destruction of normal commensal bacteria.

- Chronic anemia: iron stores are needed to maintain an adequate immune reaction.

The organism can also be sexually transmitted.

Macroscopically, white plaques of fungal hyphae develop on inflamed vaginal mucosa, and vaginal discharge is associated with severe vulval irritation. Infections are often severe in diabetics.

Dermatophytes
Infection of vulval skin with dermatophytic fungi produces a similar superficial inflammation and soreness.

Treatment
Both *Candida* and dermatophytes can be treated with topical fungicides or systemic therapy.

Figure 10.1 shows a table of the organisms that cause infections of the lower genital tract.

Dysplastic and neoplastic disorders of the vulva and vagina
Tumors of the vulva
Squamous cell carcinoma
This typically occurs in elderly women, and it may show extensive local invasion and metastases to the inguinal lymph nodes. The majority of cases appear to arise *de novo*, but some arise in epithelium in which there is severe dysplasia amounting to carcinoma in situ, known as vulval intra-epithelial neoplasia.

Vulval intra-epithelial neoplasia
This is generally seen in patients younger than those with invasive tumors. There is often coexistent evidence of HPV warty change in the affected and adjacent epithelium. Although invasive carcinoma and vulval intra-epithelial neoplasia (VIN) do occasionally coexist in elderly women, it is thought that progression of VIN to invasive carcinoma is not common.

Organisms that cause infections of the lower genital tract

Infection	Organism
Viruses	HPV HSV
Bacteria	*Gardnerella vaginalis* *Chlamydia trachomatis* (lymphogranuloma venereum) *Treponema pallidum* (syphilis)
Protozoa	*Trichomonas vaginalis*
Fungi and yeast	Dermatophytes, *Candida albicans*

Fig. 10.1 Organisms that cause infections of the lower genital tract.

Tumors of the vagina
Dysplastic
Vaginal intra-epithelial neoplasia Vaginal intraepithelial neoplasia (VAIN) is rare compared with cervical intra-epithelial neoplasia (CIN). Most cases are found in women previously treated for CIN or invasive cervical cancer.

Neoplastic
Primary malignant tumors of the vagina are extremely rare, but include squamous cell carcinomas and adenocarcinomas.

Secondary tumors are more common, particularly from malignant tumors of the cervix, endometrium, and ovary. Vaginal bleeding after hysterectomy for uterine or ovarian malignancy should always be investigated and biopsied because of the frequency of metastatic tumor in the residual vaginal vault.

Inflammation of the cervix
Acute and chronic cervicitis
Acute and chronic inflammation of the cervix is particularly common in the presence of an intrauterine contraceptive device.

Acute cervicitis
There is acute inflammation of the cervix with erosion. It is occasionally seen in herpes simplex infection, typically with herpetic disease of the vulva and vagina.

Chronic cervicitis
This chronic inflammation of the cervix is typically caused by the same organisms responsible for infective vaginitis: *Trichomonas*, *Candida*, *Gardnerella*, and the gonococci. It is characterized by a heavy plasma cell and lymphocytic infiltrate.

Endocervical polyps
These common abnormalities derived from the endocervix affect about 5% of women. Polyps protrude from the cervix through the external os, and they may cause intermenstrual bleeding from erosion and ulceration.

Macroscopically, these are smooth, rounded, or pear-shaped polyps about 1–2cm in diameter.

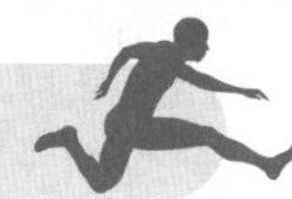

Microscopically, they are composed of endocervical stroma and glands. The surface of the polyp may show ulceration and inflammation and, if long standing, there may be surface squamous metaplasia.

Neoplasia of the cervix

Cervical intra-epithelial neoplasia

This is the preneoplastic (dysplastic) proliferation of epithelium of the transformation zone of the cervix.

Etiology—There is a strong association with HPV infection.

Risk factors are:

- Sexual intercourse: there is a very low incidence in virgins.
- Early age at first intercourse: there is a higher incidence in girls who have intercourse before the age of 17.
- Sexually transmitted diseases: there is a higher incidence in women with a history of sexually transmitted diseases.
- Smoking: there is a higher risk in women who smoke tobacco.
- Human papillomavirus: coexistence of HPV with CIN and invasive carcinoma in cone biopsy and colposcopy specimens suggests a link. DNA from HPV types 16, 18, 31, or 33 has been identified in over 90% of cervical carcinomas. Proteins produced by HPV are thought to inactivate products of tumor suppressor genes thereby facilitating tumor development. For example, the viral protein E6 of HPV subtype 16 can bind and inactivate the function of the p53 tumor suppressor protein.
- HIV infection: carcinoma of the cervix is predisposed by immunosuppression and has increased in incidence as a consequence of AIDS.

Classification

Three grades of severity are recognized. Grading depends upon the proportion of the cervical epithelium wall that is replaced by atypical cells.

- CIN I (mild dysplasia): upper two thirds of the epithelium normal, basal third atypical cells.
- CIN II (moderate dysplasia): upper half of the epithelium normal, atypical cells occupy the lower half.
- CIN III (severe dysplasia): corresponds to carcinoma in situ. Atypical cells extend throughout the full thickness of the epithelium with minimal differentiation and maturation on the surface.

Progression

CIN is associated with a risk of progression to an invasive carcinoma, the risk for CIN I being lowest, and for CIN III being the highest.

The natural history of CIN is important as it determines how often screening is required to detect progression of the disease.

Screening

The aim of screening is to detect atypical cells in the preinvasive stage of the disease by cytological examination of a smear of surface epithelial cells removed from the cervix. It has been suggested that smears repeated every 3 years are adequate for the purposes of population screening. In the U.S. it is estimated that regular attendance at screening prevents up to 90% of cervical cancer.

Management is by the local destruction of abnormal epithelium by cryotherapy, laser therapy, or cone biopsy following histological confirmation of its nature.

Cervical intra-epithelial neoplasia is the classic example of a preneoplastic condition that can be identified by screening and managed effectively to prevent development of invasive cervical carcinoma.

Squamous cell carcinoma

The vast majority of cervical carcinomas are squamous cell carcinomas arising from the transformation zone or ectocervix.

The carcinoma is preceded by the preinvasive phase of CIN (see above and Fig. 10.2). Risk factors are as for CIN.

Macroscopically, tumors demonstrate the following features (Fig. 10.2):

- Early: areas of granular irregularity of the cervical epithelium, progressive invasion of the stroma causing abnormal hardness of the cervix.
- Late: fungating ulcerated areas, which destroy the cervix.

Microscopically, lesions fall into three histological patterns:

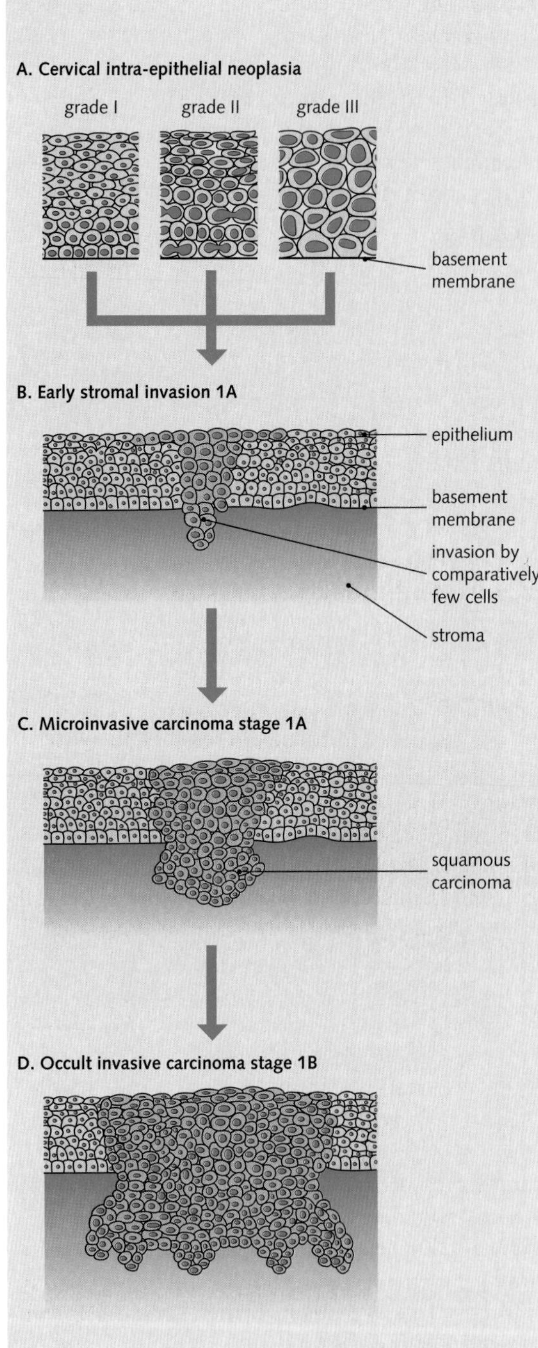

Fig. 10.2 Cervical intra-epithelial neoplasia (CIN) and invasive squamous carcinoma. (A) Increasing dysplasia of CIN grades I–III. (B) Early stromal invasion of <1 mm. (C) Microinvasive carcinoma with invasion of <3 mm. (D) Occult invasive carcinoma with invasion >500 mm^3. There is some risk of spread to the lymph nodes but the tumor is still clinically undetectable. (Adapted from Underwood, 2000.)

Stages and prognosis for carcinomas of the cervix

Stage	5-year survival (%)	Degree of local invasion
I	90	Confined to cervix
II	75	Invasion of upper part of vagina or adjacent parametrial tissues
III	30	Spread to pelvic side wall, lower vagina, or ureters
IV	10	Invasion of rectum, bladder wall, or outside pelvis

Fig. 10.3 Stages and prognosis for carcinomas of the cervix.

- Keratinizing, large cell squamous carcinoma (40%).
- Nonkeratinizing, large cell squamous carcinoma (50%).
- Nonkeratinizing, small cell squamous carcinoma (10%).

The common presenting symptom is vaginal bleeding in the early stages, but advanced neglected tumors may cause urinary obstruction due to bladder involvement.

Invasive carcinomas are managed according to the degree of local invasion and survival is related to the stage of the disease (Fig. 10.3).

Invasive carcinoma is usually managed by radical surgery and/or radiotherapy and/or chemotherapy depending on the stage of the disease. Involvement of the para-aortic lymph nodes is associated with a very poor prognosis.

Disorders of the uterus and endometrium

Inflammatory disorders

Chronic endometritis

An inflammation of the endometrium, this is typically associated with menstrual irregularities and often found in women who are being investigated for infertility.

Microscopically, there is lymphoid and plasma cell infiltration of the endometrium.

Risk factors—The majority of cases are associated with a definite clinical risk factor for developing inflammation:

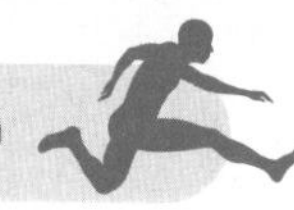

- Recent pregnancy, miscarriage, or instrumentation (50% of cases).
- Pelvic inflammatory disease, such as salpingitis (25% of cases).
- Previous use of intrauterine contraceptive devices (about 20% of cases).
- Gonococcal or chlamydial infection or tuberculosis (TB; 5% of cases).

Disorders of the endometrium

Adenomyosis

This is a condition in which the endometrium grows down to develop deep within the myometrium. This may cause enlargement of the uterus, and it is sometimes associated with menstrual abnormalities and dysmenorrhea.

Macroscopically there are small, irregular, endometrial lesions, some of which are cystic, that can be seen within the affected myometrium. Involvement of the myometrium may be diffuse (more common) or focal with deep nodules of endometrium (nodular adenomyosis).

Microscopically, islands of endometrium are found deep within muscle but in continuity with surface endometrium.

Endometriosis

There is ectopic growth of the endometrium outside the uterus that still responds to cyclical hormonal stimulation. Phases of proliferation and breakdown are associated with the development of the fibrous adhesions and accumulation of hemosiderin pigment. This affects 1 in 15 women of reproductive age.

There are numerous sites:

- Common—ovaries, fallopian tubes, round ligaments, pelvic peritoneum.
- Less common—intestinal wall, bladder, umbilicus, laparotomy scars.
- Rare—lymph nodes, lung, pleura.

Theories of origin

The pathogenesis of endometriosis remains unclear, but there are three main theories that may operate to various degrees.

- Retrograde menstruation: fragments of endometrium migrate along the fallopian tubes during menstruation.
- Metaplasia of peritoneal epithelium: differentiation of peritoneal epithelium into endometrium.
- Metastatic spread of endometrium, via the blood or lymphatic vessels.

Macroscopically, the foci of endometriosis appear as cystic and solid masses, which are characteristically dark brown because of accumulated iron pigment from repeated bleeding.

Microscopically, solid masses of endometriosis are composed of endometrial glands and stroma, fibrosis, and macrophages containing iron pigments.

Endometriosis may present with cyclical pelvic pain, dysmenorrhea, and infertility.

The complications are:

- Infertility (about 30% of cases): may be due to inability of the ovaries to ovulate; ovulation occurring into closed off areas of fibrosis; damage to tubal fimbria; kinking of tubes by adhesions; blockage of tubes by deposits of endometriosis in the wall.
- Bowel obstruction: ectopic endometrial tissue stimulates fibrosis, and it may cause fibrous adhesions between adjacent organs.
- Chocolate cysts: the whole of the fallopian tube and ovary may be converted into a cystic mass containing brown, semi-liquid material.

Endometriosis is dependent on estrogen for continued growth and proliferation, with the disease becoming inactive after oophorectomy or onset of the menopause. Thus, induction of the hypoestrogenic state by suppression of the hypothalamic–pituitary–ovarian axis with analogues of gonadotrophin-releasing hormone (GnRH) is effective in many cases.

Functional endometrial disorders

Anovulatory cycle

A menstrual cycle that is not associated with the development and release of the ovum from the ovary, this is normal and common at both the start and end of reproductive life. Several follicles may start to develop and for a time produce hormones. However, the attempt ends in atresia and the atretic follicle is absorbed.

It is associated with irregular menstruation, although the effects of excessive estrogen stimulation are manifest in the endometrium as the proliferation of glands.

Other causes of anovulation are listed in Fig. 10.4.

Non-physiological causes of anovulation		
Type	**Cause**	**Clinical feature**
Primary ovarian dysfunction	Genetic	e.g., Turner's syndrome, autoimmune
Secondary ovarian dysfunction	Disorders of gonadotrophin regulation	Hyperprolactinemia
	Gonadotrophin deficiency	Pituitary tumor Pituitary infarction Pituitary ablation
	Functional	Weight loss Exercise
	Polycystic ovary syndrome	—

Fig. 10.4 Non-physiological causes of anovulation.

Inadequate luteal phase

The irregular ripening of a follicle is associated with infertility. This may be caused by failure of the production of progesterone by the corpus luteum or by defective receptors for progesterone within the endometrium. Examination of the endometrium in the second half of the menstrual cycle shows inadequate or absent development of secretory changes.

Effects of oral contraceptives

Oral contraceptive pills cause changes in the structure of the endometrium, which is greatly reduced in bulk. Glands become small and inactive with poor development of stroma.

Menopausal changes

The menopause is the cessation of menstruation which normally occurs between 45 and 56 years of age. It occurs as a result of a lack of primordial follicles because all have been used, and because of a more refractory receptor function in the granulosa and thecal cells.

Associated endometrial changes The endometrial glands are lined by inactive cuboidal cells, and they may form large cystic spaces. There is no evidence of mitotic activity, reflecting a lack of estrogenic stimulation. The uterus becomes smaller, and it is less supported due to atrophy of the cardinal, uterosacral, and uteropubic ligaments.

Endometrial hyperplasia

Hyperplasia of the endometrium typically occurs in the third and fourth decades of life, in response to estrogenic stimulation. It presents with hemorrhage, but the severity or frequency is not related to the degree of pathological change. Certain types of endometrial hyperplasia are associated with a degree of risk for malignant change (severe/atypical hyperplasia).

Figure 10.5 shows the different types of endometrial hyperplasia.

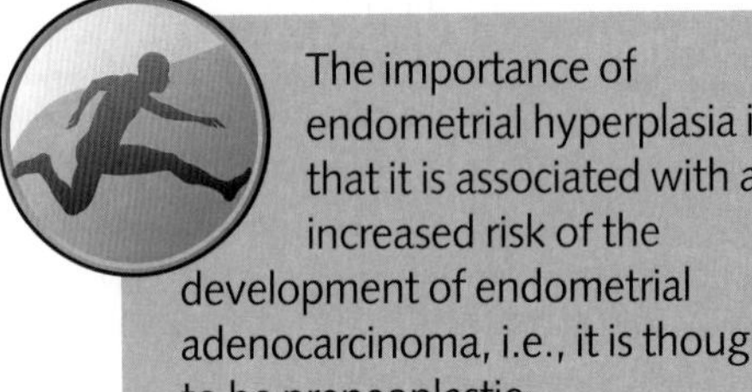

The importance of endometrial hyperplasia is that it is associated with an increased risk of the development of endometrial adenocarcinoma, i.e., it is thought to be preneoplastic.

Neoplastic disorders

Benign

Endometrial polyps

These localized overgrowths of endometrial glands and stroma are very common, and they are typically seen in the perimenopausal age range. They are caused by inappropriate proliferation of glands in response to estrogenic stimuli.

Macroscopically, they are found in the uterine fundus; their size is variable but they are usually 1–3cm in diameter. They have a firm, smooth, nodular appearance within the endometrial cavity, but occasionally prolapse through the cervical os. They may develop ulceration or undergo torsion.

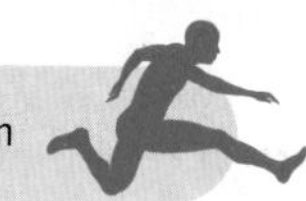

Types of endometrial hyperplasia			
Degree of hyperplasia	**Morphological features**	**Progression to adenocarcinoma (%)**	**Time taken (years) to develop into adenocarcinoma**
Mild (most common)	Cystic glandular hyperplasia with characteristic appearance of "Swiss cheese". Cells show no cytological atypia	1	10
Moderate	Crowding of glands in a back-to-back fashion. Epithelium is stratified and mitoses are relatively frequent. Cells show no cytological atypia	5	7
Severe	Cellular atypia is prominent, glands are distorted by intraglandular polypoid formations, and mitoses are frequent	30	4

Fig. 10.5 Types of endometrial hyperplasia.

Microscopically, they are cystically dilated endometrial glands in a vascular stroma.

Clinical features are associated with menstrual abnormalities and dysmenorrhea.

Fibroids (leiomyomas)

These benign, smooth muscle tumors arise in the muscle wall of the uterus. They are the most common of all tumors, affecting over half of all women over the age of 30, usually becoming symptomatic in the decade before the menopause. Their cause is unknown but risk factors include:

- Age: rare under 30 years.
- Race: more common in Afro-Caribbean populations.
- Parity: more common in nulliparous and women with low fertility.
- Genetic: often a family history.

Leiomyomas have the following features:

- Estrogen sensitive.
- Fast growing in pregnancy.
- Shrink at menopause or with antigonadotrophic hormone therapy.

Sites within the uterus (Fig. 10.6) are:

- Subserous: just beneath the peritoneum on the outer uterine surface.
- Interstitial (most common): surrounded by smooth muscle.
- Submucosal: lying immediately below the endometrium.

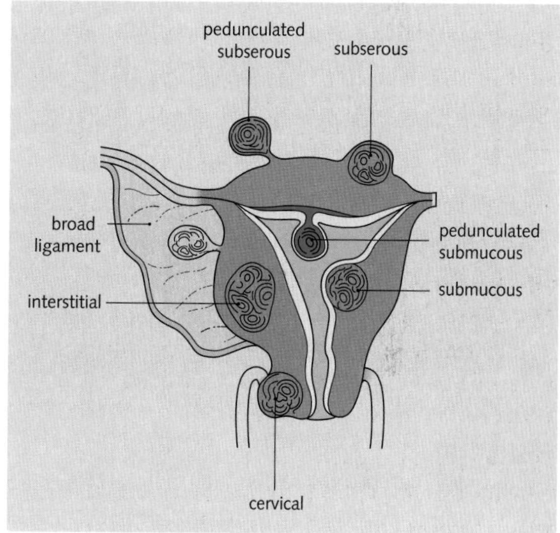

Fig. 10.6 Fibroids within the uterus.

Macroscopically, they are:

- Rounded, rubbery, pale nodules with whorled appearance on cut surface.
- Well circumscribed with pseudocapsule that may become pedunculated forming polyps.
- Size is variable. Most common are 2–4cm (but range from <1 cm up to 20–30cm in diameter).
- Typically multiple.

Microscopically, they are seen as:

- Islands of smooth muscle cells with intervening collagenous stroma.

- Lacking cellular atypia and with very few mitoses (0–3 mitoses per 10 high power fields. Note leiomyosarcomas are associated with cellular atypia and >10 mitoses per 10 high power fields).
- Several rare histological variants (e.g., myxoid).

Clinical features—Leiomyomas may present with abnormal menstrual bleeding, dysmenorrhea, and infertility.

Complications occur following ischemic degeneration, pregnancy, and compression.

Investigations are by ultrasound and laparoscopy.

Management is:

- Surgical: women who no longer wish to conceive usually undergo hysterectomy.
- Medical: uterine leiomyomas depend on estrogen for maintenance of size, therefore, the treatment of women whose families are incomplete is aimed at inducing shrinkage of fibroids with GnRH agonists, which induce hypo-estrogenism. Allows easier surgical removal by myomectomy.
- Embolization: interventional radiologists often embolize large lesions, which are slowly resorbed.

Remember that fibroids are not fibromas, but they are benign tumors of smooth muscle (leiomyomas).

Malignant

Endometrial carcinoma

Adenocarcinomas of the endometrium are common tumors, accounting for about 7% of all cancers in women. The mean age of presentation is 56 years, and 80% of women are postmenopausal.

Endometrial carcinoma is associated with:

- Hyperestrogenic state: obesity, diabetes, late menopause, prolonged use of unopposed estrogens, estrogen-secreting tumors.
- Previous pelvic irradiation.
- Lower parity.

There are two main groups—hyperestrogenic and nonhyperestrogenic tumors.

Hyperestrogenic tumors—These are associated with a generally good prognosis, and they occur in patients close to the menopause, associated with an abnormal estrogenic stimulation of the endometrium and endometrial hyperplasia. Most tumors are adenocarcinomas (60%) and are graded (I–III) according to the amount of glandular and solid pattern within the tumor. High grade tumor is associated with a worse prognosis.

Nonhyperestrogenic tumors—These are more often associated with a poor prognosis, occur in older postmenopausal women, and are not associated with estrogenic stimulation or endometrial hyperplasia.

Macroscopically, there are:

- Small tumors: diffuse, solid areas or polypoid lesions in the endometrium.
- Larger tumors: fill and distend the endometrial cavity with soft, white, friable tissue.

Microscopically, they are seen as:

- Hyperestrogenic tumors: typically well-differentiated adenocarcinomas composed of hyperplastic endometrial glandular tissue with only superficial myometrial invasion at diagnosis.
- Nonhyperestrogenic tumors: typically poorly differentiated with deep myometrial invasion.

The condition may present with postmenopausal bleeding, blood-stained discharge, and irregular bleeding.

The main route of spread is by local invasion to the fallopian tubes, ovaries, bladder, or rectum.

If venous and lymphatic invasion occurs, there may be involvement of the vagina and para-aortic nodes. Widespread hematogenous metastasis is uncommon except with papillary serous carcinomas and clear cell carcinomas.

Invasion into the myometrium is closely correlated with the prognosis—those with small invasive depth having a better prognosis than those with deeper involvement.

The prognosis of uterine carcinoma is related to stage (Fig. 10.7), as with most neoplasms.

Disorders of the ovary and fallopian tube

Inflammatory disorders and infections

Salpingitis

This is inflammation of the fallopian tube(s).

Suppurative salpingitis

Etiology—It is almost always caused by ascending infection from the uterine cavity.

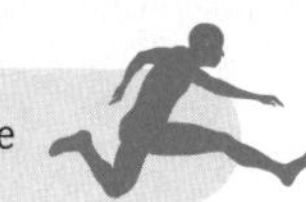

Fig. 10.7 Clinical staging of endometrial cancer.

Clinical staging of endometrial cancer			
Stage	**Proportion of cases (%)**	**Degree of invasion**	**5-year survival (%)**
I	80	Corpus of uterus only	75
II	5	Corpus and cervix	52
III	5	Invasion confined to pelvis	30
IV	10	Invasion outside pelvis or involves bladder or rectal mucosa	10

Predisposing factors are:

- Following pregnancy and endometritis.
- Intrauterine contraceptive device (IUCD) use.
- Sexually transmitted disease (*Mycoplasma*, *Chlamydia*, and gonococci).
- *Actinomyces*: colonization of the genital tract in association with use of IUDs.

Macroscopically, tubes are swollen and congested, and the serosal surface appears red and granular due to vascular dilatation.

Microscopically, tubal epithelium shows neutrophil infiltration and the lumen may contain pus.

Chronic inflammation may supervene, with sequelae of fibrosis and occlusion of the tubal lumen on resolution.

Complications are:

- Infertility—fibrosis causes distortion of mucosal plicae and occlusion of tubal lumen.
- Pyosalpinx—massive distention of tubal lumen by pus.
- Hydrosalpinx—dilatation of a fallopian tube by clear watery fluid with flattening of the mucosa. Acquired with healing of previous inflammation.

Tuberculous salpingitis

This is a tuberculous infection of the fallopian tubes.

Its etiology is the hematogenous spread of *Mycobacterium tuberculosis* from a site outside the genital tract.

Tubes develop multiple granulomas in the mucosa and wall, causing adhesions to adjacent tissues (especially ovaries). In advanced cases, tubes may develop into cavities filled with caseous necrotic material.

Pelvic inflammatory disease

Pelvic inflammatory disease (PID) is a combined infection of the fallopian tubes, ovaries, and peritoneum, and it is typically a result of ascending infection, or less commonly postoperative infection. Predisposing factors are as for suppurative salpingitis (see above).

Neisseria gonorrhoeae and *Chlamydia trachomatis* are the most common responsible organisms although anaerobic organisms are often found in pelvic abscesses.

Inflammation is initially acute, and without prompt treatment may progress to chronic PID with associated complications of tubal edema, development of adhesions within tubes, hydrosalpinx, or pyosalpinx (see above).

Clinical features are:

- Symptoms: gradual onset of pelvic pain, irregular bleeding, fever.
- Signs: abdominal tenderness and guarding; extreme tenderness of the vaginal fornices.

Treatment is by the removal of the IUD (if present) and the use of broad-spectrum antibiotics.

Cysts

Ovarian cysts

Ovarian cystic lesions are extremely common, and they can be either neoplastic or non-neoplastic. The majority of non-neoplastic cysts arise from developing Graafian follicles; a minority are derived from surface epithelium.

Follicular cysts

These unruptured, enlarged Graafian follicles are lined by granulosa cells, with an outer coat of thecal cells. Normal ovaries commonly contain one or more small cysts (<5cm in diameter), which typically disappear by the resorption of fluid. However, multiple follicular cysts are found in:

- Cystic hyperplasia of the endometrium.
- Polycystic ovary syndrome (see below).

Most cysts are clinically insignificant though some may be a cause of hyperestrogenism.

Luteal cysts (luteinized follicular cysts)

These are similar to follicular cysts, except the thecal coat is luteinized. The cyst is lined by an inner layer of large luteinized granulosa cells and an outer layer of smaller luteinized thecal cells.

Polycystic ovary syndrome (Stein–Leventhal syndrome)

This is a complex adrenal–ovarian disorder in which multiple small follicular cysts develop beneath a thickened, white ovarian capsule as a result of increased secretion of androgens from the adrenal glands or ovaries or both.

Clinical features—Patients have a persistent anovulatory state, high levels of luteinizing hormone (LH) and estrogen, and low levels of follicle-stimulating hormone (FSH) with high levels of circulating androgen. There is insulin resistance and hyperinsulinism.

Common presenting symptoms are:

- Menstrual irregularity.
- Infertility.
- Hirsutism.
- Acne.
- Occasional galactorrhea.

Complications—High estrogen levels may cause endometrial hyperplasia and increase the risk of the development of endometrial carcinoma.

Cysts of the fallopian tubes

Benign cysts of the fallopian tubes are common. There are two main types:

- Fimbrial cysts: extremely common, small, benign cysts containing clear fluid. Unilocular and typically situated at the fimbrial end of the tube.
- Cysts of Morgagni (paratubal cysts): cystic lesions situated adjacent to the fimbrial ends of the fallopian tubes and thought to be derived from remnants of the Wolffian duct.

Neoplastic disorders of the ovary

Ovarian cancer is responsible for more deaths than any other gynecological malignancy, largely because it often presents at an advanced stage. The ovarian tumor marker CA 125 is currently used routinely in the recognition of patients who have undergone treatment but have relapsed. CA 125, along with other markers, may be used in future screening programs for ovarian cancer.

Primary ovarian cancers account for 5% of all malignancies in women and of these approximately 5% have a hereditary component. In these women, mutations are found on the BRCA1 gene located on chromosome 17q. Ninety-five percent of ovarian cancer cases are sporadic and show complex genetic abnormalities including a high incidence of p53 mutation and amplification of the erb-B-2 (HER-2/neu) oncogene. There are several different tumor types.

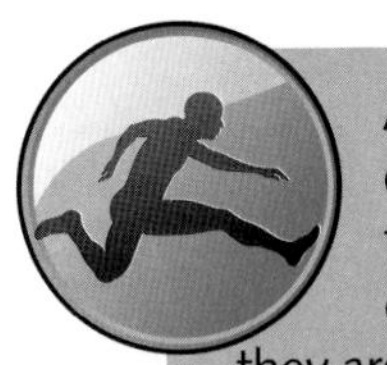

A logical way of classifying ovarian tumors is according to the normal tissue constituents from which they are derived:

- Surface epithelial tumors (70% of all cases).
- Germ cell tumors (20% of all cases).
- Sex cord and stromal tumors (10% of all cases).

Surface epithelial-stromal tumors

Epithelial tumors of the ovary comprise about 70% of all ovarian tumors and about 90% of malignant tumors. They are typically found in adult life.

The etiology is uncertain, but there is a higher incidence among women of higher social classes, and a decreased risk conferred by pregnancy and the oral contraceptive pill.

Types—Epithelial tumors are derived from surface epithelium, which in turn is derived from embryonal coelomic epithelium. Tumors with this origin can differentiate along different pathways into different types of tumors: tubal differentiation (serous tumors), endometrial differentiation (endometrial and clear cell tumors), endocervical differentiation (mucinous tumors), and transitional differentiation (Brenner tumors).

Microscopically, these tumors are classified into benign, malignant, and borderline malignancy (abnormal tissue architecture with atypical cells but no evidence of invasion). The majority behave in a benign fashion, the remainder behaving as low-grade malignant tumors.

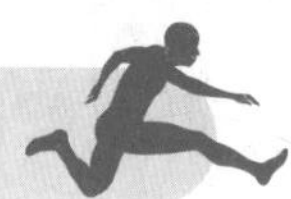

Serous tumors of the ovary

These ovarian cystic tumors of tubal differentiation contain a watery fluid; the majority (70%) are benign:

- Benign (serous cystadenoma)—thin-walled, unilocular cystic tumor lined by cuboidal regular epithelium.
- Malignant (serous cystadenocarcinoma)—characterized by pleomorphic cells and mitoses with invasion of the ovarian stroma.
- Borderline serous tumors—presence of cellular atypia but with no invasion.

Mucinous tumors of the ovary

These multilocular cystic ovarian tumors of endocervical differentiation contain gelatinous material:

- Benign (mucinous cystadenomas)—no atypical features or mitoses.
- Malignant (mucinous cystadenocarcinoma)—invasion of the ovarian stroma.
- Borderline mucinous tumors—presence of cellular atypia but with no invasion.

Endometrioid tumors

These ovarian tumors show endometrial differentiation. The vast majority are malignant (endometrioid carcinomas), accounting for 20% of all ovarian carcinomas.

The clear cell carcinoma is a variant of endometrioid carcinoma, characterized by the presence of cells with clear cytoplasm and containing abundant glycogen.

Brenner tumors of the ovary (transitional cell)

Tumors composed of nests of epithelium resembling a transitional cell epithelium of the urinary tract, these are associated with a spindle-cell stroma. The epithelial component may be benign, borderline, or malignant.

Germ cell and sex-cord stromal tumors are illustrated in Fig. 10.8.

Metastatic

The ovary is a common site of tumor metastasis, typically from the breast and gastrointestinal (GI) tract.

Krukenberg's tumor

This is an enlarged ovary with a metastatic signet ring-cell adenocarcinoma (typically of gastric origin).

Tumors of the fallopian tubes

Tumors of the fallopian tubes are extremely rare, and they can be benign or malignant.

Germ cell and sex-cord stromal ovarian tumors

Tumor	Features
Germ cell tumors	
Teratoma Benign cystic teratomas (dermoid cyst)	Cysts may be lined by structures such as the skin, hair, teeth, bone, or respiratory tract tissue
Solid teratomas	Composed of a variety of tissues including cartilage, smooth muscle, or epithelium
Dysgerminoma	Similar to seminoma of the testis
Yolk-sac tumors	Cystic, solid, and hemorrhagic; secrete α-fetoprotein
Sex-cord stromal tumors	
Granulosa cell tumors	Composed of granulosa cells derived from follicles
Sertoli–Leydig cell tumors	Mixture of cell types usually seen in the testis
Gonadoblastomas	Primitive germ cells and sex-cord stromal derivatives are present
Steroid cell tumors	Composed of cortical adrenal-like cells containing abundant lipid

Fig. 10.8 Germ cell and sex-cord stromal ovarian tumors.

Benign

Adenomatoid tumors

These are typically of the mesosalpinx.

Malignant

Malignant tumors of the fallopian tubes can be:

- Primary: adenocarcinomas; typically affect postmenopausal women. Poor prognosis due to late presentation.
- Secondary: endometrial tumors may spread up the tubal lumen, and metastatic disease in the pelvic peritoneum may involve the tubal serosa.

Disorders of the placenta and pregnancy

Ectopic pregnancies

A fertilized ovum is implanted outside the uterine cavity. This occurs in about 1 in 300 pregnancies. The fallopian tube (especially in the ampulla) is by far the most common site for this; other sites of abnormal implantation are very rare but include the peritoneal cavity, the ovary, and the cervix.

The etiology is uncertain, but ectopic pregnancies are possibly the result of some structural abnormality of the fallopian tube, e.g., scarring or adhesions resulting from previous episodes of salpingitis or endometriosis, or previous tubal surgery for contraceptive purposes, i.e., sterilization.

Pathogenesis—Following implantation, the proliferation of trophoblasts erodes the submucosal blood vessels, precipitating severe bleeding into the tubal lumen. The muscular wall of the fallopian tube is unable to undergo hypertrophy or distension, and so tubal pregnancy almost always results in the rupture of the fallopian tube and death of the fertilized ovum. This typically occurs in the early stages of pregnancy and often before the patient is even aware of being pregnant.

The types of rupture are:

- Into the lumen of the fallopian tube: common in ampullary pregnancy. Conceptus is extruded toward the fimbriated end of the tube. Mild hemorrhage into the peritoneal cavity occurs, which may collect as a clot in the pouch of Douglas.
- Into the peritoneal cavity: occurs most commonly from the isthmus of the tube, either spontaneously or as a result of pressure (e.g., straining at the stool, coitus, or pelvic examination). Hemorrhage is likely to be severe.
- Retroperitoneal (rare): rupture occurs into the potential space between the leaves of the broad ligament. Hemorrhage into the site is more likely to be controlled.

Clinical features are:

Severe lower abdominal pain: usually localized to the side of the ectopic pregnancy, but less localized if the fallopian tube ruptures.

- Vaginal bleeding: occurs after the death of the ovum, and it is an effect of estrogen withdrawal.
- Anemia: due to internal blood loss.
- Shock may occur if hemorrhage is severe and rapid (e.g., due to large vessel erosion). This is a most dangerous and dramatic consequence of tubal pregnancy.

Spontaneous abortion

Many fertilized ova fail to implant successfully, and it has been estimated that more than 40% of all conceptions fail to convert into recognizable pregnancies. Of those that survive this far, 15% terminate in a clinically recognized spontaneous abortion.

Etiology—Causes of spontaneous abortion differ at different stages of pregnancy, as shown in Fig. 10.9.

Types of spontaneous abortions

Threatened

There is bleeding from the placental site, which is not yet severe enough to terminate the pregnancy. The cervix is closed but there may be a few painful uterine contractions. The pregnancy is likely to continue.

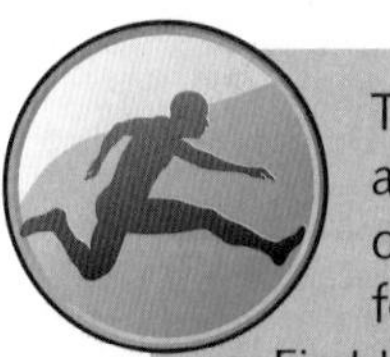

To remember the causes of abortion at different stages of pregnancy, learn the following rules of thumb:

- First trimester causes: majority are associated with abnormal fetuses.
- Second trimester causes: mainly due to uterine abnormalities.
- Third trimester causes: mainly the result of maternal abnormalities.

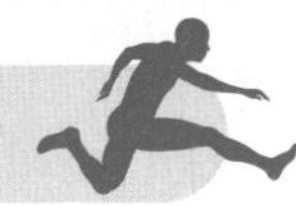

Causes of spontaneous abortion	
Time	**Cause**
First trimester	Abnormal chromosomal karyotypes, particularly Turner's syndrome Structural developmental abnormalities, e.g., neural tube defects Maternal SLE Transplacental infection, e.g., *Brucella, Listeria*, rubella, *Toxoplasma*, cytomegalovirus, and herpes
Second trimester	Chorioamnionitis Rupture of membranes Placental hemorrhages Structural abnormalities of the uterus, e.g., congenital uterine malformations Large submucosal leiomyomas Incompetence of the cervix Abnormal placentation (but more common in third trimester)
Third trimester	Uncontrolled hypertension Eclampsia Placental abnormalities, e.g., placental hemorrhage, abruption, and infarction
At any time	Endocrine abnormalities: diabetes, hypothyroidism, deficiency of progesterone or luteinizing hormone Trauma: surgical operation, blow to abdomen, or hypotensive shock

Fig. 10.9 Causes of spontaneous abortion.

Inevitable

Bleeding is slight but the cervix is usually open. Clinically the patient presents as a threatened abortion but bleeding is retroplacental and the fetus is already dead. Occasionally, products of conception may be felt in the cervical canal.

Incomplete

The fetus and membranes are expelled but the chorionic tissue remains attached and bleeding continues. Abortion must be completed by curettage.

Complete

The products of conception have been passed per vaginum and the uterus is empty. There is little bleeding, the uterus is small and the cervix closed.

Missed abortion

The embryo fails to develop or dies in utero but the products of conception are not expelled. The whole pregnancy is gradually absorbed, and often presents gynecologically as an unexplained amenorrhea. After about 12 weeks, the formation of a carnous mole (lobulated mass of laminated blood clot) is likely and after 18 weeks a macerated fetus is usually expelled.

Recurrent

This refers to three consecutive spontaneous abortions.

Pre-eclampsia and eclampsia

Pre-eclampsia

This is high blood pressure (>140/90mmHg) developing during pregnancy in a woman whose blood pressure was previously normal. It occurs in about 10% of all pregnant women. The etiology is unknown.

Risk factors are:

- Parity.
- Diabetes.
- Hypertension.
- Multiple pregnancies.
- Primigravida.
- Women over the age of 35.

It is thought to develop due to the failure of the narrow spiral arteries of the placenta to convert into low-resistance vascular sinuses.

Placental ischemia results in poor fetal growth and the liberation of substances that cause vasoconstriction and promote hypertension.

Endothelial cells of kidney arterioles become swollen, and fibrin deposition occurs in glomeruli leading to proteinuria (Fig. 10.10).

The condition may be mild or severe:

- Mild cases (majority): blood pressure is <100mmHg diastolic, with no associated proteinuria.
- Severe cases: diastolic pressure is consistently >100mmHg, with proteinuria and severe peripheral edema (pre-eclamptic toxemia syndrome).

Effects of pre-eclampsia

Reduced placental blood flow causes an increased risk of fetal hypoxia in late pregnancy, particularly during labor, with resultant perinatal mortality. The fetus may also suffer intrauterine growth retardation and have a low birth weight.

Maternal problems are less common, being largely confined to severe pre-eclampsia, which may progress into full-blown eclampsia (see below).

The disease resolves immediately after delivery.

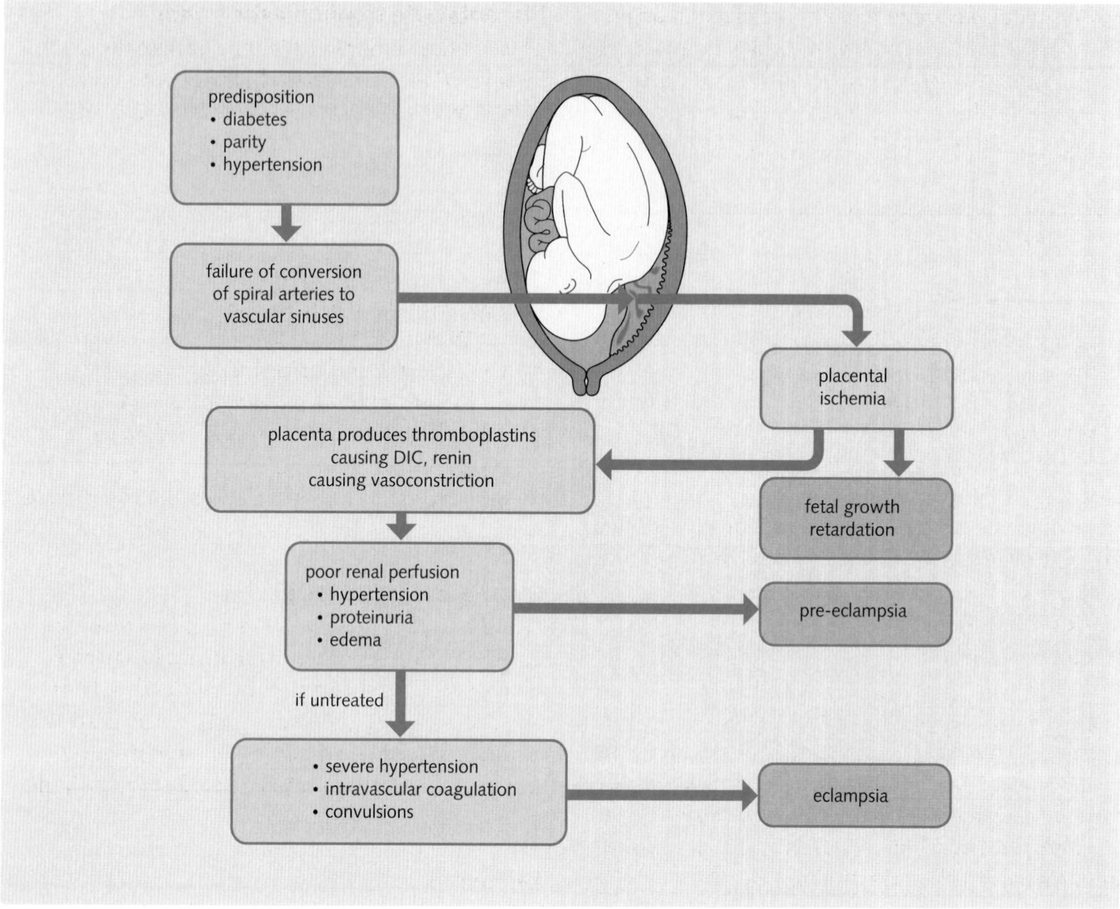

predisposition
• diabetes
• parity
• hypertension

failure of conversion of spiral arteries to vascular sinuses

placental ischemia

placenta produces thromboplastins causing DIC, renin causing vasoconstriction

fetal growth retardation

poor renal perfusion
• hypertension
• proteinuria
• edema

pre-eclampsia

if untreated

• severe hypertension
• intravascular coagulation
• convulsions

eclampsia

Fig. 10.10 Pathogenesis of pre-eclampsia.

Eclampsia

This is the occurrence of one or more convulsions not caused by other conditions such as epilepsy or cerebral hemorrhage in a woman with pre-eclampsia.

Incidence is rare; only a small proportion of patients with severe pre-eclampsia develop eclampsia.

Clinical features are severe systemic disturbance (i.e., frontal headaches, rapid and sustained rise in blood pressure, shock, anuria, and fits).

Other features may include disseminated intravascular coagulation with widespread occlusion of blood vessels, fibrinoid necrosis of vessel walls, and, in fatal cases, widespread microinfarcts in the brain, liver, kidneys, and other organs.

Fatal eclampsia is now rare because of treatment of the pre-eclamptic syndrome.

Neoplastic disorders of trophoblastic origin

Hydatidiform mole

This is the abnormal development of a gestational trophoblast leading to the formation of a benign mass of cystic vesicles derived from chorionic villi. It occurs in 1 in 2000 pregnancies in the U.S. and U.K., but it is seen more frequently in some parts of Asia, South America, and Africa.

There are two types:

- Partial: a partial mole is triploid with most containing one maternal and two paternal haploid sets of chromosomes. Cystic vesicles are found in only a part of the placenta. Fetal parts and some normal placental villi are present along with the abnormal trophoblastic tissue. There is a low risk of subsequent development of malignancy.

- Complete: a complete mole is of paternal origin and usually forms a bulky, grapelike mass that may fill the uterine cavity. No fetal parts or normal placental villi are present. There is a low risk of subsequent development of malignancy.

The pathogenesis is unknown.

Clinical features are:

- Amenorrhea followed by continuous or intermittent vaginal bleeding.
- Other symptoms of pregnancy: vomiting, preeclampsia.
- Enlarged soft uterus (often larger than dates would suggest).

Diagnosis is by elevated human chorionic gonadotrophin (hCG) excretion in urine (typically much greater than in normal pregnancies), and by ultrasound for the absence of the fetus.

Treatment is by evacuation of the uterus, with a second aspiration or curettage 2 to 4 weeks later to ensure complete removal of the mole.

Follow-up is by regular estimations of hCG for at least a year. Detection of hCG after 1 month may suggest incomplete removal and the persistence of trophoblastic disease. Untreated, this carries a risk of subsequent development of a malignant tumor of trophoblast or a choriocarcinoma.

Invasive mole (chorioadenoma destruens)

A hydatidiform mole invades through the decidua into the myometrium and associated blood vessels. Perforation of the uterus may occur, resulting in invasion of the parametrium. True malignant transformation is rare.

Choriocarcinomas

These malignant tumors of trophoblastic tissue have a propensity for invading vessel walls, and blood-borne metastases occur early to many sites, particularly the lung and brain.

They are rare in the U.S. and U.K. (at 1 per 50,000 pregnancies) but more common in Asia, South America, and Africa.

Etiology—About 50% develop from a hydatidiform mole and about 20% arise after a normal pregnancy with a variable time lag (a few months to many years).

The prognosis is excellent as the tumors respond well to cytotoxic chemotherapy (particularly if post-treatment monitoring of hCG levels is carried out).

Placental site trophoblastic tumor

This is a rare tumor in which the bulk of the tissue consists of chorionic epithelium but with very few villi. Typically benign, it may undergo malignant change.

Disorders of the breast

Inflammatory disorders and infections

Acute mastitis and breast abscess

These are uncommon, and they are usually complications of lactation. The most frequent organism is *Staphylococcus aureus*, which gains access through cracks and fissures of the nipple and areola. An abscess may form if drainage is inadequate.

Mammary duct ectasia

There is an abnormal progressive dilatation of the large breast ducts, which accumulate inspissated secretions. The etiology is unknown and it affects older women (perimenopausal age range). Patients develop a firm breast lump, which may mimic a carcinoma. There may also be blood-stained nipple discharge.

Fat necrosis

This is usually caused by trauma. Histology shows necrosis with multinucleated giant cells and later fibrosis. It may cause a discrete lump mimicking a carcinoma, sometimes with microcalcification.

Fibrocystic changes

Simple fibrocystic change

This is a generic term for a number of benign lesions in the breast that may occur together and may produce a discrete mass mimicking a carcinoma. Peak incidence is around the menopause. Etiology is unknown.

The histological changes that may be present include:

- Cysts: ranging in size from microscopic to palpable lesions 1–2cm in diameter. Cytological examination of aspirated fluid is necessary to distinguish them from carcinomas.
- Apocrine metaplasia: epithelial lining of hyperplastic ducts undergoes metaplasia to that of normal apocrine glands.
- Fibrosis: replacement of breast tissue by dense fibrous tissue.

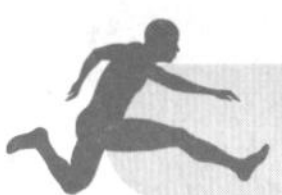

- Sclerosing adenosis: marked proliferation of specialized hormone-responsive stromal tissue and myoepithelial cells forming localized areas of irregular stellate, collagenous sclerosis in which epithelial elements are also present. Difficult to distinguish from some patterns of invasive carcinoma.
- Papillomatosis.

There is no increased risk of a carcinoma unless there is accompanying epithelial hyperplasia (see below).

Epithelial hyperplasia

This describes the proliferation of epithelial cells within ducts or lobules (ductal hyperplasia and lobular hyperplasia respectively). There are two types:

- Hyperplasia of the usual type: normal cytology and tissue architecture with no signs of malignancy.
- Hyperplasia of atypical type: biological spectrum between some abnormalities of cytology/architecture and carcinoma in situ.

The risk of subsequent invasive breast carcinoma is increased in individuals with florid usual hyperplasia, further increased in subjects with atypical hyperplasia, and much higher in those with some types of carcinoma in situ (comedo).

Epithelial hyperplasia can only be diagnosed histologically.

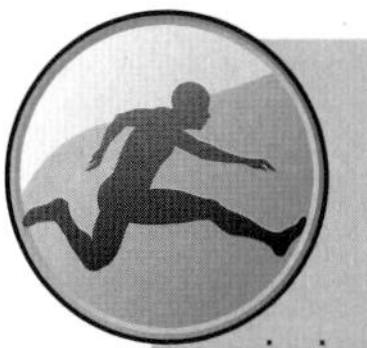

The following benign pathologies may cause discrete breast lumps or nipple discharge which mimic carcinomas:

- Duct ectasia.
- Fat necrosis.
- Fibrocystic disease (fibrosis, sclerosing adenosis, papillomatosis).
- Intraductal papilloma.
- Fibroadenoma.

Neoplasms of the breast

Fibroadenoma

This common benign tumor with a proliferation of both stroma and epithelium, occurs in young women (most frequently the 25–35 age group). It produces discrete but mobile breast lumps typically 1–4cm in size.

Phyllodes tumor

This is a tumor composed of both a stroma and epithelium, where the stroma is more cellular than fibroadenomas. It is less common than fibroadenoma and occurs in the older age group (peak incidence being 45 years of age). Clinically, the tumor presents as a breast lump.

Macroscopically, there are rubbery white lesions consisting of a whorled pattern of slit-like spaces and solid areas.

Microscopically, there is a variable appearance, classified into benign (90% of cases), or of borderline malignant potential or definitely malignant.

There is the potential for local recurrence with increasing aggressiveness, and the tumor may eventually metastasize.

Intraductal papilloma

Epithelial proliferation within ducts produces papillary structures. These generally occur in older women and may produce a blood-stained nipple discharge. Papillomas are usually solitary with no increased risk of a carcinoma. However, there is a rare condition of multiple intraductal papillomas that is premalignant.

Carcinoma

Incidence—This comprises 20% of all cancers in women, and it is the second most common cause of death in the 35–55 year age group of women, increasing with age steeply to 45 years and continuing to increase less steeply thereafter.

There is a 200-fold female preponderance, with the highest rates in America, Western Europe, and the Antipodes, and the lowest rates in Africa and Southeast Asia.

Predisposing factors are:

- Atypical epithelial proliferation.
- Mutations of BRCA 1 (chromosome 17) and 2 genes (chromosome 13) account for 5% of cases.
- Long interval between menarche and menopause.
- Older age at first pregnancy.
- Obesity and dietary factors.
- Ionizing radiation.

All breast carcinomas are adenocarcinomas derived from epithelial cells of the terminal ductal lobules.

Noninvasive carcinomas are tumors confined to ducts with no evidence of invasion through the basement membrane. Ductal carcinoma in situ (noninvasive) can become invasive. Lobular carcinoma in situ is a risk marker for developing breast cancer. Invasive carcinomas are tumors that have eroded through the basement membrane of their tissue of origin to invade surrounding stuctures.

Investigation is by ultrasound mammography, core biopsy, or fine needle aspiration cytology. Invasive carcinomas are categorized histologically:

- Invasive ductal (most common at 75%).
- Invasive lobular.
- Mucinous.
- Tubular.
- Medullary.
- Papillary.

Macroscopic features—A discrete lump with tethering to the skin or surrounding connective tissue. The macroscopic appearance of the tumor depends upon the amount and type of stroma within the carcinoma.

Spread is as follows:

- Direct: skin and muscles of the chest wall.
- Lymphatic: axillary lymph nodes, internal mammary lymph nodes.
- Blood: lungs, bone, liver, and brain.
- Transcoelomic: pleural cavities and pericardium.

Prognosis—Related to tumor grade and type (tubular—best prognosis), size of the tumor, lymph node status, and estrogen receptor status (usually responds to tamoxifen if positive).

(Proto)oncogene alterations (gene amplification) relating to C-CBB-2 (HER-2) occur in 20% of breast cancers, and they are related to poorer prognosis. This is now a target for therapy with Herceptin.

Figures 10.11–10.13 give the type, spread, and TNM staging of breast carcinoma, respectively.

Screening for breast carcinoma

There is no direct screening method equivalent to the cytology of the uterine cervix. The primary

Types of breast carcinoma

Character	Neoplasm
Non-invasive	Ductal carcinoma in situ Lobular carcinoma in situ
Invasive	Invasive ductal carcinoma (85%) Invasive lobular carcinoma (10%) Mucinous Tubular Medullary Papillary

Fig. 10.11 Types of breast carcinoma.

Spread of breast carcinoma

Spread	Area
Direct	Skin
Lymphatic	Axillary lymph nodes Internal mammary lymph nodes Supraclavicular lymph nodes
Hematogenous	Liver Lung Opposite breast Bone Brain

Fig. 10.12 Spread of breast carcinoma.

TNM staging of breast carcinoma

Tumor	Nodes	Metastases
T1 tumor 20mm or less; no fixation or nipple retraction	N0 node negative	M0 no distant metastases
T2 tumor 20–50mm, or less than 20mm with fixation	N1 axillary nodes mobile	M1 distant metastases present
T3 tumor 50–100mm, or less than 50mm with fixation	N2 axillary nodes fixed	
T4 greater than 100mm, or chest wall invasion	N3 supraclavicular nodes positive or arm edema	

Fig. 10.13 TNM staging of breast carcinoma.

screening modality is mammography, which is more effective in older women with less radiodense breast tissue. Abnormalities seen on mammograms include calcification and soft tissue deformity.

The male breast

Gynecomastia

This is the benign enlargement of breast tissue.

Etiology—Hormonal influences including increased estrogen production or receptor sensitivity. It is associated with liver disease, stilbestrol therapy for prostate carcinoma, and drugs such as chlorpromazine.

Carcinoma

Less than 1% of breast carcinomas occur in men. The condition is associated with Klinefelter's syndrome, and it is usually of the ductal type; the lobular type has not been described (there are no lobules in the male breast).

Disorders of the penis

Inflammation and infection

Viral infection

Common viral infections of the penis include genital herpes and genital warts (condyloma acuminatum).

Genital herpes

This is an acute infection of the penile mucosa by the herpes simplex virus with the formation of typical herpetic vesicles on the glans penis. The vesicles soon burst to produce shallow painful ulcers.

The virus may remain latent for many years. Recurrent herpes infections are caused by reactivation of the virus, which may be precipitated by a febrile illness, immune suppression, emotional stress, or UV light.

Condyloma acuminatum (genital warts)

These cauliflower-like warts are seen on the penis and around the perineum. They are caused by the human papillomavirus subtypes HPV6 and HPV11.

Bacterial infection

Inflammation of the glans (balanitis) and prepuce (posthitis) can be caused by a variety of bacterial organisms, the most common of which are staphylococci, coliforms, gonococci, and *Chlamydia*.

The appearance is that of marked congestion and edema with exudate on the surface of the glans. Ulceration with chronic scarring may occur if untreated.

Syphilis—primary chancre

A solitary, firm papule (typically painless) later ulcerates to form a shallow, clean-based depression with extensive surrounding induration and inguinal lymphadenopathy. The responsible organism is *Treponema pallidum*.

The most common sites are the glans and the inner side of the prepuce but occasionally also the shaft.

The condition heals spontaneously in about 2 months, or more rapidly with treatment. Untreated, it will progress to secondary syphilis (cutaneous manifestations, generalized lymphadenitis) and then tertiary syphilis (thoracic aortic aneurysms, CNS changes). The spirochetal organism is easily seen in wet preparations from the chancre, under darkfield microscopy.

Lymphogranuloma venereum (lymphogranuloma inguinale)

This venereal disease is characterized by granulomatous lesions and caused by *Chlamydia trachomatis* (serotypes L1–L3).

Clinical features are:

- Small primary lesion: develops at site of inoculation, usually transient and often unnoticed.
- Unilateral lymphadenopathy (primarily inguinal): occurs 1–2 weeks after infection. Nodes are at first discrete, but later coalesce.

The disease follows a chronic course varying from weeks to months. Healing occurs with fibrosis resulting in lymphatic blockage.

Late complications are external genitalia elephantiasis or rectal strictures due to lymphatic obstruction.

Fungi

Infection with *Candida albicans* is common in men with diabetes mellitus or recent treatment with broad-spectrum antibiotics.

Neoplastic disorders

Benign

Condyloma acuminatum

This is described above (genital warts).

Malignant

Carcinoma in situ (erythroplasia of Queyrat)

Penile carcinoma in situ is restricted to the glans, and it resembles non-specific balanitis with single or multiple, flat, red, glistening areas. There is a spectrum of changes from dysplasia to carcinoma in situ grouped together as penile intra-epithelial neoplasia. Many cases are associated with HPV infection.

The condition leads to invasive cancer unless treated vigorously with local irradiation or 5-fluorouracil cream.

Squamous cell carcinoma

This is a well-differentiated, keratinizing, invasive tumor usually seen in elderly men, occurring most commonly in uncircumcised men, and thought to be associated with a previous infection with human papillomavirus.

It presents as a warty, cauliflower-like growth that bleeds easily. It is typically slow growing, but it is often neglected because of patient embarrassment.

Disorders of the testis and epididymis

Congenital abnormalities and regression

Cryptorchidism (undescended testis)

This is a condition caused by maldescent of the testes, affecting about 5% at birth, although many descend by the first birthday.

In the embryo, the testes develop from the genital ridge high on the posterior wall.

At about 7 months' gestation, the testes migrate down the posterior abdominal wall, and they are guided by a cord (the gubernaculum) through the inguinal ring into the scrotum.

Occasionally, migration fails to occur and one (75% of cases) or both (25% of cases) testes become arrested somewhere along the route (Fig. 10.14). There are three conditions:

- Abdominal testicle: usually found just inside the internal ring.
- Inguinal testicle: in the inguinal canal.
- Retractile testicles (most common): high retractile testicle—rides up and down from the external ring to the upper part of the scrotum; low retractile testicle—can be persuaded to reach the bottom of the scrotum. Usually settles at puberty and does not need an operation.

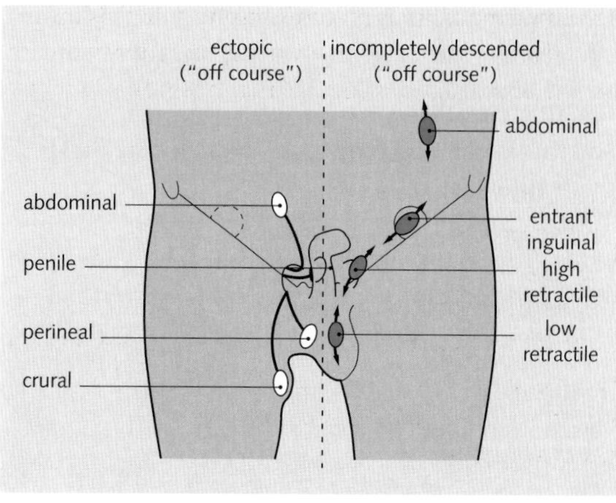

Fig. 10.14 Maldescended testes showing common sites of arrest. (Adapted from *Lecture Notes on Urology*, 5th edn, by J. Blandy, Blackwell Science, 1998.)

The complications are:

- Infertility: temperature of aberrant locations is higher than in scrotum, and prevents normal germ cell development. The testis remains small and incapable of producing effective spermatozoa.
- Malignancy: more common in an undescended testis; about 1 in 10 of all testicular tumors arise in association with cryptorchidism.
- Inguinal hernia: there is nearly always a patent tunica vaginalis that predisposes to the development of an inguinal hernia.
- Torsion of the testicle (see below).

Management is by detection and correction of testicular maldescent. This is important because of the increased risk of testicular carcinoma. Some restoration of function may be achieved by "orchidopexy" at an early stage (the testis is surgically pulled down into the scrotal sac).

Abnormalities of the tunica vaginalis

The tunica vaginalis and tunica albuginea are invested with mesothelial cells and may be the site of fluid accumulation, inflammation, or (uncommonly) tumor formation.

Hydrocoele

Fluid accumulates in the cavity bounded by the tunica vaginalis. This is the most common cause of swelling within the scrotum.

The etiology is as follows:

Congenital patency of the processus vaginalis, often with continuity into the peritoneal cavity.

Secondary to tumors, epididymitis, mumps, or acute orchitis.

Hematocoele

Blood accumulates in the cavity bounded by the tunica vaginalis.

Etiology—Trauma, torsion of the testis, hemorrhage into pre-existing hydrocoele, generalized bleeding disorders, or, rarely, due to the extension of the testicular tumor through the tunica vaginalis.

Chylocele

Obstruction to the lymphatic drainage of the tunica and cord occurs.

Hernias

Indirect inguinal hernias (described in Chapter 7) typically occur as a result of patent processus vaginalis.

Trauma and vascular disturbances

Torsion

There is twisting of a testicle on its pedicle with obstruction of venous return such that blood continues to enter the testis, but cannot leave. The testis becomes swollen and painful and, eventually, it becomes infarcted (venous infarction). In advanced torsion, the testis is almost black as a result of vascular congestion.

Early detection and surgical relief are required to save testicular viability. Surgical removal is necessary for advanced disease.

Varicocele

Variceal dilatation of the veins of the pampiniform plexus of the spermatic cord occurs.

Neoplastic disorders

Tumors of the testis, although relatively uncommon, are important since many occur in young men, and they are the most common form of malignancy in this age group.

Their incidence is uncommon (only affecting 1–2%), but with an increasing incidence in many Western countries, especially Denmark.

Typically they are seen in early adult life and particularly significant in those aged between 20 and 45.

Their etiology is unknown; maldescent of the testis is the only known risk factor.

Clinical presentations are:

- Painless unilateral enlargement of testis (majority).
- Secondary hydrocele.
- Symptoms of metastases: especially in malignant teratoma (e.g., hemoptysis from lung deposits, hepatomegaly, or retroperitoneal mass due to metastasis to para-aortic lymph nodes).
- Endocrine effects: gynecomastia, precocious puberty (typically from Leydig or Sertoli cell tumors).

There are two main groups of testicular tumors:

- Germ cell tumors (97% of cases): derived from multipotential germ cells of the testis arising as teratomas and seminomas.
- Non-germ cell tumors (3% of cases): derived from specialized and non-specialized support cells of the testis.

Note that the incidence of germ cell tumors in the testis is exactly opposite to the incidence in the ovary.

Germ cell tumors

Germ cell tumors are subdivided into:

- Seminomas: tumors showing spermatogenic differentiation.
- Teratomas: tumors retaining their totipotentiality for differentiation.
- Combined tumors: mixture of both seminomatous and teratomatous differentiation.

Seminoma

The most common malignant testicular tumor, this accounts for about 50% of all malignant germ cell tumors.

Histological types of seminoma are:

- Classic seminoma (most common subtype): characteristic feature is the presence of fibrous septa with lymphocytic infiltrate.
- Spermatocytic seminoma: larger tumor cells with some small cells resembling spermatocytes.
- Anaplastic seminoma: cells show marked pleomorphism and increased mitotic activity.
- Seminomas with trophoblastic giant cells: associated with increased blood levels of human chorionic gonadotrophin secreted by trophoblastic cells.

Teratoma

This tumor of germ cell origin is composed of several types of tissue representing endoderm, ectoderm, and mesoderm. These are more aggressive tumors than seminomas.

Teratomas are classified according to their histological pattern. There are two separate classification systems, the British system and the WHO system, which are compared in Fig. 10.15. The British classification is as follows, with basic definitions:

- Differentiated teratoma: a rare type of teratoma in which tissues are well differentiated and fully matured so that a wide range of organoid structures (e.g., skin, hair, cartilage, and bone) can be identified. Lesions are usually seen in young children, and they behave in a benign fashion.
- Malignant teratoma intermediate: partly solid and partly cystic tumor. Mixture of well-differentiated areas (resembling differentiated teratoma) and areas of malignancy with cellular pleomorphism and necrosis.
- Malignant teratoma undifferentiated: completely undifferentiated tumor with marked nuclear pleomorphism and a high mitotic rate. There is usually extensive tumor necrosis.
- Malignant teratoma trophoblastic: tumor contains areas of syncytiotrophoblast and cytotrophoblast arranged in a villous pattern. Often hemorrhagic due to vascular invasion (bloodborne metastases common); hCG and α-fetoprotein are useful markers, and they may be measured in serum or demonstrated in syncytiotrophoblast by immunocytochemistry.
- Yolk sac tumor is a highly malignant tumor derived from germ cells, and it comes in two types:
    - Pure form: more common in children especially in the first 3 years of life.
    - Mixed form: most commonly mixed with undifferentiated germ cells. Presence of yolk sac elements in association with other elements confers a worse prognosis.

The tumor makes α-fetoprotein, which can be detected in the serum or by immunohistochemical detection.

Combined germ cell tumor

Between 10 and 15% of germ cell tumors consist of a mixture of seminomatous and teratomatous elements.

Prognosis of germ cell tumors

The prognosis of testicular teratomas has improved greatly with the use of cytotoxic chemotherapy, and it is related to histological type, as well as to tumor stage. In general, germ cell tumors containing trophoblastic, yolk sac, and undifferentiated elements have the worst prognosis.

Non-germ cell tumors

Non-germ cell tumors are subdivided into:

- Sex cord and stromal tumors: interstitial (Leydig) cell tumor, Sertoli cell tumor.
- Others: mainly malignant lymphomas and metastatic tumors.

Interstitial (Leydig) cell tumor

This rare tumor arises from the interstitial or Leydig cells of the testis. It may produce androgens, estrogens, or both, causing precocious development of secondary sexual characteristics in childhood or loss of libido/gynecomastia in adults.

The majority of such tumors are benign but those over 5cm in diameter and those with mitoses may behave in a malignant fashion.

Comparison of the British and WHO classifications of teratomas

Type of differentiation	British	WHO
Somatic	Differentiated teratoma	Mature teratoma
	Malignant teratoma intermediate	Immature teratoma or mixed teratoma and embryonal carcinoma
None	Malignant teratoma undifferentiated	Embryonal carcinoma
Extra-embryonic	Yolk sac tumor	Yolk sac tumor
	Malignant teratoma trophoblastic	Choriocarcinoma

Fig. 10.15 Comparison of the British and WHO classifications of teratomas.

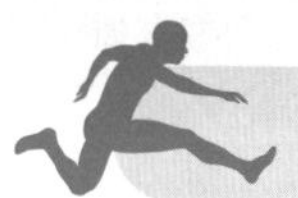

Sertoli cell tumor (androblastoma)

This well-circumscribed tumor is composed of cells resembling normal Sertoli cells of the tubules. Most lesions are benign.

Malignant lymphomas

The non-Hodgkin's-type lymphoma is usually a poorly differentiated B cell lymphoma with a diffuse pattern. These comprise about 7% of testicular tumors with a peak incidence between 60 and 80 years of age.

Metastatic tumors

The spread of other tumors to the testis may occasionally occur, particularly in acute leukemia.

Figure 10.16 provides a summary of testicular tumors.

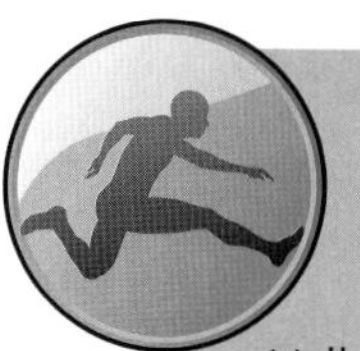

Many testicular tumors have useful cell markers:

- Trophoblastic germ cell tumors: ↑ hCG.
- Yolk sac tumors: ↑ α-fetoprotein.
- 90% of patients with malignant teratoma undifferentiated: ↑ α-fetoprotein., ↑ hCG, or both.
- 50% of patients with malignant teratoma intermediate: ↑ α-fetoprotein., ↑ hCG, or both.
- 10% of patients with seminoma: ↑ hCG.

Summary of testicular tumors	
Germ cell tumors (97% of cases)	
Seminomas	Classic seminoma Spermatocytic seminoma Anaplastic seminoma Seminomas with trophoblastic giant cells
Teratomas	Differentiated teratoma Malignant teratoma intermediate Malignant teratoma undifferentiated Malignant teratoma trophoblastic Yolk sac tumor
Combined	Mixture of seminomatous and teratomatous elements
Non-germ cell tumors (3% of cases)	
Sex-cord and stromal tumors	Interstitial (Leydig) cell tumor Sertoli cell tumor
Others	Malignant lymphomas Metastatic tumors

Fig. 10.16 Summary of testicular tumors.

Disorders of the prostate

Benign prostatic hyperplasia

Non-neoplastic enlargement of the prostate is the most common disorder of the prostate affecting almost all men over the age of 70, but it is found with increasing frequency and severity from about 45 years onwards.

The pathogenesis is uncertain, but believed to be a result of androgen–estrogen imbalance. A periurethral (central) group of prostatic glands (not the true prostatic glands at the periphery) are hormone sensitive and they undergo hyperplasia. Their continuing enlargement compresses peripheral true prostatic glands leading to their collapse, leaving only fibrous supporting stroma (Fig. 10.17).

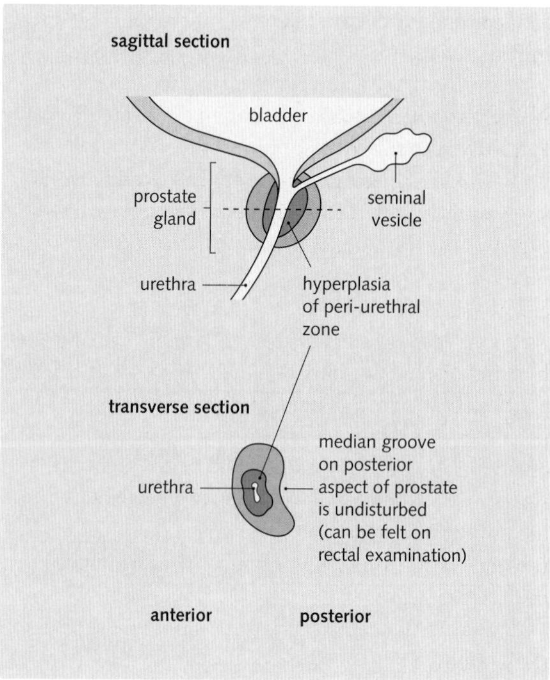

Fig. 10.17 Benign prostatic hyperplasia.

Affected lobes are:

- Two lateral lobes (majority of cases).
- Posterior lobe (uncommon) causing an obstruction of the urinary outflow tract at the internal urinary meatus at the bladder neck.

Macroscopically:

- Nodular pattern of hyperplastic glandular acini separated by fibrous stroma.
- Some nodules are cystically dilated and contain a milky fluid.
- Other nodules contain numerous calcific concretions (corpora amylacea).

Microscopically, the epithelium of hyperplastic acini (larger than normal) are lined by tall columnar epithelial cells, and they may form irregular papillary folds.

Infarction causes necrotic areas with a hemorrhagic margin. There is often muscular hypertrophy particularly in the region of the bladder neck.

Clinical presentation—Compression of the prostatic urethra by the enlarged prostate causes difficulties with micturition, mainly a delay in starting to pass urine, a poor or intermittent stream, and dribbling at the end of micturition.

Complications—Prolonged prostatic obstruction can lead to several complications which are outlined in Fig. 10.18.

Complications of benign prostatic hyperplasia	
Bladder wall	Hypertrophy of smooth muscle Trabeculation: due to prominent bands of thickened smooth muscle Diverticula: protrude between trabeculae
Bladder size	Dilatation: due to failure of bladder wall compensatory mechanisms
Ureteric changes	Dilatation of ureters
Urinary infection (cystitis)	Bladder fails to empty completely after micturition, and residual urine is liable to infection
Kidney disease	Pyelonephritis: from ascending infection Impaired renal failure Hydronephrosis Calculi

Fig. 10.18 Complications of benign prostatic hyperplasia.

Neoplastic disorders

Prostatic carcinoma

This is an adenocarcinoma of the prostate, and it is shown in Fig. 10.19. It is the second most common type of cancer in males, and its incidence is increasing. It is rare before 55 years of age with a peak incidence between 60 and 85 years.

Its etiology is uncertain, but there is probably hormonal involvement.

It arises in the true prostatic glands at the periphery of the prostate, and it is, therefore, often well established before the development of symptoms of difficulty with micturition due to urethral obstruction. Indeed, some tumors may remain silent even in the presence of widespread metastases.

Types are divided into three groups on the basis of their behaviour:

- Latent: small foci of well-differentiated carcinoma, frequently an incidental finding in

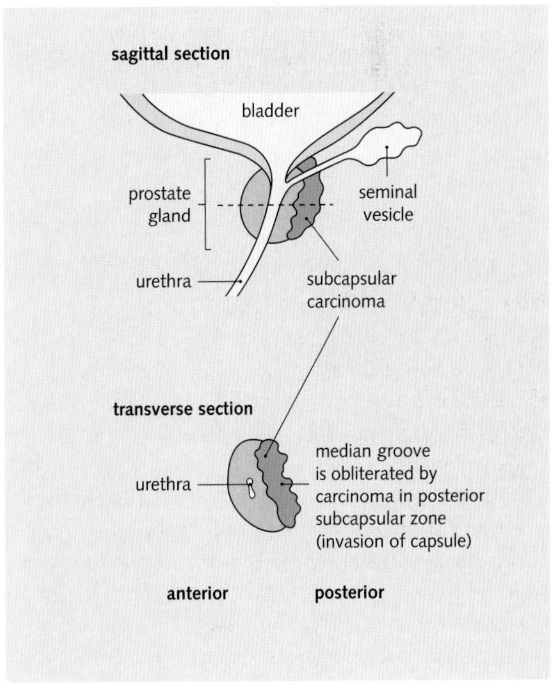

Fig. 10.19 Prostatic carcinoma.

prostatic glands of elderly men. Remain confined to the prostate for a long period.
- Invasive: invade locally and metastasize.
- Occult: not clinically apparent in primary site but present as metastatic disease.

Macroscopically, there are diffuse areas of firm, white tissue merging into fibromuscular prostatic stromal tissues. Distortion and extension outside the prostatic capsule is common producing a firm, craggy mass that can be palpated on rectal examination.

Microscopically, the majority have a differentiated glandular pattern (good prognosis); a minority have poorly differentiated sheets of cells with no acinar pattern (poor prognosis).

Spread is:
- Direct: to the base of the bladder and adjacent tissues. May cause obstruction of the urethra (difficulty in micturition) and may block the ureters, causing hydronephrosis.
- Lymphatic: to pelvic and para-aortic nodes.
- Hematogenous: most commonly to bone, but also to the lungs and liver. Bone metastases are typically sclerotic with bone production (dense on radiograph) rather than lytic with bone destruction.

Clinical features are:
- Urinary symptoms (delay in starting to pass urine, poor stream, terminal dribbling).
- Hard, craggy prostate on rectal examination.
- Bone metastases: pain (especially back pain), fracture, anemia.
- Lymph node metastases.

Sometimes the primary prostatic tumor remains small (occult carcinoma), yet it produces widespread symptomatic metastatic disease.

Diagnosis is by:
- Imaging: ultrasound, X-ray, isotope bone scan.
- Biopsy: immunohistochemical detection of prostate-specific antigen (PSA) and prostate-specific acid phosphatase (PSAP) in biopsy material.
- Serology: PSA and PSAP may also be used as serum markers for disease, levels being particularly raised when there is metastatic disease. The use of tumor markers for screening purposes has yet to be fully evaluated.
- Chemistry: bone alkaline phosphatase may be increased with metastatic disease to bone.

Treatment—Many prostatic carcinomas are dependent on testosterone for growth, and about 75% of patients benefit from a treatment which reduces androgen levels, such as orchidectomy or treatment with estrogenic drugs, or agonists of luteinizing hormone-releasing hormone may induce tumor regression.

- Name the common infections of the lower genital tract.
- Name the tumors of the vulva and vagina.
- List the risk factors for CIN and squamous cell carcinoma of the cervix.
- Describe the histological criteria for the grading of CIN I to III.
- Define endometriosis and endometritis.
- List the clinical features and complications of endometriosis.
- Define fibroids, and describe their characteristics.
- What conditions predispose to the development of salpingitis?
- Name the different types of cystic lesions that affect the ovary and fallopian tube.
- Describe the different types of ovarian surface epithelial tumor.
- What is an ectopic pregnancy? Name the types of rupture.
- List the causes and types of spontaneous abortion.
- Describe the clinical features of pre-eclampsia and eclampsia.
- List the pathologies that may cause a breast lump.
- Describe the rationale for a breast screening program.
- List the predisposing factors for the development of breast carcinoma in females.
- Name the common infections of the penis.
- Describe the malignant tumors of the penis.
- Define hydrocele, hematocele, and varicocele.
- Describe the pathology of benign prostatic hyperplasia.

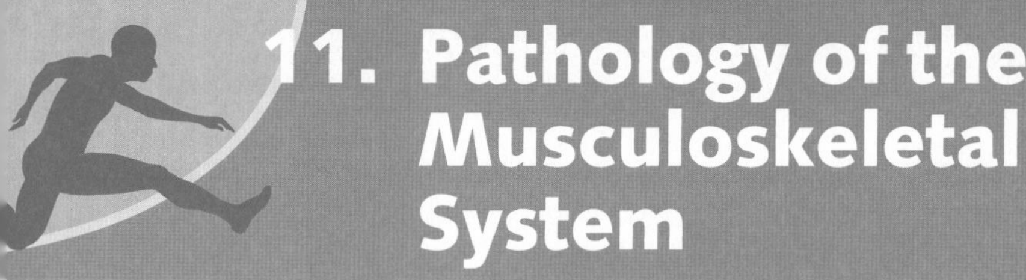

11. Pathology of the Musculoskeletal System

Disorders of bone structure

Achondroplasia

This hereditary disorder of endochondral ossification results in dwarfism due to short limbs.

Incidence—The most common cause of dwarfism, occurring in about 1 per 10,000 births.

Etiology—Autosomal dominant with a high incidence of spontaneous mutation accounting for its sudden appearance in a child with normal parents (increased incidence with paternal age). The affected gene is for fibroblast growth factor receptor.

Pathogenesis—Normal column formation of cartilage cells at epiphyseum during bone growth does not occur, resulting in diminished lengthening of cartilage bones (e.g., long bones, base of the skull, and pelvis). Periosteal bone formation is normal. Cartilage bones are, therefore, shortened but thick and strong. Membranous bone (such as the vault of the skull) is not affected.

Achondroplasia results in nonproportional dwarfism, i.e., the trunk is of normal size, but arms and legs are much shorter than normal. Other common types of dwarfism (e.g., pituitary hormone deficiency or malnutrition) are typically proportional, with all bones being affected equally.

Disorders of the bone matrix

Osteogenesis imperfecta

This heterogeneous group of rare congenital disorders is characterized by abnormal collagen formation with unusually brittle and fragile bones.

Etiology—Mutation of genes coding for type I collagen results in abnormal collagen formation in the osteoid. The pattern of inheritance can be either dominant or recessive, and it involves mutation at sites on chromosome 7 and 17.

Appearance—There is a marked variation in severity, but widespread weakness of bone results in multiple fractures frequently leading to severe deformity.

Osteoporosis

This slowly progressive disorder is characterized by reduced bone mass as a result of a relative increase in bone erosion that is not adequately counteracted by new bone formation.

Incidence—The most common metabolic bone disease. Widespread in the elderly, it is an important cause of morbidity and even mortality, the weakened bone being particularly predisposed to fracture with minimal trauma. The risk factors for osteoporosis are illustrated in Fig. 11.1.

Macroscopically—Bones are lighter in weight, less dense on radiography (Fig. 11.2) and show thinning of the cortex. Lumbar vertebral bodies are more biconcave than normal, such that the intervertebral disc space appears more spherical. Similar shaped vertebral bodies are seen in fish and consequently they are referred to as "fish vertebrae."

Microscopically—Bone trabeculae are thinner and reduced in number, and there is a decrease in the number of osteoblasts. Mineralization is not affected.

Complications are:

- Bone pain: especially in the back because of compression of vertebral bodies. Multiple compressions lead to overall loss of height, which may be compounded by uneven compression of vertebrae leading to anteroposterior bending of the spine (kyphosis).
- Fractures: reduced bone mass leads to increased fractures following minimal trauma, especially of the neck, the femur, and the wrist.

Management—Emphasis is on prevention rather than treatment, namely avoidance of risk factors, physical exercise, and adequate calcium intake.

Hormone replacement therapy (HRT) should be considered in women with low bone mass following menopause.

Mucopolysaccharidoses

This group of autosomal recessive disorders of mucopolysaccharide (glycosaminoglycans, such as

Type	Risk factors
Idiopathic	Female Early menopause Small stature Thin physique Family history Advanced age Nulliparity
Secondary-generalized	Metabolic: low calcium intake, impaired supply of protein (e.g., nephrotic syndrome or cirrhosis of liver), scurvy Assorted endocrine disorders: thyrotoxicosis, panhypopituitarism, and Cushing's syndrome Steroid therapy Cigarette smoking Alcohol abuse Reduced physical activity Aluminum antacids
Secondary-localized	Disuse atrophy: especially in neurological limb paralysis or post fracture

Fig. 11.1 Type and associated risk factors for osteoporosis.

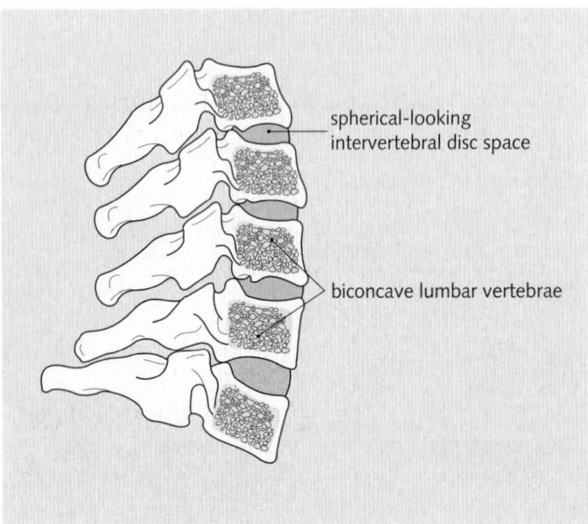

Fig. 11.2 Radiographic appearance of lumbar vertebrae in osteoporosis.

dermatan sulphate and heparin sulphate) metabolism results in abnormal substrate accumulation in cells of the brain and other tissues.

The main disorders are Hurler's syndrome (deficiency of α-L-iduronidase) and Hunter's syndrome (deficiency of iduronate sulphate sulphatase), both of which are associated with a wide variety of clinical features including stiff joints and short stature.

Disorders of osteoclast function

Osteopetrosis (marble bone disease; Albers–Schönberg disease)

This rare inherited disorder is characterized by increased density of all cartilagenous bones, especially the vertebrae, pelvic bones, and ribs.

Pathogenesis—Increased bone density is thought to be secondary to defective resorption of bone by osteoclasts.

Appearance—There is no discernible differentiation of cartilagenous bones into cortex and medulla: the cortical compact bone extends into the medulla, which is thus devoid of cancellous bone.

Effect—Bones are excessively dense, yet extremely brittle and prone to fracture. In addition to increased predisposition to fractures, the condition causes depression of marrow function and compression of cranial nerves within the base of the skull.

Paget's disease of the bone (osteitis deformans)

This chronic disease of excessive uncontrolled resorption and deposition of bone particularly affects the skull, backbone, pelvis, and long bones. It is rare before 40 years of age, but increases in incidence with age thereafter, with males more affected than females.

Etiology—Unknown, but recent evidence suggests a paramyxovirus infection of the osteoclasts. Electron microscope studies have demonstrated probable viral inclusions in the nuclei of osteoclasts.

Pathogenesis—Large, abnormal, multinucleated osteoclasts cause excessive bone erosion with destruction of trabecular and cortical bone. Each wave of bone destruction is followed by a vigorous but uncoordinated osteoblastic response, producing new osteoid to fill the defects left by the osteoclasts. However, both osteoclastic erosion and osteoblastic deposition are random, haphazard, and unrelated to functional stresses on the bone, resulting in greatly distorted bone architecture.

Morphology—Bone shows a characteristic woven, non-lamellar pattern indicative of rapid reparative deposition. There are often well marked "cement lines" visible producing the characteristic "mosaic" or "crazy-paving" appearance.

Although bone bulk is often increased, it is typically weaker than normal and more prone to fractures. X-rays reveal patchy sclerosis.

Disruption of bone architecture is followed by progressive increased vascularity in the spaces between the thickened bone trabeculae.

The effects of Paget's may be widespread (affecting many bones) or localized (confined to one area in a single bone—monostotic Paget's disease).

Most patients present with one or both of the following features:

- Bone pain: usually localized to site of most active disease.
- Bone deformity: seen only where there is extensive involvement of an entire bone or series of bones, most commonly enlargement of skull or thickening, enlargement, and bowing of tibia.

Complications—Some patients occasionally present with the complications of Paget's disease:

- Nerve compression symptoms: usually seen in association with Paget's disease of the skull, in which enlargement of the pagetic bone can lead to cranial nerve palsies (e.g., CN VIII compression results in deafness). Vertebral disease may cause kyphosis, shortening of trunk, and compression of nerves in intervertebral foramina.
- Pathological fracture: bone is increased in bulk, but it is weaker than normal and more likely to fracture with trivial trauma.
- Cardiac hypertrophy: due to increased vascularity of bones.
- Malignant tumor (1% of cases): usually osteosarcoma, which may develop in areas of long-standing active Paget's disease.

Investigations are:

- Serology: normal calcium and phosphate, increased alkaline phosphatase.
- Urine: increased urinary excretion of hydroxyproline.
- Abnormal isotope bone scans.
- X-ray: localized bone enlargement, altered trabecular pattern, and alternating areas of rarefaction and increased density.

Management is by analgesia for bone pain, and calcitonin or bisphosphonates for severe bone pain not controlled by analgesics. The latter cause inhibition of bone resorption.

Hyperparathyroidism

Elevated secretion of parathyroid hormone (PTH) stimulates osteoclastic bone resorption and inhibits osteoblastic bone deposition. This is described in more detail on p. 189.

Infections and trauma

Osteomyelitis

This infection of bone typically affects the cortex, medulla, and periosteum, and it is most commonly encountered in children under the age of 12 years. The most common causative organisms are *Staphylococcus aureus*, *Mycobacterium tuberculosis*, *Escherichia coli* (particularly in infants and the elderly), and *Salmonella* (particularly in patients with sickle-cell disease).

Infective organisms gain access to the medullary cavity of the bone by two main routes:

- Direct access through an open wound, particularly when open fractures are involved. Also important in postoperative patients who have had surgery on bones (particularly prosthetic joint replacements).
- Bloodborne spread: following bacteremia from a focus of sepsis elsewhere.

Clinical features—Abrupt onset of severe pain at the site of bone infection accompanied by fever and malaise.

Complications and sequelae:

- Resolution: with appropriate antibiotic therapy, often prolonged (6 weeks or more).
- Pathological fracture: purulent acute inflammatory exudate formed in closed compartment of marrow cavity causes compression of vessels with necrosis of medullary bone trabeculae, resulting in increased predisposition to fractures.
- Adjacent abscess: destruction of cortical bone may lead to discharge of pus into extraosseous connective tissue, and infection may track through to the skin surface producing a chronic discharging sinus.
- Chronicity: inflammation tends to become chronic because of localization of infection to a confined space of marrow cavity. Organisms may remain viable within the marrow cavity for many years. Chronicity results in extensive bone destruction, marrow fibrosis and recurrent focal suppuration (Brodie's abscess). There is also reactive new bone

formation, particularly around inflamed periosteum, leading to a thickened and abnormally shaped bone.
- Amyloidosis: long-standing chronic bone infection is a significant cause of secondary AA amyloidosis (see Chapter 12).

Diagnosis is by blood culture and isotope scan.

Management is by antibiotic therapy with surgical exploration and decompression if there is not an immediate response to the antibiotics.

Tuberculous osteomyelitis and Pott's disease

In tuberculous osteomyelitis the marrow cavity contains rapidly enlarging caseating granulomas, which destroy trabecular and cortical bone.

The mode of infection is usually by hematogenous spread from a lung focus in children or the elderly. Vertebral bodies (Pott's disease) are the most common site (affected in 50% of cases) but long bones, fingers, and joints are also involved.

Healing occurs with antituberculous chemotherapy firstly by fibrosis and subsequently by new bone formation.

Skeletal syphilis

Two types, both of which are now rare:
- Congenital: osteochondritis and periostitis.
- Acquired: periostitis and gummas.

Fractures

A fracture is a break in the continuity of bone. Note that any break, even of only one cortex, constitutes a fracture. Fractures are the most common abnormality of bone, and they are caused by physical trauma.

> There are several ways of classifying fractures: according to causation, according to pattern of fracture, or according to their relation to surrounding tissues. The third method is the simplest.

Types of fracture

Fractures can be classified into two main types according to their relation to surrounding tissues:
- Simple: without contact with external environment (i.e., skin or mucous membrane overlying bone is intact). Simple fractures are less likely to become infected.
- Compound: with direct contact between the fracture and external environment (e.g., a fracture of the tibia with laceration of overlying skin). Compound factures are more likely to become infected.

Other descriptive terms for fractures are:
- Comminuted—more than two fragments present.
- Complicated—involvement of a nerve, artery, or viscous.
- Pathological—fracture occurring in abnormal bone.
- Stress—fracture resulting from repeated application of minor force.
- Greenstick—only one cortex of the bone is fractured.

Processes of healing

Bone fractures heal by granulation tissue formation with fibrous repair, followed by new bone formation in the fibrous granulation tissue (see Chapter 3 for wound healing of the skin).

The sequence of events in healing of a simple undisplaced fracture is illustrated in Fig. 11.3.

Complications of healing

Bones show great capacity for healing, but certain complications can occur:
- Malunion: poor anatomical alignment of fractures results in deformity, angulation, or displacement.
- Delayed union: this is common, and it is said to have occurred when a fracture has not united in a reasonable time (defined as 25% longer than the average time taken for that particular type of fracture to unite).
- Nonunion: if union has not occurred within 1 year, then terminology is changed from delayed union to nonunion. The defect is typically filled with fibrous tissue—fibrous ankylosis.

Causes of complications

Efficient healing of fractures requires optimal conditions. Factors that prevent efficient healing are:
- Poor apposition of fractured bone ends.
- Inadequate immobilization.

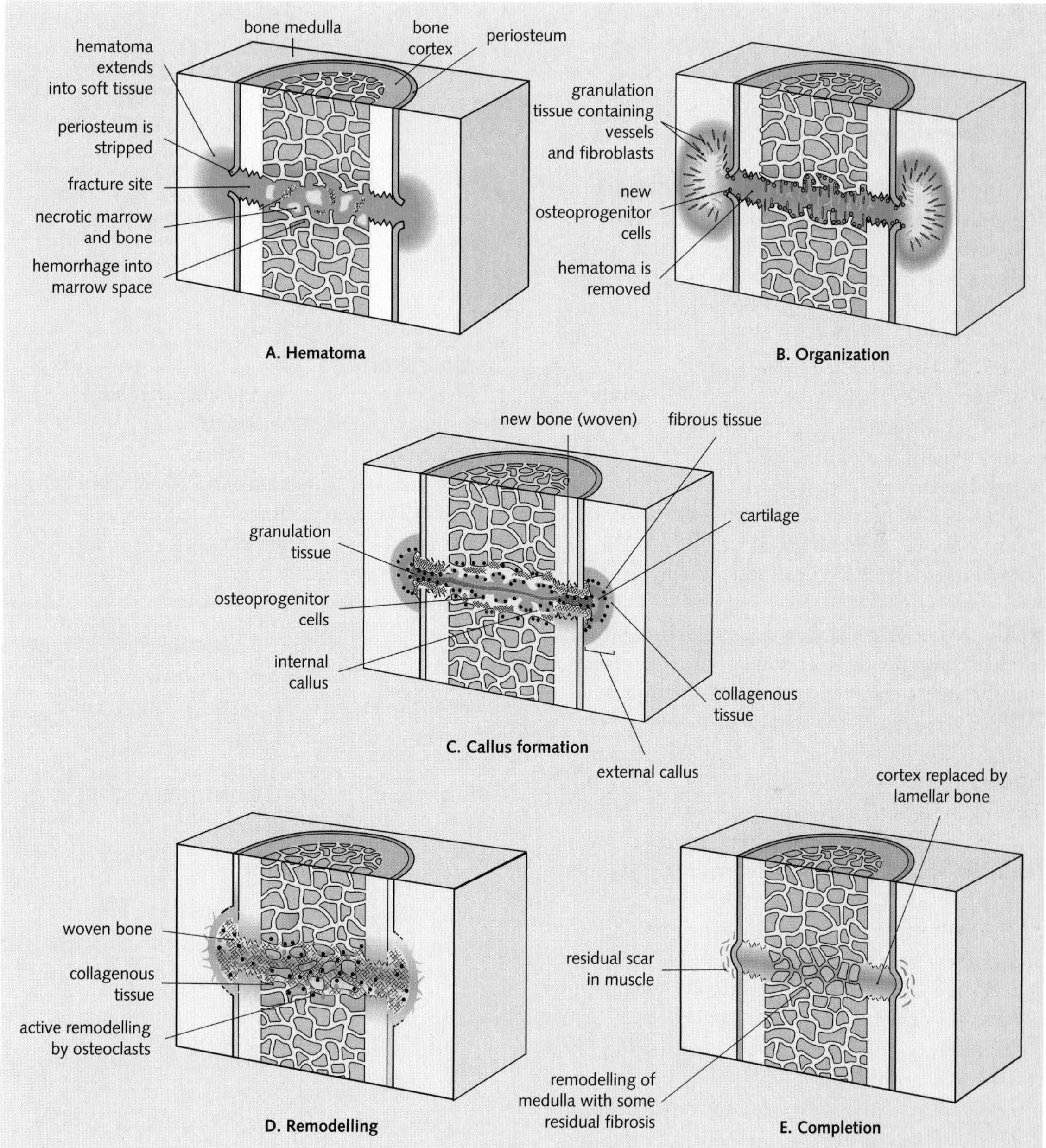

Fig. 11.3 Healing of a simple fracture. (A) Hematoma formation, due to tearing of medullary blood vessels. (B) Organization—migration of neutrophils and macrophages into fracture with organization of hematoma within about 24 hours. Capillaries and fibroblasts proliferate forming fibrovascular granulation tissue. New osteoprogenitor cells (derived from mesenchymal precursor cells) mature into osteoblasts, and they migrate into granulation tissue. (C) Callus formation—osteoblasts deposit large quantities of osteoid collagen in a haphazard way producing a woven bone pattern. Fracture is bridged on outside by external callus (may contain cartilage) and it is bridged in medullary cavity by internal callus (rarely contains cartilage). However, direct ossification may occur between fractured ends if they are closely apposed. (D) Remodelling—about 3 weeks post fracture, callus is well established and undergoes remodelling. Osteoclastic resorption and osteoblastic osteoid synthesis removes surplus calcified callus, replacing bulky, woven bone with compact, organized, lamellar bone. Process takes several months. (E) Completion—formation of new lamellar trabecular bone is complete. Bone is orientated in a direction determined by stresses to which it is exposed with mobilization. However, even after remodelling, cortical irregularities and minor marrow space fibrosis persist at site of fracture.

- Interposition of foreign bodies or soft tissues.
- Infection.
- Corticosteroid therapy.
- Poor general nutritional status.
- Poor blood supply.

Avascular necrosis (osteonecrosis)

Ischemic necrosis of cortical and trabecular bone is caused by:

- Fractures that interfere with the blood supply to certain bones (most important cause) especially affecting femoral and humeral heads, scaphoid, and talus.
- Osteoarthritis (OA) or inflammatory joint disease: osteonecrosis is seen in approximately 20% of femoral heads removed from patients who have had total hip arthroplasties.
- Vasculitis affecting extraosseous arteries.
- Obliteration of intraosseous sinusoids by thrombi, sickled erythrocytes, fat, and nitrogen emboli.
- Idiopathic: osteonecrosis occurs without obvious associated disease at a number of well-defined regional bone sites (femoral head, metatarsal head, tarsal navicular, lunate, medial femoral condyle).

Investigation is by plain radiograph, isotope bone scan with ^{99}Tc diphosphonate, and magnetic resonance imaging (MRI) or computed tomography (CT) scan.

Management is by avoiding weight bearing, analgesia for pain relief, and nonsteroidal anti-inflammatory drugs (NSAIDs) for anti-inflammatory action.

Surgery:

- Bone decompression.
- Osteotomy to reduce mechanical stresses on affected bone segments.
- Joint replacement is often required in patients with more advanced disease and secondary OA.

Tumors of the bones

Metastatic disease of the skeleton

Most common tumors in bone are blood-borne metastases from other primary sites, and tumors of hemopoietic cells located within the marrow spaces of bones, particularly leukemia.

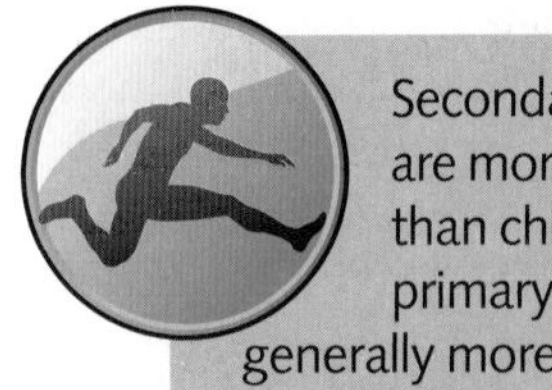

Secondary tumors of bone are more common in adults than children, whereas primary tumors of bone are generally more common in children than adults.

Carcinomas

There are five common carcinomas that have a predilection for metastasizing to bone:

- Adenocarcinoma of the breast.
- Carcinoma of bronchus (particularly small-cell, undifferentiated carcinoma).
- Adenocarcinoma of the kidney.
- Adenocarcinoma of the thyroid.
- Adenocarcinoma of the prostate.

Metastases occur most commonly in parts of the skeleton that contain vascular marrow, especially vertebral bodies, ribs, the pelvis, and upper ends of the femur and humerus.

Osteolytic vs. osteosclerotic metastases

Most metastatic tumor cells within bone marrow spaces lead to erosion of bone (osteolytic metastases). However, prostatic carcinoma (and very rarely breast carcinoma) produces metastatic deposits in which there is stimulation of new bone formation (osteosclerotic metastases) particularly in the lumbosacral vertebrae.

Clinical features:

- Bone pain: usually localized to site of deposits.
- Fractures: erosion of trabecular bone either directly, or through osteoclast-stimulated bone erosion (osteolytic metastases) → bone weakness → increased predisposition to pathological fractures.

Complications are:

- Leukoerythroblastic anemia: a result of extensive replacement of bone marrow.
- Symptoms of hypercalcemia: caused by the release of calcium from bone by osteolytic process.
- Nerve and spinal compression: particularly in vertebral metastases.

Hematopoietic malignancies

Hematopoietic malignancies found in bone (e.g., myelomas, lymphomas, leukemias) are discussed in Chapter 12.

Bone-forming tumors

Primary tumors derived from cells involved in bone formation and modelling are relatively rare.

Osteoma

Benign, smooth, rounded bone tumor is seen on the surface of long bones or skull bone. Apart from visible or palpable swelling, there are usually no symptoms.

Ivory osteoma

This cortical bone tumor is composed of densely compact bone with Haversian systems. It occurs most frequently in the vault of the skull, and it is usually asymptomatic.

Cancellous osteoma (exostosis)

This cancellous bone tumor forming an outgrowth from the end of a long bone usually rises to a point.

Osteoid osteoma and osteoblastoma

Osteoid osteoma

Causing mild bone pain that often awakes the patient at night, this typically arises between the ages of 10 and 30 years. Most commonly it affects long bones of the lower leg, but it may occur in any bone except the skull. Tumors are composed of active osteoblasts, which deposit large, irregular masses of osteoid collagen in a haphazard manner.

Radiographs characteristically show a central dense area surrounded by a halo of translucency. Excision is usually curative and lesions do not recur. X-ray of the resected segment is usually done to document complete removal.

Osteoblastoma (giant osteoid osteoma)

This large tumor with similar histological features to osteoid osteoma mainly affects the bones of the hands, feet, and vertebrae. Tumors are typically more locally aggressive, and they can recur after incomplete excision.

Osteosarcoma

This malignant tumor of osteoblasts occurs most often in adolescent children. Some cases are associated with familial cancer syndromes of retinoblastoma syndrome (defect in Rb1) and the Li–Fraumeni syndrome (defect in p53). The majority arise around the knee (the lower end of the femur or upper end of the tibia) and a minority in other long bones such as the upper end of humerus or femur.

Symptoms are bone pain increasing gradually with tumor growth, but the tumor is often well advanced at the time of diagnosis.

Spread—The tumor grows rapidly within the medullary cavity, eventually eroding through the cortical plate into soft tissue. Metastasis occurs early via the bloodstream, usually to the lung.

The prognosis is poor (5–10% 5-year survival), but it has improved with the adoption of earlier surgical treatment combined with radiotherapy/chemotherapy.

Osteosarcoma in adults is largely confined to elderly patients with a long history of active Paget's disease of the bone.

Cartilage-forming tumors

Osteochondroma

This benign tumor grows as an exophytic nodule from metaphyses of long bones. It is also known as a "cartilage-capped exostosis" as it is composed of protruberant bone covered with a cap of cartilage and an outer layer of perichondrium.

Lesions are found most commonly in the humerus, femur, and the upper end of the tibia, and they may be solitary or multiple (typically autosomal dominant condition, hereditary multiple exostoses). Chondrosarcomatous change is rare in solitary lesions but more common in hereditary multiple lesions.

Chondroma

The most common benign tumor of cartilage-forming tissue, this is composed of a scattering of benign chondrocytes embedded in a cartilaginous matrix.

Tumors are thought to originate from residual nests of cartilage cells left behind in metaphysis as bone growth proceeds. They are found most commonly in small bones of hands and feet.

They may be single ("solitary enchondroma") or multiple ("enchondromatosis"). (The term "enchondroma" is used to indicate that the tumor arises and grows within bone as opposed to osteochondroma, which grows as a nodular exophytic lesion.) A solitary chondroma rarely undergoes malignant change, but occasionally it occurs in multiple enchondromatosis.

Chondrosarcoma

This slow-growing malignant tumor often reaches a large size, eventually breaking through the periosteum into surrounding soft tissue, but usually maintaining a clearly defined border.

Macroscopically, there is a glistening white appearance, similar to that of normal cartilage.

Microscopically:

- Majority are low-grade, well-differentiated tumors that metastasize very late, and are histologically similar to benign cartilaginous tumors. Radical local surgery may be curative.
- Minority are high-grade, poorly differentiated tumors with marked pleomorphism, high mitotic activity and grow rapidly with early blood-borne metastases.

Chondroblastoma (Codman's tumor)

A rare usually benign tumor derived from chondroblasts, this typically occurs in males aged 20 years or younger. Typically it affects epiphyseal bone, especially of the knee or upper end of the humerus.

Microscopically, cells frequently show mitosis and "giant" cells.

Chondromyxoid fibroma

This rare benign tumor is composed of lobules of fibrous tissue separated by myxomatous tissue containing cells in lacunae (thus mimicking the appearance of cartilage). Typically it occurs below the age of 30 years, arising at the epiphyseal line but sparing the epiphysis.

Fibrous and fibro-osseous tumors

Fibroma

A benign tumor, this is composed of inactive, acellular, fibrous tissue. Stroma may ossify to form an ossifying fibroma. The main complication is pathological fracture.

Fibrous dysplasia

This condition results from the disorganization of tissue differentiation and the modelling of diaphyses. Shafts are usually thickened, and they may be painful. It may affect one bone (monostotic) or many (polyostotic) and deformity may be severe. Pathological fractures often occur, but they have normal healing potential. Prognosis of life is not affected.

Fibrosarcoma and malignant fibrous histiocytoma

Fibrosarcoma

This malignant tumor of fibroblasts can be classified into two types:

- Endosteal fibrosarcoma—arises within bones and gives rise to destructive lesions as it grows out. Metastasis is to both local lymph nodes and lungs. It is associated with a poor prognosis.
- Periosteal fibrosarcoma—seldom invades bone or metastasizes to distant sites. Treatment is by local excision.

Malignant fibrous histiocytoma

This high-grade malignant bone tumor contains a mixture of spindle-shaped fibroblasts with histiocytic cells, many of which are multinucleated. Fibroblasts are characteristically arranged in a cartwheel-like formation (storiform pattern). It occurs mainly in the elderly.

Other tumors

Ewing's sarcoma

A highly malignant bone tumor probably derived from primitive neuroendocrine cells, this affects children between the ages of 5 and 15 years. It has a characteristic chromosomal translocation t(11;22)(q24;q12) that results in the fusion of the FLT-1 gene from chromosome 11 with the EWS gene on chromosome 22. Areas of osteolytic bone destruction surrounded by layers of new periosteal bone give the tumor a characteristic "onion skin" appearance on X-ray. Pain, swelling, and tenderness may be associated with fever and leukocytosis (thus tumors are sometimes mistaken for osteomyelitis). Five-year survival is virtually nil despite radiotherapy and amputation.

Giant cell tumor (osteoclastoma)

Osteolytic lesions arise in the epiphyses of long bones, typically in young and middle-aged adults, and they are generally more common in women.

The tumor is composed of a mass of large multinucleated giant cells resembling large osteoclasts embedded in a supporting spindle-celled stroma. There is a gradual expansion of lesions into the metaphysis and the erosion of cortical bone, yet penetration of the periosteum or articular cartilage is rare.

Osteoclastoma is generally classed as benign, but it can recur after local removal. About 10% of cases

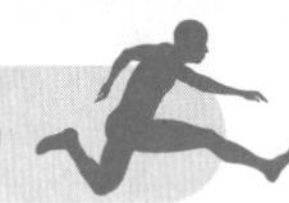

are malignant and metastasize to the lung via the bloodstream.

See Fig. 11.4 for a summary of bone tumors.

Disorders of the neuromuscular junction

Overview

Several diseases of muscle have been shown to result from disorders affecting transmission at the neuromuscular junction (NMJ).

Clinical presentation of NMJ dysfunction:

- Fatiguability: primarily affecting proximal limb muscles, extraocular muscles (causing ptosis or diplopia), and muscles of mastication, speech, and facial expression.
- Periodic paralysis: sudden reversible attacks of paralysis and flaccidity.

Summary of bone tumors

Type	Tumor	Clinical features
Metastatic (secondary)	Carcinoma of bronchus (esp. small cell) Adenocarcinomas of the breast, kidney, and thyroid Prostate	Metastases occur most commonly to vertebral bodies, ribs, pelvis, and upper ends of femur and humerus
Primary	Bone-forming tumors	Osteoma Osteoid osteoma Osteoblastoma Osteosarcoma
	Cartilage-forming tumors	Osteochondroma Chondroma Chondroblastoma (Codman's tumor) Chondrosarcoma Chondromyxoid fibroma
	Fibrous and fibro-osseous tumor	Fibroma Fibrous dysplasia Fibrosarcoma Malignant fibrous histiocytoma
	Others	Ewing's sarcoma Giant cell tumor (osteoclastoma)

Fig. 11.4 Summary of bone tumors.

Disorders can be classified into two types, pre- and postsynaptic abnormalities, depending on which of the synaptic membranes is affected.

Presynaptic abnormalities

Botulism

This rare form of food poisoning is caused by ingestion of a toxin produced by the bacterium *Clostridium botulinum*, found in imperfectly treated canned food or preserved fish contaminated with the microbe.

Pathogenesis—The toxin binds irreversibly to those presynaptic nerve terminals of axons whose impulse transmission is acetylcholine (ACh)-mediated. These include the NMJ, autonomic ganglia and parasympathetic nerve terminals. Binding of the toxin prevents the release of ACh.

Clinical symptoms are chiefly vomiting and paresis of skeletal, ocular, pharyngeal, and respiratory muscles. Antitoxin is available, but it has no effect once the toxin is bound. Recovery of transmission is achieved by terminal axonal sprouting and the formation of new synaptic contacts. Mortality can be high.

Lambert–Eaton myasthenic syndrome

This autoimmune disorder is characterized by abnormal fatiguability, and it is often found in patients with lung cancer. Autoantibodies bind to presynaptic voltage-dependent calcium channels at motor nerve terminals to cause functional loss. This in turn causes the reduced release of ACh in response to nerve stimulation. Small-cell lung carcinoma cells express calcium channels suggesting that autoantibody production is triggered by these tumor antigens.

Postsynaptic abnormalities

Myasthenia gravis

This autoimmune disease is characterized by a progressive failure to sustain a maintained or repeated contraction of striated muscle. Prevalence is about 1 in 30,000. The disease usually appears between the ages of 15 and 50 years, and females are more often affected than males.

Etiology—Autoantibodies are produced by B lymphocytes that are defectively controlled by T lymphocytes, as a result of a disorder of the thymus gland. About 15% of cases have a thymoma (see Chapter 13) and 50% of patients have thymic gland hyperplasia.

Other associations are thyrotoxicosis, diabetes mellitus (DM), rheumatoid arthritis (RA), and systemic lupus erythematosus (SLE). There is linkage with various HLA antigens such as A1, B7, and DRw3.

Pathogenesis—Autoantibodies bind to the ACh receptor located in the postsynaptic membrane of muscle motor end-plates. These antibodies prevent synaptic transmission by blocking the receptor sites.

Presentation:

- Early symptoms: intermittent ptosis or diplopia, weakness of chewing, swallowing, speaking, or moving the limbs. Movement is initially strong, but it rapidly weakens.
- Later symptoms: respiratory muscles may be involved and respiratory failure is not an uncommon cause of death. Asphyxia occurs readily as the cough may be too weak to clear foreign bodies from the airways. Muscle atrophy may occur in long-standing cases.

The disease runs a remitting/relapsing course, and relapses may be precipitated by emotional disturbances, infections, pregnancy, or severe muscular effort.

Investigations:

- Tensilon test: administration of a therapeutic trial of a short-acting, anticholinesterase drug that increases ACh concentrations in the synaptic cleft and allows transmission.
- Autoantibody screen: elevated ACh receptor antibody is found in 90% of cases.
- Thyroid function tests: to screen for associated autoimmune disease of the thyroid gland.
- PA and lateral chest radiograph/CT scan of thorax to identify thymomas.
- Electromyography (EMG) may show a characteristic decremental response.

Management:

- Medical: anticholinesterase drugs (prevent breakdown of ACh at NMJ); immunological treatment—plasma exchange (removal of antibody from the blood), intravenous immunoglobulin, immunosuppressant treatment.
- Surgical: thymectomy (may improve myasthenia in a proportion of cases).

The prognosis is variable. If the disorder is confined to eye muscles, then the prognosis for life is normal and disability slight. A prognosis of myasthenia associated with thymoma is markedly worse.

Myopathies

Definition

Myopathy is any condition that primarily affects muscle physiology, structure, or biochemistry.

Inherited myopathies

X-linked muscular dystrophy

This inherited disease of muscle is characterized by the progressive degeneration of single muscle cells over a prolonged period of time. It results in muscle fibre destruction with the development of fibrosis.

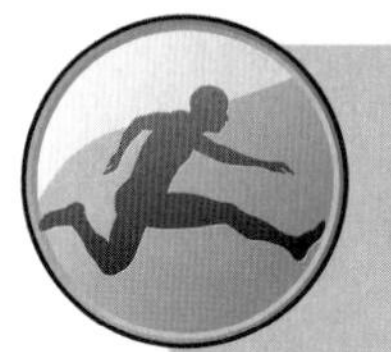

Dystrophy is a term used to describe inherited degenerative muscle diseases.

Duchenne muscular dystrophy

The pattern of inheritance is X-linked recessive (p21 region), hence the disorder is almost exclusively seen in males. This is the most common form of muscular dystrophy in childhood, affecting 1 in 3000 male births.

The disorder is due to a mutation of the gene coding for dystrophin, a protein that normally anchors the actin cytoskeleton of muscle fibres to the basement membrane via a membrane glycoprotein complex (Fig. 11.5). Lack of this protein renders fibers liable to tearing with repeated contraction.

Different degrees of severity of Duchenne dystrophy result from different mutations within the dystrophin gene:

- Severe Duchenne dystrophy: complete failure to produce dystrophin as a result of mutations causing gene frameshifts.
- Moderate to severe forms of Duchenne dystrophy: dystrophin is produced but anchorage is inefficient because of mutations in binding sites for either membrane glycoprotein complex or actin cytoskeleton.
- Mild form of Duchenne dystrophy (Becker's dystrophy): mutation in the middle rod region still

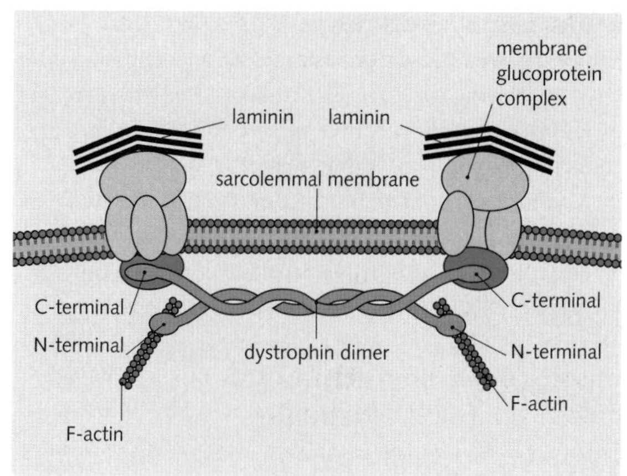

Fig. 11.5 Anchorage role of dystrophin. Dystrophin molecule is a long, rod-shaped protein, one end binding to membrane glycoprotein, the other to actin, with middle rod region.

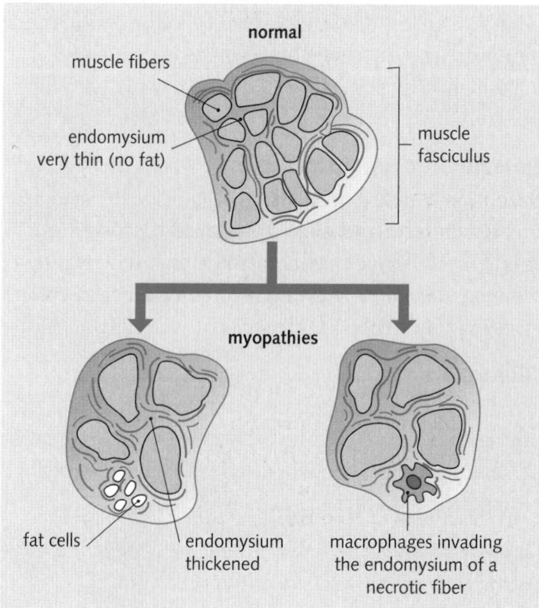

Fig. 11.6 Changes in muscle associated with Duchenne muscular dystrophy.

allows anchorage of muscle to basement membrane.

Morphological features—Muscle changes associated with Duchenne are illustrated in Fig. 11.6.

Clinical features—Childhood onset of muscle weakness is associated with a high serum creatinine kinase level (caused by muscle necrosis) and calf hypertrophy due to fatty replacement of muscle (Fig. 11.6). Cardiac muscle is also affected leading to cardiomyopathy (see Chapter 5, p. 61).

The prognosis depends on the degree of severity: for severe Duchenne it is very poor, most affected individuals dying in their late teens.

Myotonic disorders

Myotonic disorders are diseases in which there is a continuing contraction of muscle after voluntary contraction has ceased.

Myotonic muscular dystrophy

This autosomal dominant disorder is characterized by muscle weakness, myotonia (inability to relax muscles), and several non-muscle features including cataracts, frontal baldness in males, cardiomyopathy, and low intelligence.

This is the most common inherited muscle disease of adults, affecting 1 in 8000.

The genetic abnormality is an unstable CTG repeat sequence in a cAMP-dependent protein kinase located on chromosome 19. The mechanism by which this mutation causes myotonia is unknown.

Microscopically, affected muscles show abnormalities of fiber size with fiber necrosis, abundant internal nuclei, and replacement by fibrofatty tissue.

The disorder usually becomes apparent in adolescence or early adulthood with facial weakness and distal weakness in the limbs.

Prognosis—Death is commonly due to involvement of respiratory muscles in middle-age.

Acquired myopathies

Idiopathic inflammatory myopathies

There is primary inflammation of muscle with resulting fiber necrosis. The inflammatory infiltrate is mainly composed of T lymphocytes and monocytes as part of an abnormal autoimmune response. There are three main types of inflammatory myopathies.

Polymyositis

This inflammatory muscle disorder is characterized by weakness, pain, and swelling of proximal limb muscles and facial muscles, often with ptosis and dysphagia. It is the most common inflammatory muscle disorder, though still relatively rare. It occurs most frequently in adults, with females affected more than males by 3:1.

Etiology—It is a cytotoxic T cell- and macrophage-mediated autoimmunity, but the mechanism of sensitization is unknown.

Associations:

- Increased predisposition in people with HLA-B8/DR3.
- Connective tissue diseases such as SLE, rheumatoid disease, or scleroderma.
- Dermatomyositis: muscle disease is accompanied by a characteristic skin rash.
- Malignancy: particularly in association with bronchial, breast, ovarian, gastric, and nasopharyngeal carcinoma.

Microscopically, there is a lymphocytic infiltration of muscle with fiber necrosis.

Clinical features—An insidious onset in the third to fifth decade of life, with a weakness of the pelvic and shoulder girdle muscles. Progression is typically slow but it may eventually involve pharyngeal, laryngeal, and respiratory muscles leading to dysphagia, dysphonia, and respiratory failures. Spontaneous remissions with the return of muscle strength may also occur.

Investigations—Blood: increased muscle enzymes; tests for rheumatoid factor and antinuclear factor are often positive. EMG: useful for differentiating polymyositis from peripheral myopathies. Muscle biopsy: muscle necrosis and regeneration in association with inflammatory cell infiltrate. MRI: noninvasive detection of active myositis.

Treatment—It may respond to immunosuppressive treatment such as corticosteroids and azathioprine.

Dermatomyositis

Polymyositis is accompanied by periorbital oedema and a characteristic purple "heliotrope" rash on the upper eyelids. Often, there is an erythematous, scaling rash on the face, shoulders, upper arms and chest with red patches over the knuckles, elbows, and knees.

Inclusion body myositis

This slowly progressive inflammatory muscle disorder is clinically similar to polymyositis, but it occurs mainly in the elderly. By light microscopy, histological features also appear similar to polymyositis, but with electron microscopy vacuoles containing filamentous inclusion bodies can be seen within fibers.

Endocrine myopathies

There is a weakness and wasting of muscle associated with endocrine disease. The main causes are:

- Corticosteroid-induced myopathy: either iatrogenic or in Cushing's disease.
- Myopathies of thyroid dysfunction: associated with both hyperthyroidism and hypothyroidism.
- Myopathy of osteomalacia: painful myopathy often without much wasting or weakness.

Changes are usually reversible with appropriate therapy.

Toxic myopathies

Muscle damage may by incurred by a wide variety of drugs, the most common of which is alcohol. Damage to muscle is usually reversible on withdrawal of the toxic agent.

Ethanol

This may cause a spectrum of muscle diseases varying from mild, proximal weakness to severe muscle necrosis. Biopsy shows selective atrophy of type 2b fibers, which is reversible in the early stages.

Cholesterol-lowering agents

Diazocholesterol, a drug once used in the treatment of hypercholesterolemia, causes muscle spasms and weakness with myotonia. Statins, now used widely, can cause weakness and destruction of muscle, with increased CK levels.

Chloroquine

This drug is used principally in the treatment of malaria, and its use may be associated with myopathy and mild peripheral neuropathy. Damage is reversible on drug withdrawal, but recovery is slow.

L-Tryptophan

Eosinophilia myalgia has been reported with tryptophan-containing products.

Arthropathies

Osteoarthritis

Osteoarthritis is a degenerative disease of articular cartilage. It is associated with secondary changes in underlying bone resulting in pain and impaired function of the affected joint.

It is extremely common—80% of the elderly population show radiographic evidence of OA, although only around 25% of these are symptomatic.

Females are affected more than males, and the disease is often more severe in older women. It is increasingly common above 60 years of age, but it may also occur in younger age groups following any form of mechanical derangement.

OA affects joints that are constantly exposed to wear and tear, typically large weight-bearing joints (e.g., those of the hip and knee), but also small joints in the hands, particularly the thumb.

The etiology is as follows:

- Primary: no obvious causes or predisposing factors (majority of cases).
- Secondary: arising as a complication of other joint disorders, mainly inflammatory joint disease, congenital joint deformities, trauma to joints, avascular necrosis of bone.

Secondary OA is also an important component of occupational joint disease (e.g., OA of the fingers in typists and of the knee in professional football players).

Risk factors for the development of OA are:

- Ageing.
- Abnormal load on joints.
- Crystal deposition.
- Joint inflammation.

Pathological changes

Pathological changes involve cartilage, bone, synovium, and joint capsule with secondary effects on muscle (Fig. 11.7).

Early stage:

- Erosion and destruction of articular cartilage: degenerate cartilage splits along lines of fibers to produce fronds of degenerate cartilage (fibrillation). Narrowing of the joint space can be seen on radiography.
- Inflammation and thickening of the joint capsule and synovium.

Later stages:

- Sclerosis of subarticular bone: caused by constant friction of naked bone surfaces (eburnation).
- Osteophytes form around the periphery of the joint by irregular outgrowth of bone. Some may break off to form loose bodies within the joint. In distal interphalangeal joints of the fingers, osteophytes appear as small nodules (Heberden's nodes); in proximal interphalangeal joint, they are Bouchard's nodes.

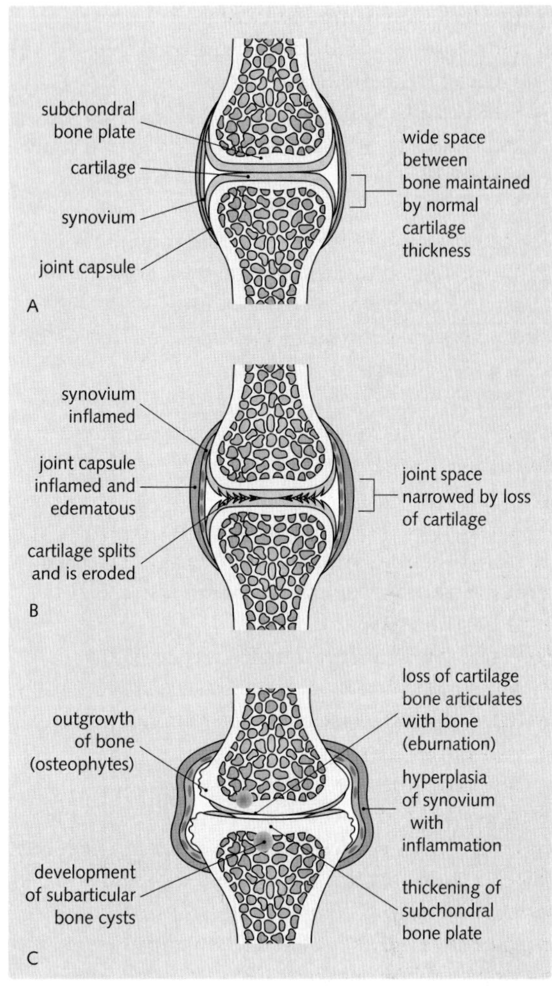

Fig. 11.7 Pathological changes in osteoarthritis (OA). (A) Normal joint. (B) Early stages of OA. (C) Later stages of OA.

- Small cysts may develop in areas where the bone is not thickened as a result of synovial fluid accumulation in underlying bone.
- Reactive thickening of synovium and joint capsule due to inflammation caused by bone and cartilage debris.
- Atrophy of muscle caused by disuse following immobility of the diseased joint.

OA can be classified according to the main presenting features as follows:

- Primary generalized OA: usually associated with development of Heberden's nodes on fingers. It is most common in postmenopausal women.

- Erosive inflammatory OA: form of OA in which there is severe inflammation and erosion of cartilage, with rapid progression.
- Hypertrophic OA: florid osteophyte formation and bone sclerosis, but with slow progression and a relatively good prognosis.

The main symptoms of OA are pain and limitation in the movement of the affected joint. Sometimes OA is associated with visible swelling (partly due to osteophytes and partly due to fluid accumulation in joint cavity and synovial fibrosis).

In OA of the cervical vertebrae (cervical spondylosis), osteophytes compressing emerging spinal nerves are responsible for much of the symptomatology.

Diagnosis—Recognized on X-ray by:

- Narrowing of joint space due to loss of cartilage.
- Presence of osteophytes, producing irregularities at bone margins.
- Cystic appearance just beneath the articular surface.
- Sclerosis: increased bone density immediately adjacent to the joint space.

Treatment:

- Lifestyle: reduction of pressure across the joint (e.g., by weight loss and/or use of walking stick in OA of the hip).
- Medical: analgesics and anti-inflammatories for pain relief; intra-articular or periarticular corticosteroid injections may also be helpful, especially with OA of the knee.
- Surgical: corrective and prosthetic surgery for advanced hip or knee disease.

Rheumatoid arthritis

Rheumatoid arthritis (RA) is an inflammatory joint disease caused by a multisystem connective tissue autoimmune disorder, rheumatoid disease (see Chapter 12). It affects about 1% of the population, females more than males by about 3:1. Onset is typically between 35 and 45 years of age, but it follows a normal distribution curve, and no age group is exempt.

Rheumatoid arthritis mainly affects peripheral synovial joints such as the fingers and wrists, but it can also affect the knees and more proximal joints.

The etiology is autoimmune, and there is an association with HLA-DR4 haplotype in most ethnic groups. The condition is characterized by the presence of circulating autoantibody that is directed against the Fc portion of native immunoglobulins (rheumatoid factor). The presence of rheumatoid factor (seropositive arthritis) distinguishes RA from several other inflammatory joint diseases (seronegative arthritis). The exact role and underlying stimulus of rheumatoid factor is uncertain (see also Chapter 12). However, immunological techniques have demonstrated it in plasma cells located in the synovium of affected joints. Interestingly there is increasing evidence to suggest that RA is a disease of both cellular and humoral immune mechanisms. For example, T helper lymphocyte populations present in rheumatoid joints are oligoclonal and they may be autoreactive.

Pathological changes

There are three main pathological changes (Fig. 11.8):

- Rheumatoid synovitis.
- Articular cartilage destruction.
- Focal destruction of bone.

Rheumatoid synovitis

The synovium becomes swollen and shows a villous pattern. Chronic inflammatory cells (mainly lymphocytes and plasma cells) increase in number within the synovial stroma, often forming an exudate which effuses into the joint space. Fibrin is deposited on the surface of the synovium. Soft tissue swelling from synovial inflammation may be marked.

Articular cartilage destruction

Vascular granulation tissue grows across the surface of the cartilage (pannus) from the edges of the joint. The articular surface shows the loss of cartilage beneath the extending pannus, most marked at joint margins.

Focal destruction of bone

Osteolytic destruction of bone occurs at the edges of the joint. Bone "erosions" can be seen on radiography, and they are associated with joint deformity.

There is also increased soft tissue swelling due to inflammation and thickening of the synovium and capsule.

Clinical features

Symmetrical polyarthritis

The insidious onset of arthritis first attacks finger joints (mainly metacarpophalangeal and proximal interphalangeal joints) followed by metatarsophalangeal joints and joints of the ankles,

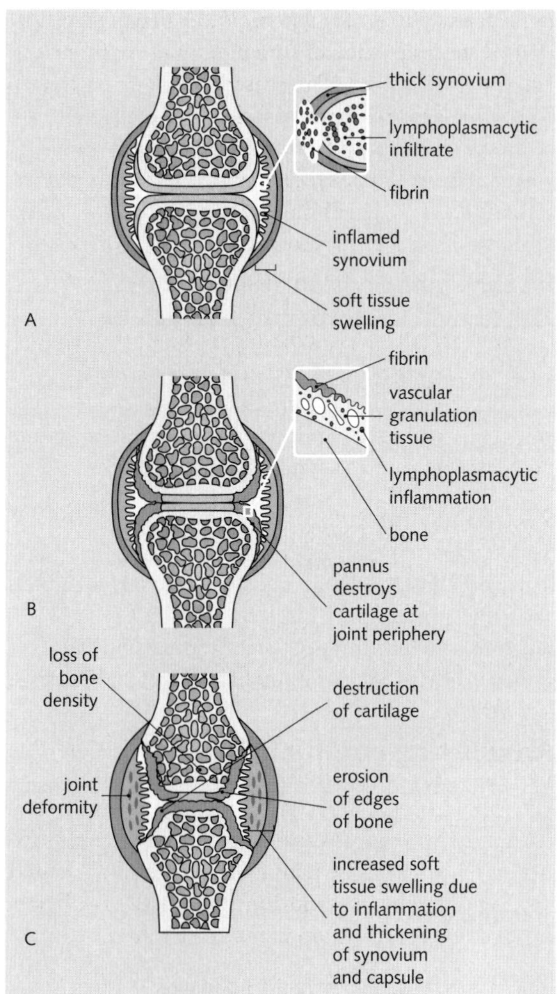

Fig. 11.8 Pathological changes in rheumatoid arthritis. (A) Rheumatoid synovitis. (B) Articular cartilage destruction. (C) Focal destruction of bone.

wrists, knees, shoulders, elbows, and hips (in decreasing order of frequency). However, the disease may also affect joints such as the temporomandibular joint and the synovial joints of the spine (particularly the upper cervical spine). Affected joints become swollen, painful, and warm, often with redness of overlying skin.

Joint deformities

As the disease progresses, muscle atrophy and joint destruction result in limitation of joint motion, joint instability, subluxation, and deformities. There are also flexion contractures of small joints of the hands and feet, knees, hips, and elbows.

Subluxation, a characteristic feature of RA, is a term used to describe a partial dislocation of any joint such that bone ends still make contact, but are misaligned.

Of the hands:

- Anterior subluxation of the metacarpophalangeal (MCP) joints with ulnar deviation of the fingers.
- "Swan neck" deformity: hyperextension of proximal interphalangeal (PIP) joint with fixed flexion at distal interphalangeal (DIP) joints.
- Boutonnière (buttonhole) deformity: fixed flexion of proximal interphalangeal joint and extension of the terminal interphalangeal joint.
- Z deformity of the thumbs: fixed flexion at metacarpophalangeal joint and hyperextension at interphalangeal joint.

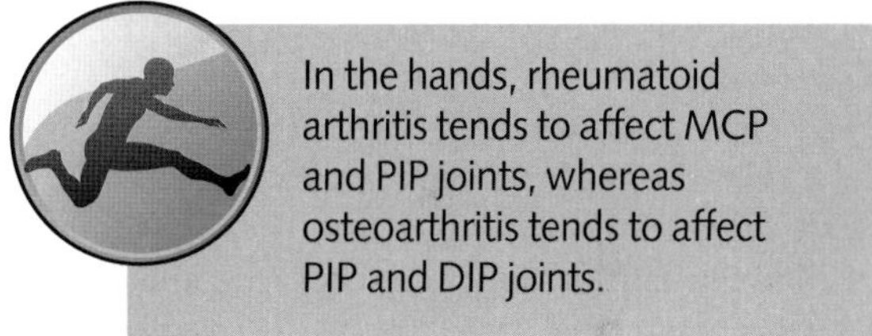

In the wrists there is often a fixed flexion deformity with a prominent, tender ulnar styloid process and pain on pronation/supination.

In the knees, Baker's cyst (cystic swelling in the popliteal fossa) is seen.

In the cervical spine, there is atlanto-axial subluxation.

Deformities are initially correctable, but permanent contractures eventually develop such that joints become completely disorganized.

Rheumatoid nodules

Joint changes are often associated with development of subcutaneous rheumatoid nodules, usually located over the extensor aspect of the forearm but occasionally found overlying other bony prominences. Nodules are composed of extensive areas of degenerate collagen surrounded by a giant cell granulomatous reaction.

Other

Other features seen in systemic rheumatoid disease are discussed in Chapter 12. Complications are:

- Secondary osteoarthritis as a result of loss of articular surface particularly in weight-bearing joints such as the knee.
- Septic arthritis: infection of the joint secondary to invasion from an ulcerated nodule or infected skin lesion.
- Amyloidosis: found in 25–30% of RA patients at autopsy.
- Carpal tunnel syndrome.
- Ruptured extensor tendons of the hand.

Investigations and diagnosis

Investigations include the following:

- Radiography: periarticular osteoporosis, loss of articular cartilage (joint space), erosions, subluxation, and ankylosis.
- Serology: rheumatoid factors (IgG- or IgM-type immunoglobulins that react with the Fc portion of IgG).
- Synovial fluid analysis: useful in the differential diagnosis of inflammatory and degenerative arthropathies.

Diagnosis of RA is made with four or more of the following criteria (American Rheumatism Association, 1988 revision):

- Morning stiffness (>1 hour), of at least 6 weeks' duration.
- Arthritis of three or more joint areas, of at least 6 weeks' duration.
- Arthritis of hand joints, of at least 6 weeks' duration.
- Symmetrical arthritis, of at least 6 weeks' duration.
- Rheumatoid nodules.
- Rheumatoid factor.
- Radiological changes.

Treatment

Treatment involves the use of:

- Anti-inflammatories.
- Immunosuppression: penicillamine, gold, azathioprine, salazopyrine.
- Surgery for advanced painful disease in any joint.

Prognosis

The course of RA is variable:

- 25% remain fit for all normal activities.
- 40% have moderate impairment of function.
- 25% are quite badly disabled.
- 10% become wheelchair patients.

The worst prognosis is associated with high titers of rheumatoid factor, early appearance of erosions, rheumatoid nodules, systemic manifestations, and HLA-DR4.

Juvenile form of rheumatoid arthritis

This accounts for approximately 15% of cases of juvenile chronic arthritis. It may begin before 16 years of age. Clinical features are identical to those of adults, and tests for rheumatoid factor are positive. Prognosis is worse than for adults.

Sjögren's syndrome

This autoimmune disorder is characterized by dryness in both eyes and mouth due to impaired tear and saliva production caused by chronic inflammatory infiltrates in both lacrimal and salivary glands. The disorder is present in 15% of all RA cases.

Ankylosing spondylitis

This inflammatory arthritic disorder is characterized by a rigid spine due to ossification of the spinal joints and ligaments. The condition begins in the lumbar vertebral spine and sacroiliac joints, extending upwards to involve thoracic and cervical vertebrae. There may also be involvement of peripheral joints, mainly the hips and knees.

It affects <1% of the population in the U.S., typically presenting in late adolescence and young adults (age 15–30 years of age), and in males more than females by 2:1.

The etiology is unknown, but more than 90% of men with ankylosing spondylitis have the HLA-B27 antigen (less than 10% of the normal population have this antigen), which suggests an autoimmune disorder.

Morphological changes—Chronic inflammation of vertebral ligaments slowly heals by dense fibrosis and ossification to form a rigid shell which links the periphery of the vertebral bodies. Eventually the vertebral column becomes fused, inflexible and rigid ("bamboo spine").

Symptoms are typically an insidious onset of recurring episodes of low back pain and stiffness sometimes radiating to the buttocks or thighs. Symptoms are characteristically worse in early morning and after inactivity.

Systemic manifestations include aortic valve incompetence (as a result of rheumatoid aortitis), recurrent iritis, and chronic inflammatory bowel disease.

On investigation, the erythrocyte sedimentation ratio (ESR) is raised or normal, serology is negative for rheumatoid factor, and X-ray shows typical bamboo spine.

The disease progresses slowly but unremittingly.

Management is by:

- Lifestyle: regular physiotherapy and exercise (e.g., non-weight-bearing sports such as swimming) to maintain as full mobility as possible and to prevent deformity.
- Medical: NSAIDs (for symptomatic relief); radiotherapy (if response to drug therapy is unsatisfactory, but this carries a small risk of leukemia).
- Surgery for associated hip disease.

Fig. 11.9 gives a comparison of joint diseases.

Arthritis in association with other systemic disease

Reiter's syndrome

This inflammatory syndrome is characterized by the triad of arthritis, urethritis, and conjunctivitis. It complicates 0.8% of urethral infection in males, and 0.2% of cases of dysentery. It occurs in males more than females by 20:1, and the usual age of onset is 20–40 years of age.

Classification is on the basis of etiology:

- Genital type: usually follows nonspecific (nongonococcal) urethritis, or, less commonly, cystitis or prostatitis.
- Intestinal or postdysenteric type: in some parts of the world it may follow dysentery or occasionally nonspecific diarrhea, occurring 10–30 days after intestinal manifestations.

The underlying pathological mechanism is unknown but probably autoimmune.

Clinical features are:

- Arthritis, usually affecting knee or ankle. Clinically and histologically, arthritis resembles rheumatoid arthritis with chronic inflammatory synovitis.
- Dysuria and penile discharge.
- Conjunctivitis (in 30% of cases).

Prognosis—The first attack typically resolves spontaneously within 6 months. However, 50% of patients relapse and some have continued relapsing

Comparison of joint diseases

	Osteoarthritis	Rheumatoid disease	Ankylosing spondylitis
Affected age group	Elderly	Any age	Onset usually before 30 years
Rheumatoid factor	Negative	Positive	Usually negative
Sex	Females > males	Females > males	Males > females
HLA association	None known	HLA-DR4	HLA-B27
Hands	Heberden's nodes (DIP) Bouchard's nodes (PIP)	Ulnar deviation of MCP joints Swan neck deformity Boutonnière deformity Z thumbs Prominent ulnar styloid process	—
Affected joints	Mainly hip, knees, and spine	Any	Mainly spine
Joint pathology	Erosion of cartilage Osteophytes	Destruction of joints	Bony ankylosis
Synovial pathology	Slight synovial hyperplasia	Florid synovial hyperplasia; pannus	—
Associated diseases	—	Rheumatoid disease Sjögren's syndrome Interstitial lung fibrosis	Aortic valve incompetence Uveitis Inflammatory bowel disease

Fig. 11.9 Comparison of joint diseases. (DIP, distal interphalangeal; PIP, proximal interphalangeal; MCP, metacarpophalangeal.)

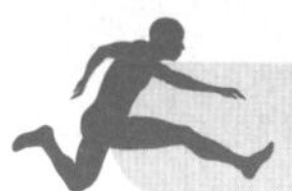

of chronic arthritis with attacks recurring at regular intervals, causing disability but seldom deformity. In a minority of cases, there is development of severe spondylitis and features very similar to ankylosing spondylitis.

Psoriatic arthritis

About 5% of psoriasis patients develop arthropathy which characteristically involves the distal interphalangeal joints (see Chapter 14).

Arthritis associated with gastrointestinal disease

Bacterial gastroenteritis

This arises post infection with *Salmonella*, *Yersinia*, or *Campylobacte*r. HLA-B27 antigen is present in 80% of affected patients.

Inflammatory bowel disease

Arthritis is seen at some stage in up to 20% of patients with ulcerative colitis and Crohn's disease. Typically it involves knee joints, but occasionally also ankles, elbows, and small digital joints. Sacroiliitis and ankylosing spondylitis are also much more frequent in patients with inflammatory bowel disease.

Behçet's syndrome

This syndrome of unknown etiology is characterized by the triad of oral ulceration, genital ulceration, and iritis, but it is also accompanied by arthritis in 60% of cases.

Arthritis may be chronic or episodic, and it is usually polyarticular. It most commonly affects the knees and ankles, but occasionally affects the elbows, wrists, and small joints of the hands or feet.

Others

Neuropathic (Charcot's) joint disease

This joint disease occurs secondary to the loss of pain and position sense within the joint, which is swollen and deformed, but not painful. Possible causes of loss of joint sensation include diabetic neuropathy, tabes dorsalis, syringomyelia, leprosy, and cauda equina lesions (e.g., myelomeningocele).

Sarcoid arthritis

Arthritis occurs in 10% of patients with sarcoidosis, with onset typically in the first year of the disease. It may be of two types:

- Early acute transient type: polyarticular symmetrical arthritis typically affecting knees and ankles, and usually associated with erythema nodosum.
- Chronic persistent type: polyarticular associated with chronic sarcoidosis.

Chronic hemodialysis

There is an increased predisposition to septic arthritis (see below).

Crystal arthropathies

These diseases are characterized by deposition of crystals in joints and soft tissues. Affected patients usually present with an episode of acute arthritis, inflammation being caused by the deposition of the crystals, sometimes called a "chemical arthritis." With time, inflammatory changes lead to the development of chronic arthritis with features of osteoarthritis (secondary osteoarthritis).

Nomenclature

The term "gout" is used as a clinical description of joints affected by crystal deposition. This term is then refined by demonstrating the type of crystal involved. There are two main types of crystal arthropathies: urate gout ("true gout" or just "gout") and calcium pyrophosphate gout ("pseudogout").

Gout

This acute inflammatory crystal arthropathy is caused by the deposition of urate crystal in joints and soft tissues as a result of hyperuricemia. It affects 0.3% of the population, and it is largely confined to men (90%) although some women develop the condition post menopausally. It can present at any time between the ages of 20 and 60 years of age.

Etiology—Uric acid is normally derived from the breakdown of purines, and it is excreted in the urine. Increased concentrations of serum uric acid (hyperuricemia) can result in gout.

There are two main causes of hyperuricemia:

- Underexcretion of uric acid (most common): of uncertain origin but clinically associated with hyperlipidemia, renal failure, lactic acidosis (alcohol, exercise, starvation, vomiting), and thiazide diuretics.
- Overproduction of uric acid (least common): a result of either high cell turnover (e.g., leukemia, chemotherapy, severe psoriasis, post trauma, surgery, or severe systemic illness), or rare congenital enzyme defects of purine metabolism.

However, it should be noted that the majority of patients who have a raised blood uric acid level will never develop gout or any of its complications. The condition has a familial tendency, and it is believed to be polygenically inherited.

Pathogenesis—Gout affects the joints, soft tissues, and kidney, as discussed below.

Joints—Urate crystals are deposited in certain joints, forming white powdery deposits on the surface of articular cartilage, beneath which degenerative changes can be seen. Crystal deposition stimulates an acute inflammatory reaction leading to the excruciating pain, edema, and redness seen in the acutely inflamed joint. Microscopically, neutrophil polymorphs can be seen to phagocytose urate crystal in the joint fluid.

Soft tissues—Uric acid crystals are also deposited in the soft tissues around joints, where their presence excites a foreign body, giant cell reaction. These soft tissue masses may enlarge to produce a palpable mass composed of white chalky material (tophi), especially around the pinna of the ear.

Kidney—Urate crystals deposited in the kidney may lead to an interstitial nephritis and to renal calculi composed of uric acid. Precipitation of urates in renal tubules may produce acute tubular necrosis and acute renal failure in leukemic patients, with massive purine release after chemotherapy.

Characteristics of gout are:

- Intermittent attacks of excruciating pain, edema, and redness (acute gouty arthritis).
- Monoarthropathy (90%); polyarthropathy (two or more affected joints; 10%).
- Metatarsophalangeal joint of the big toe is most commonly affected (75%), but gout occasionally affects the ankle, or less commonly the knee and hip.

Recurrent attacks affecting the same joint eventually lead to articular cartilage destruction, chronic synovial thickening, and secondary osteoarthritis—chronic gouty arthritis.

Diagnosis:

- Clinical features (as above).
- Raised serum urate level (>0.480μmol/L in adult males; >0.390μmol/L in adult females).
- Presence of crystals of sodium urate in aspirated synovial fluid from joint (detected with polarizing light).

Management—Analgesia for acute attacks: NSAIDs (e.g., indometacin) and colchicine. Preventative measures required for patients with recurrent attacks of gouty arthritis or associated renal disease:

- Allopurinol: suppresses uric acid synthesis by inhibiting xanthine oxidase.
- Uricosuric agents (e.g., probenecid).
- Diet: excessive purine intake and overindulgence in alcohol should be avoided.

Prognosis—Some patients have only a single attack or suffer another only after an interval of many years. More often there is a tendency toward recurrent attacks that increase in frequency and duration so that, eventually, attacks merge and the patient remains in a prolonged state of subacute gout.

Pseudogout

This acute inflammatory crystal arthropathy is caused by deposition of calcium pyrophosphate crystals in articular cartilage and joint spaces. It is most common in the elderly and in males more than females.

The etiology can be sporadic, metabolic, or familial.

Sporadic

In the vast majority of cases, the cause of pyrophosphate deposition is unknown, but it is probably an age-related phenomenon.

Metabolic

In patients under the age of 60 years, the disease is often associated with hyperparathyroidism, hemochromatosis, or other less common metabolic or endocrine disorders.

Familial

In a minority of patients, the disease is inherited as an autosomal dominant disorder.

Pathogenesis—crystals are deposited in the articular cartilage of joints (chondrocalcinosis) where they often remain entirely asymptomatically. However, if crystals are shed into the joint space, patients develop an acute arthritis similar to that seen in urate gout. This shedding of crystals may be precipitated by trauma or intercurrent illness, or it may be spontaneous.

With time, damage to cartilage leads to the development of secondary osteoarthritis.

Clinical features—As with gout, the affected joint becomes suddenly painful, warm, swollen, and tender. However, the most commonly affected joint is the knee (>50% of cases), followed by the wrist, shoulder, and ankle. The duration of the attack can vary from days to weeks, and recurrent attacks are uncommon.

Diagnosis is by X-ray—cartilaginous calcification is usually obvious on X-ray—and by the presence of calcium pyrophosphate dihydrate crystals in aspirated synovial fluid from the joint (detected with polarizing light).

Intra-articular corticosteroids are the most effective treatment for acute pseudogout (anti-inflammatory drugs and colchicine are less effective than in true gout).

Infective (septic) arthritis

This inflammation of a joint is caused by infection—typically bacterial. This may affect any age group, but children and young adults are the most commonly affected. In older adults, most cases are associated with penetrating injury. Males are affected more often than females by 2:1. The knee and hip are the most common sites.

Etiology—A wide range of bacteria may be responsible, but *Staphylococcus aureus*, streptococci and *Hemophilus* are the most important.

Risk factors are DM, RA, joint puncture, or surgery and immunosuppressive treatment.

Bacteria gain access to a joint by:

- Local trauma: well-recognized complication of penetrating injury such as open fractures, insertion of surgical prosthesis, and non-sterile, intra-articular injection of steroids for established autoimmune arthritis.
- Spread from adjacent infective foci.
- Bloodstream: less common, but an important route in gonococcal infective arthritis in teenagers and young adults. Intravenous (IV) drug users are particularly likely to develop septic arthritis associated with Gram-negative bacteremia.

Clinical features—There is an abrupt onset of severe pain, tenderness, swelling, and erythema. The majority of cases affect a single joint only, but some cases of gonococcal arthritis and arthritis in intravenous drug abusers may affect more joints.

Complications—Untreated, it proceeds rapidly to joint destruction often with osteomyelitis, sinus formation, ankylosis, and dislocation of the hip.

Diagnosis—Radiographs are normal at first, but useful to exclude fractures or other bony injury. Later in the course of the disease, features of periarticular osteoporosis, joint space narrowing, periostitis, and articular erosions may become apparent. Examination and culture of aspirated joint space fluid is essential for identification of the causative organism.

Treatment is by antibiotic therapy (IV or IM (intramuscular)).

The prognosis for recovery without joint damage is directly related to the speed with which antibiotic therapy is instituted.

Other types of infective arthritis

Tuberculous arthritis

Now rare, this is the result of bloodstream spread from pulmonary tuberculosis (TB). It produces a persistent arthritis with typical caseating granulomatous lesions. The hip and knee are most commonly involved in children, whereas in adults the vertebral column is most often affected.

Infective arthritis in syphilis and brucellosis is now rare.

Lyme disease

This arthritis is due to the spirochaete *Borrelia burgdorferi*. It occurs in outbreaks in the U.S. and Europe. (For more on Lyme disease, see Chapter 13.)

Virus-associated arthritis

Many different viral infections are associated with a transient arthritis or at least distinct pain within joints. Examples include rubella, viral hepatitis, and infectious mononucleosis.

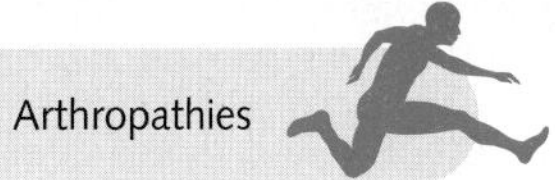

- List the risk factors for osteoporosis.
- What are the complications of osteoporosis?
- Describe the morphology of affected bone in Paget's disease.
- What are the complications of pyogenic osteomyelitis?
- Explain what is meant by simple and compound fractures.
- Describe bone healing, and name the factors that prevent efficient healing.
- List the causes of avascular necrosis.
- List the five common carcinomas that metastasize to bone.
- Name the bone-forming tumors.
- Describe the different cartilage-forming tumors.
- Name the presynaptic abnormalities of the NMJ.
- Define Lambert–Eaton myasthenic syndrome.
- Describe the pathogenesis and clinical presentation of myasthenia gravis.
- Define the terms "myopathy," "dystrophy," and "myotonia."
- Explain the molecular basis and clinical details for Duchenne muscular dystrophy.
- Describe the three types of idiopathic inflammatory myopathies.
- Define and comment on osteoarthritis (OA) and rheumatoid arthritis (RA).
- What is ankylosing spondylitis? Describe the morphological changes that occur in the spine.
- Name the types of crystals involved in gout and pseudogout.
- What are the risk factors for the development of infective arthritis?

12. Pathology of the Blood and Immune Systems

Autoimmune disease

Systemic disease

Autoimmune diseases that cause damage in many tissues and organs, involving a number of systems, are termed "multisystem" or "systemic" autoimmune diseases (Fig. 12.1).

Systemic lupus erythematosus

This inflammatory disorder of connective tissues is associated with autoantibodies to DNA and other nuclear components. Many tissues are affected, but synovial joints, skin, kidneys, and the brain are the major target organs (Fig. 12.2).

Systemic lupus erythematosus (SLE) affects about 30 per 100,000 of the U.S. population, and it presents most commonly in the young and middle-aged with a peak incidence between 20 and 30 years of age. Females are more affected than males by about 8:1.

Incidence is higher in Black people and Asians than in Caucasians.

The etiology is unknown, but there is a strong familial tendency. Drugs (hydralazine, phenytoin, procainamide), chemicals, and unidentified viral infections have all been postulated as the sensitizing stimulus to autoantibody production.

Pathogenesis—Antibodies are produced against components of both nucleic acids and cytoplasmic phospholipids:

- Anti-dsDNA: antibody against double-stranded DNA (most frequently detected).
- Anti-ssDNA: antibody against single-stranded DNA.
- Anti-DNA histone: antibody to a protein (histone) packaged with DNA in chromosomes.
- Antibodies to other nuclear components: anti-Ro, anti-La, and anti-Sm.
- Antiphospholipid (cardiolipin): causes thrombotic tendency, recurrent abortions, and false positive test for syphilis.
- Red cell antibodies: cause autoimmune hemolytic anemia.
- Rheumatoid factors: antibodies directed against self-IgG antibodies.
- Cell- or organelle-specific antibodies (e.g., mitochondrial, smooth muscle, gastric parietal cell).

None of these antibodies is specific for SLE, and most have been detected in other connective tissue disorders or in diseases with an immunological basis.

Microscopically, fibrinoid necrosis is typically seen in vessels of affected organs, especially small arteries, arterioles and capillaries.

The disease commonly presents with malaise, weight loss, fever, marked musculoskeletal symptoms, and a rash. However, the range of features that may occur is vast as demonstrated in the list below.

The American Rheumatism Association's list of diagnostic criteria for SLE

This is listed in order of specificity:

- Discoid skin rash: round (discoid), red, scaly, telangiectatic plaques, usually on the face and scalp and less commonly on the hands.
- Neurological disorder: most common feature is nonorganic psychiatric disorder of unknown cause, which on autopsy is often found to be associated with either acute neutrophilic or lymphocytic vasculitides in the brain. A variety of symptoms (e.g., grand mal epileptic seizures) are due to infarction and neuronal loss, a result of vascular occlusion attributed to the action of antiphospholipid antibodies on platelet aggregation.
- Malar skin rash: symmetrical erythematous rash on the cheeks and the bridge of the nose (butterfly rash).
- Skin photosensitivity: development of a rash of either malar or discoid patterns in sun-exposed areas. Caused by immune complex deposits on the dermal side of the basement membrane.
- Oral ulceration: red erosions closely resembling oral lichen planus.
- Renal abnormality (lupus nephritis): severity varies from minor abnormalities such as asymptomatic proteinuria to severe glomerular disease leading to renal failure (see Chapter 8).
- Evidence of immunological disorder.

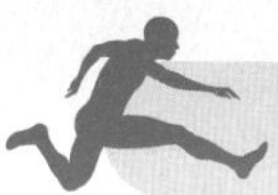

Summary of systemic autoimmune diseases			
Disorder	**Sex ratio**	**Type of autoimmunity**	**Clinical features**
SLE	8F:1M	Antibodies directed against components of nucleic acids and cytoplasmic phospholipids	Skin rashes, neurological disorders, glomerulonephritis, hematological disorders, etc.
Rheumatoid disease	3F:1M	Rheumatoid factors: autoantibodies directed against native IgG	Chronic polyarthritis, subcutaneous nodules, vasculitis, interstitial pulmonary fibrosis, splenomegaly, etc.
Polymyositis and dermatositis	3F:1M	Cell-mediated autoimmunity	Weakness, pain, and swelling of proximal limb muscles and facial muscles Ptosis and dysphagia Dermatomyositis (= additional features of erythematous, scaling rash)

Fig. 12.1 Summary of systemic autoimmune diseases.

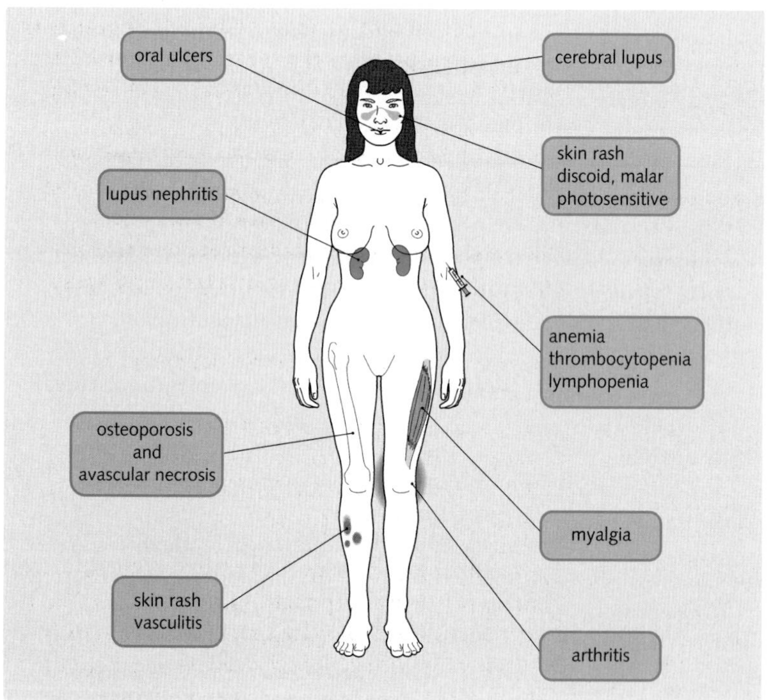

Fig. 12.2 Multisystem manifestations of systemic lupus erythematosus (SLE).

- Hematological disorders: normocytic hypochromic anemia, autoimmune hemolytic anemia, reduced peripheral white cell count (usually due to lymphopenia), thrombocytopenia (sometimes associated with antiplatelet antibodies), predisposition to thrombosis (especially if there are anticardiolipin/lupus anticoagulant antibodies).
- Serosal inflammation: pleurisy, pericarditis.
- Presence of antinuclear antibodies: cluster of antibodies that are aimed against nuclei (see above).

- Arthritis, bone disease and/or myalgia: often misdiagnosed as rheumatoid arthritis, beginning in the fingers, wrists, and knees. Bone disease usually presents as disproportionately severe osteoporosis for the patient's age. Myalgia in the form of skeletal muscle pain is common, and it is thought to be caused by a lymphocytic vasculitis.

Diagnosis is based on a combination of clinical features and the result of laboratory investigation, primarily the identification of autoantibodies, especially those directed against nuclear DNA. The condition is frequently under-diagnosed.

Treatment is by systemic corticosteroid therapy for acute and life-threatening manifestations of SLE. Immunosuppressive drugs are reserved for patients with severe diffuse proliferative glomerulonephritis who are not responding adequately to steroid therapy.

The disorder follows a protracted course of relapses and remissions. Renal, central nervous system (CNS) and cardiac lesions are the most important prognostically. With treatment, in excess of 90% of patients can be anticipated to survive for 10 years.

Rheumatoid disease

This multisystem autoimmune connective tissue disease primarily affects the joints (rheumatoid arthritis) but also the skin, lungs, blood vessels, eyes, and the hemopoietic and lymphoreticular systems.

It affects about 1% of the U.S. population. Onset is typically between 35 and 45 years of age, but it follows a normal distribution curve, and no age group is exempt. Females are more affected than males by about 3:1.

The etiology is unknown, although there is a genetic predisposition and an association with the HLA-DR4 haplotype.

Pathogenesis—Circulating autoantibodies termed "rheumatoid factors" are present which react with the Fc portion of IgG antibodies. The most common type of rheumatoid factor is of the IgM type, which can form pentamer complexes with circulating IgG. Immune complex deposition then leads to complement activation via the classical pathway, which triggers an inflammatory cascade.

Clinicopathological features

Joints This symmetrical polyarthritis is characterized by the destruction of articular cartilage and its replacement by chronic inflammatory pannus (see Chapter 11 for full coverage).

Rheumatoid arthritis is a common disease and often appears in the clinical examinations as either a long or short case.

Skin Subcutaneous rheumatoid nodules can often be seen, usually located over the extensor aspect of the forearm but occasionally found overlying other bony prominences. Nodules are composed of extensive areas of degenerate collagen surrounded by a giant cell granulomatous reaction.

Lungs Pulmonary involvement causes interstitial pneumonitis and fibrosing alveolitis, which eventually leads to a pattern of interstitial pulmonary fibrosis. Also, patients may develop lesions similar to the subcutaneous rheumatoid nodule, both within the lungs and on the pleural surfaces. These rheumatoid granulomas are particularly common in patients who already have industrial lung disease caused by inhaling various types of silica; the association of coalminer's lung with rheumatoid granulomas in seropositive miners is called Caplan's syndrome.

Blood vessels There is the development of vasculitis which is either:

- Acute neutrophilic vasculitis, presenting with purpura and occasional foci of ulceration.
- Lymphocytic vasculitis, producing a more low-key erythematous patchy rash.

Eyes Dry eye syndrome (keratoconjunctivitis sicca) is caused by lymphocytic inflammation of both lacrimal and mucus glands. Lack of tears leads to secondary inflammation of the cornea. In addition, scleritis may occur because of degeneration of collagenous tissue in the eye, and in severe cases this progresses to perforation of the globe—scleromalacia perforans (rare).

Hemopoietic and lymphoreticular systems Anemia of chronic disorders is common in rheumatoid disease, and a minority of patients develop hypersplenism or lymphadenopathy. Felty's syndrome describes a syndrome of splenomegaly,

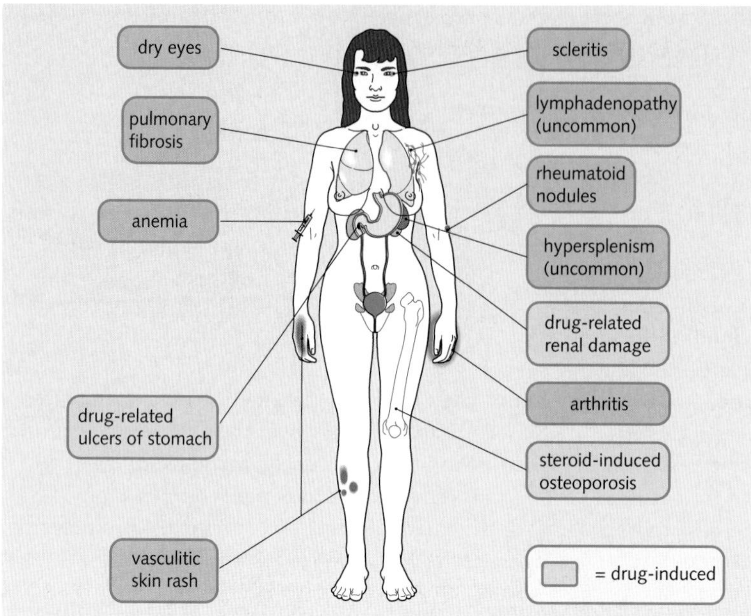

Fig. 12.3 Clinical features of rheumatoid disease.

lymphadenopathy, anemia, and leukopenia with rheumatoid arthritis. Sepsis is an important and common cause of death in these patients.

Fig. 12.3 shows a diagram of the clinical features of rheumatoid disease.

Diagnosis:

- Clinical features (Fig. 12.3).
- Radiography: periarticular osteoporosis, loss of articular cartilage (joint space), erosions, subluxation, and ankylosis.
- Serology: presence of rheumatoid factors. Two tests—Rose–Waaler test (based on the ability of IgM rheumatoid factor to agglutinate sheep red cells that have been coated with rabbit antisheep antibody); and latex agglutination test (rheumatoid factor agglutinates latex particles that have been coated with human IgG; less specific than the Rose–Waaler test).
- Anemia: normochromic normocytic.
- Erythrocyte sedimentation ratio (ESR) and CRP levels: both are typically elevated.

Treatment is by:

- Analgesia and anti-inflammatories.
- Immunosuppressive therapy: penicillamine, gold, azathioprine, salazopyrine.
- Surgery for advanced painful disease in any joint.

Treatment for rheumatoid disease may itself cause pathology (i.e., steroid-induced osteoporosis, analgesic-related ulceration of the stomach, and drug-induced renal disease).

Course and prognosis are variable. Studies of patients with disease of such severity as to require hospitalization showed that within 10 years:

- 25% have complete remission.
- 40% have only moderate impairment of function.
- 25% will be more severely disabled.
- 10% will be severely crippled.

Mortality is greatly increased in patients with functional impairment; the 5-year survival for severely disabled rheumatoid arthritis (RA) patients is reduced by 50%.

Organ-specific or cell-type specific disease

Autoimmune diseases involving a single organ or cell-type are known as organ-specific or cell-type specific autoimmune diseases (Fig. 12.4).

> Although organ-specific autoimmune diseases specifically affect one organ, they frequently occur together. For example, Addison's disease is often associated with autoimmune gastritis.

Organ-specific autoimmune diseases		
Disease	**Associated autoantibody**	**Comment**
Graves' disease	LATS (long-acting thyroid stimulator) or thyroid-stimulating immunoglobulin (TSI)	Hyperthyroidism
Hashimoto's disease	Anti-thyroid hormones	Hypothyroidism
Type 1 diabetes mellitus	Anti-islet β-cell antibody	Insulin-responsive hyperglycemia
Addison's disease	Antiadrenal antibodies	Hypoadrenocorticalism
Autoimmune gastritis	Anti-intrinsic factor and antiparietal cell antibodies	Pernicious anemia
Vitiligo	—	Hypopigmentation
Myasthenia gravis	Antiacetylcholine receptor antibody	Muscle fatigue

Fig. 12.4 Organ-specific autoimmune diseases.

Hashimoto's thyroiditis

Organ-specific autoimmune disease eventually causes hypothyroidism as a result of antibody-mediated destruction of the thyroid gland (see Chapter 9, p. 186).

Graves' disease

An organ-specific autoimmune disorder, this results in thyrotoxicosis due to overstimulation of thyroid-stimulating hormone (TSH) receptors of the thyroid gland by autoantibodies (see Chapter 9, p. 187).

Type 1 diabetes mellitus

Type 1 (insulin-dependent) diabetes mellitus is an organ-specific autoimmune disorder characterized by hyperglycemia, which is responsive to insulin. Disorder is caused by antibody-mediated destruction of the insulin-secreting cell population of the pancreas (see Chapter 9, p. 196, for full coverage).

Note that although type 1 diabetes mellitus is an organ-specific autoimmune disorder (i.e., the autoimmune mechanism attacks only one system—the endocrine pancreas), the effects of hyperglycemia are multitudinous, affecting many systems. Consequently diabetes mellitus is also classified as a multisystem disease.

Addison's disease

This rare condition of chronic adrenal insufficiency is most commonly caused by the autoimmune-mediated destruction of the adrenal cortex (see Chapter 9, p. 195). It is often associated with autoimmune thyroid disease, autoimmune gastritis, and other endocrine organ autoimmune diseases.

Autoimmune gastritis

Chronic inflammation of the gastric mucosa caused by the autoimmune destruction of gastric parietal cells, with or without intrinsic factor, results in the development of pernicious anemia.

Vitiligo

The autoimmune destruction of melanocytes causes patchy loss of pigmentation (see Chapter 13, p. 309).

Myasthenia gravis

The autoimmune destruction of acetylcholine receptors occurs at the neuromuscular junction (see Chapter 11, p. 237).

Diseases of immunodeficiency

Immunodeficiency can be defined as the occurrence of, or increased susceptibility to, severe and prolonged infection caused by a specific defect in the immune system. Primary immunodeficiencies are a rare group of diseases, which usually result from genetic defects in one or more of the effector components of the immune system, and they are, therefore, present from birth. More than 95 inherited immunodeficiency disorders have now been identified. Secondary immunodeficiencies are disorders that result from extrinsic or environmental causes and are acquired. There are many origins of secondary immunodeficiencies.

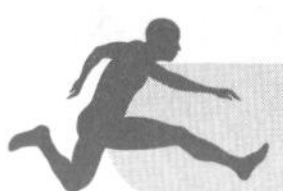

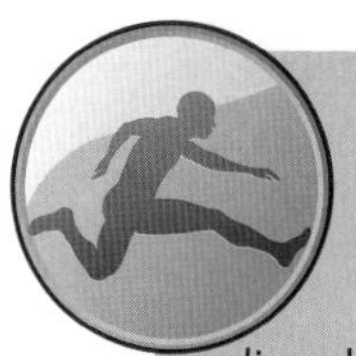

The type of infection associated with diseases of immune deficiency depends on the category of immune disorder:

- B cell deficiencies (defective antibody response): increased susceptibility to opportunistic infections caused by extracellular organisms.
- T cell deficiencies (defective cell-mediated immunity): increased susceptibility to opportunistic infections caused by intracellular organisms.
- Mixed B and T cell deficiencies (defective antibody response and cell-mediated immunity): increased susceptibility to most infections.

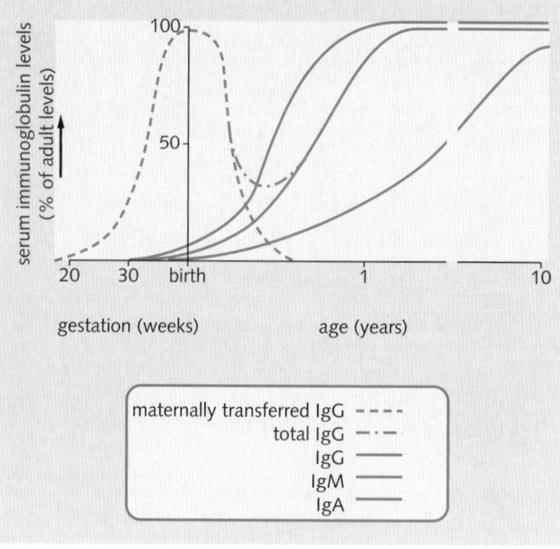

Fig. 12.5 Serum immunoglobulin levels in the neonate. (Adapted from Introduction to *Clinical Immunology*, by M. Haeny, Butterworths, London, 1985.)

Primary immunodeficiencies

Transient physiological agammaglobulinemia of the neonate

This natural transient trough in antibody levels, usually occurs between 3 and 6 months of age, is caused by falling levels of maternally derived IgG prior to the appearance of the infant's own antibody (IgM followed by IgG and IgA); detailed in Fig. 12.5. It can be more prolonged and more severe in premature infants.

X-linked agammaglobulinemia of Bruton

In this X-linked recessive disorder, affected males present with recurrent infections from between 4 months and 2 years of age (maternal IgG protects against earlier infection). Pre-B cells are unable to differentiate into mature B cells because of a lack of an enzyme called Bruton's tyrosine kinase (located on chromosome Xq22). The disease is characterized by:

- Deficiency of B cells and plasma cells.
- Negligible levels of immunoglobulins.
- Small lymph nodes and absent tonsils.

T cell numbers and functions are normal, and, therefore, infections are primarily bacterial.

Treatment is with long-term immunoglobulin replacement therapy and the rigorous use of antibacterial agents.

Common variable immunodeficiency

This acquired form of agammaglobulinemia is characterized by an increased susceptibility to infections—especially bacterial—presenting most often in the third decade of life. It is also known as late-onset hypogammaglobulinemia.

Its etiology is unknown, but it may follow viral infection (e.g., Epstein–Barr virus (EBV)).

Although not hereditary it is commonly associated with MHC haplotypes HLA-B8 and HLA-DR3.

Pathogenesis is variable, and it can be caused by any of the following:

- Intrinsic B cell defect which produces malfunctioning, immature B cells.
- Immunoregulatory T cell imbalance, hence B cells fail to differentiate due to lack of T helper cells or due to overactivity of T suppressor cells.
- Autoantibodies to T or B cells.

The disease is more common and more variable than the X-linked form (hence the name); however, the pattern of infection is similar, chiefly affecting the lungs, sinuses, and gastrointestinal (GI) tract.

Treatment is as for X-linked deficiency.

Isolated IgA deficiency

The most common form of immunodeficiency, this affects 1 in 700 Caucasians (but it is very rare in other ethnic groups). Most cases are sporadic, but some patients have family members with varied forms of antibody deficiency.

Circulating B cells bearing surface IgA are immature, and they fail to differentiate into IgA-secreting plasma cells.

Patients are prone to sinopulmonary infections and bowel colonization with *Giardia*, *Salmonella*, and other enteric pathogens.

It is associated with an increased incidence of autoimmune diseases and allergies.

DiGeorge syndrome (thymic hypoplasia)

This rare, congenital disorder is caused by the arrested development of the third and fourth branchial arches, resulting in an almost complete absence of the thymus and parathyroid gland. The genetic defect has been mapped to chromosome 22q11.

Immunoglobulin levels are normal, but affected individuals have decreased circulating levels of T lymphocytes, resulting in impaired cell-mediated immunity.

Patients typically develop a triad of infections, namely candidiasis, pneumocystis pneumonia, and persistent diarrhea.

The syndrome is also characterized by hypocalcemia (due to hypoparathyroidism) and associated with abnormalities of the great vessels (e.g., transposition or Fallot's tetralogy).

Treatment requires transplantation of thymic tissue.

Severe combined immunodeficiency

This inherited deficiency of lymphocytic stem cells is characterized by:

- Deficiency of both T and B cells.
- Negligible circulating immunoglobulins.
- Greatly reduced cell-mediated immunity.
- Hypoplastic thymus.

The condition can be X-linked (gamma chain of interleukin-2 receptor at Xq13-21.1) or an autosomal recessive disorder. It presents during the first few months of life with a failure to thrive and persistent infections. In addition infants are at risk from graft-versus-host disease. One example of this occurs when maternal T cells cross the placenta; another involves T cells in non-irradiated blood products.

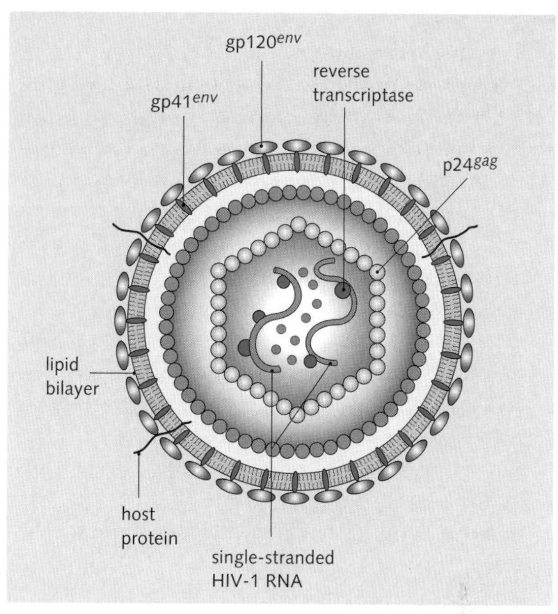

Fig. 12.6 Structure of the human immunodeficiency virus (HIV)-1.

Death usually occurs within the first 2 years of life from multiple infections, although a bone marrow transplant can be an effective cure in some cases.

Secondary immunodeficiencies

Secondary immunodeficiencies are those that result from extrinsic or environmental causes, as listed in Fig. 12.9 below. The pathologies of most of these diseases are covered in other chapters.

Acquired immune deficiency syndrome

Acquired immune deficiency syndrome (AIDS) is caused by infection with the human immunodeficiency virus (HIV). It is characterized by a profound defect in cell-mediated immunity with lymphopenia and diminished T lymphocyte responses.

The usual cause is HIV-1 (Fig. 12.6) although another strain of the virus (HIV-2) has also been associated with AIDS in Africa.

Routes of transmission are threefold: sexual contact, blood-borne (transfusions or contaminated needles), and maternal (placental or via breast milk). Over 30 million people worldwide are now infected with HIV.

Pathogenesis

HIV is an enveloped RNA retrovirus that binds to CD4 receptors present on T helper cells and various cells of the monocyte/macrophage system via its cell surface heterodimer of glycoproteins, gp 120/gp 41.

- Following cell entry, the virus loses its coat and utilizes its enzyme, reverse transcriptase, to make viral DNA, which is inserted into the host chromosome.
- Viral replication is initially repressed by intracellular factors and by cell-mediated immunity mediated by $CD8^+$ cytotoxic T cells, and so the virus can remain latent (i.e., dormant) for months or even years.
- Activation of latently infected T cells triggers viral replication, and infectious virus particles are released, resulting in the infection of more $CD4^+$ cells.

Eventually, there is depletion of T helper cells, which results in a severely impaired cell-mediated immunity, with a high risk of multiple opportunistic infections.

There is a correlation between the fall in the CD4 cell count and increasing viral antigen levels (Fig. 12.7).

Clinical features

The clinical outcome of HIV infection has been classified into four stages (Fig. 12.8).

The duration of each stage is highly variable—some patients pass directly through stages II and III to AIDS-related conditions or even to fully developed ("full blown") AIDS, while others remain in the earlier stages for months or years. A small proportion of HIV-infected patients do not develop clinical AIDS.

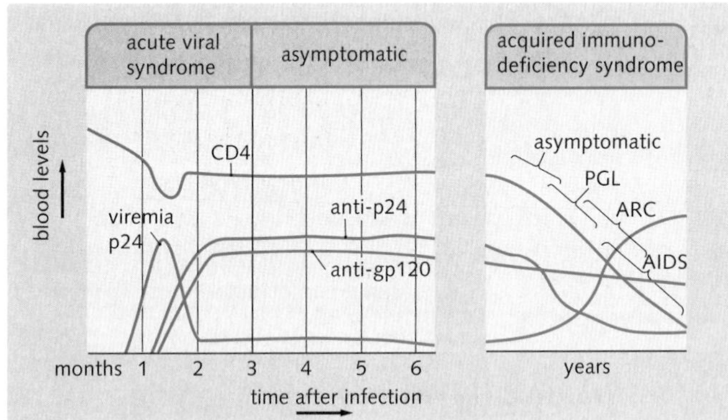

Fig. 12.7 CD4 count, viral antigen (p24) and antibody levels following HIV infection. (p24, nucleocapsid protein; PGL, persistent generalized lymphadenopathy; ARC, AIDS-related complex; AIDS, acquired immune deficiency syndrome.)

Classification of HIV infection	
Stage I	Initial infection; can be either: • symptomatic seroconversion: mononucleosis-like syndrome, mild meningoencephalitis • asymptomatic seroconversion
Stage II	Chronic asymptomatic infection: lab tests typically normal but may have anemia, neutropenia, thrombocytopenia, low CD4 lymphocytes, lymphopenia, and hypergammaglobulinemia
Stage III	Persistent generalized lymphadenopathy: with or without lab test abnormalities as in stage II
Stage IV	AIDS-related complex: generalized lymphadenopathy with persistent fever, weight loss, unexplained diarrhea, CNS manifestations, and hematological abnormalities including thrombocytopenia, leukopenia, and anemia Fully developed AIDS: • wide spectrum of opportunistic infections including *Pneumocystis carinii*, toxoplasmosis, *Cryptococcus*, cryptosporidiosis, atypical mycobacteria, herpes simplex or zoster, oral hairy leukoplakia, histoplasmosis, candidiasis, cytomegalovirus, *Salmonella* • secondary cancers, e.g., Kaposi's sarcoma, non-Hodgkin's lymphoma, squamous carcinoma of the mouth or rectum

Fig. 12.8 Classification of HIV infection.

The reasons for these variations in the course of the disease are poorly understood, and the factors that determine progression from one stage into the next remain unclear.

Prognosis and treatment

The prognosis for AIDS patients is improving for those who have access to HAART (highly active antiretroviral therapy). HAART is a combination of three drugs, including a reverse transcriptase and a protease inhibitor. In addition, antimicrobial therapy is given with the aim of preventing or treating infection (prophylactic antibiotics or antifungals). Unfortunately many AIDS patients in developing countries have a very poor prognosis because these expensive therapies are unavailable.

Fig. 12.9 gives a summary of immune deficiencies.

Amyloidosis

Definition and chemical nature of amyloid

Amyloidosis is the deposition of abnormal extracellular fibrillar protein, amyloid, in different tissues. Amyloid is composed of a meshwork of rigid, straight fibrils formed from precursor peptides (immunoglobulin light chains, serum amyloid protein A, peptide hormones) lined up in an antiparallel, β-pleated sheet structure. The β-pleated sheet structure is important because enzymes in the body are incapable of digesting such large molecules in this form. It is detected histologically as a bright pink hyaline material, and it takes up certain stains, the best known being Congo red.

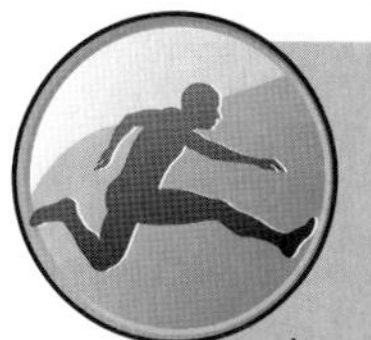

It is important to note that the physical arrangement of the constituent amino acids makes a protein an amyloid rather than any specific amino acid sequence.

There are many different types of amyloid, each being formed from different precursor amino acids. The precursors themselves are often fragments of larger proteins.

Summary of immune deficiencies

Category	Deficiency	Example
Primary	B cell (antibody deficiency)	Transient hypogammaglobulinemia of infancy X-linked agammaglobulinemia Acquired common variable hypogammaglobulinemia Selective IgA or IgG subclass deficiencies
	T cell	Thymic hypoplasia (DiGeorge syndrome)
	Mixed B and T cell	Severe combined immune deficiency
Secondary	B cell (antibody deficiency)	Myeloma Protein deficiency
	T cell	AIDS Hodgkin's disease Non-Hodgkin's lymphoma Drugs, e.g., steroids, ciclosporin, azathioprine
	Mixed B and T cell	Chronic lymphocytic leukemia Post-bone marrow transplantation Post-chemotherapy/radiotherapy Chronic renal failure Splenectomy

Fig. 12.9 Summary of immune deficiencies.

Amyloid formation

Amyloid formation occurs because of the production of either:

- Abnormal amounts of normal precursor peptide (common), such as immunoglobulin light chains in multiple myeloma or serum amyloid A protein in acute phase response. It may be a result of overproduction, reduced degradation, or reduced excretion of protein.
- Normal amounts of abnormal (amyloidogenic) peptide (rare), due, for example, to transthyretin or gelsolin polymorphisms.

Macrophages are then thought to process the precursor proteins to form amyloid fibrils.

Amyloid also contains a serum glycoprotein called serum amyloid P protein (pentraxin family), which is thought to assist in its polymerization.

Classification of amyloidosis

Clinically, amyloidosis presents with organ involvement that is either:

- Systemic: may involve many tissues as it is particularly deposited in the blood vessel walls and basement membranes. Usually fatal, death generally occurring from renal or cardiac disease.
- Localized: affects only one organ or tissue. Rarely, it may be found without any obvious predisposing cause. The skin, lungs, and urinary tract are the most frequent sites.

In both cases, the progressive accumulation of amyloid leads to cellular dysfunction by preventing the normal processes of diffusion through extracellular tissues, and by physical compression of functioning parenchymal cells.

Systemic amyloidosis

Reactive systemic amyloidosis This amyloid is composed of protein A and is termed the AA type. It is derived from serum amyloid A, which is synthesized in the liver and is one of several acute phase reactant proteins, so named because of their increased serum concentration in response to a variety of diseases.

Reactive amyloidosis always has a predisposing cause, which is invariably a chronic inflammatory disorder:

Chronic infections (e.g., tuberculosis).

- Hodgkin's disease.
- Rheumatoid arthritis.
- Bronchiectasis.
- Chronic osteomyelitis.

AA-type amyloid is deposited in many organs but it has a predilection for the liver, spleen, and kidney. It results in hepatosplenomegaly with or without renal vein thrombosis and nephrotic syndrome.

Myeloma-associated amyloidosis This amyloid is composed of immunoglobulin light chains (and/or parts of their variable regions) and is termed AL type. Immunoglobulin light chains are formed by proliferating plasma cells usually in association with:

- Multiple myeloma.
- Waldenström's macroglobulinemia.
- Heavy chain disease.
- Primary amyloidosis.

Primary amyloidosis is a myeloma-associated amyloidosis that occurs in the absence of any clinically obvious myeloma. It is caused by a clinically occult plasma cell tumor, and it is accompanied by the presence of a monoclonal immunoglobulin band on serum electrophoresis. It is also known as benign monoclonal gammopathy.

AL-type amyloid is deposited in many organs including the tongue, skin, heart, nerves, kidneys, liver, and spleen, and it has a predilection for connective tissue within these organs.

Patients may present with heart failure, macroglossia, peripheral neuropathy, carpal tunnel syndrome, or renal failure.

Hemodialysis-associated amyloidosis This amyloidosis is associated with long-term hemodialysis for chronic renal failure. Amyloid material deposited in the affected tissues appears to be β_2-microglobulin, and the amyloid is termed AH type (H for hemodialysis).

Clinical features include arthropathy and carpal tunnel syndrome.

Hereditary amyloidosis Hereditary forms of amyloidosis are rare, and they include familial Mediterranean fever (AA type) and familial neuropathic forms (AF, prealbumin, type).

Localized amyloidosis

Alzheimer's disease The most common example of amyloid deposition occurs in the nervous system, in both Alzheimer's disease and in normal ageing (cerebral angiopathy). The amyloid (Aβ) is composed of peptide fragments termed β-protein or A4 protein, both of which are derived from a normal, neuronal membrane protein—Alzheimer precursor protein (APP).

Endocrine amyloidosis Amyloid material is often found in the stroma of peptide hormone-producing tumors. It is particularly characteristic of medullary carcinoma of the thyroid, a tumor of the calcitonin-producing interfollicular C cells. In this instance, the amyloid contains calcitonin precursor molecules arranged in a β-pleated sheet configuration.

In type 2 diabetes, the excessive secretion of amylin by the β-cells of the pancreas is associated with its deposition as islet amyloid.

Senile amyloidosis Minute deposits of amyloid usually derived from serum transthyretin (prealbumin) are found in the heart and in the walls of blood vessels in many organs of elderly people. However, significant signs or symptoms of amyloidosis occur in only a few cases.

Disorders of white blood cells

Leukopenia

Leukopenia is defined as a reduction in circulating leukocytes. The classification of leukocytes is shown in Fig. 12.10.

For a quick review of leukocyte (white blood cell) classification, see Fig. 12.10.

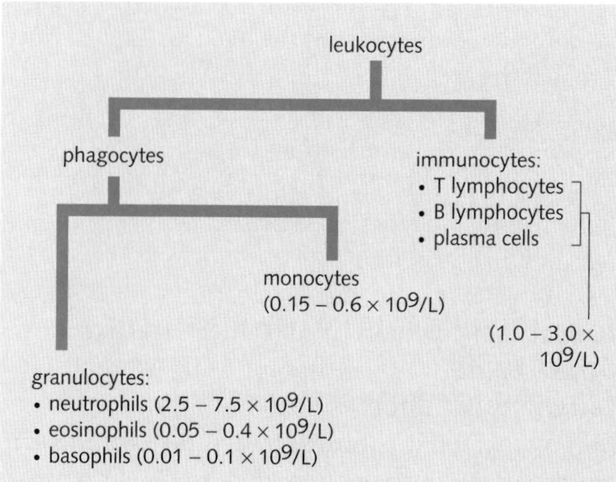

Fig. 12.10 Classification of leukocytes.

Neutropenia

Neutropenia, a deficiency of neutrophil granulocytes, is the most important form of leukopenia. The lower limit of normal neutrophil count is $2.5–7.5 \times 10^9$/L. Levels of less than these values are classified as neutropenia.

Neutropenia may be selective or part of a general pancytopenia. The causes of both types are listed in Fig. 12.11.

Clinical features depend on the degree of neutropenia:

- Mild: usually asymptomatic.
- Moderate to severe ($<0.5 \times 10^9$/L): associated with a progressive increase in risk and severity of infections.
- Levels of $<0.2 \times 10^9$/L are associated with a high mortality from overwhelming infections.

Infections are predominantly bacterial and are usually opportunistic, most commonly Gram-positive skin organisms (e.g., *Staphylococcus* and *Streptococcus*) or Gram-negative gut bacteria (e.g., *Pseudomonas*, *Escherichia coli*, *Proteus*).

They can be either localized (e.g., of the mouth, throat, skin, or anus) or generalized (i.e., septicemias). The latter may be rapidly fatal.

Treatment is of the underlying cause and with antimicrobial therapy.

Reactive proliferation of white cells

Leukocytosis

Leukocytosis is defined as an increase in numbers of circulating white blood cells.

Types of leukocytosis

The types of leukocytosis are:

- Polymorphonuclear leukocytosis (neutrophilia): increased numbers of neutrophils (most common cause of leukocytosis).
- Monocytosis: increased numbers of the monocyte/macrophage cells.
- Eosinophil leukocytosis (eosinophilia): increased numbers of eosinophils.
- Basophil leukocytosis (basophilia): increased numbers of basophils.
- Lymphocytosis: increased numbers of T and/or B lymphocytes.

Leukocytosis can be:

- Primary: caused by bone marrow disease (e.g., leukemias, lymphomas–described later in this chapter).

Causes of neutropenia		
Type	**Cause**	**Clinical features**
Selective neutropenia	Reduced granulopoiesis	Congenital: Kostmann's syndrome—autosomal recessive disease presenting in the first year of life with life-threatening infections Cyclical: rare syndrome characterized by recurrent severe but temporary neutropenia with a periodicity of 3–4 weeks Nutritional: B_{12} or folate deficiency Racial: African races
	Accelerated granulocyte removal	Immune: • autoimmune • systemic lupus erythematosus • Felty's syndrome • hypersensitivity and anaphylaxis Infectious: • viral, e.g., hepatitis, influenza, HIV • fulminant bacteria, e.g., typhoid, miliary tuberculosis
	Drug-induced neutropenia	Drug-induced damage of either neutrophils or precursor marrow cells can occur via direct toxicity or immune-mediated mechanisms in susceptible individuals; examples of such drugs include: • anti-inflammatory: phenylbutazone, cyclophosphamide • antibacterial: chloramphenicol, cotrimoxazole, sulfasalazine • anticonvulsants: phenytoin • antithyroids: carbimazole • hypoglycemics: tolbutamide • phenothiazines: chlorpromazine, thioridazine • psychotropics and antidepressants: clozapine, imipramine • miscellaneous: gold, penicillamine
Part of general pancytopenia	Reduced granulopoiesis	Bone marrow failure, megaloblastic anemia
	Accelerated granulocyte removal	Splenomegaly

Fig. 12.11 Causes of neutropenia.

- Secondary: caused by the normal response of bone marrow to abnormal conditions (e.g., infection). Also known as reactive leukocytosis (Fig. 12.12).

Lymphadenitis

This inflammation of lymph nodes is usually caused by infection, and it is characterized by a painful swelling of the affected nodes as a result of:

- Increased blood flow.
- Macrophage activation and increased cell number.
- Lymphocyte activation and increased cell number.

Additional changes depend on the type of lymphadenitis:

- Acute nonspecific lymphadenitis—typically caused by acute infections (e.g., infectious mononucleosis, rubella, pertussis, mumps). Bacterial infection commonly involves infiltration of node by neutrophils. Most commonly affected lymph nodes are those in the neck associated with tonsillitis.
- Chronic nonspecific lymphadenitis—typically caused by chronic infections (e.g., brucellosis, tuberculosis, syphilis, hepatitis). Additional changes include increased plasma cells and granuloma formation.

Neoplastic proliferation of white blood cells

Malignant lymphomas

In this group of lymphoproliferative diseases normal lymphoid tissue is replaced by abnormal cells of lymphoid origin, forming solid malignant tumors of the lymph nodes.

Causes of reactive leukocytosis	
Cause	**Clinical features**
Neutrophilia ($>7.5 \times 10^9$/L)	Acute infections Hemorrhage/hemolysis Inflammation and tissue necrosis Metabolic disorders Myeloproliferative diseases Neoplasia Steroid therapy Strenuous exercise
Monocytosis ($>0.8 \times 10^9$/L)	Chronic infections, e.g., tuberculosis Brucellosis, malaria, inflammatory disorders, e.g., rheumatoid disease, SLE, Crohn's disease, neoplasia
Eosinophilia ($>0.44 \times 10^9$/L)	Allergy, e.g., asthma Parasites, e.g., tapeworms Skin disease, e.g., eczema, psoriasis Neoplasia, especially Hodgkin's disease Miscellaneous, e.g., polyarteritis nodosa, sarcoidosis
Basophilia ($>0.1 \times 10^9$/L)	Myxedema Chickenpox Myeloproliferative disorders
Lymphocytosis ($>3.5 \times 10^9$/L)	Acute infections, e.g., infectious mononucleosis Chronic infections, e.g., tuberculosis, brucellosis, hepatitis

Fig. 12.12 Causes of reactive leukocytosis.

All lymphomas are broadly classified as either Hodgkin's disease or non-Hodgkin's lymphomas.

Hodgkin's disease

The most common type of lymphoma, Hodgkin's disease (HD) is characterized by the painless enlargement of one or more groups of lymph nodes, and the presence of large binucleate cells (Reed–Sternberg cells) within them.

It affects 3 per 100,000 in the U.S., males more so than females by almost 2:1. It can occur at any age, but there are two peaks of incidence—one in young adults (20–30 years old) and the other in late middle-age.

The etiology of Hodgkin's disease is obscure, as is the origin of the malignant Reed–Sternberg (RS) cells. However, RS cells form only a small percentage of the total population of the affected node, the majority being composed of reactive lymphocytes, plasma cells, histiocytes, and eosinophils.

Ann Arbor staging system of Hodgkin's disease	
Stage	**Comment**
I	Involvement of single lymph node region (I) or of single extralymphatic organ or site (hence Ie)
II	Involvement of two or more lymph node regions, with all lesions confined to the same side of the diaphragm (II), or localized involvement of an extralymphatic site and one or more lymph node regions confined to one side of the diaphragm (IIe)
III	Involvement of lymph node regions on both sides of the diaphragm (III) which may also involve the spleen (IIIs), localized extralymphatic sites (IIIe) or both (IIIse)
IV	Widespread involvement of extralymphoid sites such as the liver, lung, and bone marrow with or without lymph node involvement

Fig. 12.13 Ann Arbor staging system of Hodgkin's disease. Suffix A indicates the absence of systemic symptoms; suffix B indicates the presence of systemic symptoms. For example, stage IIIeB denotes involvement of lymph nodes on both sides of the diaphragm accompanied by localized involvement of an extralymphatic site with systemic symptoms.

Hodgkin's disease often presents clinically as the enlargement of accessible nodes, most often in the upper half of the body (e.g., cervical or axillary). The disease is initially localized to a single peripheral lymph node region, but it spreads in a fairly consistent pattern to adjacent nodes via the lymphatics and then, following splenic involvement, to other organs via the bloodstream.

One third of patients have systemic symptoms, notably weight loss, and pyrexia. Symptoms are due to:

- Lymph node enlargement producing mediastinal compression and lymphedema.
- Hematology: normochromic–normocytic anemia, neutrophilia, eosinophilia, lymphopenia (advanced disease), raised ESR.
- Immunology: depression of T cell function and susceptibility to infection.

The stage (extent of spread) of the disease is an important determinant in lymphoma treatment and prognosis. The staging system currently used is known as the Ann Arbor staging system, named after the location at which it was first proposed (Fig. 12.13).

Diagnosis of Hodgkin's disease can only be made on examination of biopsied lymph nodes:

Macroscopically: affected lymph nodes are enlarged, with a smooth surface, and the lymph node capsule is rarely breached (cf. non-Hodgkin's lymphomas).

Microscopically: four subtypes of Hodgkin's disease are recognized and classified according to the Rye classification system (Fig. 12.14).

Treatment is dependent on the stage of the disease, either localized (radiotherapy) or generalized (systemic chemotherapy). Approximately 75% of patients treated for Hodgkin's disease survive for at least 5 years.

The prognosis of patients with Hodgkin's disease declines with advancing stages and the presence of systemic symptoms.

Non-Hodgkin's lymphomas

Non-Hodgkin's lymphomas (NHLs) include all lymphomas other than Hodgkin's disease. They are predominantly diseases of middle and later life, with males affected more than females.

The etiology of NHLs is poorly understood, but several factors have been implicated:

- Immunosuppression: increased incidence in primary immunosuppressive diseases (e.g., X-linked agammaglobulinemia).
- Viral infection with lymphotropic viruses (e.g., EBV, HTLV-1, HIV).
- Toxic chemicals.
- Radiation.

Chromosomal translocations are a feature of many types of lymphoma, for example:

- Burkitt's lymphoma: translocation 8:14. Also associated with EBV infection.
- Follicular B cell lymphoma: translocation 14:18.
- Small or large cell diffuse lymphomas: associated with translocation 11:14.

These translocations cause a neoplastic transformation as a result of the transfer of an oncogene or oncogene-regulatory gene to an abnormal site resulting in the increased expression of that oncogene.

In malignant lymphomas, the tumor represents a clone of cells whose maturation is fixed at a particular stage of development.

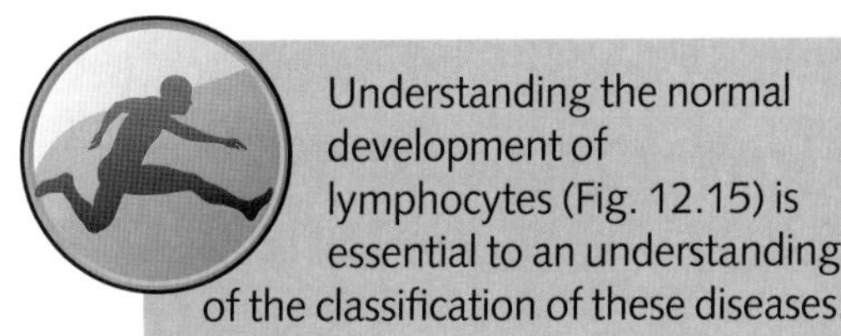
Understanding the normal development of lymphocytes (Fig. 12.15) is essential to an understanding of the classification of these diseases.

The vast majority (over 90%) of NHLs are B cell lymphomas, which are derived from follicle center cells. These tumors have either follicular or diffuse architecture.

Clinical manifestations of NHLs are similar to those of Hodgkin's disease, but they are more varied because of their heterogeneous nature. The majority present with asymmetric painless enlargement of lymph nodes in one or more peripheral lymph node regions. However, extranodal presentation is more frequent than in HD, with 20% of all NHLs originating within extranodal sites.

Common primary extranodal sites include the orbit, nasopharynx, tonsil, GI tract, skin, and bone.

Systemic symptoms are less prominent than in HD although fever is a feature of extensive disease.

Several classification systems are used for NHLs.

One relatively simple classification, based on the Kiel system (Fig. 12.16), considers the following:

Rye classification of Hodgkin's disease

Type	Characteristic
Nodular sclerosis (60%–70%)	Thick bands of collagen encircle abnormal tissue; lacunar cells (variants of Reed–Sternberg—RS—cell) are often numerous; good prognosis
Mixed cellularity (15%)	Numerous RS cells and intermediate numbers of lymphocytes, plasma cells, and eosinophils; poor prognosis
Lymphoctye predominant (10%)	Numerous lymphocytes, few RS cells and a scattering of unusual Hodgkin's cells— "popcorn" cells (so named due to their excessively lobulated nuclei); increased risk of development of non-Hodgkin's B cell lymphoma; otherwise good prognosis
Lymphocyte depleted (2%)	Dominance of RS cells but sparse lymphocytes with or without diffuse fibrosis; worst prognosis

Fig. 12.14 Rye classification of Hodgkin's disease.

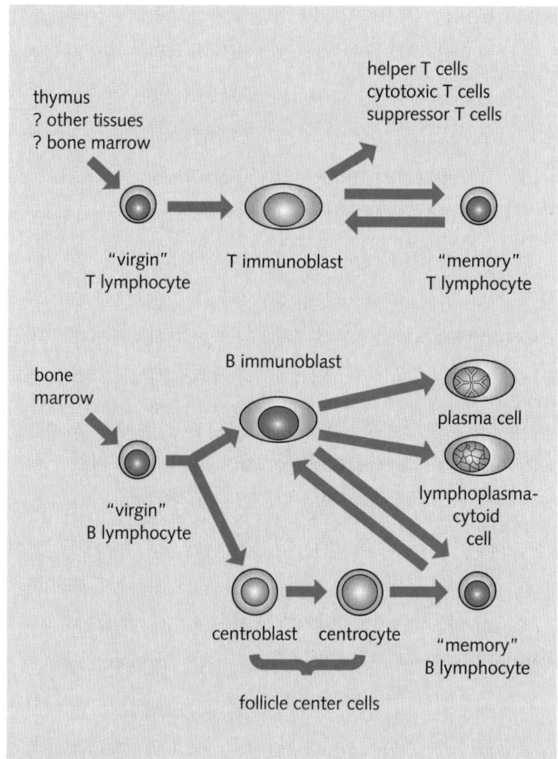

Fig. 12.15 Normal lymphocyte development. (Adapted from *Essential Haematology*, 3rd edn, by V. Hoffbrand and J. Pettit, Blackwell Science, 1993.)

- Degree of malignancy: low grade (associated with well-differentiated, relatively inactive cell types—progress over years); high grade (associated with primitive actively proliferating cells—progress over weeks or months).
- Tumor architecture: follicular or diffuse.
- Functional cell type: either T cell or B cell.
- Specific cell type or size (e.g., centroblastic or immunoblastic, large or small cell).

A similar staging system to that used in HD may be used, but it is less clearly related than the histological type to the prognosis.

Treatment is by single or combination chemotherapy with which some patients show long-term remission if not cure. Bone marrow transplantation is under evaluation.

The prognosis depends on the type of lymphoma and varies widely from highly proliferative and rapidly fatal diseases (e.g., immunoblastic lymphoma) to indolent and well-tolerated malignancies with a mean survival of about 7 years (e.g., follicular centrocytic lymphoma).

Leukemias

Leukemias are neoplastic proliferations of white blood cell precursors in the bone marrow.

Classification of NHLs based on the Kiel system

Grade	B cell	T cell
Low grade malignancy	Follicular: • centrocytic • centroblastic–centrocytic Diffuse: • lymphocytic: chronic lymphocytic and hairy cell leukemia • lymphoplasmacytoid • plasmacytic: multiple myeloma • centrocytic • centroblastic–centrocytic	Lymphocytic Small cerebriform cell: • mycosis fungoides • Sézary's syndrome Lymphoepithelioid Angioimmunoblastic T zone Pleomorphic small cell
High grade malignancy	Diffuse: • centroblastic • immunoblastic • anaplastic • lymphoblastic • "Burkitt-type": small, non-cleaved cell	Pleomorphic medium or large cell (HTLV-1) Immunoblastic Anaplastic Lymphoblastic

Fig. 12.16 Classification of non-Hodgkin's lymphomas (NHLs) based on the Kiel system.

Classification—Leukemias are classified into two broad groups according to the ability of the leukemic cells to differentiate. The ability to differentiate also reflects the rate of disease progression.

- Acute: characterized by numerous immature "blast" cells (leucocyte precursors), and rapid disease progression.
- Chronic: characterized by large numbers of precursor cells that are more differentiated than blast cells, and associated with slower disease progression.

These groups are then further classified into two main groups depending on neoplastic cell types:

- Myeloid leukemia (cells of granulocytic series).
- Lymphocytic leukemia (cells of the lymphoid series).
- Etiology—In the majority of cases, the cause of leukemia is unknown. However, certain factors are known to initiate leukemic transformation:
- Genetics: slight familial tendency (high concordance in monozygotic twins); chromosome abnormalities (both quantitative and qualitative) are present in about 50% of patients; increased incidence in Down syndrome.
- Ionizing radiation: excessive exposure in therapy (e.g., for ankylosing spondylitis, malignant disease); nuclear explosions/accidents as at Hiroshima and Chernobyl.
- Drugs: prolonged chemotherapy (e.g., with alkylating agents).
- Immune status: increased incidence in immunosuppressed individuals.
- Viruses (e.g., HTLV-I causes adult T cell leukemia/lymphoma; HTLV-II is associated with hairy cell leukemia).

Common features of leukemias

The common features of leukemias are bone marrow failure, gout, and metastasis.

Bone marrow failure Overproduction of leukocyte precursor cells causes the suppression of normal blood cell production, thus:

- Deficiency of red cell production leads to anemia.
- Deficiency of platelet production (thrombocytopenia) leads to hemorrhage.
- Deficiency of normal leukocyte production (granulocytes and lymphocytes) leads to failure to control infection.

Gout Increased cell turnover leads to increased uric acid synthesis, which may result in gout.

Metastasis There is infiltration of organs such as the liver, spleen, lymph nodes, meninges, and gonads by the leukemic cells.

Acute leukemia

In acute leukemia, blast cells (lymphoblasts or myeloblasts) fail to differentiate properly and proliferate in an uncontrolled manner.

There are two main types: acute lymphoblastic leukemia (ALL) and acute myeloblastic leukemia (AML). These are further subclassified according to cytological features of the blast cells. There are three subtypes for ALL (L_1–L_3) based on the degree of uniformity of cell size and vacuolation. There are eight subtypes for AML (M_0–M_7) based on the degree of cytoplasmic granularity.

See Fig. 12.17 for a table with the features of ALL and AML.

Clinical features of both AML and ALL are similar. They commonly present with symptoms of anemia (e.g., tiredness, malaise) and their course is typified by a series of overwhelming infections and mucosal hemorrhage.

Onset is frequently rapid, and progression to death from anemia, hemorrhage, or infection occurs within weeks if no treatment is given.

The clinical course is less catastrophic in childhood ALL. Hematological investigations reveal:

- Anemia: normocytic, normochromic.
- Leukocytosis, although leukopenia may be an occasional feature, despite massive marrow infiltration with blast cells.
- Neutropenia—overt infections.
- Thrombocytopenia—petechiae, purpura, epistaxis, bleeding gums, GI hemorrhage, cerebral hemorrhage.

Involvement of other organs:

- Skeleton (bone pain, especially in children): probably caused by osteolytic lesions.
- Lymphadenopathy.
- Hepatomegaly and splenomegaly: usually slight.
- Symptoms and signs secondary to CNS infiltration.

Management:

- Repeated courses of combination chemotherapy.
- Intensive blood transfusions.
- Antimicrobial agents.

Features of acute lymphoblastic and acute myeloblastic leukemia		
	Acute lymphoblastic leukemia (ALL)	Acute myeloblastic leukemia (AML)
Epidemiology	Mainly (>90%) affects children of <14 years with highest incidence at 3–4 years Second increase in incidence occurs around middle-age	Occurs at all ages and is the most common form of leukemia in adults
Proliferating cell type	Neoplastic lymphoblasts (lymphocyte precursor cells)	Neoplastic myeloblast (granulocyte/monocyte precursor cell)
Degree of differentiation	Blast cells show no differentiation	Blast cells usually show some evidence of differentiation to granulocytes
Prognosis	Children aged 2–9 years: 50–75% cure rate Adults: 35% cure rate with chemotherapy; 50% with allogeneic bone marrow transplant	20–25% cure rate with standard chemotherapy 50% with allogeneic bone marrow transplant

Fig. 12.17 Features of acute lymphoblastic and acute myeloblastic leukemia.

- Bone marrow transplantation: encouraging results in younger patients but largely depends on availability of suitable tissue matched donor.

For the prognosis see Fig. 12.17.

Chronic leukemias

Chronic myeloid leukemia There is neoplastic proliferation of an abnormal myeloid clone of leukocyte precursors in the bone marrow.

Over 95% of cases are characterized by the presence of a karyotypic abnormality—the Philadelphia chromosome—within the hemopoietic stem cells. This involves reciprocal translocation of part of the long arm (q) of chromosome 22 with the long arm of chromosome 9. The Philadelphia chromosome-positive cases are referred to as chronic granulocytic leukemia (CGL).

Chronic myeloid leukemia (CML) occurs in all age groups but most frequently between the ages of 40 and 60 years. The disease has a mild chronic phase characterized by anemia and massive splenomegaly. However, in over 70% of cases, the disease enters a more aggressive phase due to the emergence and dominance of a more malignant clone of myeloid cells.

Clinical features of the aggressive phase are much more severe; they bear a close resemblance to those of acute leukemia (usually AML), and they are rapidly fatal.

Hematological investigation reveals leukocytosis and normocytic anemia. Note that in contrast to acute leukemias, neutropenia, lymphopenia, and thrombocytopenia are not common in the chronic phase, and infection and bleeding are not typical.

There is often massive splenomegaly due to infiltration by CGL cells, and hepatomegaly is also frequently present.

Treatment is by:

- Chemotherapy.
- Interferon therapy.
- Bone marrow transplantation.

Prognosis—CGL is a fatal disorder with a mean survival of about 4 years. However, a minority of patients do survive for 10 years or more.

Chronic lymphocytic leukemia This chronic lymphoproliferative disorder is characterized by the proliferation of an abnormal lymphoid clone of leukocyte precursors in the bone marrow.

Chronic lymphocytic leukemia (CCL) is the most common leukemia of adults comprising about 30% of all leukemias, with males affected more than females by 2:1.

Clinical features—A slowly progressive disease of the elderly that follows a predictable course over a period of years; this is summarized in Fig. 12.18. Features are similar to a low-grade lymphoma but with predominant blood and bone marrow involvement.

This disease is much less aggressive than other leukemias.

Hematological changes are:

- Leukocytosis: small, nonfunctional lymphocytes of B cell origin.

Clinical features and staging of chronic lymphocytic leukemia according to the RAI classification	
Stage	**Feature(s)**
0	Lymphocytosis of blood and marrow
I	Lymphocytosis and enlarged nodes
II	Lymphocytosis and enlarged liver or spleen
III	Hemoglobin <11 g/dL, with features of stages 0, I, or II
IV	Platelet count <100 × 10^9/L, with features of stages 0, I, II, or III

Fig. 12.18 Clinical features and staging of chronic lymphocytic leukemia according to the RAI classification.

- Anemia and thrombocytopenia are late developments.
- Secondary autoimmune hemolytic anemia develops in 10% of cases.

The lymph nodes, liver, and spleen are characteristically involved, and normal architecture may become completely effaced by the infiltrating cells.

Survival for more than 10 years from diagnosis is common, and, as CLL is a disease of the elderly, death is often from an unrelated cause. However, anemia, hemorrhage, and infection may become life-threatening in the later stages.

In younger subjects, a more aggressive course of CLL may develop with massive glandular enlargement and severe infections secondary to a compromised immunity.

Myelodysplastic syndromes

This group of acquired neoplastic disorders of the bone marrow is characterized by increasing bone marrow failure with quantitative and qualitative abnormalities of all three myeloid cell lines (red cell, granulocyte/monocyte, and platelets) due to a defect of stem cells. They are also known as refractory anemias.

In most cases, the disease arises *de novo* and the etiology is likely to be as for the leukemias. However, in a significant proportion of cases, the disease is secondary to treatment with chemotherapy (with or without radiotherapy) for a previous neoplastic disease.

The hallmark of the disease is ineffective hemopoiesis resulting in pancytopenia despite a marrow of either normal or increased cellularity.

Bone marrow contains morphologically abnormal cells including ring sideroblasts and hypogranular white cells, often with abnormal chromosomes.

The disease has tendency to progress to acute leukemia, and it is, therefore, considered "preleukemic."

Clinical features—More than half the patients are over 70 years old, and more than 75% are over 50; males are affected more often than females.

Symptoms are generally sequelae of cytopenia and include anemia, infection, and hemorrhage. Disease progression is slow, but there is a tendency for it to transform into acute myeloid leukemia.

Diseases are subclassified depending on the presence of ring sideroblasts and the proportion of leukemic-type blast cells in the bone marrow (Fig. 12.19).

Treatment is largely supportive, by blood transfusion and treatment of the infection.

Morbidity and deaths are largely attributable to the refractory cytopenias either directly (e.g., from hemorrhage) or indirectly (e.g., from transfusion-related hemosiderosis).

In a minority of patients deaths are related to leukemic transformation.

Hairy cell leukemia

This rare, B cell leukemia is characterized by variable numbers of "hairy" cells in the blood, bone marrow, liver, and other organs. Hairy cells are so named because of their characteristic irregular outline caused by cytoplasmic projections or "hairs."

The disease has a peak incidence at 40–60 years old, males more so than females by 4:1.

It is characterized clinically by features of pancytopenia and splenomegaly.

The disorder typically runs a chronic course and remission is common with chemotherapy or interferon treatment. Splenectomy is also useful in management.

Myeloproliferative disorders

These are autonomous proliferations of one or more myeloid cells (erythroid, granulocytic, megakaryocytic) with differentiation to mature forms (Fig. 12.20).

Progression from one disorder to another within the group is common.

Classification of myelodysplastic syndromes (MDS)			
Type of MDS	Peripheral blood	Bone marrow	Median survival (months)
Refractory anemia (RA)	Blasts <1%	Blasts <5%	50
RA with ring sideroblasts (RARS)	Blasts <1%	Blasts <5% Ring sideroblasts >15% of total erythroblasts	50
RA with excess blasts (RAEB)	Blasts <5%	Blasts 5–20%	10
RAEB in transformation (RAEB-t)	Blasts >5%	Blasts 20–30% or Auer rods present	5
Chronic myelomonocytic leukemia (CMML)	Blasts <1% Monocytes $>1.0 \times 10^9$/L	Blasts 5–20% Promomonocytes	10

Fig. 12.19 Classification of myelodysplastic syndromes (MDS).

Myeloproliferative disorders and their basic features			
Disorder	Principal proliferations	Bone marrow morphology	Clinical features
Polycythemia rubra vera	Erythroblasts	Increased cellularity, especially erythroid	Erythrocytosis with increased Hb and PCV Often neutrophilia and thrombocytosis Pruritus (related to basophilia) Thrombosis or hemorrhage Splenomegaly
Myelofibrosis	Fibroblasts	Increased deposition of collagen/reticulin; bone marrow difficult to aspirate	Leukoerythroblastic blood picture Anemia with tear-drop poikilocytes Hepatosplenomegaly
Chronic granulocytic leukemia	Myeloblasts	Increased cellularity, especially myeloid	Leukoerythroblastic blood picture Anemia, neutrophilia, basophilia Splenomegaly
Essential thrombocythemia	Megakaryoblasts	Increased megakaryocytes	Thrombocytosis Thrombosis or hemorrhage Occasional splenomegaly

Fig. 12.20 Myeloproliferative disorders and their basic features. (Hb, hemoglobin; PCV, packed cell volume.)

Polycythemia rubra vera This idiopathic condition is characterized by an above normal increase in red cell concentration, usually with concomitant increases in hemoglobin concentration and hematocrit. Red cell mass may be as high as 80mL/kg (normal range: males 25–35mL/kg, and females 22–32mL/kg).

The disorder has a prevalence of 1 per 100,000 in the U.S. and typically it affects the middle-aged, males more so than females.

Progression of this disease is chronic but about 20% of cases evolve into myelofibrosis, and another 5–10% into acute leukemia.

Onset is usually insidious and nonspecific (e.g., malaise, fatigue, headache, and dizziness). The principal symptoms are caused by vascular engorgement, increased hematocrit, and thrombosis, with or without hemorrhage. Splenomegaly is common, and hepatomegaly is occasional.

Treatment is by venesection or myelosuppression with chemotherapy or use of radioactive ^{32}P.

Treated patients have a mean survival of about 13 years.

Note that most cases of polycythemia are not due to polycythemia rubra vera but are secondary to conditions resulting in chronic hypoxia (p. 284). Splenomegaly and pancytosis are not usually features of these conditions.

Myelofibrosis This condition is characterized by a proliferation of fibroblasts in the bone marrow and gross marrow fibrosis, with a corresponding massive extramedullary hemopoiesis in the liver and spleen. It is also known as myelosclerosis.

The condition is a chronic disorder of late and middle age, and it may arise *de novo* (with unknown etiology), or as an end-stage of other myeloproliferative disorders, in which case the reactive fibrosis is thought to be stimulated by factors released from proliferating pathological megakaryocytes.

The disease is usually slowly progressive. However, in about 10% of patients transformation to acute leukemia occurs.

Clinical features are:

- Blood film: typically leukoerythroblastic; erythropoiesis is ineffective leading to anemia with marked anisocytosis and tear-drop poikilocytes.
- Splenomegaly is invariable.
- Hepatomegaly is common.
- Increased bone density due to sclerosis (hence the alternative name).

Symptoms are usually caused by anemia and massive splenomegaly. Systemic symptoms (e.g., fever, weight loss) are usually late features.

Treatment is generally supportive, and with careful management median survival is about 5 years.

Primary (essential/idiopathic) thrombocythemia This condition is characterized by increased platelet production due to a clonal myeloproliferative disorder. It is most commonly seen in patients over 50 years of age. Its features are:

- Large, atypical platelets with increased platelet count, often $>1000 \times 10^9$/L.
- Combined pathological hemorrhages and thromboembolic episodes.
- Iron-deficiency anemia due to chronic blood loss is an occasional feature.
- Spleen may be enlarged but it is usually normal or reduced in size because of thromboembolic infarction.

Treatment with chemotherapy and antiplatelet drugs (e.g., aspirin) is effective and median survival with treatment is 8–10 years.

Proliferation of plasma cells

Myeloma

Multiple myeloma

This diffuse, neoplastic, monoclonal proliferation of plasma cells throughout the red marrow typically affects the elderly, with almost all cases occurring after the age of 40.

Pathogenesis—Proliferating plasma cells produce a monoclonal immunoglobulin or light chain, referred to as the "M component" or paraprotein (NB: The "M" stands for myeloma not IgM).

The M component is usually IgG (>60%) but may be IgA (20%) or immunoglobulin light chain (κ—kappa—being more frequent than λ—lambda).

(IgD and IgE are unusual, and IgM-producing plasma cells are a feature of a different type of plasma cell neoplasm: Waldenström's macroglobulinemia).

The presence of a single type of immunoglobulin is reflected in the electrophoretic pattern which shows normal levels of α- and β-globulins but a dramatic increase in the levels of γ-globulins (Fig. 12.21).

Renal impairment Whole immunoglobulins are too large to pass through the glomerular filter but in two thirds of cases of IgG and IgA myelomas, monoclonal free light chains are also produced, which are small enough to enter the urine, where they are called Bence Jones proteins.

During passage through the tubules, the protein precipitates as "casts," causing damage to the tubular epithelial cells, with concomitant formation of surrounding giant cells—"Bence Jones or myeloma kidney."

Light chains that pass through capillaries are incorporated into amyloid (systemic amyloidosis; p. 259) by mechanisms not yet fully elucidated, causing damage to many organs, including the kidneys.

Raised blood uric acid (from increased cell turnover) worsens renal impairment, as does increased blood calcium from bone osteolysis.

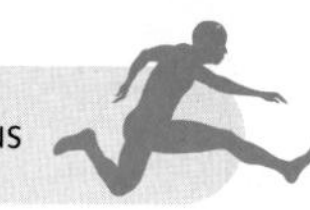

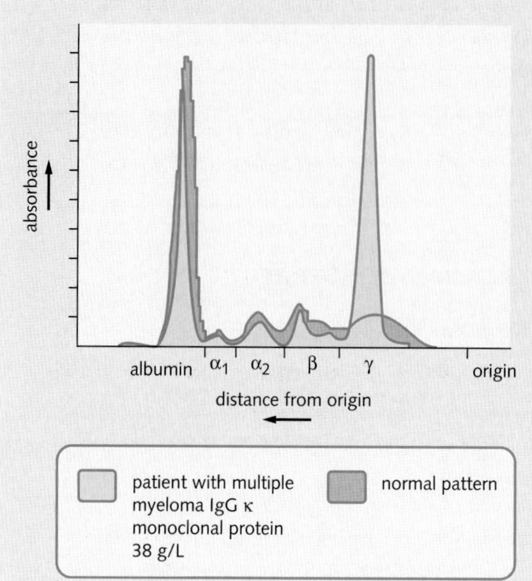

Fig. 12.21 Serum electrophoresis showing characteristic gamma band of multiple myeloma. (Adapted from *Essential Haematology*, 3rd edn, by V. Hoffbrand and J. Pettit, Blackwell Science, 1993.)

Bone changes These are as follows:

- Hypercellular marrow with a large proportion of abnormal plasma cells, especially in the skull, ribs, vertebrae, and pelvis.
- Osteolysis of medullary and cortical bone due to increased numbers of bone-resorbing osteoclasts: thought to be stimulated by activation factors (e.g., interleukins) produced by the malignant plasma cells.
- Osteolytic lesions are seen as "punched out" defects in the bones, the skull showing this appearance particularly well.
- Generalized osteoporosis may result in pathological fractures or vertebral compression.

Hematological findings These are as follows:

- Anemia: usually normochromic, normocytic.
- Marked rouleaux formation (red cells pile together adhering by their rims forming cylinders).
- Raised blood viscosity (depending on the type of immunoglobulin).
- Reduced concentration of unaffected immunoglobulins: "immune paresis."
- Abnormal plasma cells: occasionally seen in peripheral blood.
- Neutropenia and thrombocytopenia: common features in late stages.

Clinical features are:

- Bone pain (especially backache and pathological fractures).
- Features of anemia: lethargy, weakness, dyspnea, pallor, tachycardia.
- Repeated infections: related to deficient antibody production and, in advanced disease, to neutropenia.
- Abnormal bleeding tendency: M component may interfere with platelet function and coagulation factors; thrombocytopenia occurs in advanced disease.
- Features of renal failure and/or hypercalcemia.

Treatment involves chemotherapy and radiotherapy. Median survival is about 2 years with treatment.

Solitary myeloma

This rare disease is characterized by discrete solitary tumors of proliferating monoclonal plasma cells, usually in the bone.

Proliferation does not occur in parts of the skeleton beyond the primary lesion, and marrow aspirates distant from the primary tumor are usually normal.

The associated M component usually disappears following radiotherapy to the primary lesion. However, a minority of cases progress to multiple myeloma.

Disorders of the spleen and thymus

Splenomegaly

The spleen serves as the site of filtration and phagocytosis of the following:

- Effete cells and cell debris, especially red cells.
- Microorganisms.
- Abnormal or excess material derived from metabolic processes.

Splenomegaly (enlargement of the spleen) is a common physical sign, and it may have many causes, the main types of which are summarized in Fig. 12.22.

A palpable spleen is at least twice its normal size, and it is vulnerable to traumatic rupture (e.g., in glandular fever or malaria).

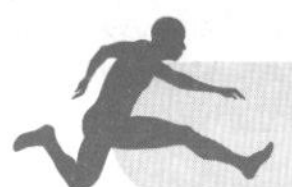

Causes of splenomegaly	
Cause	**Comments**
Infections	Bacterial, e.g., typhoid, tuberculosis, brucellosis, infective endocarditis Viral: infectious mononucleosis Protozoal: malaria, leishmaniasis, trypanosomiasis, toxoplasmosis
Congestion	Due to persistent elevation of splenic venous blood pressure, the cause of which may be: • prehepatic: thrombosis of hepatic, splenic, or portal vein • hepatic: long-standing portal hypertension associated with cirrhosis • posthepatic: raised venous pressure of inferior vena cava, e.g., due to right-sided heart failure, which is transmitted to the spleen via the portal system
Storage diseases	Heritable enzyme deficiencies, which result in storage of material in splenic macrophagic cells, e.g., Gaucher's disease, Niemann–Pick disease, and Tay–Sachs disease
Neoplasia	Primary: rare Secondary: • lymphomas: Hodgkin's disease and non-Hodgkin lymphomas • leukemias: especially chronic leukemias • metastases: splenic metastases from solid tumors, e.g., carcinomas or sarcomas, are rare • extramedullary hemopoiesis, e.g., in myeloproliferative diseases and diseases with diffuse marrow replacement by tumor
Hematological disorders	Hematological anemias, e.g., hereditary spherocytosis, β-thalassemia, autoimmune hemolysis Autoimmune thrombocytopenia: destruction of antibody-coated platelets in spleen results in accumulation of foamy histiocytes in sinuses
Immune disorders	Felty's syndrome: follicular hyperplasia in spleen associated with hypersplenism and rheumatoid disease Sarcoidosis: spleen infiltrated by granulomas Amyloidosis: spleen infiltrated with amyloid

Fig. 12.22 Causes of splenomegaly.

Effect of splenomegaly

Regardless of the cause, enlargement of the spleen may result in the development of hypersplenism, i.e., a decrease in the circulating numbers of erythrocytes, leukocytes, and platelets (pancytopenia), resulting from the destruction or pooling of these cells by the enlarged spleen.

Hypersplenism is often accompanied by a compensatory response—hyperplasia of the bone marrow.

Splenectomy leads to clinical and hematological improvement.

Congestive splenomegaly

This is enlargement of the spleen caused by any condition that leads to a persistent elevation of splenic venous blood pressure. Causes of raised splenic venous pressure are outlined in Fig. 12.23.

A quick review of splenic venous anatomy is helpful in understanding the causes of raised splenic venous pressure (Fig. 12.23).

Morphological features—Sinusoids of the spleen are initially distended with red cells. Fibrosis eventually occurs, and sinusoids then appear ectatic and empty.

The cut surface of the spleen has a purple-red colour with an inconspicuous white pulp, and it is often flecked with firm, brown nodules (called Gamna–Gandy nodules) that represent areas of healed infarction.

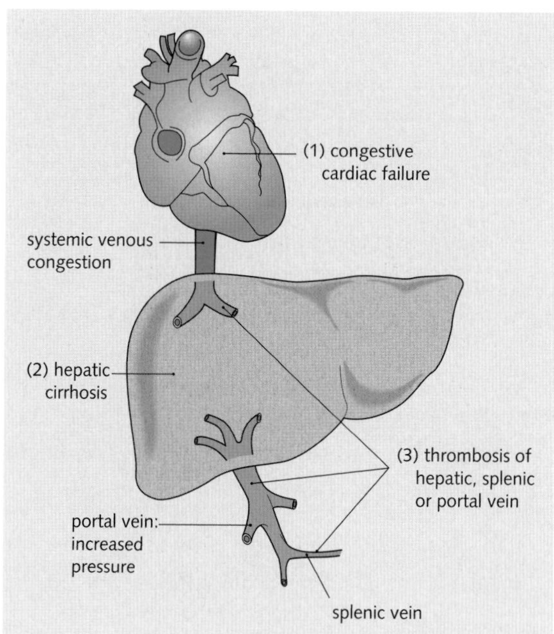

Fig. 12.23 Causes of raised splenic venous pressure.

Foci of extramedullary hemopoiesis are an occasional feature and are thought to be secondary to local hypoxia.

Splenic infarcts

Splenic infarction follows occlusion of the splenic artery or its branches and it may be caused by:

- Emboli that arise in the heart (most common).
- Local thrombosis (e.g., in sickle cell diseases, myeloproliferative disorders, and malignant infiltrates).

Infarcts may be single or multiple and are generally wedge-shaped and pale.

Rupture of the spleen

Rupture of a normal spleen usually occurs following a considerable abdominal trauma, particularly as occurs in some automobile accidents.

Spontaneous rupture of an abnormal enlarged spleen may occur, particularly in infectious mononucleosis, malaria, or splenic hemopoietic proliferations such as myelofibrosis.

A massive intraperitoneal hemorrhage usually follows splenic rupture, necessitating emergency splenectomy.

Disorders of the thymus

The thymus is composed of lymphoid cells and specialized epithelial cells, and it is known as the "primary" lymphoid organ. It is concerned with the development and processing of the long-lived T lymphocytes prior to their distribution to lymphoid tissues and to a circulating pool of T lymphocytes.

Thymic activity is maximal in fetal and childhood stages; regression is rapid after puberty.

Developmental disorders

Thymic hypoplasia and aplasia

These occur due to the developmental failure of either:

- Epithelial tissue—thymus is completely absent or is represented by a fibrous streak (e.g., DiGeorge syndrome (p. 257) and Nezelof's syndrome).
- Lymphoid tissue—severe combined immunodeficiency syndromes, ataxia telangiectasia and reticular dysgenesis.

Both types of developmental disorders result in T cell deficiency associated with a disordered, cell-mediated immune response.

Thymic cysts

These are cysts lined with thymic tissue, and they occur in the neck or anterior mediastinum. Usually congenital, they may be acquired due to degeneration within the thymus gland or within thymic neoplasms.

Thymic hyperplasia

This is a rare condition in which lymphoid follicles (germinal centers) composed of B cells develop in the thymic medulla. It is often accompanied by an increase in the size of the thymus, and it is associated with autoimmune disease, especially myasthenia gravis; in some cases autoantibodies are thought to be produced by the lymphoid tissue.

Thymomas

These rare tumors are derived from thymic epithelial cells, and they may be benign or malignant. Most arise within the thymus, but ectopic thymomas occasionally arise in the soft tissues of the neck, the hilum of the lung, and other sites within the mediastinum or rarely the thyroid.

Histologically, thymomas are composed of uniform epithelial cells variably admixed with reactive lymphoid cells.

They are associated with a variety of disorders including myasthenia gravis and non-organ specific autoimmune diseases.

Benign thymomas

The majority (80–90%) of thymomas are benign, well-circumscribed, encapsulated, lobulated tumors. Most are asymptomatic but some present with local disease caused by the compression of adjacent mediastinal structures:

- Respiratory passages—dyspnea and cough.
- Esophagus—dysphagia.
- Great veins—cyanosis and suffusion of the face.

The remainder present with autoimmune disease. Complete surgical excision is curative.

Malignant thymomas

Around 10–20% of thymomas are malignant and invade the local tissues. There are two types:

- Type 1: histologically indistinguishable from benign thymomas but invade the local tissues (e.g., pericardium, lungs, pleura). Rarely spread outside the thorax.
- Type 2: rare malignant thymomas histologically distinct from benign and from type 1 thymomas (e.g., squamous cell carcinoma, oat cell carcinoma). Poor prognosis.

Disorders of red blood cells

Abnormalities of red cell size and shape

Many hematological and systemic disorders are associated with specific abnormalities of red cell size (anisocytosis) and/or abnormal red cell shape (poikilocytosis).

> It is useful to know the red cell abnormalities associated with specific diseases because they are readily detected microscopically and they are of diagnostic importance.

A diagrammatic representation of some of the variations in red cell size and shape, and the disorders that cause them is shown in Fig. 12.24.

A Anisocytosis

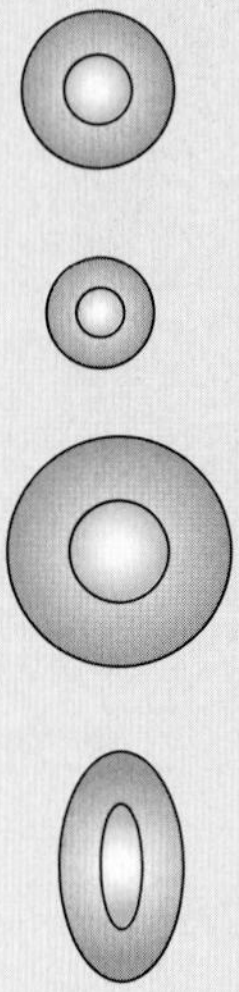

Type	Clinical features
normocyte	
microcyte	• iron deficiency • thalassemia
round macrocyte	• liver disease • alcohol abuse • hypothyroidism
oval macrocyte	• megaloblastic anemia

B Poikilocytosis

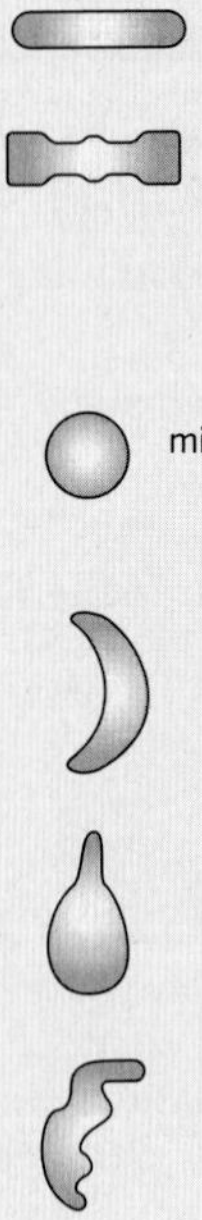

Type	Clinical features
pencil cell	• iron deficiency
target cell	• iron deficiency • megaloblastic anemia • hemoglobinopathy • liver disease • hyposplenism
microspherocyte	• hereditary spherocytosis • immune hemolytic anemia • burns
sickle cells	• homozygous sickle cell disease
tear-drop cell	• myelofibrosis • marrow infiltration
schistocyte	• microangiopathic hemolytic anemia

Fig. 12.24 Diagrammatic representation of (A) abnormalities in red cell size (anisocytosis) and (B) abnormalities in red cell shape (poikilocytosis). (Adapted from Underwood, 2000.)

Anemia

Anemia may be defined as a state in which the blood hemoglobin level is below the normal range for the patient's age and sex. The normal hemoglobin range in males is 12.5–18.0g/dL and in females is 11.5–16.0g/dL. The causes of anemia are shown in Fig. 12.25.

Blood loss

Acute blood loss

Following acute blood loss, a state of cardiovascular collapse may occur, and the shock syndrome is often the predominant feature.

On cessation of hemorrhage, the plasma volume begins to be restored, and anemia becomes apparent.

Causes of anemia	
Cause	**Clinical features**
Increased red cell loss, lysis, or pooling	Blood loss Hemolysis: • intrinsic abnormalities of red cells: hereditary: membrane defects, enzyme defects, hemoglobinopathies acquired: paroxysmal nocturnal hemoglobinuria • extrinsic abnormalities of red cells: antibody-mediated red cell destruction mechanical trauma to red cells Hypersplenism
Impaired red cell production	Deficiency of hematinics: • megaloblastic anemias: lack of B_{12} or folate • iron-deficiency anemia Dyserythropoiesis (production of defective cells): • anemia of chronic disorders • myelodysplasia • sideroblastic anemia Hypoplasia of marrow (failure to produce cells): • aplastic anemia • red cell aplasia Invasion of marrow by malignant cells: • leukemias • myeloproliferative diseases • non-hematological malignancies

Fig. 12.25 Causes of anemia.

The blood picture is:

- Normocytic and normochromic anemia.
- Polychromatic erythrocytes and reticulocytes, reflecting increased hemopoiesis.
- Transient leukocytosis and thrombocytosis.

Plasma proteins and other biochemical constituents are restored rapidly (in 2–3 days). Full red cell restoration may take up to 6 weeks.

Chronic blood loss

Chronic blood loss is the most common cause of iron-deficiency anemia. The main causes of chronic hemorrhage are:

- Diseases of the gastrointestinal tract: particularly peptic ulceration, carcinoma of the stomach, and carcinoma of the colon.
- Menorrhagia.
- Lesions in the urinary tract.

Patients with unexplained iron-deficiency anemia require careful screening for an occult cause of blood loss.

Hemolytic anemias

In all hemolytic anemias, the basic pathological change is a reduction in the lifespan of the red cells due to an increased rate of destruction—hemolysis. The effects of increased hemolysis are:

- Anemia: normocytic with increased reticulocytes in the blood.
- Erythroid hyperplasia of bone marrow.
- Splenomegaly.
- Unconjugated hyperbilirubinemia, which may lead to the development of pigment gall stones, jaundice (kernicterus in neonates).
- Hemoglobinuria: leading to tubular damage in the kidney.

The etiology of hemolytic anemias can be broadly classified into:

- Intrinsic abnormalities of red cells: hereditary defects, acquired defects.
- Extrinsic abnormalities of red cells: antibody-mediated red cell destruction, mechanical trauma to red cells.

Hereditary defects of the red cell

Hereditary defects of the red cell can be classified into:

- Cell membrane defects: hereditary spherocytosis and hereditary elliptocytosis.

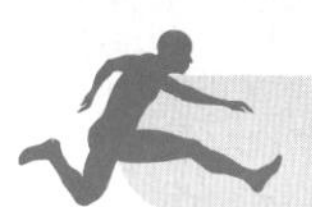

- Enzyme deficiencies: deficiency of glycolytic enzymes or hexose monophosphate shunt enzymes.
- Hemoglobinopathies (e.g., thalassemias and sickle cell disease).

Hereditary spherocytosis and hereditary elliptocytosis

Hereditary spherocytosis is the most common cause of hereditary hemolytic anemia in the U.S. It is an autosomal dominant condition caused by an abnormality of the cytoskeletal-associated membrane protein—spectrin.

The cells are spherical, of reduced deformability, and abnormally fragile.

Reduced deformability of the spherical red cells causes their retention in the splenic microcirculation where they undergo metabolic stress caused by a lack of glucose and acidosis. Increased fragility of metabolically stressed cells causes spontaneous lysis or premature phagocytosis by the splenic macrophages.

Blood film shows:

- Increased microspherocytes, which are more deeply stained with loss of the central pallor of normal erythrocytes.
- Increased polychromatic cells and reticulocytes.

The general clinical features of chronic hemolysis are present. Splenectomy is performed to prevent hemolysis.

Hereditary elliptocytosis is similar to spherocytosis, but the red cells are elliptical. This is caused by abnormalities of the cytoskeletal-associated membrane proteins ankyrin, spectrin, or band 42 protein.

This condition is not as severe as hereditary spherocytosis, and it does not usually cause anemia or jaundice.

Enzyme deficiencies

In erythrocytes, 90% of glucose is metabolized anaerobically to lactate via the Embden–Meyerhof glycolytic pathway (pathway is similar to regular glycolysis except that the end product is lactate not pyruvate); 10% of glucose is used in the hexose monophosphate shunt (also known as the pentose phosphate pathway) to increase the levels of NADPH to those required for the reduction of glutathione. Reduced glutathione is essential for maintaining hemoglobin (Hb) in the reduced (ferrous) state (Fig. 12.26).

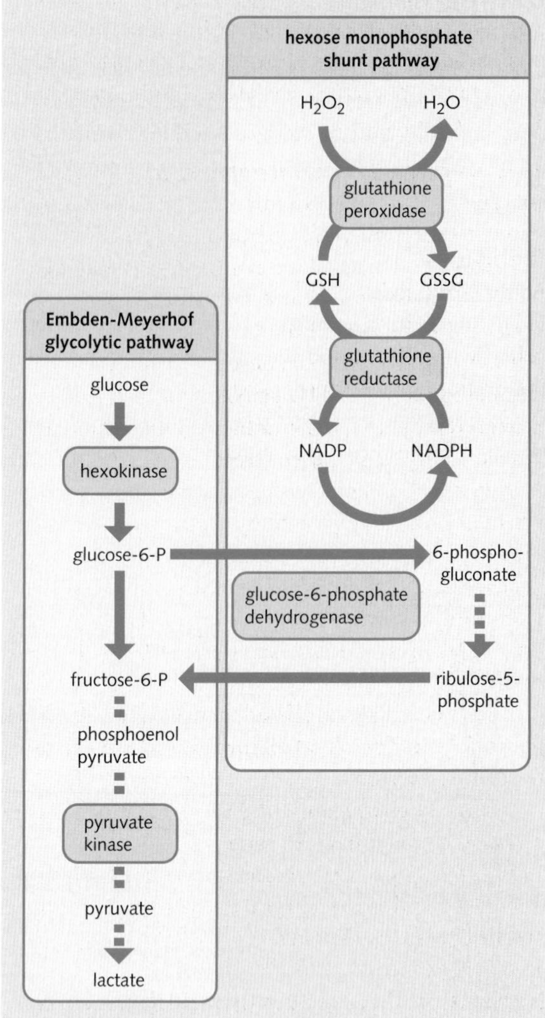

Fig. 12.26 Metabolic pathways of the red cell. (H_2O_2, hydrogen peroxide; GSH, GSSG, reduced and oxidized glutathione; NADP, NADPH, oxidized and reduced nicotinamide-adenine-dinucleotide phosphate; glucose-6-P, glucose-6-phosphate; fructose-6-P, fructose-6-phosphate).

Deficiencies of glycolytic enzymes Pyruvate kinase deficiency is a rare, autosomal recessive defect which results in congenital chronic hemolytic anemia. Red cells become rigid due to reduced ATP formation, and they are removed by the spleen.

Anemia is generally mild, but blood film shows raised poikilocytosis and distorted "prickle cells."

Clinically, jaundice is usual and gallstones are frequent.

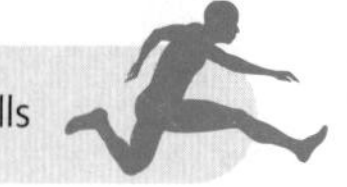

Many other enzymopathies of glycolytic enzymes exist but they are extremely rar (e.g., deficiencies of hexokinase, glucose phosphate isomerase, and phosphofructokinase). The effects are similar to pyruvate kinase deficiency.

Deficiencies of hexose monophosphate shunt enzymes The most common deficiencies are glucose-6-phosphate dehydrogenase (G6PD) deficiency and glutathione synthetase deficiency.

G6PD deficiency is an X-linked recessive condition especially common among people of African or Mediterranean descent. It results in a decreased ratio of NADPH/NADP, which leads to impaired reduction of glutathione, and an increased susceptibility to oxidative stress.

Spontaneous anemia is rare but hemolytic crises are frequently precipitated by infections, ingestion of fava (broad) beans, or the administration of certain drugs (quinine, phenacetin, aspirin).

Blood film during hemolytic crises shows raised poikilocytosis with bite-shaped defects ("bite" cells) or surface blebs ("blister" cells), and Heinz bodies (red cells containing oxidized, denatured hemoglobin). The blood picture is normal between hemolytic episodes.

Female heterozygotes have the advantage of being resistant to Falciparum malaria.

A deficiency of glutathione synthetase leads to defective synthesis of glutathione causing a similar syndrome to G6PD deficiency.

Hemoglobin abnormalities (hemoglobinopathies)

Hemoglobinopathies are caused by either:

- Decreased α- or β-globin synthesis: the α- and β-thalassemias.
- Synthesis of abnormal hemoglobin (e.g., sickle cell disease, unstable hemoglobins).

Anemias resulting from hemoglobinopathies are usually a combined result of both dyshemopoiesis and hemolysis.

Thalassemias Normal adult hemoglobin (HbA) is composed of two α-globin chains and two β-globin chains ($\alpha_2\beta_2$). In thalassemia, one or more of the genes responsible for synthesis of α- or β-globin chains is abnormal, resulting in α- or β-thalassemia, depending on which chain is affected.

The disease is inherited, and it is common in the Mediterranean, the Middle and Far East, and South-East Asia, where carrier rates of 10–15% are found.

α-Thalassemia—Mainly caused by deletion (rather than mutation) of parts of the α-globin genes. Normal individuals have four copies of the α-globin gene, two copies on each chromosome 16. There are, therefore, four possible degrees of α-thalassemia, depending on how many genes are abnormal (Fig. 12.27).

Hemolysis is less severe in α-thalassemia than in β-thalassemia.

β-thalassemia—Caused by a mutation of the β-globin gene(s) leading to either reduced (β^+) or absent (β^0) synthesis of the β-globin chain. Normal individuals have two copies of each β-globin gene (one on each chromosome 11). There are, therefore, two possible degrees of β-thalassemia:

- Thalassemia minor: heterozygous trait associated with mild anemia.
- Thalassemia major: homozygous syndrome associated with severe hemolytic anemia.

Sickle-cell disease This is caused by an abnormal form of hemoglobin, HbS ($a_2\beta S_2$), caused by a point mutation (resulting in the substitution of valine for glutamate) in the gene coding for the β-globin chain.

The disease is common in west and central Africa, the Mediterranean, and the Middle East. Carriage of the gene may confer some protection against falciparum malaria.

HbS polymerizes at low oxygen saturations, causing an abnormal rigidity and deformity of red cells, which assume a sickle shape (Fig. 12.28). As a result, deoxygenated red cells undergo aggregation (causing vascular occlusion of small vessels) and hemolysis (due to increased fragility).

Heterozygous vs. homozygous state Heterozygous condition—Sickle cell trait in which only 30% of the hemoglobin is HbS, resulting in no significant clinical abnormality.

Homozygous condition—Sickle cell disease in which more than 80% of the hemoglobin is HbS, the rest being HbF and HbA. It is associated with serious clinicopathological features.

Fig. 12.29 shows a table with the pathogenesis and clinical features of sickle-cell disease.

"Crises" of sickle-cell disease In addition to the effects of aggregation and hemolysis, sickle-cell disease is characterized by various "crises" that occur after the age of 1 or 2 years, when HbF levels have fallen and the proportion of HbS has increased. These are of three main patterns:

Thalassemia disorders

Type of thalassemia		**Globin chains present**	**Clinicopathological features**
β-thalassemia	Thalassemia minor	Heterozygous $\beta^0\beta$ Heterozygous $\beta^+\beta$	Moderate reduction in HbA Compensatory increase in HbA_2 ($\alpha_2\delta_2$) Mild anemia with hypochromic cells
	Thalassemia major	Homozygous $\beta^0\beta^0$ Homozygous $\beta^+\beta^+$ or occasionally $\beta^+\beta^0$	Hypochromic microcytic anemia Severe hemolysis with hepatosplenomegaly Marrow hyperplasia causing skeletal deformities Iron overload from repeated transfusions
α-thalassemia	Silent carrier	-α/αα	Asymptomatic with normal hematology or slightly reduced MCV
	α-thalassemia trait	--/ααor α-/α-	Asymptomatic but mild hemolytic anemia with some microcytic cells
	Hemoglobin H disease	--/α-	Excess β-chains form tetramers: HbH Moderate hemolytic anemia with hypochromia and microcytosis Splenomegaly
	Hydrops fetalis	--/--	Death *in utero*

Fig. 12.27 Summary of the thalassemia disorders.

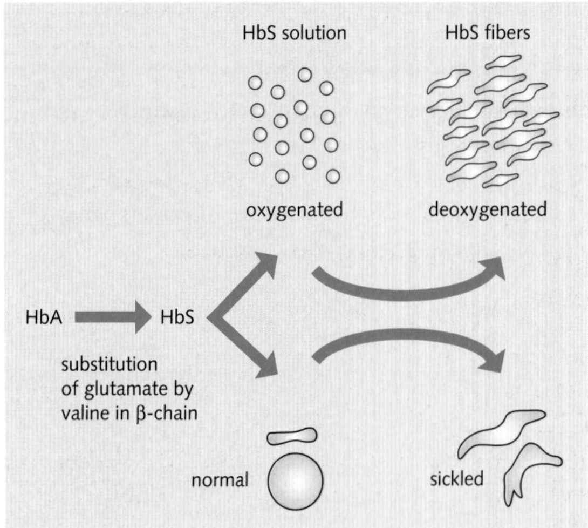

Fig. 12.28 Aggregation of sickle-cell hemoglobin in conditions of low oxygen.

Pathogenesis and clinical features of sickle-cell disease

Pathogenesis	**Clinical features**
Vascular occlusion	Cerebral infarction Retinopathy → blindness Pulmonary infarction → acute respiratory distress Cor pulmonale Hematuria and polyuria Splenic atrophy → hyposplenism → infections Bone necrosis → osteomyelitis Leg ulcers
Chronic hemolysis	Anemia Jaundice and gallstones Hemochromatosis (due to iron overload in transfused patients)

Fig. 12.29 Pathogenesis and clinical features of sickle-cell disease.

- Sequestration crises: sudden pooling of red cells in the spleen may develop in the early years of the disease causing a rapid fall in hemoglobin concentration, which can lead to death.
- Infarctive crises: due to obstruction of the small blood vessels. Commonly affected tissues are bone (especially femoral head), the spleen (leading to splenic atrophy), and skin (leg ulcers).
- Aplastic crises: splenic infarction predisposes to infection leading to depression of red cell production and exacerbation of pre-existing anemia.

ABO blood group system			
Genotype	Phenotype	Antibodies	Frequency of phenotype in U.S.
OO	O	Anti-A, -B	Most common
AA or AO	A	Anti-B	Common
BB or BO	B	Anti-A	Rare
AB	AB	None	Most rare

Fig. 12.30 ABO blood group system.

Treatment is by the avoidance of factors known to precipitate crises, especially hypoxia. Blood transfusions are necessary during crises.

Mean survival figures are variable reflecting differing standards of medical care. However, death in infancy or childhood is usual in underdeveloped countries.

Unstable hemoglobins Hereditary abnormalities in globin chains result in the decreased stability of the hemoglobin molecule with hemolytic anemia of variable severity. Examples are hemoglobins Köln and Zurich.

Acquired defects of the red cell

Paroxysmal nocturnal hemoglobinuria

This rare disorder of young adults is caused by a clonal abnormality of erythrocytes, which renders them abnormally sensitive to lysis by complement. The cells lack the enzyme required for the synthesis of phosphatidyl inositol, which usually anchors several proteins to the red cell membrane. This may arise *de novo* or follow an episode of aplastic anemia. Venous thrombosis is a frequent complication.

Hemosiderinuria is conspicuous in all cases. However, nocturnal hemolysis with or without hemoglobinuria is present in only about 25% of cases.

Antibody-mediated red cell destruction

Isoimmune

Incompatible ABO blood transfusion This classic example of red cell hemolysis is caused by iso-antibodies (Fig. 12.30).

For example, if donor blood is group A (i.e. cells contain A antigen) and recipient blood is group O (cells do not possess A or B antigens but plasma contains both anti-A and anti-B antibodies), then anti-A antibodies of the recipient will cause agglutination and hemolysis of donor red blood cells.

Clinical and pathological effects:

- Massive intravascular hemolysis leading to collapse, hypotension, and pain in the lumbar region.
- Hemoglobinuria is common, and renal failure may ensue.
- Disseminated intravascular coagulation may be triggered by red cell lysis.

The effects may be precipitated with only a few milliliters of incompatible red cells.

Transfusion-induced hemolysis due to incompatibility of the rhesus system is generally milder, since antibodies to the rhesus system are not complement fixing.

Hemolytic disease of the newborn (HDN) This hemolysis of red blood cells in rhesus (Rh)-positive fetuses is caused by the placental passage of maternal anti-rhesus IgG antibodies from rhesus-negative mothers. It is particularly associated with D antigen of the rhesus blood group.

The pathogenesis is as follows:

- First pregnancy: Rh-positive fetus in Rh-negative mother with no antibodies—healthy baby. However, if fetal red blood cells enter maternal circulation during breach of placental barrier (e.g., at birth or miscarriage), then isoimmunization of mother will occur.
- Subsequent pregnancies: anti-Rh antibodies acquired by mother during previous pregnancy cause HDN in Rh-positive fetuses.

HDN is categorized into three groups according to severity.

1. Congenital hemolytic anemia: mild anemia and jaundice, usually self-limiting.
2. Icterus gravis neonatorum: rapidly developing severe anemia and jaundice. May result in brain damage due to kernicterus, hepatosplenomegaly due to extramedullary hemopoiesis, or death from severe anoxia.
3. Hydrops fetalis: death *in utero* associated with severe anoxia and cardiac failure.

The incidence of HDN has been reduced by the prophylactic removal of fetal cells entering the maternal circulation by the injection of anti-D before isoimmunization can occur.

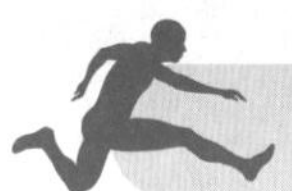

Autoimmune hemolytic anemia

This is the most common type of hemolytic anemia, caused by the immune destruction of red blood cells by the host's own antibodies. It may be idiopathic, secondary to other diseases, or drug related.

It is divided into two main groups according to the temperature at which hemolytic reactions occur.

"Warm" antibody type

Autoantibody is IgG and most reactive at 37°C, leading to chronic anemia with microspherocytes. Red cell destruction occurs in the spleen.

Clinical features are those of hemolytic anemia: pallor, jaundice, and splenomegaly (Fig. 12.31).

"Cold" antibody type

Autoantibody is IgM and is most reactive at 4°C, but it can still bind complement and agglutinate red cells at 30°C, the temperature of peripheral tissues (hands, feet, nose, and ears). There is destruction of red cells by Kupffer's cells of the liver.

Clinical features are of anemia and of blueness and coldness of the fingers, toes, nose, and ears, occasionally progressing to ischemia and ulceration. Disorder is chronic and usually mild (Fig. 12.32).

Fig. 12.33 is a summary of antibody-mediated hemolytic anemias.

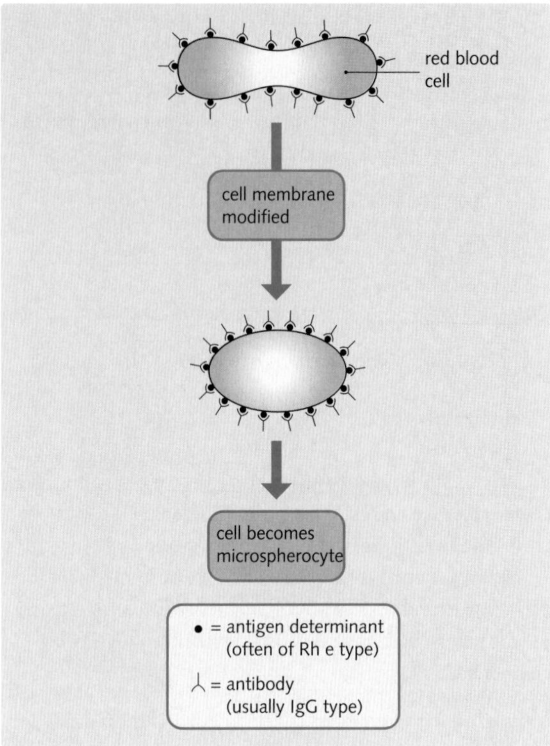

Fig. 12.31 "Warm" antibody type hemolysis. The red cell membrane is modified, and becomes a microspherocyte with consequences similar to hereditary spherocytosis: early sequestration in the spleen, etc. (Adapted from *Pathology Illustrated*, 4th edn, by A. Govan, P. Macfarlane, and R. Callander, Churchill Livingstone, 1995.)

Mechanical trauma to red cells

Mechanical damage to red cells may lead to reduced lifespan and hemolysis.

There are several groups of mechanical hemolysis, as described below.

Microangiopathic hemolytic anemia

Hemolysis is caused by physical trauma to erythrocytes as they are forced through narrow areas in the vasculature. It is commonly present in:

- Disseminated intravascular coagulation: red blood cells are damaged on fibrin strands deposited in the small blood vessels.
- Hemolytic uremic syndrome.
- Thrombotic thrombocytopenic purpura (TTP).

Blood film shows the presence of schistocytes, helmet cells, and crenated cells.

Macroangiopathic hemolytic anemia

This is caused by physical trauma to erythrocytes as they are forced through prosthetic heart valves. Blood film is as above.

Splenic sequestration

Splenic sequestration of red cells causes their premature hemolysis resulting in hypersplenism (p. 272).

Malaria

Hemolysis is common in malaria; *Plasmodium* spp. enter the erythrocytes where they multiply and mature to form schizonts, which eventually escape by rupturing the erythrocytes. Extreme splenomegaly is often present.

Chemical

Snake bites, spider bites, scorpion stings, and chemicals are occasionally causes of hemolysis.

Hypersplenism

There is a decrease in the numbers of circulating erythrocytes, leukocytes, and platelets (pancytopenia) as a direct result of their destruction or pooling by an enlarged spleen (p. 272).

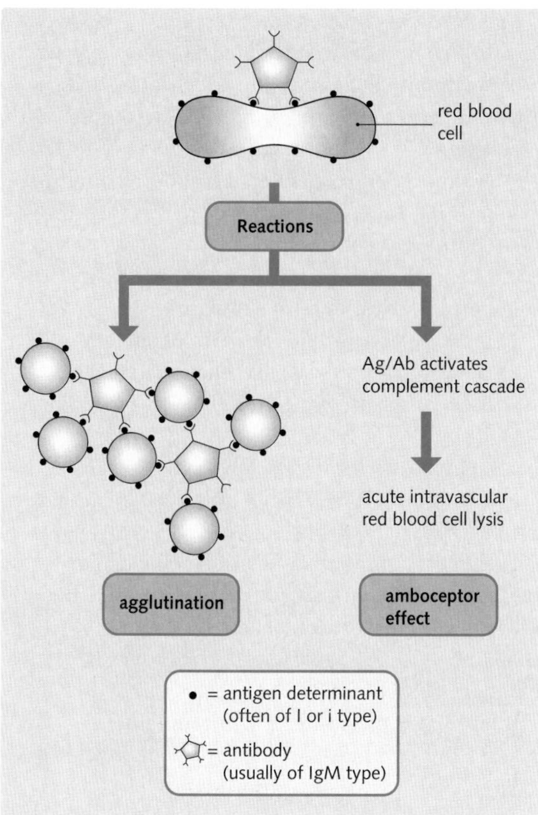

Fig. 12.32 "Cold" antibody type hemolysis. The antibody combines with red blood cells resulting in agglutination (clinically presenting as painful hands and feet) or the amboceptor effect (clinically presenting as paroxysmal cold hemoglobinuria—hemoglobinemia and hemoglobinuria). (Adapted from *Pathology Illustrated*, 4th edn, by A. Govan, P. Macfarlane, and R. Callander, Churchill Livingstone, 1995.)

Hematinic deficiency

There is a deficiency of those dietary factors required for either hemoglobin synthesis or erythrocyte production.

Megaloblastic anemia

This type of anemia is the result of impaired DNA synthesis in marrow precursor cells, and it is caused by a deficiency of vitamin B_{12} or folic acid (folate).

In the marrow, lack of B_{12} or folate causes the development of abnormally large red cell precursors (megaloblasts), which develop into abnormally large red cells (macrocytes).

Bone marrow becomes hypercellular with megaloblasts— macrocytic anemia, neutropenia, and thrombocytopenia. Defective cells are prematurely destroyed—hemolytic anemia.

Note that the effects of B_{12} and folate deficiency occur in most organs of the body, but they are prominent where cell turnover is rapid, e.g., in the marrow and mucous membranes of the alimentary tract and genitalia.

Vitamin B_{12} (cobalamin)

The source is animal products (e.g., meat and eggs).

Requirements are 1 μg per day but up to several years' supply are stored in the liver.

Absorption—Vitamin B_{12} is normally absorbed from the diet by binding to intrinsic factor (IF), which is secreted by gastric parietal cells. The B_{12}–IF complex binds to cells in the terminal ileum, where B_{12} is absorbed. The causes of vitamin B_{12} deficiency are as follows:

Summary of antibody-mediated hemolytic anemias

Isoimmune	Autoimmune	
	"Warm" antibody type (autoantibody is IgG class)	"Cold" antibody type (autoantibody is IgM class)
Transfusion reactions Hemolytic disease of the newborn	Idiopathic (50%) Secondary: • chronic lymphatic leukemia • lymphoma related • systemic lupus erythematosus and other autoimmune disorders • viral infections • drug related, e.g., methyl-dopa, penicillin, quinidine	Idiopathic Secondary: • lymphoma related • infectious mononucleosis • mycoplasma pneumonia

Fig. 12.33 Summary of antibody-mediated hemolytic anemias.

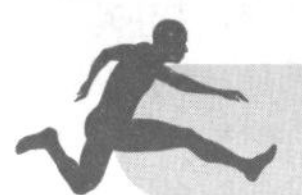

- Pernicious anemia: most common cause of B_{12} deficiency, and in females more than males. Caused by autoimmune atrophic gastritis resulting in lack of production of IF and malabsorption of B_{12}. Corrected by injections of vitamin B_{12}.
- Congenital: lack of IF.
- Surgical gastrectomy: results in loss of IF.
- Surgical removal of the terminal ileum: loss of B_{12} absorption site.
- Disease of terminal ileum (e.g., Crohn's disease): loss of B_{12} absorption site.
- Bacterial overgrowth: compete for B_{12}.
- Malnutrition: rare but occasionally seen in veganism.

The effects of vitamin B_{12} deficiency are as follows:

- Megaloblastic anemia, with associated neutropenia and thrombocytopenia.
- Lesions of the nervous system: myelin degeneration of posterior and lateral columns of spinal cord—subacute combined degeneration of the cord (see Chapter 14).
- Malabsorption: due to mucosal changes—weight loss.

Treatment is by correction of the underlying cause (if possible), and/or injections of vitamin B_{12}.

Folic acid

Sources are vegetables, cereals, meat, and eggs.

Requirements are up to 200μg per day and only 50–100 days' supply is stored in the liver.

- Absorption—Folic acid is normally absorbed from the diet in the jejunum. The causes of folate deficiency are as follows:
  - Malnutrition (e.g., from anorexia, alcoholism, poverty, overcooking of food). This is the most common cause of deficiency.
  - Malabsorption (e.g., celiac disease, dermatitis herpetiformis, Crohn's disease).
  - Increased requirements (e.g., pregnancy and lactation, hemolysis, malignancy, extensive psoriasis or dermatitis).

Drugs may cause malabsorption (e.g., anticonvulsants) or may block utilization (e.g., methotrexate).

The effects of folate deficiency—Blood and bone marrow changes are identical to those in B_{12} deficiency. However, deficiency of folate is not associated with the neurological features of B_{12} deficiency (Fig. 12.34).

Treatment is by oral folic acid supplements, resulting in a complete reversal of the pathological features, even in malabsorption states.

Iron-deficiency anemia

Iron deficiency is the most common cause of anemia.

Iron is abundant in meat, vegetables, eggs, and dairy foods.

Comparison of vitamin B_{12} and folate deficiency

	Vitamin B_{12} deficiency	Folate deficiency
Source	Animal produce	Most foods
Requirements	1μg/day (heat stable, body stores = several years)	Minimally 50μg/day (heat labile, body stores = months)
Nutritional deficiency	Uncommon (only in vegans)	Common
Time of onset	Slow (years)	Over several weeks
Area of absorption	Absorbed in terminal ileum and requires intrinsic factor	Absorbed in jejunum (and duodenum)
Disease causing deficiency	Gastric or terminal ileal disease may cause deficiency	Jejunal disease may cause deficiency
Drug involvement	No	May be drug related (anticonvulsants or antimetabolites)
Neurological involvement	Neurological lesions frequent	No

Fig. 12.34 Comparison of vitamin B_{12} and folate deficiency.

Requirements are:
- In men and postmenopausal women: 1 mg per day.
- In menstruating women: 2mg per day.
- In pregnancy: 3mg per day.
- In children: 1.5mg per day.

Absorption is via the duodenum and upper jejunum in the ferrous (Fe^{2+}) form.

The causes of iron deficiency are:
- Chronic blood loss: most common cause (e.g., diseases of the GI tract, menorrhagia, lesions of the urinary tract).
- Increased requirements (e.g., in childhood and pregnancy).
- Malabsorption due to gastrectomy, celiac disease.
- Malnutrition.

The effects of iron deficiency in blood film are:
- Hypochromic microcytic erythrocytes.
- Low numbers of reticulocytes for the degree of anemia.
- Poikilocytosis (especially "pencil" cells).
- Anisocytosis.

Laboratory findings are as follows: reduced total serum iron, reduced serum ferritin, and reduced transferrin saturation, but with a greatly increased total iron binding capacity.

Clinical features are:
- Anemia: lethargy, dyspnea, headache, palpitations.
- Angular cheilitis: fissures at angles of mouth.
- Atrophic glossitis (smooth tongue).
- Esophageal webs.
- Hypochlorhydria.
- Koilonychia (spoon nails).
- Brittle nails.
- Pica (indiscriminate eating of non-nutritious substances such as grass, stones, or clothing).

Treatment is of the underlying cause and iron supplements.

Dyserythropoiesis

This group of disorders is characterized by the production of defective red cells. The pathogenesis of associated dyserythropoiesis is poorly understood.

Anemia of chronic disease

Chronic disorders are a common cause of anemia, being second only to iron-deficiency.

It may develop in patients with:
- Non-organ specific autoimmune diseases (e.g., rheumatoid disease and SLE).
- Chronic infective diseases (e.g., tuberculosis, malaria, and schistosomiasis).
- Neoplasia: lymphoma and some carcinomas.

Blood film—Mainly normocytic and normochromic but a mild degree of microcytic, hypochromic anemia.

Laboratory findings are a reduced serum iron and reduced serum iron-binding capacity, with an increased or normal serum ferritin (cf. iron-deficiency anemia).

The disorder may be due to the failure of macrophages to transfer their iron stores to the bone marrow. Circulating red cells have a reduced life-span, and the marrow shows a lack of response to erythropoietin.

Myelodysplasia

This acquired neoplastic disorder is caused by a defect of the stem cells, and it is characterized by progressive bone marrow failure with quantitative and qualitative abnormalities of all three myeloid cell lines (red cell, granulocyte/monocyte, and platelets) (p. 268).

Sideroblastic anemia

This anemia caused by defective heme synthesis results in the accumulation of excess iron in the cytoplasm of the red blood cell progenitors in the form of hemosiderin, forming cells termed ring sideroblasts.

There are two groups of the disease:
- Primary sideroblastic anemia: myelodysplastic syndrome.
- Secondary sideroblastic anemia: drug-, toxin-, and neoplasia-related.

Hypoplasia

This anemia is due to the failure of red cell production by the bone marrow.

Aplastic anemia

A severe life-threatening disease caused by failing bone marrow stem cells, this is characterized by pancytopenia. The marrow is hypocellular, and it is replaced by fat.

It may be idiopathic or secondary to:
- Radiation.
- Antineoplastic chemotherapy.

- Drugs: chloramphenicol, gold, NSAIDs.
- Toxins: benzene.
- Viruses: papovavirus, HIV-1.
- Fanconi's anemia.

Red cell aplasia

This anemia is caused by the suppression of red cell progenitor cells. In contrast to aplastic anemia, other blood cells are not affected. There are three main types:

- Self-limited red cell aplasia: occurs after parvovirus infection or exposure to certain toxins.
- Chronic acquired red cell aplasia: autoimmune and it may be associated with thymomas (p. 274).
- Chronic constitutional red cell aplasia: due to a hereditary defect in progenitor cells.

Marrow infiltration (myelopthisic anemia)

Extensive infiltration of the bone marrow may cause the obliteration of normal hemopoietic elements. It is caused by:

- Leukemias.
- Myelofibrosis.
- Disseminated carcinomas.
- Disseminated lymphomas.

Patients develop leukoerythroblastic anemia characterized by circulating erythroblasts and primitive white cells. Extramedullary hemopoiesis commonly develops.

Polycythemia

Polycythemia (erythrocytosis) is defined as a sustained increase in red cell numbers, usually with a corresponding increase in hemoglobin concentration and hematocrit.

Relative polycythemia

This occurs when the hematocrit reading is raised due to a decrease in plasma volume, usually as a result of fluid loss. This is not "true" polycythemia.

Absolute polycythemia

Primary

Primary polycythemia occurs in a rare condition termed polycythemia rubra vera, which is one of the myeloproliferative disorders (p. 268).

Secondary

Most cases of polycythemia are secondary to conditions resulting in:

- Chronic hypoxia (common)—"appropriate" polycythemia (e.g., high altitude, cyanotic heart disease, respiratory disease (such as chronic bronchitis, emphysema), smoking, hemoglobinopathy (resulting in defective release of O_2 to tissues)).
- Renal tumors and ischemia (rare)—"inappropriate" polycythemia (e.g., renal carcinomas or cysts, renal artery stenosis).

Both chronic hypoxia and renal tumors/ischemia result in increased erythropoietin production, which stimulates the bone marrow production of red cells.

See Fig. 12.35 for a comparison table of the main features of primary and secondary polycythemia.

Disorders of hemostasis

Definitions

Purpura

This skin rash results from bleeding into the skin from capillaries. It is caused either by defects in

Comparison of main features of primary and secondary polycythemia

	Primary	Secondary
Prevalence	Rare	Common
Cause	Unknown	Hypoxia Renal tumors/ischemia
Erythropoietin	Normal or decreased	Increased
Blood film	↑ RBGs (may be hypochromic) ↑ leukocytes ↑ megakaryocytes	↑ RBCs (normochromic)
Splenomegaly	Common	None

Fig. 12.35 Comparison of the main features of primary and secondary polycythemia. (RBCs, red blood cells.)

capillaries or by defects or deficiencies of blood platelets. Individual small purple spots of the rash are called petechiae.

Ecchymosis

This bruise presents as a bluish-black mark on the skin resulting from the release of blood into the tissues either through injury or through the spontaneous leaking of blood from the vessels.

Hematoma

This accumulation of blood within the tissues clots to form a solid swelling.

Abnormalities of the vessel walls

This heterogeneous group of conditions is characterized by easy bruising and spontaneous bleeding from small vessels. The underlying lesions are of two main types:

- Abnormal perivascular connective tissue which leads to inadequate vessel support.
- Intrinsically abnormal or damaged vessel wall.

Hemorrhages are mainly in the skin, causing petechiae, ecchymoses, or both. In some disorders there is also bleeding from the mucous membranes.

Infections

Some bacterial and viral infections cause purpura as a result of either vascular damage by the organism or through immune complex formation (e.g,. measles, dengue fever, or meningococcal septicemia).

Drug reactions

A variety of drugs may sometimes cause vasculitic reactions.

Scurvy and Ehlers–Danlos syndrome

Vitamin C is required for the hydroxylation of proline as a step in collagen synthesis. In both Ehlers–Danlos syndrome (an inherited disorder of collagen synthesis) and scurvy (vitamin C deficiency) capillaries are fragile because of defective collagen synthesis.

Perifollicular petechiae, bruising, and mucosal hemorrhages are common.

Steroid purpura

Long-term steroid therapy or Cushing's syndrome results in purpura caused by defective vascular supportive tissue.

Henoch–Schönlein purpura

This immune complex (type III) hypersensitivity reaction is usually found in children, and it often follows an acute infection. It is characterized by red wheals and a purple rash on the buttocks and lower legs due to bleeding into the skin from inflamed capillaries and venules.

Arthritis, hematuria, and GI symptoms may also occur.

It is a self-limiting condition, but occasionally patients develop renal failure.

Osler–Weber–Rendu syndrome (hereditary hemorrhagic telangiectasia)

This rare, autosomal dominant disorder is characterized by multiple dilatations of small vessels (telangiectasia) that appear during childhood and become more numerous in adult life.

Telangiectasia develops in the skin, mucous membranes, and internal organs and frequently bleeds spontaneously or following relatively mild trauma. Recurrent GI tract hemorrhages and epistaxis may cause chronic iron-deficiency anemia.

Disordered platelet function

Reduced platelet count (thrombocytopenia)

Decreased production

This is the most common cause of thrombocytopenia (normal platelet count 150–400 × 10^9/L).

Generalized disease of bone marrow Aplastic anemia—This severe, life-threatening disease is caused by failing bone marrow stem cells and characterized by pancytopenia. The marrow is hypocellular and is replaced by fat.

Marrow infiltration—Extensive infiltration of bone marrow may cause the obliteration of normal hemopoietic elements.

Specific impairment of platelet production
Selective megakaryocyte depression may result from either drug toxicity (alcohol, cytotoxics) or viral infections (measles, HIV).

Ineffective megakaryopoiesis

- Megaloblastic anemia (folate or B_{12} deficiency) is characterized by decreased numbers of platelets or increased numbers of megakaryocytes.
- Paroxysmal nocturnal hemoglobinuria: may cause ineffective megakaryopoiesis.

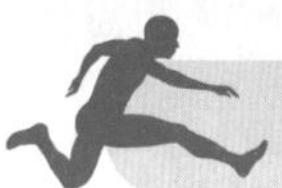

Decreased platelet survival

Immune destruction—autoimmune thrombocytopenic purpura The destruction of antibody-coated platelets by the reticuloendothelial system, especially the spleen, results in spontaneous or post-traumatic hemorrhage at various sites:

- Skin: petechiae and ecchymoses.
- Mucous membranes (e.g., epistaxis, bleeding gums, menorrhagia, hematuria, melena).
- CNS: may be fatal.

This is often associated with anemia (secondary to hemorrhage).

Clinical types are:

- Acute: often in children and usually self-limiting with spontaneous resolution. May be post-infective (e.g., measles).
- Chronic: usually in adults, mainly idiopathic but occasionally symptomatic of CLL or lymphoma, or it may occur in association with other autoimmune disease (e.g., rheumatoid arthritis, SLE).
- Drug induced (e.g., quinine, heparin, sulfonamides).

Nonimmune destruction This is mainly through thrombotic thrombocytopenic purpura (TTP) and hemolytic-uremic syndrome (HUS).

HUS and TTP are thought to represent the same disease process but with different distributions of thrombotic lesions.

Thrombocytopenia occurs due to abnormal platelet activation and consumption. Platelets adhere to the endothelium of capillaries and precapillary arterioles where they undergo aggregation and release, with fibrin deposition, which results in microvascular occlusive platelet plugs and microangiopathic hemolytic anemia (p. 280).

Etiology—The underlying cause of the disorder is obscure but the following pathogenetic factors have been implicated:

- Immune-mediated vessel damage.
- Platelet hyperaggregation due to deficiency of an IgG inhibitor of platelet-agglutinating factor in normal plasma.
- Diminished production of prostaglandin by vessel walls.
- Excess of high-molecular-weight multimers of von Willebrand's factor, which interact with platelet agglutinating factor, causing platelet adhesion to vascular endothelium.

In TTP, occlusive plugs lead to widespread ischemic organ damage, especially of the brain and kidney, resulting in neurological abnormalities and progressive renal impairment. In HUS, organ damage is limited to the kidney.

Disseminated intravascular coagulation can also cause widespread consumption of platelets results in simultaneous thrombosis and hemorrhage (p. 289).

Splenic sequestration

Thrombocytopenia is common in splenomegaly due to platelet "pooling" by the spleen. Unlike red cells, platelets tolerate splenic stasis without injury and so platelet lifespan is unaffected.

Dilutional thrombocytopenia

Platelets are unstable at 4°C and so transfusion with massive amounts of stored blood may cause abnormal bleeding. The effect can be minimized by replacement with specific screened products (e.g., fresh frozen plasma and platelet concentrates).

See Fig. 12.36 for a summary of the causes of thrombocytopenia.

Causes of thrombocytopenia

Cause	Clinical features
Decreased platelet production	Generalized disease of bone marrow: • aplastic anemia, marrow infiltration Specific impairment of platelet production: • drugs: alcohol, thiazides, cytotoxics • infections: measles, HIV Ineffective megakaryopoiesis: • megaloblastic anemia and paroxysmal nocturnal hemoglobinuria
Decreased platelet survival	Immune destruction: • autoimmune thrombocytopenic purpura Non-immune destruction: • thrombotic thrombocytopenic purpura/hemolytic–uremic syndrome • disseminated intravascular coagulation
Splenic sequestration	—
Dilutional thrombocytopenia	—

Fig. 12.36 Causes of thrombocytopenia.

Defects of platelet function

Congenital

Defective adhesion (Bernard–Soulier syndrome)

This rare disease causes life-threatening hemorrhages. The platelets are deficient in glycoprotein receptors (glycoprotein Ib/IX), which are essential for the binding of von Willebrand's factor. The platelets are larger than normal, and there is defective adherence to exposed subendothelial connective tissues and defective platelet aggregation. There is also a variable degree of thrombocytopenia.

Defective aggregation—thromboesthenia (Glanzmann's disease)

This failure of primary platelet aggregation is due to a deficiency of membrane receptors (glycoproteins IIb and IIIa) for fibrinogen binding.

Defective secretion (storage pool disease)

A common, mild defect of platelet function, this causes easy bruising and bleeding after trauma. It is caused by a deficiency of "dense granules" within the platelets, which normally store ADP. The decreased storage pool of ADP prevents the secondary wave of platelet aggregation.

Acquired

Aspirin

Aspirin therapy is the most common cause of defective platelet function, and it produces an abnormal bleeding time.

Aspirin inhibits cyclooxygenase, causing an impairment in thromboxane A_2 synthesis, which is necessary for the release reaction and aggregation. After a single dose the effects last 7–10 days.

Bleeding tendency is mild, with increased skin bruising and bleeding after surgery. The use of aspirin may contribute to GI hemorrhage associated with acute mucosal erosions, and it may be life-threatening.

Uremia

In uremia, defects may be caused by an abnormal arachidonate metabolism with reduced synthesis of thromboxane. Platelet interactions with subendothelium are abnormal and bleeding may be severe.

Clotting factor abnormalities

Hereditary factor abnormalities

Von Willebrand's disease

This is the most common of the hereditary coagulation disorders. It is an autosomal dominant disorder of abnormal platelet adhesion associated with low factor VIII activity. The primary defect is a reduced synthesis of von Willebrand's factor, which has two main functions:

- Promotes platelet adhesion.
- Carrier molecule for factor VIII, protecting it from premature destruction.

The disease is characterized by operative and post-traumatic hemorrhage, mucous membrane bleeding (e.g., epistaxes, menorrhagia), and excessive blood loss from superficial cuts and abrasions.

Bleeding episodes are treated with intermediate-purity factor VIII concentrates that contain both von Willebrand's factor and factor VIII.

Hemophilia A (factor VIII deficiency)

A common hereditary disorder of blood coagulation, this is characterized by the absence or low levels of plasma factor VIII.

Its inheritance is X-linked, but 33% of patients have no family history and the disorder presumably results from spontaneous mutation; it affects 1 per 10,000 in the U.S.

Blood clotting time is prolonged, and in severe disease, the blood is incoagulable.

The disease is characterized by frequent episodes of spontaneous hemorrhage into a major joint, especially knees, hips, elbows, and shoulders. Without factor replacement therapy, bleeding continues until the intra-articular pressure rises sufficiently to prevent further hemorrhage.

Resolution of acute haemarthrosis occurs slowly with recurrent bleeds producing massive synovial hypertrophy, erosion of joint cartilage and bone, and changes of severe osteoarthritis.

Bleeding into muscles, retroperitoneal tissues, urinary tract, and epistaxes also occurs.

Operative and post-traumatic hemorrhage is life threatening, both in severely and mildly affected patients.

Mild, moderate and severe forms of the disease are recognized depending on the residual clotting factor activity (Fig. 12.37).

Treatment—Control can be achieved by intravenous clotting factor replacement. Note that the transmission of hepatitis C and HIV occurred in some hemophiliacs prior to the introduction of cloned factor VIII.

Hemophilia B (factor IX deficiency)

Inheritance, clinical features and treatment of factor IX deficiency are identical to those of hemophilia A.

Classification of hemophilias			
Category	**Frequency**	**Coagulation factor activity (% of normal)**	**Clinical features**
Severe	40%	<1%	Frequent spontaneous bleeding episodes from birth Degenerative joint disease
Moderate	10%	1–5%	Post-traumatic bleeding Occasional spontaneous episodes Bruising
Mild	50%	5–20%	Post-traumatic bleeding may be subclinical

Fig. 12.37 Classification of hemophilias.

Common hereditary clotting factor abnormalities			
	Hemophilia A	**Factor IX deficiency**	**Von Willebrand's disease**
Deficiency	Factor VIII	Factor IX	Von Willebrand factor → factor VIII deficiency
Inheritance	X-linked	X-linked	Dominant
Prevalence in U.S.	1 in 10,000	1 in 50,000	1 in 5000
Main sites of hemorrhage	Muscle, joints: post trauma or post surgery	Muscle, joints: post trauma or post surgery	Mucus membranes, post trauma and operation

Fig. 12.38 Common hereditary clotting factor abnormalities.

However, factor IX deficiency is less common, the incidence being only about one fifth of that of hemophilia A. This is also known as Christmas disease.

The features of the most common hereditary clotting factor deficiencies are summarized in Fig. 12.38.

Other deficiencies

Hereditary deficiencies of most of the other coagulation factors have also been described, but they are extremely rare.

Acquired factor abnormalities

Acquired disorders of coagulation are far more common than the inherited disorders, and multiple clotting factor deficiencies are usual.

Vitamin K deficiency

Vitamin K is essential for the γ-carboxylation and hence activation of factors II, VII, IX, and X and proteins C and S (inhibitors). The deficiency is associated with decreased activity of these proteins leading to coagulopathies. This may present in the newborn or in later life.

Vitamin K is obtained from green vegetables and bacterial synthesis in the gut. It is a fat soluble vitamin, and it requires bile for its absorption.

Causes of vitamin K deficiency:

- Inadequate diet.
- Malabsorption (e.g., obstructive jaundice (reduced bile), celiac disease).
- Drugs: warfarin (a vitamin K antagonist).

Neonates are particularly susceptible to vitamin K deficiency because of their lack of gut bacteria and low concentrations of the vitamin in breast milk. The combined effect of vitamin K deficiency and low levels of clotting factors due to liver immaturity may produce a life-threatening disease: hemorrhagic disease of the newborn.

Treatment is by vitamin K supplementation of all newborns.

Causes of disseminated intravascular coagulation	
Problem	**Cause**
Infections	Septicemia, viral infections (purpura fulminans), malaria
Malignancy	Mucin-secreting adenocarcinomas, acute promyelocytic leukemia
Obstetric complications	Amniotic fluid embolism, premature separation of placenta, eclampsia
Hypersensitivity reactions	Anaphylaxis, incompatible blood transfusion
Widespread tissue damage	Burns, major accidental trauma, major surgery, shock, intravascular hemolysis, dissecting aortic aneurysm
Liver disease	Various causes

Fig. 12.39 Causes of disseminated intravascular coagulation.

Liver disease

This is commonly associated with coagulation defects due to:

- Impaired absorption of vitamin K caused by biliary obstruction, producing decreased activation of factors II, VII, IX, and X and proteins C and S.
- Reduced synthesis of clotting factors and of fibrinogen, and increased amounts of plasminogen activator in severe hepatocellular disease.
- Thrombocytopenia from hypersplenism associated with portal hypertension.
- Dysfibrinogenemia: functional abnormality of fibrinogen found in many patients with liver disease.
- Qualitative platelet disorders.

Disseminated intravascular coagulation

This condition is characterized by increased coagulation, which leads not only to widespread thrombosis, but also to hemorrhage due to consumption of platelets and coagulation factors. Thus both thrombosis and hemorrhage are a feature of this disorder.

The disorder may cause a severe hemorrhagic syndrome with high mortality or may run a milder, more chronic course.

Etiology—This is shown in Fig. 12.39.

Pathogenesis—The causes listed in Fig. 12.39 activate the coagulation system in small vessels throughout the body via:

- Release of procoagulant material into circulation (e.g., obstetric disorders, certain malignancies, liver disease, severe falciparum malaria, and hemolytic transfusion reactions).
- Widespread endothelial damage (e.g., septicemia, certain viral infections, severe burns, or hypothermia).
- Platelet aggregation: some bacteria, viruses, and immune complexes may have a direct effect on platelets.

The main effects of DIC are:

- Vascular occlusion results in organ dysfunction (from ischemic damage) and microangiopathic hemolysis.
- Consumption of platelets, clotting factors, and fibrinogen causes hemorrhage.
- Activation of fibrinolytic system results in increased fibrin degradation products, which themselves have anticoagulant effect causing hemorrhage.

Treatment is of the underlying cause, with clotting factor and platelet replacement.

Thrombosis

Thrombosis is the formation of a solid mass of blood constituents—thrombus—within the vascular system during life. It is not to be confused with a clot, which occurs in non-flowing blood.

Thrombosis can affect both arteries and veins.

Arterial thrombosis

This is most commonly superimposed on an atheroma. As the plaque enlarges, it causes turbulent blood flow, which results in the loss of intimal cells. The exposure of vessel collagen predisposes to platelet activation. Turbulence itself will predispose to fibrin deposition and platelet clumping. The greatest degree of turbulence occurs at the downstream side of the forming thrombus and, consequently, thrombi grow in the direction of the blood flow (propagation). An arterial thrombosis may result in tissue infarction and ischemia.

Venous thrombosis

Many venous thrombi begin at damaged valves that produce turbulence. Furthermore, blood stasis during surgery or due to immobilization may result in the formation of a deep vein thrombosis (risk of pulmonary embolism). However, some thrombi form at sites with no known predisposing factors. Often thrombi grow by successive deposition of alternating bands of white platelets and red blood cells. These patterns are known as the lines of Zahn. A thrombosed vein may cause an inflammatory response (thrombophlebitis) or a vein that is inflamed may thrombose (phlebothrombosis).

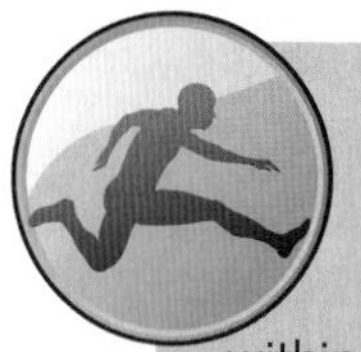

A thrombus is different from a clot! A clot is defined as blood coagulated outside the vascular system, or within the vascular system after death.

Virchow's triad

Factors that predispose to thrombosis can be classified into three main groups, collectively known as Virchow's triad:

- Changes in the blood constituents.
- Changes in the intimal surface of the blood vessel.
- Changes in the pattern of blood flow.

Questions about Virchow's triad are extremely common in examinations.

Hypercoagulability

Primary (hereditary) Hereditary defects of hypercoagulability lead to a lifelong tendency to thrombosis (thrombophilia), and they usually affect the venous system:

- Antithrombin III deficiency: autosomal dominant condition characterized by recurrent venous thromboses usually starting in early adult life. Primary defect is a deficiency of antithrombin III, which usually neutralizes thrombin and other activated clotting factors.
- Protein C deficiency: most common form of hereditary thrombophilia. Autosomal dominant condition resulting in failure of neutralization of activated factors V and VIII. Protein S is a cofactor for protein C, therefore, protein S deficiencies produce a similar pathology.
- Abnormal factor V: point mutation in the factor V gene, which results in factor V protein that is resistant to neutralization by protein C.
- Defective fibrinolysis: rare causes of thrombophilia resulting from defects of fibrinogen (dysfibrinogenemia) or of plasminogen.

Secondary (acquired) Defects are as follows:

- Malignancy: patients with carcinoma of the breast, lung, prostate, pancreas, or bowel have an increased risk of venous thrombosis.
- Blood disorders, such as. increased viscosity (especially polycythemia rubra vera), and thrombocytosis lead to an increased risk of venous thrombosis.
- Estrogens: associated with raised plasma levels of various clotting factors leading to an increased risk of venous thrombosis.
- Antiphospholipid antibody leads to the interaction of the antibody with phospholipid-bound proteins involved in coagulation and causes prolongation of clotting times in vitro, with a paradoxical increased risk of venous and arterial thrombosis. Often found in patients with autoimmune disease, especially SLE.
- Cholesterol: partly genetic, partly acquired (diet/life-style), leads to an increased risk of arterial thrombosis.

Endothelial injury

Direct injury to the endothelium as seen in trauma and inflammation may lead to thrombosis. Damage to the endothelium also occurs in association with atheroma.

Alterations to blood flow

Alterations are:

- Stasis: allows platelets to come in contact with endothelium, and slow flow prevents blood from diluting activated coagulation components.
- Turbulence: may cause physical trauma to endothelial cells, and loss of laminar flow may bring platelets into contact with endothelium.

- Describe the clinical manifestations of systemic lupus erythematosus (SLE).
- Name the common organ-specific autoimmune diseases.
- Describe the life cycle and stages in infection of the human immunodeficiency virus (HIV).
- Describe immunodeficiency disorders.
- Define amyloidosis, and describe amyloid formation.
- Name the most common type of leukopenia. What are its causes and effects?
- Describe the morphological features and cellular composition of affected lymph nodes in Hodgkin's disease.
- Explain the classification basis of leukemia.
- Describe the common clinical features of leukemia.
- List the myeloproliferative disorders, and describe their basic features.
- Describe the pathogenesis of multiple myeloma.
- List the causes of splenomegaly.
- Name four developmental disorders of the thymus.
- Describe the different types of thymoma.
- Describe the classification of anemia.
- Name the common hemoglobinopathies, and describe their basic pathology.
- Describe the types of anemia caused by hematinic deficiency.
- Describe the various etiologies of vessel wall abnormalities.
- What are the most common hereditary and acquired clotting factor abnormalities?
- What are the components of Virchow's triad, and how do they cause thrombosis?

13. Pathology of the Skin

Terminology of skin pathology

Macroscopic appearances

Macule

This localized, flat area of altered skin color can be hyperpigmented as in a freckle, hypopigmented as in vitiligo, or erythematous as in a capillary hemangioma.

Papule

A small, raised, solid lesion of the skin, this is generally defined as being less than 5mm in diameter.

Nodule

This is similar to a papule but greater than 5mm in diameter. It may be solid or edematous, and it can involve any layer of the skin.

Plaque

An extended papule which forms a plateau-like elevation of skin, a plaque is usually more than 20 mm in diameter but rarely more than 5mm in height.

Wheal

This is similar to a papule or plaque but transitory and compressible. It is caused by dermal edema, red or white in color, and usually signifies urticaria.

Blister

This fluid-filled space within the skin is caused by the separation of cells and the leakage of plasma into the space.

Vesicle

This small blister (less than 5mm in diameter) contains clear fluid within or below the epidermis.

Bulla

This is similar to a vesicle but larger than 5mm in diameter.

Pustule

A small, pus-containing blister, a pustule commonly indicates infection, but not always (e.g., those seen in psoriasis are not infected).

Scale

This thickened horny layer of keratin forms readily detached fragments of skin. Scaling is caused by disturbances in the processes of keratinization, and usually indicates inflammation of the epidermis (Fig. 13.1A).

Lichenification

There is a thickening of the epidermis with exaggeration of the normal skin creases caused by abnormal scratching or rubbing of skin (Fig. 13.1B).

Excoriation

This is caused by the destruction or removal of the surface of the skin usually by scratching, but also by chemical application or other means.

Onycholysis

This is the separation of part or all of a nail from its bed. It may occur in psoriasis and in fungal infections of the skin and nail bed, and it is more common in women.

Microscopic appearances

See Fig. 13.2 for a diagrammatical representation of normal skin and normal epidermis.

Hyperkeratosis

Thickening of the outer horny layer of the skin (stratum corneum) occurs.

Parakeratosis

There is excessive keratin, in which nuclear remnants persist (a histological sign of increased epidermal growth).

Acanthosis

The thickening of the epidermis is caused by an increased number of prickle cells in the stratum spinosum (prickle cell layer).

Dyskeratosis

There is an abnormal premature keratinization of cells in the prickle cell layer.

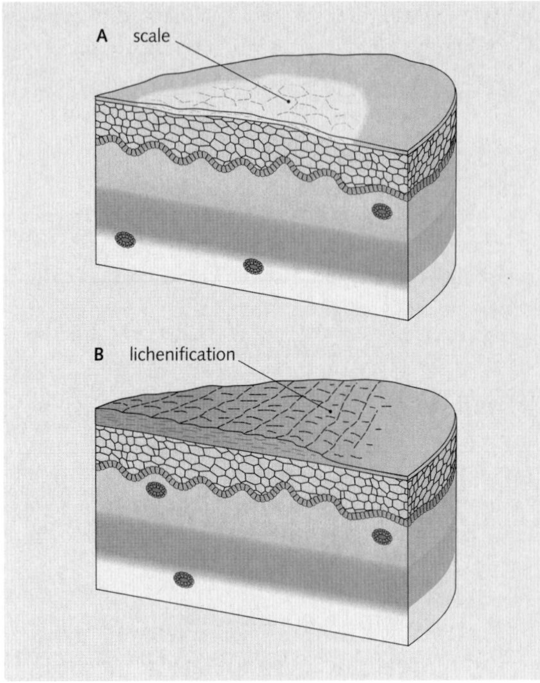

Fig. 13.1 Basic lesions of the skin showing scale and lichenification.

Acantholysis

The loss of cellular cohesion and separation of epidermal keratinocytes are due to the rupture ofintercellular bridges. Bulla formation often results.

Spongiosis

Epidermal edema causes partial separation of keratinocytes.

Vacuolization

This is the formation of intracellular, fluid-filled spaces (vacuoles).

Papillomatosis

In this condition many papillomas (finger-like projections) grow on an area of skin or mucus membranes.

Lentiginous

This describes skin whose increased pigmentation is a result of increased numbers of melanocytes.

Exocytosis

Migratory inflammatory cells appear in the epidermis.

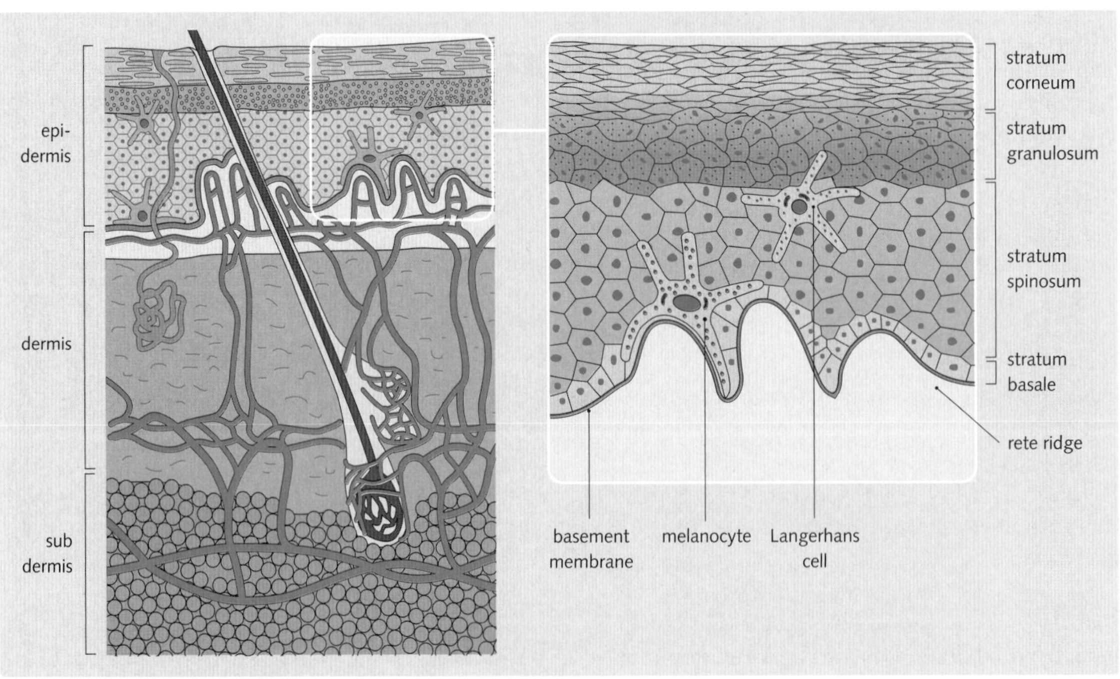

Fig. 13.2 Normal skin and epidermis.

Erosion

This is the loss of all or part of the epidermis that does not extend into the dermis, but which heals without scarring.

Ulceration

A full thickness defect (epidermis and dermis) of the skin forms.

> The vocabulary of dermatology is quite distinct from that of other specialities. Learning the common dermatological terms is essential in order to correctly describe different skin disorders.

Inflammation and skin eruptions

Psoriasis

Definition

Psoriasis is a chronic, noninfectious, inflammatory disease of the skin characterized by erythematous plaques covered with thick, silvery scales.

It affects about 2% of the population in the U.S., and it can start at any age, but the peak onset is in the second and third decades of life.

The etiology of psoriasis is unclear; however, about 35% of patients show a family history. It is associated with HLA haplotypes CW6, B13, and B17.

Environmental factors are thought to trigger the disease in genetically susceptible individuals. Triggers and exacerbating factors include infection (group A *Streptococcus*), drugs, ultraviolet light, alcohol abuse, and stress.

Pathogenesis:

- Epidermal cell proliferation rate is increased 20-fold or more.
- Epidermal turnover time is greatly reduced.
- Keratinocytes are normal, but the stem cell number is increased.

Thus, there is an increase in skin turnover and the granular layer is often absent. Epidermal cells are immature, and there is accumulation of abnormal keratin, which results in scale. Characteristic histological features are:

- Long rete ridges separated by a markedly edematous papillary dermis in which there are large numbers of dilated capillaries.
- Scale: composed of flakes of thickened surface keratin, which contain remnants of nuclei (parakeratosis).
- Neutrophil polymorphs migrate through the epidermis and may be trapped beneath the thickened horny layer.

Precipitating factors—A number of factors have been identified that can precipitate psoriasis:

- Köebner's phenomenon: trauma to skin (e.g., scratch, surgical scar, or burn).
- Infection: streptococcal sore throat may precipitate psoriasis.
- Drugs: β-blockers, lithium, and antimalarials can precipitate or worsen psoriasis.

Psoriasis most commonly affects the extensor surfaces of the knees and elbows, the trunk, and the scalp (Fig. 13.3). Nail involvement is frequent. Pitting and thickening of the nail may be followed by onycholysis.

Several types of psoriasis exist, which are of variable appearance and behavior (see Fig. 13.4).

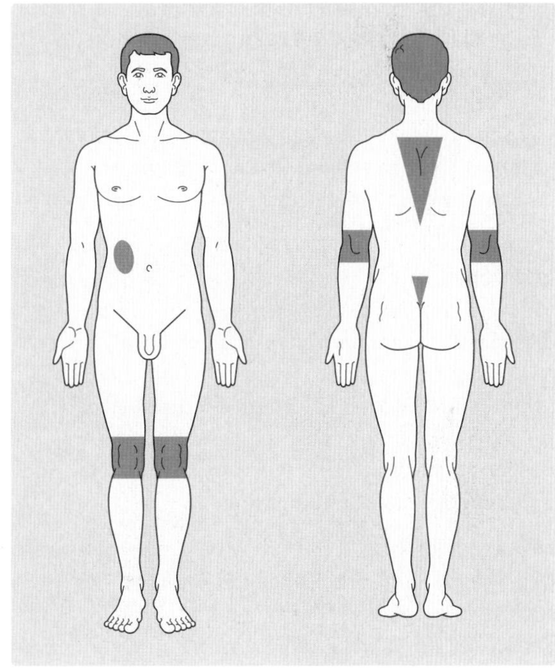

Fig. 13.3 Common sites of psoriasis.

Types of psoriasis	
Type	**Features**
Plaque	Most common type. Disc-shaped, erythematous plaques covered with white silvery scale
Guttate	Symmetrical "drop-like" lesions. May be associated with streptococcal infection in the young
Flexural	Smooth erythematous plaques, often glazed
Localized	Scalp, palmoplantar pustulosis, napkin (nappy area in infants), and acrodermatitis of Hallopeau (nails) types
Generalized	Rare, but potentially life threatening

Fig. 13.4 Types of psoriasis.

Complications

Psoriatic arthropathy

About 5% of psoriasis patients develop arthropathy, which takes one of four forms:

- Distal arthritis—the most common form. Affects the distal interphalangeal joints of the hands and feet, causing "sausage-like" swelling of the digits.
- Rheumatoid-like arthritis—polyarthropathy similar to rheumatoid disease, but less symmetrical and with negative test for rheumatoid factor.
- Mutilans arthritis—progressive deformity of the hands and feet caused by erosion of the small bones. Often associated with severe psoriasis.
- Ankylosing spondylitis/sacroiliitis—in HLA-B27-positive patients.

Erythroderma

This rare complication of psoriasis (and other disorders) is characterized by a generalized reddening, flaking, and thickening of all, or nearly all, of the skin surface. It is accompanied and often preceded by pyrexia, malaise, and shivering. Associated systemic effects are potentially fatal, and inpatient treatment is required.

Management

Management of psoriasis includes topical therapy such as tar preparations, dithranol, topical corticosteroids, and keratolytics. Systemic therapies such as photochemotherapy, retinoids, and methotrexate are used in severe cases.

Eczema and contact dermatitis

Definitions

Eczema and dermatitis are non-infective inflammatory conditions of the skin. They are not diseases, but are reactive conditions occurring in response to certain stimuli, many of which are unknown. They can be acute or chronic.

Acute and chronic forms

Acute eczema/dermatitis

Acute eczema/dermatitis is characterized by:

- Erythema: caused by chronic inflammatory cell infiltrate (lymphocytes) around dilated vessels in the upper dermis.
- Spongiotic, fluid-filled vesicles: caused by epidermal edema (leakage of fluid from the dilated vessels) with separation of keratinocytes (spongiosis).
- Erythematous lesions are itchy (histamine release), and vesicles may weep and crust.

Chronic eczema/dermatitis

Scratching of the itchy, acute-stage lesions causes secondary changes, which result in the chronic form of the condition. It is characterized by:

- Thickening of the prickle cell layer (acanthosis).
- Thickening of the stratum corneum (hyperkeratosis).
- Elongation of the rete ridges and dermal collagenization.
- Dilation of dermal vessels and infiltration of the dermis with inflammatory cells.

Characteristic thickening, which occurs as a result of scratching, is termed lichenification (see above).

Atopic eczema

This chronic form of eczema is often associated with a strong family history of other atopic diseases such as asthma and hay fever. Uncontrollable itching is common, and the condition follows a remitting relapsing course.

Although 10–15% of the population are atopic, only about 5% of these individuals will develop atopic eczema.

The etiology of atopic eczema and other atopic diseases is not well understood; however, the strong family history associated with these conditions suggests at least a partial genetic cause for the disease.

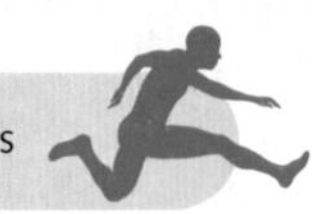

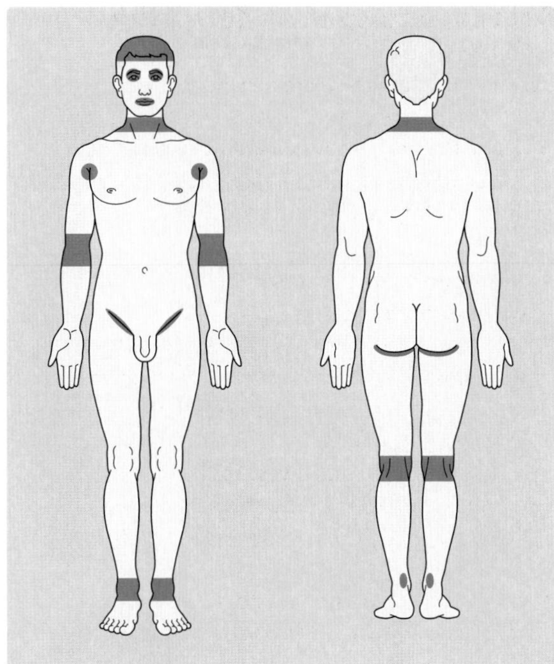

Fig. 13.5 Distribution of atopic eczema.

The pathogenesis is as follows:

- Individuals prone to atopy have higher circulating levels of IgE antibodies than non-atopic individuals.
- On exposure to certain allergens, IgE-mediated, type I hypersensitivity reactions are triggered, causing large-scale mast-cell degranulation with the release of histamine and other inflammatory mediators.
- In the skin, this type of hypersensitivity reaction results in the histological changes of acute eczema, which on scratching becomes chronic eczema.

Atopic eczema presents at an early age, with 60% presenting before 1 year and 90% by 5 years.

The appearance of atopic eczema varies between different age groups (see below and Fig. 13.5):

- Infancy: babies develop the typical acute form of eczema on the face and hands, often with secondary infection.
- Childhood: progression from acute to chronic condition. Usually involves the antecubital and popliteal fossae, neck, wrists, and ankles.
- Adults: chronic condition with lichenified (and sometimes nodular) lesions. The hands are most commonly affected but a few adults also develop the chronic, severe form of generalized atopic eczema, which is often precipitated by stressful situations.

The complications are:

- Bacterial infection: typically with *Staphylococcus aureus*.
- Viral infection: increased susceptibility to the development of viral warts, molluscum contagiosum, and to secondary infection with herpes simplex (eczema herpeticum).
- Growth retardation: may occur in children with severe eczema. The cause is unknown.
- Cataracts: rare; may occur in young adults in association with severe atopic eczema.

The treatment for atopic eczema is topical therapy (emollients, topical steroids, and antibiotics), systemic therapy (antihistamines and antibiotics) and dietary manipulation (useful for food allergies).

Contact dermatitis

Contact dermatitis is a form of dermatitis precipitated by exogenous agents (Fig. 13.6). It can be classified into:

- Irritant contact dermatitis: the most common form. Caused by contact of the skin with water, abrasives, acids, alkalis, solvents, or detergents.
- Allergic contact dermatitis: caused by a type IV hypersensitivity reaction to allergens such as nickel.

Lesions are localized to the site of contact, and they are most common on the hands and face.

Management is by identification and reduction in contact of the offending allergen/irritant (e.g., by protective gloves) and by topical therapy (e.g., steroids).

Other forms

Seborrheic dermatitis

This is a common, chronic inflammatory condition in which the skin is reddened and covered by thick, waxy, or white scale. The eruption often occurs in the sebaceous gland areas of the scalp and face, although other areas may also be involved.

The etiology is unknown, but genetic factors and overgrowth of the yeast commensal *Pityrosporum ovale* have been implicated.

There are four common patterns in the clinical presentation (as shown in Fig. 13.7):

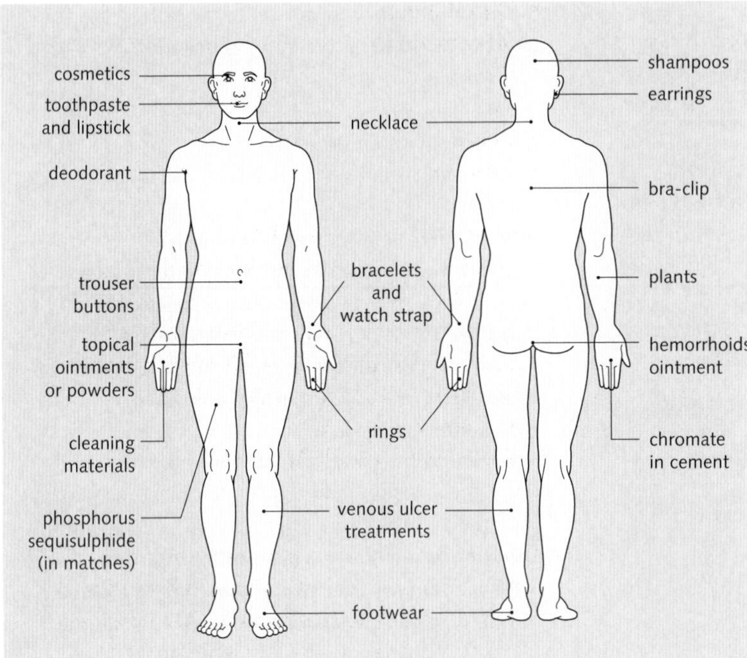

Fig. 13.6 Distribution and causes of contact dermatitis.

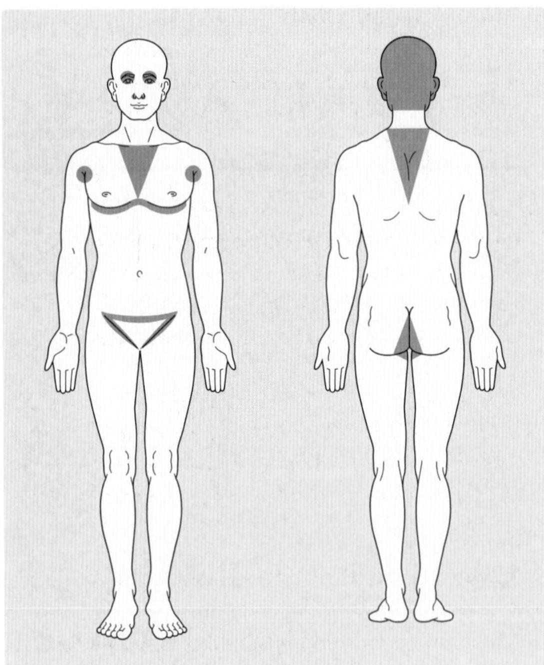

Fig. 13.7 Distribution of seborrheic dermatitis.

- Scalp and facial involvement: affects the side of the nose, scalp margin, eyebrows, and ears and excessive dandruff is usually present. Most common in young males.
- Petaloid: affects presternal area.
- *Pityrosporum folliculitis*: erythematous follicular eruption with papules or pustules typically affecting the back.
- Flexural: involvement of the axillae, groins, and submammary areas, often secondarily colonized by *Candida albicans*.

The management is as follows:

- Medicated shampoos for scalp lesions.
- Topical antifungals for facial, truncal, and flexural involvement.
- Topical hydrocortisone.

Discoid (nummular) eczema

A condition of unknown etiology, this is characterized by "coin-shaped," symmetrical, eczematous lesions, which typically affect the limbs of middle-aged or elderly men. Secondary bacterial infection is common.

Venous (stasis) eczema

This typically affects the legs of middle-aged or elderly women, and it is associated with underlying venous disease. It may present with hemosiderin pigmentation around the ankles or with fibrosis of the dermis and subcutaneous tissue and ulceration. It is also known as gravitational eczema.

Hand dermatitis and pompholyx

This common, acute or chronic eczema may appear as a vesicular eruption known as pompholyx—with "sago-like" vesicles on the sides of the fingers and on the palms.

Pompholyx is caused by the formation of eczematous vesicles that cannot rupture the thick, horny layer of the skin on the hands. The vesicles therefore persist and cause intense itching until the skin eventually peels. Onset is usually in young adults, especially in warm weather, and is often recurrent.

Asteatotic eczema (eczema craquelé; winter eczema)

This dry eczema with cracking of the skin appears as a fine, "crazy-paving" pattern of fissuring, commonly affecting the limbs and trunk of the elderly. Causes are the overwashing of patients in institutions, a dry winter climate, hypothyroidism, or the use of diuretics.

Lichen striatus

A rare, self-limiting linear eczema of unknown etiology; it typically affects the limbs of adolescents.

Dermatitis and eczema essentially describe the same reactive condition, i.e., they are histopathologically identical, and the terms are often used interchangeably. However, eczema is used to describe the reaction that occurs in response to an endogenous stimulus, whereas dermatitis is used to describe the reaction that occurs in response to an exogenous stimulus.

Infections and infestations

Bacterial infections

Normal skin microflora

The skin is colonized by numerous microorganisms known as microflora or commensals (see Chapter 4), which may number as many as 0.5 million per cm^2. Some examples are:

- *Staphylococcus epidermidis*.
- *S. aureus*.
- Diphtheroids.
- Streptococci.
- *Pseudomonas aeruginosa*.
- Anaerobes.
- *Candida* and *Torulopsis*.
- *Pityrosporum*.

Overgrowth of normal flora

Some diseases are caused by an overgrowth of normal flora:

- Erythrasma: dry, scaly, reddish-brown eruption caused by corynebacteria. Usually asymptomatic, but it can be treated with topical or oral antibiotics.
- Trichomycosis axillaris: overgrowth of corynebacteria, which form yellow concretions on axillary hair.
- Pitted keratolysis: overgrowth of micrococci, which digest keratin causing malodorous and pitted erosions with depressed discolored areas. Occurs with occluding footwear and sweaty feet.

Staphylococcal infections

Impetigo This highly contagious superficial skin infection is caused by either streptococci, staphylococci, or both. The clinical features of impetigo are as follows:

Generally occurs in children and spreads rapidly through populations (e.g., in schools).

Characterized by the development of large, thin-walled bullae, often on the face, which leave areas of yellow crusted exudate ("honey crusts").

Commonly confused with herpes simplex or fungal infections.

The management of impetigo is by the removal of crusts with saline soaks and the application of topical antibiotics; widespread infection can be treated with systemic antibiotics. It is also important to trim the child's fingernails.

Ecthyma This is a full-thickness infection of epidermis by *S. aureus*.

The clinical features of ecthyma are as follows:

- Characterized by circumscribed, ulcerated, and crusted infected lesions that eventually heal with scarring.
- Occurs most commonly on the legs, usually as aresult of an insect bite or neglected minor injury.
- May also be seen in drug addicts due to the use of contaminated needles.

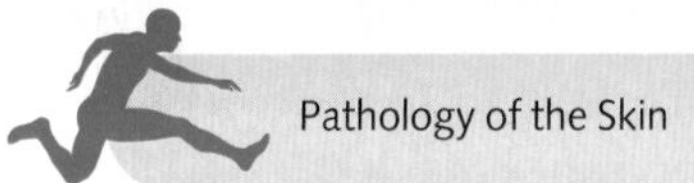

The management of ecthyma is by systemic and topical antibiotics.

Folliculitis This infection of multiple hair follicles is usually caused by *S. aureus*.

The clinical features of folliculitis are:

- Characterized by the production of tiny pustules located in the necks of hair follicles (superficial folliculitis).
- In men, it commonly affects the beard area (sycosi barbae).
- In women, it commonly affects the legs after hair removal by shaving or waxing.

A furuncle (boil) is a deep infection of a follicle resulting in an expanding collection of pus that destroys the follicle and extends into the surrounding dermis.

A carbuncle is a deep abscess formed in a group of follicles with multiple drainage channels, resulting in a painful suppurating mass; it may cause systemic symptoms.

The management of folliculitis is through systemic and topical antibiotics.

Carbuncles often need surgical drainage.

Staphylococcal scalded skin syndrome An acute toxic illness usually of infants, this is characterized by the shedding of sheets of skin, and it is caused by the potent exotoxin (exfoliatin) produced by a specific strain of *S. aureus*.

The clinical presentation is as follows:

- Extensive disruption of the epidermis, with widespread confluent blistering and denuded erythematous areas resembling scalding of the skin.
- Condition may follow impetigo.

Management—It is a serious condition requiring hospital admission and systemic antibiotic treatment.

Streptococcal infections

Erysipelas This acute, erythematous, spreading infection of the dermis is caused by *Streptococcus pyogenes*.

The clinical presentation is as follows:

- Usually affects the face or the lower leg and appears as a painful red swelling.
- Lesion is usually well demarcated, and it is often edematous and tender.
- Often preceded by fever and flu-like symptoms.
- Streptococci usually gain entry to the skin via a fissure (e.g., behind the ear or between the toes, especially with so-called "athlete's foot").

Severe infection requires parenteral antibiotic treatment, usually penicillin. Less severe cases can be treated with oral antibiotics.

Necrotizing fasciitis A deep-spreading infection of the fat, fascia, and muscle, this is caused by *S. pyogenes*.

The condition presents as an ill-defined erythema typically affecting the leg, and associated with a high fever. Infected tissues become rapidly necrotic.

It usually occurs in otherwise healthy subjects after minor trauma.

Management is by extensive emergency surgical debridement (removal of dead tissue); systemic antibiotics are essential.

TB, which may have cutaneous manifestations, is rare in the U.S. However, approximately 3 million people in developing countries die annually from TB!

Spirochetal infections

Syphilis Syphilis is a chronic infectious disease caused by the spirochete *Treponema pallidum*, and it is usually transmitted by sexual intercourse. It typically involves three stages: primary, secondary, and tertiary.

Skin lesions may be seen in all stages, but predominant skin manifestations present during the secondary stage.

Secondary syphilis

This is an inflammatory response in the skin and mucous membranes to the disseminated spirochete.

The clinical presentation is as follows:

- Presents about 4–12 weeks after the onset of primary chancre (primary stage).
- Characterized by a non-itchy, pink or copper-colored papular eruption on the trunk, limbs, palms, and soles, and it is often accompanied by lymphadenopathy and general malaise.

- Other signs are moist warty papules (condylomata lata) in the anogenital area, buccal erosions, and diffuse patchy alopecia.
- Untreated, the eruption resolves in 1–3 months.

Management is by intramuscular penicillin, contact tracing of sexual partners, and assessment for other venereal diseases.

Nonvenereal treponemal infections Rare in the U.S. but endemic in tropical and subtropical areas, these are transmitted by direct contact:
- Yaws—Central Africa, Central America, and South East Asia (*Treponema pertenue*).
- Pinta—Central America (*T. carateum*).
- Endemic syphilis (bejel)—Middle East (*T. pallidum*).

Lyme disease This cutaneous and systemic infection is caused by the spirochete *Borrelia burgdorferi* and spread by certain ticks. The majority of cases develop a slowly-extending erythematous rash at the site of the tick bite. Intermittent systemic symptoms include fever, malaise, headache, neck stiffness, and muscle and joint pain.

Other bacterial infections

Anthrax This rare infection is caused by *Bacillus anthracis* associated with farm animals, particularly cattle.

A hemorrhagic bulla forms at the site of inoculation, and it may be followed by vasculitis and a necrotizing, hemorrhagic inflammation of the skin.

The disease has a variable clinical course, but death can occur if it is not rapidly diagnosed and treated. The pulmonary form should be considered as prima facie evidence of bioterrorism.

Gram-negative infections Gram-negative bacilli, such as *Pseudomonas aeruginosa*, can readily infect burns, ulcers, or other moist skin lesions. They can also cause folliculitis and cellulitis (infection of subcutaneous tissues).

Fig. 13.8 provides a summary of bacterial skin infections.

Summary of bacterial skin infections	
Causative bacteria	**Associated skin disease**
Commensal overgrowth	Erythrasma, trichomycosis axillaris, pitted keratolysis
Staphylococci	Impetigo, ecthyma, folliculitis, scalded skin syndrome
Streptococci	Erysipelas, impetigo, necrotizing fasciitis
Mycobacteria	TB (lupus vulgaris, scrofuloderma, warty tuberculosis), leprosy
Spirochetes	Secondary syphilis, yaws/bejel/pinta, Lyme disease
Others	Anthrax, Gram-negative infections

Fig. 13.8 Summary of bacterial skin infections.

Viral infections

Viral warts (verrucae)

These common, benign, hyperkeratotic, papillomatous growths on the skin are caused by infection with human papillomavirus (HPV).

Keratinocytes in the stratum granulosum (granular layer) beneath the wart are often vacuolated due to the viral infection.

Clinical presentation

Common warts Firm, dome-shaped, horny papules (1–10mm across), usually multiple, warts are found mainly on the hands, but they may also affect the feet, face, and genitalia.

Plantar warts These occur on the soles of the feet, and they are often covered by callus (hyperkeratosis). Pressure causes inward growth, which results in tenderness.

Plane warts Flat, skin-colored papules usually found on the face, these are usually multiple. They resist treatment but eventually resolve spontaneously.

Genital warts These affect the genitalia and the perianal region. The warts may be small or may coalesce into large, cauliflower-like, warty growths called condylomata acuminata. Affected women have an increased risk of developing cervical cancer.

Management

Hand and foot warts frequently disappear spontaneously. Resistant varieties are treated with topical "wart paints" (salicylic acid, lactic acid, gluteraldehyde, etc.) or with cryotherapy. Genital warts generally require cryotherapy or curettage and cautery with a local anesthetic.

Molluscum contagiosum

This presents as discrete, multiple, pale papules with a central depression. It is caused by a DNA poxvirus.

Clinical presentation—It mainly affects children or young adults. The most commonly affected areas are the face, neck, and trunk.

The virus is transmitted by contact, including sexual transmission, or on towels.

Untreated, the papules disappear in 6–9 months.

The treatment is by curettage, cryotherapy, or by expressing the content of papule (which contains a cheesy material) under local anesthetic.

Herpes simplex

A common, acute vesicular eruption of the skin or mucus membranes, this is caused by infection with herpes simplex virus (HSV).

Pathologically:

- HSV blisters are highly contagious and they are transmitted through direct contact.
- Virus penetrates the epidermis or mucus membrane, and it replicates within the epithelial cells.
- Following primary infection, the virus enters a latent stage within infected cells.
- Reactivation can occur at any time, even years after initial infection.
- Recurrence is thought to be precipitated by respiratory infection, sunlight, or local trauma.

Clinical presentation—There are two types of HSV:

- HSV type 1—Primary infection usually occurs in childhood and causes the common cold sore, present on or around the lips. Epithelial infection may be accompanied by fever, malaise, or local lymphadenopathy, and it lasts for about 2 weeks.
- HSV type 2—This is mainly associated with genital herpes and is sexually transmitted.

However, both type 1 and 2 viruses can cause genital herpes and cold sores, depending on the site of the initial infection.

Complications are:

- Secondary bacterial infection: usually staphylococcal.
- Eczema herpeticum: atopic eczema may be complicated by herpes simplex infection. Potentially fatal.
- Disseminated herpes simplex: occasionally occurs in the newborn or in immunosuppressed patients.
- Chronic herpes simplex: common in patients with human immunodeficiency virus (HIV) infection.
- Herpes encephalitis: serious complication of HSV infection.
- Erythema multiforme: immune-mediated disease characterized by erythematous lesions on the hands and feet.

Management is by topical acyclovir (used for mildfacial or genital herpes simplex) and oral acyclovir (prescribed for severe episodes of HSV infection).

Herpes zoster (shingles)

This acute, vesicular eruption occurs in a dermatomal distribution and is caused by the reactivation of latent varicella zoster virus.

Following an attack of chickenpox, the virus remains dormant in the dorsal root ganglion of the spinal cord. On reactivation (the causes of which are unknown), the virus migrates down the sensory nerve to affect one or more dermatomes on the skin. The clinical presentation is as follows:

- Usually presents as densely grouped vesicles and erythema on one dermatome.
- Thoracic dermatomes are most commonly affected, except in the elderly, in whom the ophthalmic division of the trigeminal nerve is particularly common.
- Vesicles become pustular and form crusts, which separate in 2–3 weeks to leave scarring.
- Vesicular blisters contain virus, which when shed may cause chickenpox in contacts with no previous exposure.
- Associated with pain, tenderness, or paraesthesia in the dermatome. This may also precede the eruption by 3–5 days.
- Local lymphadenopathy is common.

Complications are:

- Secondary bacterial infections.
- Ophthalmic scarring: corneal ulcers and scarring may occur following shingles of the ophthalmic division of the trigeminal nerve.
- Motor palsy: rare; viral involvement may spread from the posterior horn of the spinal cord to the anterior horn to infect motor nerves resulting in palsies or paralysis of individual muscles or muscle groups.
- Disseminated herpes zoster: may occur in the immunosuppressed leading to potentially fatal varicella pneumonia or encephalitis.

- Postherpetic neuralgia: occurs in one third of those over 60 years old, but infrequently in patients under 40 years old. Pain usually subsides within 12 months.

Management of mild shingles is by symptomatic treatment with rest, analgesia, and calamine lotion.

Severe cases are treated with oral acyclovir, which, if taken within 48 hours of onset, decreases the duration and the intensity of the disease, and it may prevent postherpetic neuralgia.

Fungal infections

Dermatophyte infections

Dermatophytes are filamentous (hyphal) fungi, which reproduce by spore formation. They commonly inhabit the keratin of the skin, hair, and nails producing superficial mycoses (Fig. 13.9).

Dermatophytes are collectively termed "ringworm," but they comprise three genera:

- *Microsporum* (e.g., *M. canis*).
- *Trichophyton* (e.g., *T. rubrum* and *T. interdigitale*).
- *Epidermophyton* (e.g., *E. floccosum*).

Management is by topical therapy for minor fungal infections, with systemic therapy for widespread involvement or disease of the nails or scalp. Humid and sweaty conditions, including occlusive footwear, should be minimized.

Candida albicans

Candida albicans is a yeast-type fungus, and it is a commensal of the vagina and alimentary canal. It commonly produces opportunistic infections; predisposing factors may be humidity, obesity, diabetes, and oral antibiotic therapy.

Clinical presentation—In infection, hyphal forms of C. *albicans* are seen, and the infection is termed candidosis (or candidiasis).

Candidosis

Genital This is especially common in the vagina ("thrush") where white-yellowish plaques on the inflamed mucus membranes produce itching/discomfort, and sometimes a white vaginal discharge. It can be spread by sexual intercourse; males develop similar changes on the penis. Broad-spectrum antibiotic treatment may favor overgrowth of *Candida*, due to suppression of endogenous bacterial flora.

Oral White plaques adhere on the tongue or inside the cheeks.

Intertrigo A superficial inflammation of two skin surfaces that are in contact (e.g., between the thighs

Dermatophyte infections and their clinical effects		
Affected area	**Commonest organism**	**Clinical presentation**
Tinea corporis (trunk and limbs)	*Trichophyton verrucosum, Microsporum canis, T. rubrum*	Single of multiple ring lesions with scaling and erythema, especially at the edges
Tinea pedis (athlete's foot)	*T. rubrum, T. interdigitale, Epidermophyton floccosum*	Redness, erosion, and scaling which is often interdigital, but diffuse involvement of skin also occurs Common in young men; increased predisposition by communal washing, swimming baths, occlusive footwear, and hot weather
Tinea capitis (scalp/hair)	*M. canis, M. audouinii, T. tonsurans, T. schoenleinii*	Hair loss and scaling Usually affects children
Tinea cruris (groin)	*T. rubrum, E. floccosum, T. interdigitale*	Red, scaly rash with brown patches; more common in men and often seen in athletes ("jock itch")
Tinea manuum (hand)	*T. rubrum*	Unilateral diffuse powdery scaling of the palm
Tinea unguium (nails)	*T. rubrum, T. interdigitale*	Thick, crumbling nails more commonly affecting toenails Incidence of onychomycosis increases with age

Fig. 13.9 Dermatophyte infections and their clinical effects.

or under the breasts) is often aggravated by C. *albicans* infection. Interdigital clefts are commonly affected in wetworkers.

Paronychia The nail-fold becomes inflamed and swollen, the cuticle is lost, and the nail may be ridged transversely. It is often seen in wetworkers.

Systemic This occurs in the immunosuppressed, producing red nodules on the skin with small, satellite pustules.

Mucocutaneous This is a rare (and sometimes inherited) disorder of immune deficiency. It causes chronic C. *albicans* intertrigo and nail and mouth infections.

Management Management is by:

- Topical therapy: for body folds, oral, and genital *Candida*.
- Systemic therapy: short course useful for recurrent or persistent candidosis (reduces bowel carriage), long-term treatment for mucocutaneous candidiasis.

Infestations

Insect bites

These are a cutaneous inflammatory reaction to insect parts or to injected foreign substances. Common culprits include garden insects (gnats, etc.), insects of household pets (fleas, mites), and bedbugs (inactive within furniture during the day but emerge at night).

Bites are usually grouped on a limb, and lesions vary from itchy wheals to quite large bullae depending on the insect and the type of immune response elicited.

Secondary bacterial infection of excoriated insect bites is common.

It can be managed by the elimination of the cause, if within the household, and with topical hydrocortisone or calamine lotion.

Pediculosis (lice)

Lice are blood-sucking insects that, using their well-adapted legs and claws, attach to, and lay eggs (nits) in, hair and clothing of humans. There are two types:

- Pubic louse (*Pediculosis pubis*): sexually transmitted and mostly found in young adults (colloquially known as "crabs").
- Body louse: associated with poor social conditions. Spread is by infested bedding or clothing. A variant, the head louse, is quite common in school children and is spread by head to head contact (*Pediculosis capitis*).

Clinical presentation—Intense itching caused by bites results in excoriation and commonly in secondary bacterial infection.

Lice are found in the seams of clothes, and their eggs can often be seen on hair shafts.

Scabies

Scabies is caused by the burrowing of the female mite *Sarcoptes scabei* through the stratum corneum where she lays her eggs. After a few days the eggs hatch into larvae, which moult and mature in the epidermis. The new mites mate in the stratum corneum; the male dies, and the fertilized female burrows and continues the cycle.

Clinical presentation—Very itchy, raised lesions, often red and scaling, typically arise on the sides of fingers, palms, nipples, and genitalia.

Linear tracks (the burrows), about 1 cm long, are often seen, and the mite itself is occasionally visible as a white dot at the end of the burrow.

Itching causes excoriation that frequently results in secondary bacterial infection. Untreated, the condition becomes chronic.

Management—Scabies is transmitted by direct transfer, and, therefore, all contacts require treatment.

Treatment is with topical scabicides applied to the whole body.

Tropical skin infections and infestations

Leprosy

This chronic granulomatous disease is caused by *Mycobacterium leprae*.

Leprosy is rare in the U.S., but it occurs in tropical and subtropical areas with about 10 million patients worldwide.

Transmission is thought to occur by the inhalation of nasal droplets, after which the incubation period may be many years.

The clinicopathological features of leprosy (a.k.a. Hansen's disease) are dependent on the degree of hypersensitivity response (delayed type IV) instigated against the infection by the host.

The spectrum of disease ranges from tuberculoid (strong, cell-meditated immunity) to lepromatous (weak, cell-mediated immunity) forms.

Clinical presentation—*M. leprae* has a predilection for nerves (see Chapter 14) and the skin. Fig. 13.10 shows the skin involvement in the lepromatous and tuberculoid forms of leprosy.

Management is by triple therapy antibiotic treatment continued for at least 2 years.

Leishmaniasis

A common disease in the tropics and subtropics caused by the protozoan *Leishmania*, this is transmitted by sand flies. Three forms of the disease exist, caused by different species of *Leishmania* (Fig. 13.11).

Management—Cutaneous leishmaniasis often heals spontaneously. However, other forms require pentavalent antimony compound intravenously for 10–21 days. Liposomal amphotericin B and fluconazole have proved to be promising alternatives to the highly toxic antimony treatment.

Filariasis

This tropical disease is caused by the nematode worms *Wuchereria bancrofti* and *Brugia malayi*. The worms, which are transmitted by various

Skin involvement in lepromatous and tuberculoid forms of leprosy	
Lepromatous form	**Tuberculoid form**
Minimal immune response (occurs in patients with low cellular immunity)	Vigorous T cell mediated (delayed) hypersensitivity
Bacteremia occurs to peripheral sites	Bacteremia rare
Many skin lesions with symmetrical distribution	Few skin lesions with asymmetrical distribution
Macules, papules, plaques, and nodules	Raised, red plaques with hypopigmented center Sensation is often impaired within the plaque
Typically involves arms, legs, buttock, and face	Often affects the face
Progression causes a thickened, furrowed appearance of face (leonine facies) with eyebrow loss	Progression is slow: combined effect of extensive destruction of tissue by immune response and repeated trauma to desensitized areas results in severe disfigurement, especially to hands and feet
Untreated, this form is lethal due to the impaired immune response	Eventually heals spontaneously

Fig. 13.10 Skin involvement in lepromatous and tuberculoid forms of leprosy.

Different types ofleishmaniasis			
Type of leishmaniasis	**Endemic areas**	**Protozoan**	**Clinical presentation**
Visceral (kala azar)	Asia, Africa, and South America	*Leishmania donovani*	Affects lymphatic system, spleen, and bone marrow, causing splenomegaly, hepatomegaly, anemia, and disability; patchy pigmentation may occur on face, hands, and abdomen
Cutaneous	Mediterranean coast, Middle East, and Asia	*L. tropica*	Characterized by "oriental sore," a red–brown nodule that appears at site of inoculation and which either ulcerates or spreads slowly to form crusty plaque
Mucocutaneous	Central and South America	*L. braziliensis*	Characterized by a skin lesion similar to that of oriental sore but is followed by necrotic ulcers which cause deformity of nose, lips, and palate

Fig. 13.11 Different types of leishmaniasis.

mosquitoes, cause inflammation and eventual blockage of the lymph vessels. The net result is gross edema of the surrounding tissues—elephantiasis—especially of the legs or scrotum.

Larva migrans

Also known as "creeping eruption," this is caused by the larvae of nematode hookworms. Larvae burrow through the skin, leaving intensely itchy tracks in their wake. Treatment is with topical tiabendazole, although the larvae eventually die spontaneously after a few weeks, as they cannot complete their life cycle in humans.

Deep mycoses

These systemic diseases are usually caused by dimorphic fungi. They include:

- Blastomycosis—wart-like ulcers on the face, neck, and limbs.
- Histoplasmosis—lung disease plus granulomata of the skin or tongue.
- Mycetoma—chronic granulomata on the foot.
- Sporotrichosis—chronic subcutaneous skin infection.

Onchocerciasis

This is endemic disease of Africa and Central America caused by the nematode worm *Onchocerca volvulus*, which is transmitted to humans by a biting fly. The worms cause an itchy papular eruption on the skin, which progresses to form fibrous nodules with lichenification and pigmentary change. Microfilariae also invade the eye, resulting in total or partial blindness (called "river blindness" in Africa).

Disorders of specific skin structures

Sweat and the sebaceous structures

Acne vulgaris

This inflammatory disorder of the pilosebaceous glands is characterized by comedones (blackheads and whiteheads), papules, pustules, cysts, and scars. It is extremely common in adolescents, the peak age for clinical acne being 18 years.

Pathogenesis—The cause of acne is uncertain, but the androgen-sensitive sebaceous glands show a hyperresponsiveness to testosterone that results in the following sequence of events:

- Increased sebum excretion.
- Hyperkeratosis of pilosebaceous ducts.

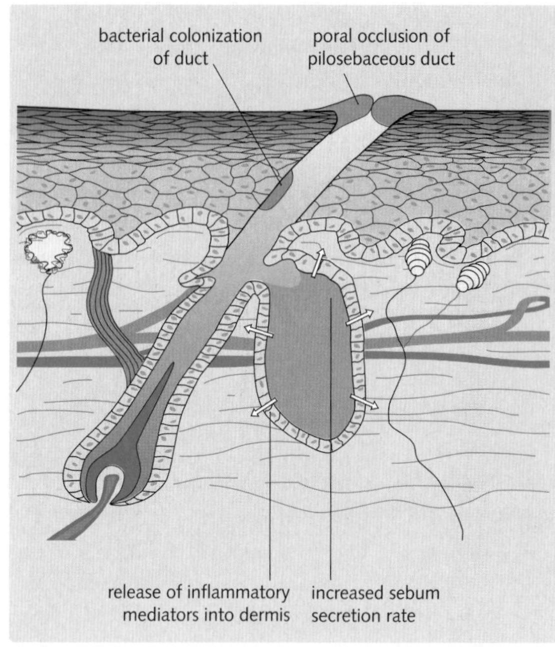

Fig. 13.12 Pathogenesis of acne.

- Blockage of pilosebaceous units with excess keratin and sebum, causing comedo formation.
- Colonization of ducts with *Propionibacterium acnes*.
- Release of inflammatory mediators.

Fig. 13.12 gives a diagrammatical representation of the pathogenesis of acne.

Clinical presentation—Comedones (singular = comedo) are of two types:

- Open as in blackheads: dilated pores with dark plugs of keratin and sebum.
- Closed as in whiteheads: small cream-colored, dome-shaped papules.

The colonization of ducts with *P. acnes* causes the evolution of comedones into inflammatory papules, pustules, or cysts, which often form scars on healing. This may persist until the early 20s and even into the fifth decade of life in a few patients, especially in women.

There is a predilection for areas that have many sebaceous glands—the face, shoulders, back, and upper chest.

Management of acne is shown in Fig. 13.13.

Management of acne vulgaris		
Type	**Treatment**	**Comment**
Topical treatment (mild acne)	Benzoyl peroxide	Reduces numbers of *Propionibacterium acnes* but may cause irritation
	Tretinoin	Reduces number of non-inflamed lesions but may cause irritation
	Antibiotics	Used in treatment of mild or moderate acne
Systemic treatment (moderate or severe acne)	Antibiotics	e.g., Tetracyclines or erythromycin for a minimum of 4 months
	Antiandrogens	Usually combined with an oestrogen and prescribed to females over a period of 6–12 months; suppresses sebum production and is also a contraceptive
	Retinoids	Isotretinoin: reduces sebum excretion, inhibits *P. acnes* and is anti-inflammatory; 4–6 month course; very effective but side effects common

Fig. 13.13 Management of acne vulgaris.

Rosacea

This chronic inflammatory disease of the face is characterized by erythema, telangiectasia, and pustules.

The etiology of rosacea is unknown.

Telangiectatic dilatation of the upper dermal vessels is common, and it causes erythema. Fragments of the mite *Demodex folliculorum* are commonly found in follicles, but its role in the pathogenesis is unclear.

Follicular pustules often develop in the markedly dilated hair follicles.

Rupture of the follicles leads to the development of a florid, lumpy form of rosacea, the result of a giant cell granulomatous reaction in response to follicular content release.

Clinical presentation—It typically affects the middle-aged or elderly, with a slightly higher incidence in women. It may persist for years, and it is often complicated by:

- Rhinophyma—hyperplasia of sebaceous glands and connective tissue of the nose.
- Eye involvement—blepharitis (inflammation of the eyelids) and conjunctivitis.

The condition is exacerbated by sunlight and topical steroids.

Management is by oral antibiotic treatment (e.g., tetracycline or erythromycin). Plastic surgery is required for rhinophyma.

Hair disorders

Alopecia

This is commonly classified into three main types: diffuse nonscarring, localized nonscarring, and scarring (cicatricial).

Diffuse nonscarring

There is a diffuse reduction in hair density. The patient usually notices excessive numbers of hairs on the pillow, brush, or comb.

The causes of diffuse nonscarring alopecia are:

- Male pattern/androgenic alopecia: inherited, androgen-dependent hair loss. Extremely common in men, but it also occurs in women, becoming more pronounced after the menopause.
- Endocrine related: hypo- and hyperthyroidism, pituitary or adrenal underactivity. Androgen-secreting tumors in women can produce male pattern baldness.
- Nutrition related: iron or zinc deficiency, malnutrition—especially kwashiorkor (protein deficiency).
- Telogen effluvium: hair follicles, which are usually out of phase, can, under certain circumstances, become synchronized into the resting phase (telogen) and then be shed in unison 3 months later. The causes of synchronization are high fever, childbirth, surgery, drugs, or stress.
- Drug induced (e.g., with cytotoxics, heparin, warfarin, carbimazole, colchicine, and vitamin A).

Localized nonscarring

There is patchy hair loss. The causes are:

- Alopecia areata: common condition associated with autoimmune disorders in which the growth phase of hair is prematurely arrested.
- Infections (e.g., with scalp ringworm or secondary syphilis).
- Trauma/traction.

It typically presents in the second or third decade of life with bald patches on the scalp, but the eyebrows and beard can also be affected, and the nails may show pitting.

The course is unpredictable, varying from the progressive enlargement of bald patches to the regrowth of hair (more common).

A poor prognosis is indicated if the onset is prepubertal, associated with atopy, or shows extensive involvement.

Rarely, complete scalp alopecia (totalis) or loss of all bodily hair (universalis) occurs.

Scarring (cicatricial) alopecia

This is caused by scarring of the scalp with the destruction of hair follicles.

The causes of scarring are:

- Irradiation/burns (chemical or thermal).
- Infection (e.g., shingles of the ophthalmic division of the trigeminal nerve, kerion, or tertiary syphilis).
- Lichen planus/lupus erythematosus: erythema, scaling, and follicular changes may result in scarring.
- Pseudopelade: end stage of an idiopathic or unidentified destructive inflammatory process in the scalp.

Excess hair

Hirsutism

This is the growth of coarse, pigmented hair with an androgenic distribution in a female.

Fig. 13.14 shows the etiology of hirsutism.

Etiology of hirsutism	
Idiopathic	Most common form; probably due to increased hypersensitivity of end-organ to androgens
Iatrogenic	e.g., Androgens, progestogens
Virilizing tumors	e.g., Ovarian or adrenal tumors
Endocrine disorders	Congenital adrenal hyperplasia, Cushing's syndrome, acromegaly

Fig. 13.14 Etiology of hirsutism.

Hypertrichosis

Excessive growth of hair in a non-androgenic distribution is less common than hirsutism. It can be:

- Localized (e.g., on melanocytic nevi or following topical steroid usage).
- Generalized: fine terminal hair appears on the face, limbs, and trunk. Mostly drug induced, but it can also be caused by anorexia nervosa (or malnutrition), porphyria, cutanea tarda, or underlying malignancy.

Others

Hairshaft defects

These are rare, usually inherited, brittle hair conditions.

Dandruff

This is caused by excessive exfoliation of fine scales from an otherwise normal scalp.

Tinea capitis

Infection of the scalp with dermatophyte (p. 303); may cause scarring alopecia.

Nail disorders

Congenital disease

Congenital conditions are as follows:

- Racket nails: most common congenital nail defect characterized by broad, short, thumb nails.
- Nail–patella syndrome: nails (and patellae) are absent or rudimentary.
- Pachyonychia congenita: thickened, discolored nails present from birth.

Trauma

Traumatic conditions are as follows:

- Subungual hematoma: bleeding under the nail following trapping of a finger- or toenail.
- Splinter hemorrhages: almost always occur with infective endocarditis, but they may also be trauma-induced.
- Ingrowing toenails: usually caused by ill-fitting shoes.
- Onychogryphosis: big toenails become thickened and horn-like, usually in response to trauma.

- Brittle nails: usually due to repeated exposure to detergents and water.

Nail involvement in the dermatoses

These are:

- Alopecia areata: pitting and roughness of nail surface.
- Psoriasis: pitting, nail thickening, onycholysis, brown patches, subungual hyperkeratosis.
- Eczema: pitting and transverse ridging.

Infections

Infections are:

- Tinea unguium: fungal infection of the nails (Fig. 13.15).
- Chronic paronychia: C. *albicans* infection of the nails, common in wetworkers (p. 304).
- Acute paronychia: typically, a bacterial infection of the nails usually caused by staphylococci.

Tumors of the nails

The tumors are:

- Viral warts: common around the nail-fold.
- Periungual fibroma: associated with tuberous sclerosis (see Chapter 14).
- Myxoid cysts: mucous cysts adjacent to the nail-fold that probably arise from folds of synovium.
- Malignant melanoma: subungual malignant melanoma, which produces a pigmented longitudinal streak in a nail, and may cause its destruction.

Nail changes in systemic disease

Fig. 13.15 gives examples of nail changes and their possible causes.

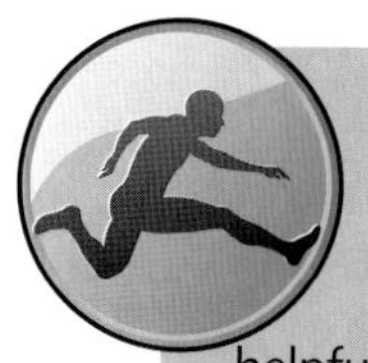

Systemic disorders often cause specific nail changes. A thorough examination of the nails can often be helpful in the diagnosis of a disease.

Disorders of pigmentation

Hypopigmentation

Vitiligo

This common disorder is characterized by the appearance of symmetrical white or pale macules on the skin, which are caused by the patchy loss of pigmentation.

Pathogenesis—Autoimmune disease ofmelanocytes is often associated with otherautoimmune diseases, such as pernicious anemia, thyroid disease, and Addison's disease.

The etiology is unknown, but about 30% of patients have a family history.

Clinical presentation—It affects about 1% of all races, but it is more conspicuous in dark-skinned races.

Onset is usually between 10 and 30 years of age, and it may be precipitated by injury or sunburn.

It commonly affects the hands, wrists, knees, neck, and areas around orifices (e.g., mouth), and it has an unpredictable course ranging from progression to repigmentation (rarely).

Vitiligo is managed with camouflage cosmetics and sunscreens (to reduce contrast between pigmented and non-pigmented skin). Topical steroids occasionally induce repigmentation in darker skins. PUVA (psoralen and UV-A) is occasionally beneficial.

Albinism

This is a rare (1 in 20,000) autosomal recessive disease characterized by the lack of pigmentation in the skin, hair, and eyes. Melanocyte numbers are normal, but melanin production fails because of a deficient or defective enzyme—tyrosinase.

The skin is white, or pink, the hair is white, and pigmentation is lacking in the eye. It is associated with poor sight, photophobia, and nystagmus. Albinos have an increased risk of skin tumors on exposure to UV light.

Prenatal diagnosis is possible.

Phenylketonuria

This autosomal recessive inborn error of metabolism is caused by a deficiency of phenylalanine hydroxylase, which normally converts phenylalanine to tyrosine.

Patients also have fair hair and skin because of impaired melanin synthesis (tyrosine is a precursor of melanin). The concentration of phenylalanine and its metabolites is increased, and this causes damage to the neonatal brain. Untreated, mental retardation and choreoathetosis develop, although a low phenylalanine diet can prevent neurological damage.

The prevalence is 1 per 10,000, and it is detected by routine screening tests.

Nail changes and their possible causes		
Nail change	**Description**	**Possible causes**
Beau's lines	Transverse ridges	Severe illnesses that affect nail growth, e.g., pneumonia or myocardial infarction
Brittle nails	Easily broken nails	Repeated exposure to water/detergent, iron deficiency, hypothyroidism, ischemia of digits
Color change	Black transverse bands Blue Blue-green Brown Brown patches Brown longitudinal streak Red-brown streaks (splinter hemorrhages) White spots White (leakonychea) Yellow Yellow nail syndrome	Cytotoxic drugs Hematoma, cyanosis, antimalarials *Pseudomonas* infection Fungal infection, cigarette stains, chlorpromazine, gold, Addison's disease Psoriasis Melanocytic naevus, malignant melanoma, Addison's disease Infective endocarditis, trauma Trauma to nail matrix (not calcium deficiency) Hypoalbuminemia Psoriasis, tinea unguium, jaundice, tetracycline Defective lymphatic drainage
Clubbing	Swelling of nail with loss of angle between nail-fold and nail plate normal clubbed	Respiratory: pulmonary tuberculosis, bronchiectasis, empyema, lung cancer, fibrosing alveolitis Cardiovascular: infective endocarditis, congenital heart disease Other less common diseases, e.g., asbestosis, Crohn's disease, ulcerative colitis, cirrhosis
Koilonychia	Concave (spoon-shaped) nails	Iron deficiency anemia Repeated exposure to detergents
Nail-fold telangiectasia	Reddened nail-folds caused by dilated capillaries	Inflammatory connective tissue disorders including SLE, systemic sclerosis, and dermatomyositis
Onycholysis	Separation of part or all of nail from its bed	Psoriasis, tinea unguium, trauma, thyrotoxicosis, tetracyclines
Pitting	Small holes in nail-bed	Psoriasis, eczema, alopecia areata, lichen planus
Ridging	Transverse	Beau's lines, eczema, psoriasis, chronic paronychia
	Longitudinal	Secondary to trauma

Fig. 13.15 Nail manifestations of disease and deficiency disorders.

Summary of causes of hypopigmentation		
	Cause	Example
Generalized hypopigmentation	Genetic	Albinism and phenylketonuria
Patchy hypopigmentation	Endocrine	Hypopituitarism (↓ ACTH and ↓ MSH)
	Infective	Leprosy, yaws, pityriasis versicolor
	Postinflammatory	Cryotherapy, eczema, psoriasis, morphea, pityriasis alba
	Chemical	Substituted phenols, hydroquinone
	Other	Vitiligo, lichen sclerosus, halo nevus

Fig. 13.16 Summary of causes of hypopigmentation.

A summary of the causes of hypopigmentation is given in Fig. 13.16.

Hyperpigmentation

Freckles and lentigines

Freckles

Freckles are small, light brown macules that darken on exposure to sunlight. They contain normal numbers of melanocytes, but melanin production is increased. They are common in childhood, especially in fair skinned children. No treatment is required.

Lentigines

Lentigines (also known as lentigos) are similar in appearance to freckles, but they are more scattered and they do not darken in the sun. They contain increased numbers of melanocytes and may develop in childhood, but they are more common in a sun-exposed, elderly skin. They respond to cryotherapy.

Chloasma (melasma)

This photosensitivity reaction in pregnant women (or in women taking oral contraceptives) causes the appearance of symmetrical, ill-defined brown patches on the face. These are caused by estrogen-induced melanocyte stimulation.

Sunscreens and cosmetic camouflage can help mask the brown patches, which usually improve spontaneously.

Drug-induced pigmentation

This can be caused by stimulation of melanogenesis or by drug deposition in the skin. Drugs commonly responsible include amiodarone, bleomycin, psoralens, chlorpromazine, and minocycline.

Other causes

Addison's disease

This is characterized by hypoadrenalism with overproduction of adrenocorticotrophic hormone (ACTH) by the pituitary. ACTH stimulates melanogenesis resulting in hyperpigmentation of mucosae and flexures.

Addisonian-like pigmentation is also seen in Cushing's syndrome, hyperthyroidism, and acromegaly.

Peutz–Jeghers syndrome

This rare, autosomal dominant disorder is characterized by perioral lentigines and intestinal polyps.

Fig. 13.17 provides a summary of the causes of hyperpigmentation.

Blistering disorders

Blisters are fluid-filled spaces within the skin caused by the separation of two layers of tissue and the leakage of plasma into the space. The type of blister formed (Fig. 13.18) depends on the level of separation, and it can be:

- Subcorneal—bullous impetigo or pustular psoriasis.
- Intra-epidermal—acute eczema, herpes simplex/zoster, pemphigus, friction blisters.
- Subepidermal—pemphigoid, dermatitis herpetiformis, cold and thermal injury.

Pemphigus

This rare but potentially fatal group of autoimmune disorders is marked by successive outbreaks of blisters on the skin and in the mouth.

Pathogenesis—Patients have circulating IgG autoantibodies that bind to intercellular junctions in the epidermis. Binding of IgG activates complement, and adjacent keratinocytes are induced to release

Summary of causes of hyperpigmentation	
Cause	**Problem**
Genetic	Inherited: freckles, neurofibromatosis (café-au-lait spots), Peutz-Jeghers syndrome Acquired: lentigines
Endocrine	Chloasma, Addison's disease, Cushing's syndrome, hyperthyroidism, and acromegaly
Metabolic	Biliary cirrhosis (jaundice), hemochromatosis (iron deposition), porphyria
Nutritional	Carotenemia (orange discoloration), malnutrition/malabsorption, pellagra
Postinflammatory	Eczema, lichen planus, systemic sclerosis
Drugs	e.g., Estrogens, amiodarone, bleomycin, psoralens, chlorpromazine, and minocycline
Other	Acanthosis nigricans, malignant melanoma, nevi, argyria (deposition of silver), chronic renal failure

Fig. 13.17 Summary of causes of hyperpigmentation.

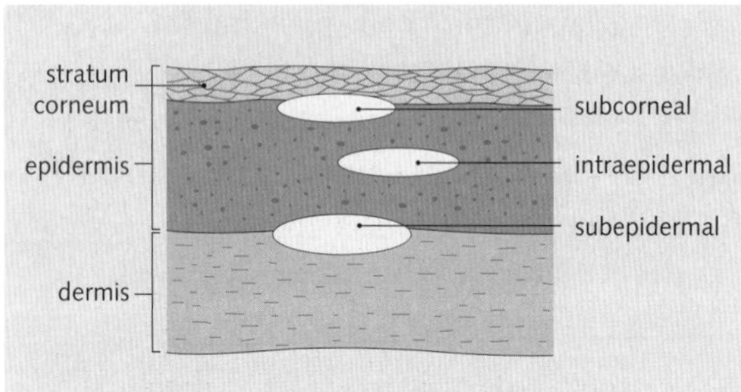

Fig. 13.18 Location of blisters within the skin.

proteolytic enzymes. Cellular adhesion is lost (acantholysis), and an intra-epidermal separation occurs.

This is also associated with other organ-specific autoimmune disorders such as myasthenia gravis.

Clinical presentation—The most common form is pemphigus vulgaris, which typically affects middle-aged people. Oral erosions precede cutaneous blistering in 50% of cases. Flaccid, superficial blisters develop over the scalp, face, back, chest, and flexures.

If left untreated, the blistering is progressive and ultimately fatal (due to the loss of electrolytes and protein). It is managed with systemic steroids and other immunosuppressive agents.

Bullous pemphigoid

This is a chronic, itchy blistering disorder of the elderly.

Pathogenesis—An autoimmune disorder, in which IgG antibodies are deposited at the basement membrane.

Inflammatory cells attracted by complement activation release proteolytic enzymes resulting in subepidermal bullae formation.

Clinical presentation—Large, tense blisters commonly appear on the limbs, trunk, and flexures, but they are occasionally localized to one site, often the lower leg. Oral lesions occur in only 10% of cases. An urticarial eruption may precede the onset of blistering.

The disease is self limiting in about 50% of cases, and it is managed with systemic steroids and other immunosuppressants.

Dermatitis herpetiformis

This presents as a rare eruption of symmetrical itchy blisters on the extensor surfaces.

Etiopathogenesis—The etiology is unknown but associated with celiac disease (gluten hypersensitivity). It is characterized by granular IgA at the dermal papillae of normal-looking skin, and villus atrophy of the small intestine.

It usually presents in the third or fourth decade of life, with males more often affected than females by 2:1. There are groups of small, intensely itchy vesicles on the knees, elbows, scalp, buttocks and shoulders.

Despite villus atrophy in most patients, symptoms of gastrointestinal (GI) disturbances are uncommon. It should be managed with a gluten-free diet with or without dapsone.

A summary of blistering disorders is given in Fig. 13.19.

Summary of blistering disorders			
Disorder	**Type of bullae**	**Autoimmunity**	**Clinical features**
Pemphigus vulgaris	Intra-epidermal	IgG deposited on intercellular junctions	Flaccid, superficial bullae More common in middle-aged High mortality
Bullous pemphigoid	Subepidermal	IgG deposited on basement membrane	Large, tense bullae More common in elderly Self-limiting in about 50% of cases
Dermatitis herpetiformis	Subepidermal	IgA deposited on dermal papillae	Small, itchy vesicles Usually presents in 3rd or 4th decade; males > females Associated with celiac disease

Fig. 13.19 Summary of blistering disorders.

Blistering diseases are rare but important as they can be severe, and they are potentially fatal. Pemphigus vulgaris is the most life threatening type of blistering disorder.

Tumors of the skin

Benign tumors of the skin

Epidermal tumors

Seborrheic keratosis

This common, benign tumor of basal keratinocytes typically occurs on the trunk, face, and arms of the elderly. The etiology of these tumors is unknown:

- Warts are often greasy looking (hence seborrheic), but they are not associated with seborrhea nor with sebaceous glands.
- Usually multiple, and vary in size from a few mm to several cm.
- Progress from lightly pigmented, small papules to darkly pigmented, warty nodules.
- Often have a "pasted on" appearance with well-defined edges.

Microscopically, all lesions show basal cell proliferation, hyperkeratosis, and a variable degree of pigmentation.

Actinic keratosis

This presents as roughened, scaly brownish-to-red lesions, usually less than 1 cm across, which bleed when rubbed. They typically arise on sun-exposed areas, especially the face, scalp, and hands, of the middle-aged and elderly.

Histologically, they show hyperkeratosis and parakeratosis, abnormal keratinocytes with loss of maturation, and a mild to moderate degree of pleomorphism and mitotic figures.

The lesions are considered as premalignant, with 20% of them evolving into squamous cell carcinoma.

Actinic keratosis is also known as solar keratosis or senile keratosis.

Skin tags

These common, benign, pedunculated polyps, a few mm in length, typically affect the elderly or middle-aged, and they have a predilection for the neck, axillae, groin, and eyelids. They consist of a fibrovascular core with an epidermal covering.

Their etiology is unknown, but they are often found in obese individuals.

Cysts

These benign, keratin-filled, firm, skin-colored cysts are normally 1–3cm in diameter.

Common types are epidermal cysts (derived from the epidermis) and pilar cysts (derived from the outer root sheath of the hair follicle). These are often incorrectly grouped together as sebaceous cysts.

Milia

These small, white, keratin cysts, normally 1–2mm in diameter, often affect the eyelids and the upper cheeks. They are common in children, but they can appear at any age. (Milia is the plural of milium.)

Dermal tumors

Dermatofibroma (histiocytoma)

This firm, reddish-brown nodule of about 5–10mm in diameter is common in young adults, females more than males, and usually appears on the lower legs.

Histologically, it consists of intertwining bands of collagen fibres formed by proliferating fibroblasts, with reactive hyperplasia and hyperpigmentation of overlying epidermis. It can be mistaken for a melanocytic nevus or malignant melanoma.

Pyogenic granuloma

A benign, rapidly-growing, bright-red nodule arising mainly on the fingers or face, this typically develops at a site of trauma (e.g., a thorn prick), and it is more common in young adults and children. It is neither pyogenic nor granulomatous, but it is a well-circumscribed dermal lesion of proliferating capillaries and inflammation that closely resembles a hemangioma.

Excision and histological examination are required to rule out malignant melanoma.

Keloid

This is an excessive proliferation of connective tissue occurring in previously injured skin, but extending beyond the margin of the original injury. Characteristics are:

- Firm, smooth, erythematous nodules occurring mainly over the upper back, chest, or ear lobes.
- More common in people of African or Mediterranean descent.
- Highest incidence in second to fourth decades of life.

Treatment is by steroid injection into the keloid.

Campbell De Morgan's spot (cherry angioma)

Small, bright red papules (about 1–2mm diameter) composed of benign capillary proliferations commonly arise on the trunk in elderly or middle-aged patients.

Lipoma

A soft, subcutaneous tumor of mature adipocytes, this is often multiple, and mostly found on the trunk, neck, and upper extremities.

Chondrodermatitis nodularis

This small painful nodule on the upper rim of the pinna occurs usually in elderly men. It is caused by inflammation of the underlying cartilage, and it is not a neoplasm. Excision is curative.

Fig. 13.20 provides a summary of benign skin tumors.

Nevi

Definition

Nevi are benign, colored lesions on the skin formed from a proliferation of one or more of the normal constituent cells of the skin. Though often congenital (birthmarks), they may be acquired.

Melanocytic nevi

These consist of benign collections or nests of melanocytic cells, and they are the most common type of nevus (also known as "moles"). They present in most Caucasians, but they are less prevalent in those with Down syndrome and in people of color.

The etiology of nevi development is unknown, but it seems to be an inherited trait in many families:

- About 1% of nevi are congenital.
- Majority develop during childhood or adolescence; numbers reach a peak at puberty, and they have a tendency to decline during adult life.
- A few new nevi develop during the third and fourth decade of life, especially if provoked by excessive sun exposure or pregnancy.

Nevi can be classified according to the position of the nevus cells within the skin as follows:

Summary of benign skin tumors

Tumor type	Example
Benign epidermal tumors	Viral wart Actinic keratosis Seborrheic keratosis Milia Cysts Skin tags
Benign dermal tumors	Dermatofibroma Melanocytic nevus Cherry angioma Pyogenic granuloma Keloid Lipoma Chondrodermatitis nodularis

Fig. 13.20 Summary of benign skin tumors.

- Junctional nevi: flat macules consisting of rounded nests of melanocytes in the lower epidermis at the dermo-epidermal junction.
- Compound nevi: papules or nodules with an irregular surface, which consist of junctional nests of melanocytes combined with an intradermal mass of melanocytic cells.
- Intradermal nevi: dome-shaped papules/nodules composed entirely of melanocytic cell clusters within the upper dermis (no junctional component present).

These different types of nevi are thought to arise by progression from junctional to intradermal (Fig. 13.21).

Other variants are:

- Congenital nevi: usually over 1 cm in diameter; they may be protuberant or hairy, and they have a risk of malignant change.
- Blue nevi: steely blue intradermal nevus, usually solitary, and most commonly found on the extremities.
- Halo nevi: white halo of depigmentation surrounds nevi. Represents involution of nevus by immune destruction. Mainly seen in children and adolescents.
- Becker's nevi: rare, unilateral lesion on upper back or chest. Initially hyperpigmented, it later becomes hairy. More common in adolescent males.
- Familial dysplastic nevus syndrome: familial condition characterized by large numbers of atypical and "dysplastic" nevi. Affected individuals have a greatly increased risk of developing malignant melanoma.

The majority of nevi are entirely benign, but malignant changes can occur. Junctional components of junctional or compound nevi carry the highest risk for malignancy. Invasion is preceded by nuclear pleomorphism with increased mitoses and cellular atypia. Clinically, malignant nevi appear larger than normal, and they have an irregular edge, surface, and pigmentation.

The management is as follows:

- Increase public awareness about significance of change in pigmented lesions.
- Problematical nevi or nevi with an increased risk of malignant change are excised and sent for histological examination.

Vascular nevi

These common nevi, are usually congenital or developed soon after birth. They are composed of small dermal blood vessels. There are four main types:

- Salmon patch—most common type (present in about 50% of neonates), typically on neck or eyelids. Usually fade quickly.
- Port wine stain nevus—irregular red/purple macule, which often affects one side of the face.
- Capillary hemangioma (strawberry nevus)—red nodular lesion, which develops during the first few weeks of life, reaches its maximum size in the first 12 months, and then involutes. Most cases have regressed by 5–7 years of age.
- Cavernous hemangioma—similar to strawberry nevus but composed of larger and deeper channels and presents as a nodular swelling. Regression is not as complete.

The treatment is by camouflage cosmetics or laser treatments for port wine stains. Strawberry nevi are usually left to involute.

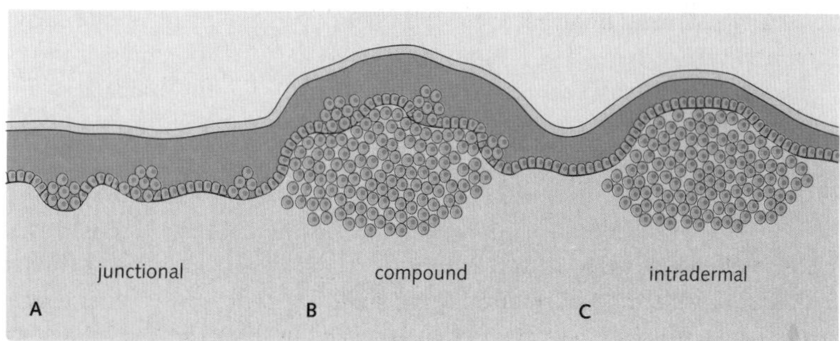

Fig. 13.21 Types of melanocytic nevi.

Summary of nevi	
Type of nevus	**Comments**
Melanocytic	Very common, usually multiple, pigmented, and benign Consist of nests of melanocytic cells Classified into junctional, compound, and intradermal Types are congenital, blue, halo, Becker's, and dysplastic
Vascular	Common, usually congenital, composed of small dermal blood vessels Types are salmon patch, port wine stain, capillary hemangioma ("strawberry"), cavernous hemangioma
Epidermal	Warty, pigmented, and often linear
Connective tissue	Rare, skin-colored, collagenous nevi

Fig. 13.22 Summary of nevi.

Epidermal nevi

These warty, pigmented and often elongated nevi are usually congenital or develop in early childhood. Most are a few cm long, but they can be extensive.

Treatment is by excision, but recurrence is common.

Connective tissue nevi

Rare, skin-colored papules composed of coarse collagen bundles in the dermis, these are common in tuberous sclerosis.

Fig. 13.22 provides a summary of nevi.

Malignant melanoma (melanocarcinoma)

This malignant tumor of melanocytes usually arises in the skin. Incidence in the U.S. is 10 per 100,000 per year, but it is rising steadily. Females are more often affected than males by 2:1.

It occurs in all races, but it is more common in caucasoids, with an incidence that is proportional to geographical latitude, suggesting an effect of UV radiation. The most common site in males is on the back, but in females it is the lower leg.

The etiology is unknown, but repeated exposure to UV radiation is thought to play an important role.

Major risk factors for the development of malignant melanoma (with decreasing risk) are:

- Familial dysplastic nevus syndrome.
- Multiple melanocytic nevi (50 nevi over 2mm in diameter).
- Congenital nevus.
- Previous malignant melanoma.
- Immunosuppression.
- Fair skin.

Classification

Four main types of malignant melanoma are recognized.

Superficial spreading malignant melanoma

A flat tumor with variable pigmentation and irregular edges, this is the most common type, accounting for 50% of all cases. There is a female preponderance, and it is most common on the lower leg.

Lentigo malignant melanoma

A nodular lesion arising in a pre-existing lentigo maligna, this typically occurs in sun-damaged skin of the face in elderly patients. It comprises about 15% of cases.

(The lentigo maligna is similar to a benign lentigine but it is generally larger, at over 2cm, and it has atypical melanocytes.)

Acral lentiginous malignant melanoma

This resembles the lentigo malignant melanoma, but it affects the palms, soles, and nail-beds (subungual melanoma). It comprises 10% of U.S. cases, but it is the most common form of malignantmelanoma in oriental people. It is often diagnosed late and consequently has poor survival figures.

Nodular malignant melanoma

A pigmented nodule that may grow rapidly and ulcerate, this accounts for 25% of melanomas, and it is more common in males, typically arising on the trunk.

Staging and prognosis of malignant melanoma

Local invasion of the malignant melanoma is assessed using the Breslow method (Fig. 13.23). The Breslow thickness is the measured thickness in mm (on a histological section) from the granular layer of the epidermis to the deepest identifiable melanoma cell.

The Breslow thickness is directly related to the risk of metastasis (Fig. 13.24). Tumors are divided into one of three prognostic groups—good, intermediate, or poor—depending on their Breslow thickness.

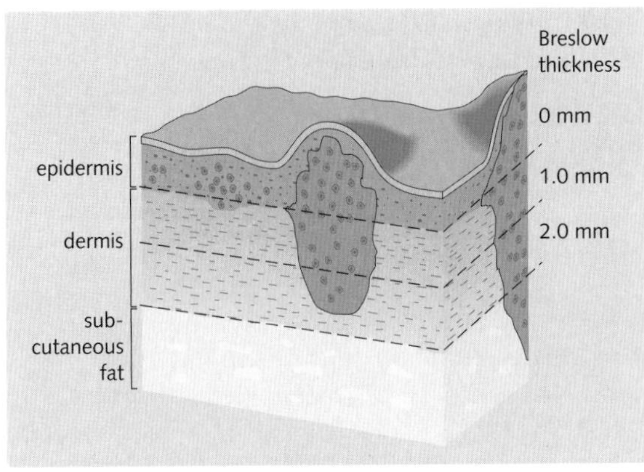

Fig. 13.23 Staging of malignant melanomas.

Diagnosis—One or more of following changes observed or reported in a nevus or pigmented lesion may suggest malignant melanoma:

- Size: usually increased.
- Shape: irregular outline.
- Color: irregular pigmentation.
- Inflammation: at the edge of lesion.
- Crusting: oozing or bleeding lesion.
- Itchiness: a common symptom.

The differential diagnosis of malignant melanoma includes:

- Benign lentigine.
- Benign melanocytic nevi.
- Dermatofibroma.
- Hemangioma.
- Pigmented basal cell carcinoma.
- Seborrheic wart.

Management is by surgical excision with regular follow-up to detect recurrence, which may be:

- Local: at edge of excised site.
- Lymphatic: in regional lymph nodes or in lymphatics between tumor and nodes.
- At distant sites: due to hematogenous spread.

Malignant epidermal tumors

Basal cell carcinoma (rodent ulcer)

A malignant tumor that arises from the basal keratinocytes of the epidermis, this is the most common form of skin cancer, typically seen on the face in elderly or middle-aged subjects, with a male preponderance.

Tumors are locally very invasive, but they almost never metastasize.

Risk factors for the development of basal cell carcinoma include:

- Repeated UV exposure: tumors are more common in light-skinned races, with increasing incidence toward the Equator.
- X-ray irradiation.
- Chronic scarring.
- Genetic predisposition.

Tumors are typically composed of basophilic cells that invade the dermis, as well-defined lobules and islands of cells.

Clinical presentation—They typically occur on sun-exposed sites, commonly around the nose, inner canthus of the eyelids, and the temple.

Tumors grow slowly but relentlessly and they may destroy underlying cartilage, bone, and soft tissue structures.

There are three main types of basal cell carcinoma:

- Nodular: most common form. Skin-colored nodule, which may show numerous telangiectatic vessels and a glistening pearly edge. Often has central ulceration with an adherent crust.
- Superficial (or multicentric): flat, red plaque often with an irregular rim-like edge, and light pigmentation. Often multiple, and occasionally seen on the trunk.
- Morpheic: flat, thickened, whitish yellowish plaque with indistinct edges. These may have focal areas of ulceration.

Five-year survival rates for malignant melanomas of different Breslow thickness

Prognosis	Breslow thickness (mm)	5-year survival rate (%)
Good	<1.0	93
Intermediate	1–3.5	67
Poor	>3.5	31

Fig. 13.24 Five-year survival rates for malignant melanomas of different Breslow thickness.

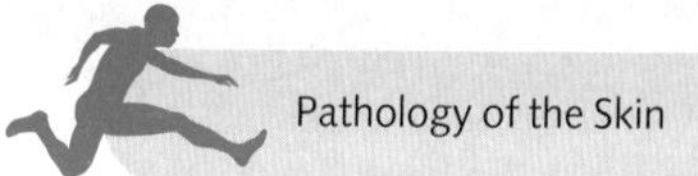

Management—Complete excision is usually the best treatment, but it is not always possible. Radiotherapy is often used for non-excisable tumors. Recurrence is about 5% at 5 years for most methods of treatment.

Squamous cell carcinoma

This malignant tumor is derived from keratinocytes of the upper layers of the epidermis, and typically seen on the face in elderly or middle-aged subjects, with a male preponderance. Tumors are locally invasive and they may also metastasize.

Its etiology is related to:

- Chronic sunlight exposure.
- Chemical carcinogens (e.g., tar, arsenic, and machine oil).
- X-ray radiation.
- Chronic ulceration and scarring.
- Smoking (lip lesions).
- Common wart virus with immunosuppression.
- Genetic (e.g., xeroderma pigmentosum).

Histologically, tumors consist of disorganized keratinocytes with typical malignant cytology, which destroy the dermo-epidermal junction and form invading strands into the dermis. Foci of keratinization are seen within the tumor.

The clinical presentation is:

- Dome-shaped nodules, which usually arise in sun-exposed sites such as the face, neck, forearm, or hand.
- Nodules typically develop into roughened keratotic areas, ulcers, or horns.
- Often difficult to distinguish from keratoacanthomas.
- Less aggressive form may arise within actinic keratosis as a small papule, which progresses to ulcerate and then crust over.
- More aggressive forms may arise at the edge of chronic skin ulcers (rare).

Management—The treatment of choice is surgical excision. Radiotherapy can be used for carcinomas of the face or scalp in the elderly.

There are only two skin neoplasms in which metastasis is a common feature:

- Malignant melanoma tumor of melanocytes, which metastasizes early.
- Squamous cell carcinoma tumor of upper epidermal keratinocytes, which metastasizes late.

Both are epidermal in origin.

Intra-epidermal carcinoma (Bowen's disease)

This carcinoma in situ typically occurs on the lower leg in elderly women. Its predisposition is associated with previous exposure to arsenicals. It is characterized by:

- Slowly extending, pink or lightly pigmented, scaly plaques up to several cm in size.
- Atypical keratinocytes throughout whole thickness of the epidermis with prominent nuclear pleomorphism, and large numbers of mitoses.

Carcinomas usually remain in situ for many years, but they have the capacity to transform into squamous cell carcinomas.

Other tumors of the skin

Keratoacanthoma

This benign, self-limiting tumor typically arises on the face of elderly people. It grows very rapidly, changing from a small, red papule to a large, domed nodule with raised edges and a central mass of keratin within a few weeks. It resembles a squamous cell carcinoma, but it does not invade deeply and never metastasizes.

The majority spontaneously regress within a few months.

Mycosis fungoides (cutaneous T cell lymphoma)

This rare, slowly progressive (years) tumor of CD4+ (T helper) lymphocytes evolves in the skin. No fungal infection is involved, despite the name. There are four stages:

- Premycotic phase: erythematous eczematoid lesions. May persist for 10 or more years.
- Infiltrative phase: plaques develop, typicallyaffecting the trunk. This stage may last for years.
- Fungoid phase: tumor nodules or ulcers develop within the plaques. Has a mean survival time of 2.5 years.
- Systemic disease: involvement of lymph nodes or internal organs.

Dermatofibrosarcoma

This is a locally invasive dermal tumor of proliferating myofibroblasts with low-grade malignancy. It is similar in appearance to dermatofibromas but more aggressive in nature, and characterized by protuberant nodules on the epidermis. It has a tendency to recur following excision.

Kaposi's sarcoma

This malignant disorder is characterized by bluish-brown plaques or nodules formed from a proliferation of small blood vessels and spindle cells in the dermis.

Intradermal hemorrhage with hemosiderin deposition occurs within the nodules.

It commonly occurs in association with acquiredimmune deficiency syndrome (AIDS) but is also endemic in certain African regions withcytomegalovirus. The lesions may be single ormultiple, and they have a tendency to metastasize.

- Describe the histological changes that occur in psoriasis.
- Describe the histological changes that occur in eczema/dermatitis.
- Name the bacterial groups that commonly cause skin disease.
- Describe the skin conditions caused by each category of bacteria.
- Outline the clinical presentation of four common viral skin diseases.
- Name the body sites that can be infected by dermatophytes.
- Describe the pathogenesis of acne and its distribution on the body.
- State the three main categories of alopecia and their causes.
- What are the causes of excess hair?
- List the causes of generalized and patchy hypopigmentation.
- Describe the differences between freckles and lentigines.
- Categorize the causes of hyperpigmentation.
- What are the main characteristics of pemphigus vulgaris?
- Compare and contrast the pathogenesis of pemphigus and pemphigoid.
- Describe the pathogenesis and clinical presentation of dermatitis herpetiformis.
- Name the benign tumors of the epidermis and dermis.
- Describe the classification of melanocytic nevi.
- State the main risk factors for the development of malignant melanoma.
- What are the four clinical types of malignant melanoma?
- Describe the malignant tumors of the epidermis.

14. Pathology of the Nervous System

Disorders of the central nervous system

Common pathological features

Intracranial herniation

Intracranial herniation is the movement of part of the brain from one space to another with resultant damage. It usually occurs following a critical increase in intracranial pressure caused by an expanding lesion (e.g., tumor or hematoma). However, it may be inadvertently precipitated by withdrawing cerebrospinal fluid (CSF) at lumbar puncture.

Fig. 14.1 shows a diagrammatical representation of the sites of intracranial herniation.

Cerebral edema

This is an abnormal accumulation of fluid in the cerebral parenchyma. It is usually the result of breakdown of the blood–brain barrier, and it may occur following damage initiated by several different causes:

- Ischemia (e.g., from infarction).
- Trauma (e.g., from head injury).
- Inflammation encephalitis or meningitis.
- Cerebral tumors (primary or secondary).
- Metabolic disturbances (e.g., hyponatremia or hypoglycemia).

The condition results in cerebral swelling, and it is associated with raised intracranial pressure.

Treatment is by minimizing the formation of edema by use of osmotic agents or steroids.

Hydrocephalus

Hydrocephalus is an increase in the volume of CSF within the brain resulting in the expansion of the cerebral ventricles. It can occur by one of three mechanisms:

- Obstruction to flow of CSF (most common form).
- Impaired absorption of CSF at arachnoid villi (rare).
- Overproduction of CSF by choroid plexus neoplasms (very rare).

Obstructive hydrocephalus is either congenital or acquired.

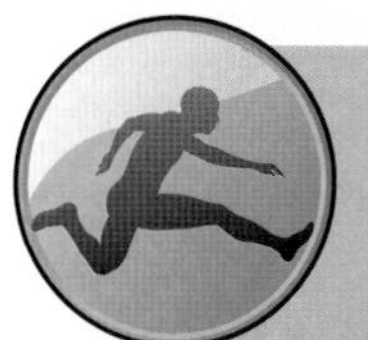

Obstructive hydrocephalus is by far the most common form of hydrocephalus. It is commonly subdivided into:

- Noncommunicating hydrocephalus—obstruction within the ventricular system leading to blockage of CSF flow from the ventricles to the subarachnoid space.
- Communicating hydrocephalus—extraventricular obstruction within subarachnoid space.

Congenital hydrocephalus

This occurs in 1 per 1000 births. The principal causes are congenital malformations, for example:

- Arnold–Chiari malformation (see p. 323).
- Congenital stenosis of the cerebral aqueduct.
- Atresia of the foramina of Magendie and Luschka (Dandy–Walker syndrome).
- Some genetic causes associated with X-linked inheritance.

Acquired hydrocephalus

This may result from any lesion that obstructs the CSF pathway such as:

- Tumors—especially if located in the posterior fossa, as the fourth ventricle aqueducts are easily obstructed.
- Scarring—postinflammatory fibrosis of the meninges at exit foramina, following meningitis or subarachnoid hemorrhage.
- Hemorrhage—intraventricular or in the posterior fossa.

Diagnosis

Severe forms of congenital hydrocephalus may be diagnosed antenatally via ultrasound. Less severe forms may present with considerably enlarged heads at birth.

In acquired hydrocephalus, enlargement of the head is prevented by the inability of the skull to expand, but this leads to massive dilatation of the

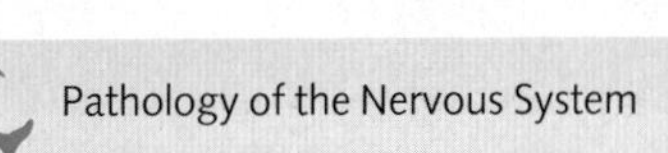

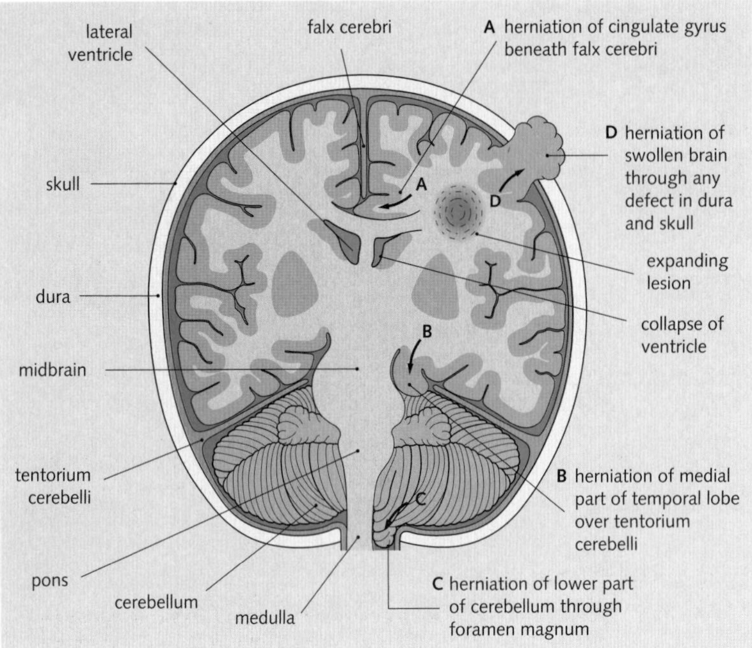

Fig. 14.1 Sites of intracranial herniation. (A) Herniation of the cingulate gyrus beneath the falx cerebri. (B) Herniation of the medial part of the temporal lobe over the tentorium cerebelli. (C) Herniation of the lower part of the cerebellum through the foramen magnum. (D) Herniation of swollen brain through any defect in the dura and skull.

ventricles resulting in increased intracranial pressure.

Associated features are dementia with gait disturbances and incontinence.

Treatment and management

A ventricular shunt with one-way valve system can be inserted to drain CSF into the peritoneum.

Prognosis

Untreated patients may suffer irreversible brain damage, and the condition is often fatal.

Special types of hydrocephalus

Secondary or compensatory hydrocephalus

Here, an increase in CSF occurs as a compensatory measure following loss of brain tissue (e.g., due to infarction or atrophy). There is no associated increase in CSF pressure.

Normal pressure hydrocephalus (intermittent pressure hydrocephalus)

This is a rare condition of progressive dementia associated with ventricular dilatation. Random sampling shows normal CSF pressure, but continuous monitoring reveals intermittent increases.

Malformations, developmental disease, and perinatal injury

Neural tube defects and posterior fossa abnormalities

The etiology of central nervous system (CNS) malformations includes genetic factors, maternal infections, toxicity, metabolic factors, and irradiation *in utero*. Neural tube defects are the commonest congenital abnormalities of the CNS, and they are caused by defective closure of the midline structures over the neural tube. Screening for neural tube defects can be performed with ultrasound or by measurement of α-fetoprotein in the maternal serum or amniotic fluid. This is raised in 90% of cases. Posterior fossa abnormalities are the second most common development abnormality of the CNS. Fig. 14.2 illustrates the types of congenital abnormalities.

Syringomyelia and hydromyelia

Syringomyelia is a rare condition in which a cyst (syrinx) develops within the spinal cord, usually posterior to the central canal (Fig. 14.3). The cavity is lined by gliosis (astrocytes). It is most common in the cervical spinal cord, but it may extend into the medulla (syringobulbia).

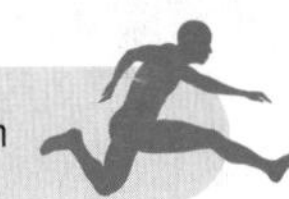

Fig. 14.2 Types of congenital abnormality.

Types of congenital abnormality	
Condition	**Features**
Neural tube defects with cranial involvement	
Anencephaly	Absence of the cranial vault and failure in the development of the cerebral hemispheres
Encephalocele	Ossification defects in the bones of the skull results in herniation of the brain and meninges. Most common form is occipital
Neural tube defects with spinal involvement	
Spina bifida occulta	Abnormal development of the vertebral arches but the cord and meninges are normal. Usually asymptomatic
Spina bifida cystica	Presents as either meningomyelocele (90% of cases) or meningocele (10% of cases). Abnormal development of the vertebral arches results in cystic outpouching
Posterior fossa abnormalities	
Arnold–Chiari malformation	Prolongation of the cerebellum downwards through the foramen magnum often resulting in obstructive hydrocephalus
Dandy–Walker malformation	Obstruction of the foramina of Luschka and Magendie (exit of the fourth ventricle) results in the formation of a cyst-like structure between the cerebellar hemispheres

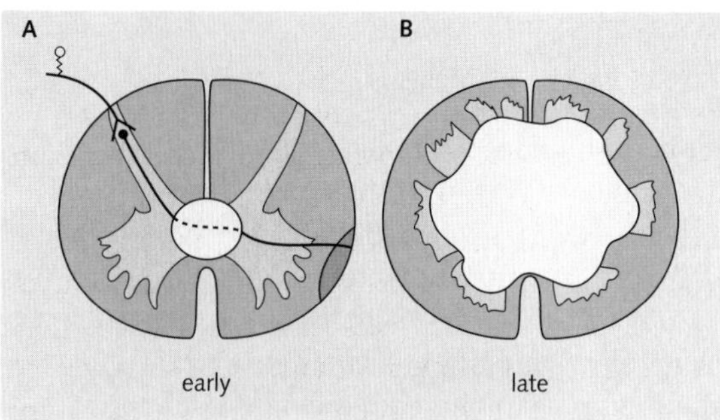

Fig. 14.3 Syringomyelia. (A) Early effects: damage to the decussating sensory fibers, with loss of temperature and touch in local segments. (B) Late effects: destruction of grey matter and gradual affection of long tracts with loss of local reflexes, severe sensory loss, and spastic paralysis.

Hydromyelia is the term used to denote cases in which the dilatated central canal contains CSF, and is lined by ependyma.

The causes of these conditions are either:

- Acquired (majority of cases)—secondary to trauma or ischemia or occurring in association with tumors of the spinal cord.
- Congenital—may be associated with maldevelopment of the cord or other developmental abnormalities of the craniocervical junction, especially in Arnold–Chiari syndrome.

The clinical manifestations are muscle weakness and atrophy in the upper limbs due to compression of the anterior horn cells. There is loss of the sensations of pain and temperature, but preservation of those of position and vibration, due to damage to nerve fibers crossing the cord in the lateral spinothalamic tracts.

Surgery may arrest or alleviate symptoms by decompression or by draining the fluid in the cystic cavity.

Perinatal injury

Cerebral palsy

Cerebral palsy describes brain malformation or damage affecting motor areas of the brain. It is the leading cause of crippling handicap in children, affecting 2 per 1000 live births. Damage may occur during fetal life, may be birth related, or may occur postnatally (Fig. 14.4).

Causes of cerebral palsy
Cerebral malformation Cerebrovascular accident Hypoglycemia Hypoxia Infection Kernicterus (bilirubin-induced brain damage) Poisoning Toxins Trauma (peri- and postnatal)

Fig. 14.4 Types of cerebral palsy and their associated characteristics.

Types of cerebral palsy and their associated characteristics

Type	Characteristics
Spastic cerebral palsy (70%)	Hypertonia, ankle clonus, and extensor plantar response
Dystonic (athetoid) cerebral palsy (10%)	Irregular, involuntary muscle movements
Ataxic cerebral palsy (10%)	Hypotonia, weakness, uncoordinated movements, and intention tremor
Mixed cerebral palsy (10%)	—

Fig. 14.5 Causes of cerebral palsy.

The different types of cerebral palsy are outlined in Fig. 14.5.

Ischemia and hypoxia

Ischemia and hypoxia are major causes of severe perinatal brain damage. Perinatal hypoxia is usually due to asphyxiation associated with the trauma of birth, whereas perinatal ischemia is commonly caused by intracranial hemorrhages.

Premature infants are highly susceptible to developing intracranial hemorrhages because of disturbances in the cerebral circulation possibly caused by *in-utero* hypoxia/ischemia.

In full-term infants, intracranial hemorrhages with the formation of small hematomas may occur during difficult deliveries, although this is less common now because of improved obstetric care.

Mortality is high; one third of survivors may develop cerebral palsy, epilepsy, or mental retardation.

Traumatic injuries to the central nervous system

Skull fractures

Skull fractures occur in approximately 80% of fatal cases of head injuries. The most common are linear fractures of the vault of the skull (62%); such fractures may extend into the base of the skull causing cranial nerve laceration.

The other types of skull fracture are:

- Penetrating—increased risk of infection due to tearing of the dura.
- Compound—increased risk of infection due to laceration of the scalp and tearing of the dura.
- Depressed—increased incidence of epilepsy.
- Comminuted (fragmented)—increased incidence of massive brain damage.

Parenchymal damage

Concussion

This is an abrupt transient loss of consciousness due to temporal neuronal dysfunction following a relatively slight impact. It is caused by an enormous, but short-lived, increase in pressure within the cranium at time of impact. Full recovery usually ensues, although repeated concussion may result in permanent brain damage.

Contusions and lacerations

A contusion is a bruise with extravasation of blood but with the pia-arachnoid intact. A laceration is where the pia-arachnoid is torn.

Both are focal types of brain damage occurring at the moment of injury, caused by striking the brain against adjacent bone. They are most common at the frontal and occipital poles and mainly affect the crests of gyri. Both lesions are characteristically hemorrhagic.

Types of contusion:

- Fracture contusion—occurs at the site of fracture.
- Coup contusion—occurs at point of impact in absence of fracture.
- Contrecoup contusion—occurs diametrically opposite to the site of impact.
- Herniation contusion—occurs when the hippocampi or cerebellar tonsils (or both) are impacted and bruised by the free edge of the tentorium and foramen magnum, respectively.

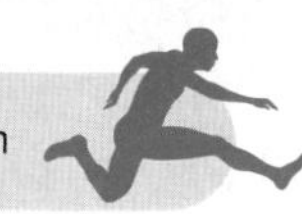

- Gliding contusion—occurs at the superior margins of the cerebral hemispheres; usually caused by interference of the dura with a rotational movement of the brain.

Diffuse axonal injury

The condition is produced as a result of rotational movements of the brain within the skull during angular acceleration or deceleration. It often occurs in the absence of any skull fracture or cerebral contusions.

There are two main features:

- Small hemorrhagic lesions in the corpus callosum and the dorso-lateral quadrant of brainstem (macroscopic).
- Widespread tearing of axons (microscopic).

This type of injury occurs in almost 50% of patients with a severe head injury, and in almost all fatal head injuries. It is associated with head injuries involving vehicular accidents.

Traumatic vascular injury

Bleeding from craniocerebral trauma is often associated with high mortality, and it may take place in one or more of the potential spaces surrounding the brain, e.g., extradural and subdural.

Extradural (epidural) hemorrhage

This type occurs in 2% of all head injuries and in 15% of fatal cases. Hemorrhage occurs between the skull and dura, and gradually stripping dura from bone forming a large, saucer-shaped hematoma (Fig. 14.6).

This injury is almost always the result of skull fracture, usually a linear fracture of the thin squamous part of the temporal bone, which contains the middle meningeal artery (a branch of the maxillary artery).

It is associated with a post-traumatic lucid interval of several hours followed by a rapid increase in intracranial pressure.

Subdural hemorrhage

Hemorrhage occurs between the dura and the outer surface of the arachnoid membrane. It is usually caused by a rupture of the small bridging veins or the venous sinuses. The resulting hematoma is often extensive because of the loose attachment of the dura and arachnoid membranes.

Subdural hemorrhage may be acute or chronic.

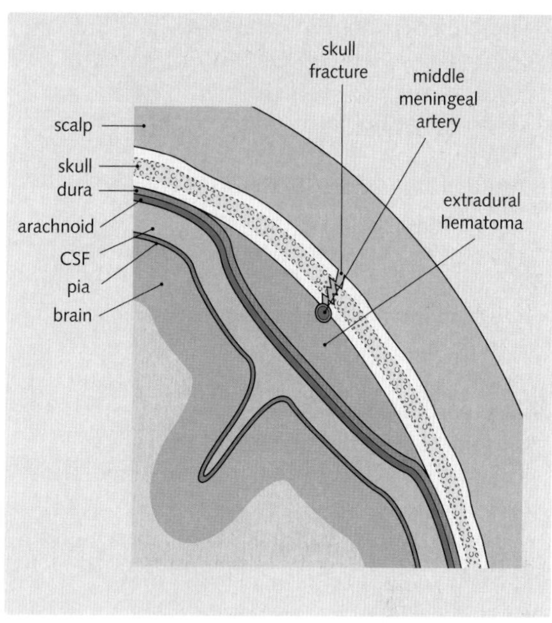

Fig. 14.6 Extradural hemorrhage. (Redrawn from *Pathology* by A. Stevens and J. Lowe, Mosby.)

Acute subdural hemorrhage is associated with:

- Severe head injury, subarachnoid hemorrhage, and cerebral contusions.
- A rapid increase in intracranial pressure.

Chronic subdural hemorrhage has the following characteristics:

- More common in the very young and elderly.
- Usually occurs as a result of minimal trauma, or as a result of cerebral atrophy (in the elderly), which causes a gradual widening of the subdural space leading to rupture of the bridging veins.
- Blood typically accumulates slowly over a period of days or weeks.
- Presents with personality change, memory loss, and confusion.

Subarachnoid hemorrhage

Arterial rupture is usually secondary to superficial contusions or lacerations of the brain. Small amounts of blood can be disposed of by arachnoid granulations. Larger hemorrhages cause arachnoid fibrosis leading to meningeal irritation and raised intracranial pressure. It can also occur as a result of hypertension, aneurysms, embolisms, or infarction.

Intracerebral hemorrhage

This is caused by direct rupture of the intrinsic cerebral vessels at the time of injury.

Resulting hematomas are classified into three types:

- Solitary—occur in association with cortical contusions; common in temporal and frontal poles.
- Multiple—associated with severe contrecoup lesions; often fatal.
- Burst lobe—intracerebral or intracerebellar hematoma in continuity with subdural hematoma; most common in temporal and frontal lobes; rapidly fatal.

Spinal cord injuries

Most spinal injuries occur in males aged under 40 years. Road traffic accidents account for more than 80% of such injuries.

There are two types of spinal cord injuries—open and closed.

Open injuries

These are rare, and they are a result of direct trauma to the spinal cord and nerve roots. They can be either perforating (i.e., with extensive disruption and hemorrhage) or penetrating (i.e., with incomplete cord transection—Brown–Séquard's syndrome).

Closed injuries

These are in the majority, and they are associated with fracture or dislocation of the spinal column causing compression of the cord by distortion of the spinal canal.

Primary damage:

- Contusions.
- Nerve fiber transection.
- Hemorrhagic necrosis.

Secondary damage:

- Extradural hematoma.
- Infarction.
- Infection.
- Edema.

The consequences depend mainly on the site and severity of the lesion. Cervical lesions result in tetraplegia; lower thoracic lesions result in paraplegia.

Cerebrovascular disease

Cerebrovascular disease is the third leading cause of death in the U.S.

Stroke is a common outcome of cerebrovascular disease, and it is defined as a sudden event in which a neurological deficit occurs over minutes or hours and lasts for longer than 24 hours.

If CNS disturbance lasts for less than 24 hours, then the condition is termed a transient ischemic attack.

The incidence is 1 or 2 per 1000 per year, but it is much higher in the elderly, affecting males more than females.

Causes of stroke are:

- Cerebral infarction (80%).
- Intracerebral hemorrhage (10%).
- Subarachnoid hemorrhage (10%).

Pathological effects occur because of extensive hypoxic neuronal damage. The area of brain affected can be readily localized since the blood supply of the brain has a fairly constant anatomic distribution. Fig. 14.7 shows the territories of the major arteries.

Clinical features of stroke depend on localization and the nature of the lesion. Risk factors are atheroma, heart disease, hypertension, and diabetes mellitus.

Hypoxia, ischemia and infarction

Cerebral infarction is the process whereby a focal area of necrosis is produced in the brain in response to a decreased supply of oxygen (and glucose) in the territory of a cerebral arterial branch.

There are two main causes of infarction:

- Hypoxia—the reduction of oxygen supply to tissues despite an adequate blood supply, e.g., following respiratory arrest.
- Ischemia—blood supply to tissues is absent, or severely reduced, usually as a result of constriction or obstruction of a blood vessel.

Ischemia accounts for the majority of cases of cerebral infarction.

Mechanisms of ischemia

Ischemia may be caused by:

- Vascular diseas (e.g., thrombosis, embolic occlusion, or vasculitis).
- Cardiac disease (e.g., prolonged hypotension or cardiac embolism)
- Trauma (head injury leading to vascular occlusion, dissection, or rupture).

Infarcted tissue becomes swollen and soft with the loss of definition between gray and white matter. The infarcted tissue undergoes liquefactive necrosis

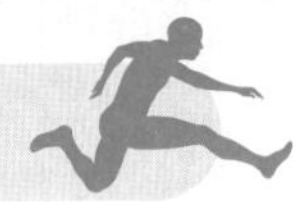

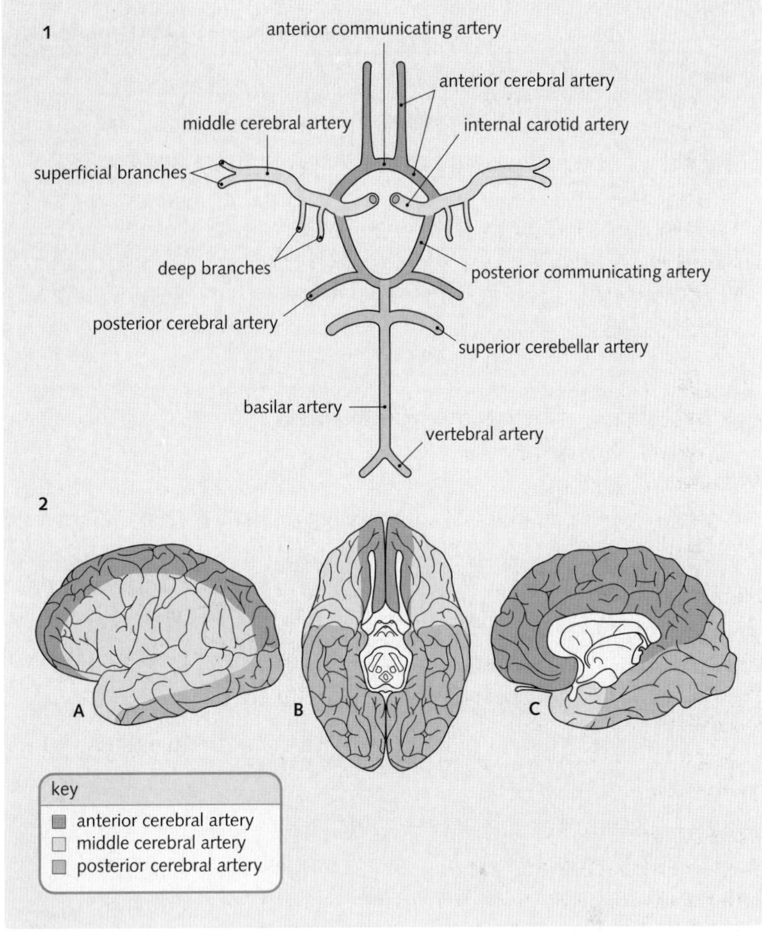

Fig. 14.7 Territories of the major arteries. (1) Main cerebral arteries forming circle of Willis. (2) Their territories: (A) Lateral view. (B) Inferior view. (C) Medial view. (Reproduced from *Anderson's Pathology*, Damjanov, ed, Mosby.)

and shows microglial macrophage infiltration. Eventually, the necrotic tissue is completely phagocytosed to leave a fluid-filled cystic cavity with a gliotic wall. Fig. 14.8 shows the macroscopic and microscopic pathological features of cerebral infarction.

Strokes caused by cerebral infarction clinically present with slowly evolving signs and symptoms.

Atraumatic hemorrhage

Intracerebral hemorrhage The majority of intracerebral hemorrhages are thought to arise from Charcot–Bouchard microaneurysms associated with hypertension and diabetic vascular disease. These hemorrhages occur most frequently in the basal ganglia (80%), brainstem, cerebellum, and cerebral cortex.

The resulting hematoma acts as a space-occupying lesion leading to increased intracranial pressure and herniation. The clinical picture is often indistinguishable from a cerebral infarction, but the raised intracranial pressure commonly gives rise to sudden headache, vomiting, and impairment of consciousness. Mortality is about 80%.

Subarachnoid hemorrhage This can occur at any age, but it is an important cause of death and disability in the 20–40 year age group. The majority of subarachnoid hemorrhages are caused by saccular berry aneurysms, which develop at proximal branch points in the major cerebral vessels on the circle of Willis (Fig. 14.9).

These aneurysms occur in 1–2% of the population, but they are more common in the elderly and hypertensives.

The clinical picture is one of sudden onset of severe headache accompanied by neck pain/stiffness and vomiting. Only 30–40% survive for a few hours; among those who survive longer, there is a 30% mortality rate within the first month.

Pathological features of cerebral infarction		
Time	**Macroscopic**	**Microscopic**
Before 24h	No naked eye abnormalities	Some neuronal damage
After 24h	Softening and swelling (edema) of affected tissue	Line of demarcation between normal and abnormal myelin in white matter
After a few days	Necrotic tissue	Infiltrating macrophages Proliferating astrocytes and capillaries
After weeks/months	Fluid-filled cystic cavity with gliotic wall	Necrotic tissue removed Thickened capillary walls Only astrocytes remain

Fig. 14.8 Pathological features of cerebral infarction.

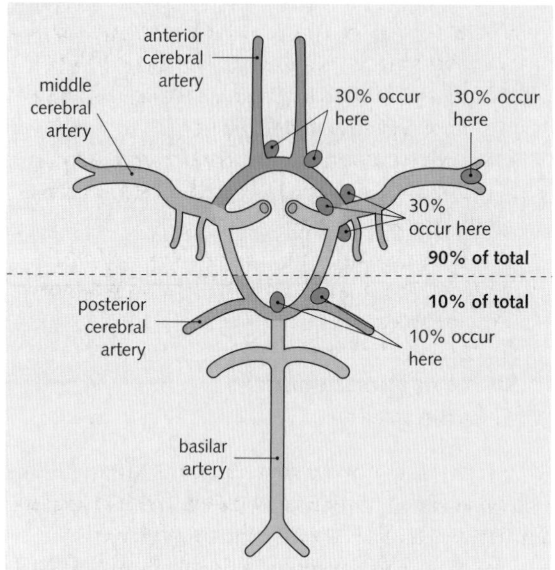

Fig. 14.9 Berry aneurysms—approximate frequency and distribution. The dotted line separates anterior from posterior circulation. (Redrawn from *Anderson's Pathology*, Damjanov, ed, Mosby.)

Hypertensive cerebrovascular disease

Systemic hypertension can affect the CNS resulting in neurological dysfunction, thus:

- Atheroma of the larger cerebral vessels leads to a loss of autoregulation of cerebral blood flow.
- Aneurysms, both saccular and microaneurysms, may cause spontaneous intracerebral hemorrhage.
- Encephalopathy—pathogenesis is uncertain but damage to the blood–brain barrier leads to forced cerebral hyperperfusion.

Infections of the central nervous system

Bacterial meningitis

Meningitis refers to inflammation of the meninges. There are two classes: leptomeningitis with inflammation centred on the subarachnoid space, and pachymeningitis with inflammation centered on the dura.

There are four possible mechanisms of meningeal infection:

- Direct spread: from penetrating trauma (e.g., compound skull fractures) or adjacent focus of infection (e.g., sinusitis, middle ear, or mastoid infection).
- Bloodborne spread: from septicemia or septic emboli from other infections such as bacterial endocarditis.
- Iatrogenic infection: following the introduction of organisms into CSF at lumbar puncture.
- Congenital abnormalities (e.g., meningomyeloceles).

Acute pyogenic (bacterial) meningitis

This is infection of the leptomeninges—pia and arachnoid mater—and the CSF, which diffusely affects the whole meninges and subarachnoid space.

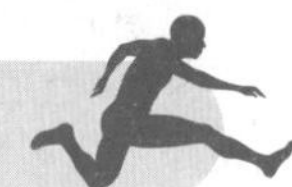

Fig. 14.10 Meningitis-causing bacteria.

Meningitis-causing bacteria			
Neonates	**Infants**	**Young adults**	**Elderly**
Escherichia coli *Group B Streptococcus* *Listeria monocytogenes*	*Neisseria meningitidis* *Hemophilus influenzae* *Streptococcus pneumoniae*	*N. meningitidis* *S. pneumoniae*	*S. pneumoniae* *N. meningitidis* *L. monocytogenes*

Organisms that typically cause this condition vary between age groups (Fig. 14.10).

The clinical features are headache, drowsiness, vomiting, fever, petechial rash, and neck stiffness.

The complications are:

- Ventriculitis.
- Intracerebral abscess (see below).
- Cerebral infarction.
- Subdural empyema.
- Epilepsy.
- Disseminated intravascular coagulation (DIC).
- Adrenal hemorrhage.

Diagnosis and management—The CSF is cloudy due to increased numbers of neutrophils (>1000 cells/mm^3). CSF protein levels increase and glucose concentrations fall. Treatment is with vigorous antibiotic therapy.

Prognosis—Mortality ranges from 3% for *Hemophilus influenzae* to 60% for *Streptococcus pneumoniae*, and it is highest in the very young and the elderly.

Aseptic (viral) meningitis

This is the most common cause of meningitis. It is a benign and self-limiting illness, usually less severe than bacterial meningitis. It may occur as a complication of viral infection, e.g., mumps or measles.

Common causative organisms

The common causative organisms are enteroviruses (e.g., echoviruses, coxsackie viruses, and polioviruses) and mumps virus.

The illness clinically presents with acute onset of headache, irritability, and rapid development of meningeal irritation.

Diagnosis and management—The CSF is clear and colorless. It contains excess lymphocytes but normal glucose and protein. Treatment involves control of symptoms only.

Prognosis—Complete recovery usually occurs without specific therapy.

Brain abscess

A brain abscess is a severe focal infection of the brain and is typically 1–2cm across. It starts as an area of cerebritis—inflammation of the brain parenchyma—and develops into a pus-filled cavity walled off by gliosis and surrounded by cerebral edema. It often results in raised intracranial pressure.

The etiology of brain abscesses is as follows:

- Middle ear infection (60%)—temporal lobe and cerebellar abscesses.
- Frontal sinusitis (20%)—frontal lobe abscess.
- Bacteremia/septicemia (10%)—usually frontal lobe abscess.
- Penetrating skull trauma.
- Secondary to meningitis.
- Unknown causes.

Common causative organisms are *Viridans streptococcus*, *Staphylococcus aureus*, and *Klebsiella*, but it may also be caused by fungal infection.

The clinical presentation is similar to that of acute bacterial meningitis but focal neurological signs, epilepsy, and fever are common manifestations.

Complications include:

- Meningitis.
- Intracranial herniation.
- Focal neurological deficit.
- Epilepsy.

Treatment is with antibiotic therapy at an early stage, with surgical aspiration or excision of the capsule.

Prognosis—Overall mortality is about 10%.

Subdural empyema

This is a collection of pus in the subdural space and it is relatively uncommon. In adults it usually results from frontal sinusitis, whereas in infants it is usually secondary to meningitis.

Clinically, patients with subdural empyema are usually very ill. The pus spreads rapidly on the surface of a hemisphere, producing hemiparesis, raised intracranial pressure, fits, and meningism.

Chronic meningoencephalitis

Tuberculous meningitis

This is meningitis due to infection by *Mycobacterium tuberculosis*. It is rare in the U.S. but a major problem in developing countries.

The disorder is almost always secondary to tuberculosis elsewhere in the body; infection usually reaches the CNS via the bloodstream.

Pathogenesis—Granulomatous inflammation affects the basal meninges, large arteries and cranial nerves.

It presents clinically with slow-onset, subacute meningitis. It may be accompanied by isolated cranial nerve palsies.

Hydrocephalus may result from impaired reabsorption of CSF or obstruction of CSF outflow from the fourth ventricle.

CSF shows an initial increase in polymorphs, then an increase in lymphocytes.

Prognosis—Untreated, the disease is usually fatal. Intensive treatment with antituberculous drugs lowers mortality to 15–20%.

Chronic meningitis

This is a rare condition, which usually occurs in the middle-aged and elderly. *Neisseria meningitidis* is the most common cause. The patient can be unwell for weeks or even months with recurrent fever, sweating, joint pains, and transient rash.

Neurosyphilis

This is caused by invasion of the CNS by *Treponema pallidum* weeks, months, or years after initial infection. Meningitic illness occurs in only approximately 25% of cases of syphilis. It is usually mild or even asymptomatic, but it may be severe with transient cranial nerve palsies and convulsions.

Lyme disease

This disorder is caused by the tick-borne spirochete *Borrelia burgdorferi*. It is a systemic illness characterized by skin lesions and neurological features.

Viral encephalitis

This is a virally induced diffuse inflammation of the brain, which is usually concomitant with inflammation of the meninges. It is a common complication of many viral illnesses. Common causative viruses are:

- Arboviruses.
- Herpes simplex virus I and II.
- Measles.
- Cytomegalovirus.
- Polio and enterovirus.
- Rabies.
- Human immunodeficiency virus (HIV).

Most cases are mild and self-limiting. However, some cases (e.g., those involving herpes simplex virus type I and rabies) result in extensive tissue destruction and may be fatal.

Mortality for the more severe type is 50%, and the majority of survivors have severe, permanent brain damage. Rabies is virtually 100% fatal.

Fungal infections

These are relatively rare and occur mainly in the immunosuppressed (e.g., associated with chemotherapy, steroid treatment, acquired immune deficiency syndrome—AIDS), but some organisms (e.g., *Cryptococcus neoformans*) can produce disease in the absence of immunosuppression.

The spread can be hematogenous (e.g., from the lungs, which is the most common) or direct (e.g., from the nose and paranasal sinuses, which is rare).

Causative organisms are:

- *Cryptococcus neoformans*—fungal meningitis.
- *Aspergillus fumigatus*—fungal abscesses usually accompanied by pulmonary infection.
- *Candida albicans*—fungal abscesses.
- Phycomycosis—thrombosis and associated infarction; commonly affects uncontrolled diabetics.

Protozoal infection

Toxoplasmosis

This is caused by infection with *Toxoplasma gondii*. It may be acquired by eating poorly-cooked infected meat or food contaminated with feline feces. It has two forms: congenital and acquired.

The incidence of congenital toxoplasmosis shows geographical variation, ranging from 1 per 4000 births in the U.S. to 1 per 100 births in France. This geographical variation is probably due to the habit of eating raw or rare meat in France. The organism may be transmitted to the fetus through the placenta during maternal infection.

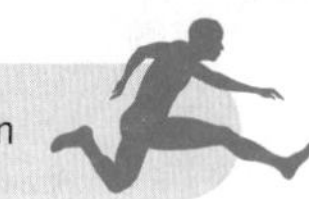

Congenital infection can cause:

- Abortion or stillbirth.
- Severe brain damage leading to early death.
- Moderate brain damage and chorioretinitis; compatible with life but with permanent disability.

Acquired toxoplasmosis is the most common opportunistic infection of the CNS in adults with AIDS. It results in:

- Necrotizing cerebritis.
- Chronic abscesses.
- Meningoencephalitis.

However, in healthy subjects, it rarely causes cerebral symptoms.

Other protozoan organisms that may cause infection of the CNS are:

- Amoebae.
- *Plasmodium falciparum*.
- Trypanosomes.

Progressive multifocal leukoencephalopathy

Multifocal destruction of oligodendrocytes results in demyelination with minimal inflammation and minimal damage to axons. It is caused by the DNA JC papovavirus, and it occurs in association with underlying diseases such as AIDS, chronic lymphocytic leukemia, carcinoma, and systemic lupus erythematosus.

Patients present with progressive dementia. The disease is progressive and death usually occurs within a few months.

Subacute sclerosing panencephalopathy

This subacute encephalitis occurring in children is due to persistent measles infection. It presents with progressive neurological dementia, and death usually occurs within two years of onset.

Spongiform encephalitis (Creutzfeldt–Jakob disease)

This is rapidly progressive dementia, ataxia, and myoclonus, and it is rare in the U.S. (at 1 per 1,000,000 per year). The infectious agent is not precisely known, but it is most likely to be non-nucleic acid transmission by prion (or proteinaceous infectious agent) protein (see page 34). The condition has an incubation period of up to 30 years but it is always fatal, usually within 6 months of onset.

A recently described variant in the U.K. appears to be the human manifestation of bovine spongiform encephalopathy ("mad cow disease").

Demyelination and degeneration

Demyelinating diseases

This group of diseases has a common factor of primary damage to myelin of nerves while the axons and nerve cells remain relatively intact.

Multiple sclerosis

Multiple sclerosis (MS) is the most common demyelinating disorder of the CNS, affecting 50 per 100,000 in the U.S. Peak incidence is between 20 and 40 years with a slight female predominance.

MS is characterized by relapsing and remitting episodes of immunologically mediated demyelination within the CNS. Recovery from each episode of demyelination is usually incomplete, leading to progressive deterioration. There is an association between the disease and certain HLA antigens (A3, B7, DR2, and DQ1). However, the etiology is unknown. Current theories are:

- Myelin abnormality.
- Autoimmune disorder.
- Toxin damage.
- Viral infection of the CNS (e.g., measles).

Pathogenesis—Acute demyelination occurs in the central white matter in discrete areas known as plaques. Abnormalities are confined to the CNS; the peripheral nervous system (PNS) is usually spared. Common sites are the optic nerve, brainstem, cerebellum, periventricular regions, and cervical spinal cord.

Fig. 14.11 gives a list of the clinical manifestations of MS and their causes.

Diagnosis and management—Clinical evaluation and computed tomography (CT) and magnetic resonance imaging (MRI) scans can show areas of demyelination within the brain. CSF examination shows increased lymphoid cells and oligoclonal bands of IgG. There is no specific treatment but corticosteroids may accelerate remission in relapse. Beta-interferon has also been used to some success.

The disease's progress is variable. In about 5% of patients, the disease is rapidly progressive and fatal within 5 years. However, others may survive for more than 20 years with only minor disability.

Clinical manifestations of MS and their causes	
Manifestations	**Causes**
Early clinical symptoms	
• blurring of vision	Optic nerve disease
• incoordination	Cerebellar peduncle disease
• abnormal sensation	Disease of long ascending sensory tracts
Late stages	
• blindness, paraplegia, and incontinence	Spinal tract involvement
• ataxia	Spinal and cerebellar involvement
• intellectual dysfunction	Loss of hemispheric white matter

Fig. 14.11 Clinical manifestations of multiple sclerosis (MS) and their causes.

Degenerative disorders

Cortical

Alzheimer's disease This is the most common cause of dementia in Western countries. In the U.S. it affects 5% of people over 65 years, and 15% of people over 80 years; females more than males. Also of significance is the subgroup of early onset patients (40–60 years). Genetic studies have shown that there is an increase in incidence of sporadic cases in individuals with ApoEe4 genotype on chromosome 19. The amyloid precursor protein (APP) gene on chromosome 21 has been implicated in the familial cases.

However, the etiology and pathogenesis are unknown. Some cases (5%) are familial, but most (95%) are sporadic. Current theories involve:

- Infectious agents.
- Toxins (e.g., aluminum).
- Traumatic injury.

Macroscopically, there is marked atrophy, especially of the frontal lobes; the brain is reduced in weight to 1000g or less (normal average = 1400g). There is a loss of cortical gray and white matter.

Histological hallmarks are as follows:

- Senile plaques—composed of an extracellular core of amyloid protein (10–150nm diameter) surrounded by dystrophic neurites; occur most frequently in the hippocampus, cerebral cortex, and deep grey matter.
- Neurofibrillary tangles—abnormal tangles of insoluble cytoskeletal-like proteins (paired helical filaments) that form within the neurons of the brain.
- Neuropil threads—distorted, twisted and dilated dendritic processes and axons of cerebral cortex found around amyloid plaques.

Clinically, there is failure of memory and disturbance of emotions.

Prognosis—Progressive physical decline with poor food intake and inability to walk. Death is commonly due to the development of pneumonia.

Basal ganglia

Parkinsonism This term is used to refer to patients whose clinical presentation is one of akinetic rigidity and resting tremor. The causes are:

- Parkinson's disease.
- Postencephalitic parkinsonism.
- Neuroleptic drugs.
- Cerebral anoxia.

Parkinson's disease This is characterized by rest tremor, slowness of voluntary movement, and rigidity. It occurs in 1 per 1000 adults but 1 per 200 over the age of 65. The etiology is unknown.

Pathogenesis:

- The disorder shows degeneration of pigmented dopaminergic neurons of the substantia nigra, the locus caeruleus, and several other brainstem nuclei.
- Degeneration of these cells causes disease by reducing the amount of dopamine in the corpus striatum.
- Surviving cells in the substantia nigra contain eosinophilic spherical inclusions (Lewy bodies), which contain cytoskeletal filaments.

The disease can be symptomatically treated with drugs, such as L-dopa, that correct neurotransmitter imbalance. Eventually, there is failure of response to treatment, and patients die from wasting and poor nutritional intake.

Motor neuron disease A progressive neurodegenerative disease characterized by the

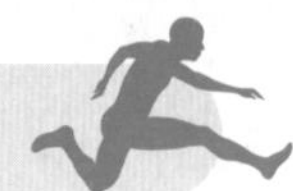

Fig. 14.12 Additional types of degenerative disease.

Additional types of degenerative disease	
Degenerative disorder	**Features**
Pick's disease	Progressive dementia with severe memory and speech loss. Atrophy of cortex in areas of the frontal and temporal lobes. Surviving neurons contain Pick's bodies
Huntington's disease	Autosomal dominant disorder (trinucleotide repeat, chromosome 4) characterized by chorea and progressive dementia. Cerebral atrophy in the caudate nucleus and putamen
Friedreich's ataxia	Autosomal recessive spinocerebellar disease. Degeneration of the posterior columns, corticospinal, and spinocerebellar tracts

selective loss of motor neurons from the spinal cord, brainstem, and motor cortex. Its prevalence is 5 per 100,000 of the population, with male incidence greater than female. In the U.S., motor neuron disease is known as Lou Gehrig's disease.

The majority of cases are sporadic but 5% of cases are familial—mutation of superoxide dismutase gene.

It eventually progresses to severe paralysis with loss of swallowing and respiration, leading to death in 2–3 years.

Other degenerative disorders are considered in Fig. 14.12.

Metabolic disorders and toxins

Vitamin deficiencies

Vitamin B_1 (thiamine) deficiency

This is common in chronic alcoholics, resulting in:

- Wernicke's encephalopathy: memory impairment, ataxia, visual disturbances, and peripheral neuropathy.
- Korsakoff's psychosis: confused state, memory loss, and confabulation.

If both occur, it is known as Wernicke–Korsakoff syndrome.

Vitamin B_{12} (cyanocobalamin) deficiency

This produces weakness and paraesthesia in the lower limbs resulting from subacute combined degeneration of the spinal cord (Fig. 14.13). Replacement therapy at an early stage reverses the degenerative process, but long-standing cases show irreversible axonal damage with reactive gliosis.

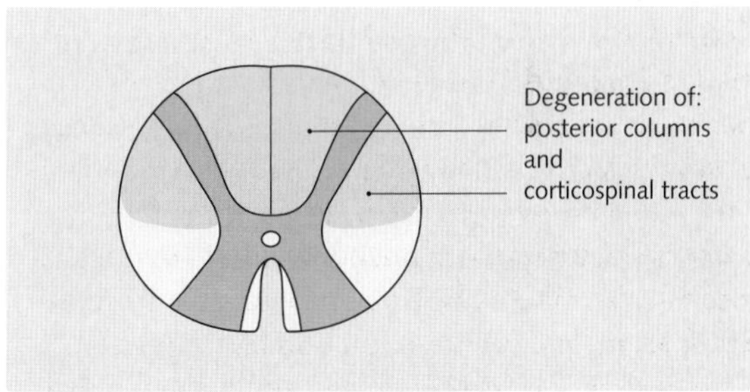

Fig. 14.13 Subacute combined degeneration of the spinal cord. Degeneration of posterior columns leads to sensory loss (vibration and proprioception) causing ataxia. Degeneration of corticospinal tracts leads to upper motor neuron damage causing spastic paralysis.

Iodine deficiency

Severe iodine deficiency causes hypothyroidism; it is the most important endocrine disorder to affect the CNS in children. In the fetus, severe iodine deficiency causes cretinism characterized by dwarfism, mental defect, and spastic diplegia. This can be prevented by iodine supplements during pregnancy.

Toxins

Carbon monoxide

Carbon monoxide (CO) binds irreversibly to hemoglobin, rendering erythrocytes incapable of oxygen transport. CO poisoning, therefore, results in brain damage due to hypoxia. This poisoning may be accidental or associated with attempted suicide.

The amount of carbon monoxide-bound hemoglobin (HbCO) with corresponding clinical symptoms are as follows:

- 20%—Dyspnea and slight headache.
- 30%—Severe headache, fatigue, and impaired judgment.
- 60–70%—Loss of consciousness.
- 70%—Rapidly fatal.

Pathogenesis—Hypoxia results in neuronal necrosis with a predilection for globus pallidus. Other selectively vulnerable regions are the hippocampus, and cerebral and cerebellar cortices.

Methanol

Methanol is highly toxic to the CNS. It is lipid soluble, so it readily diffuses into the CSF and aqueous humor in concentrations higher than in plasma.

Methanol is metabolized into formic acid and formaldehyde. It is the formaldehyde that is thought to be the mediator of toxic effects. There are two types of methanol poisoning:

- Acute—sudden death with multiple hemorrhagic lesions in the cerebral hemispheres.
- Chronic—atrophy of retinal ganglion cells with secondary degeneration of the optic nerve.

Ethanol

The consequences of excessive ethanol intake on the CNS are manifold (Fig. 14.14).

Neoplasms of the central nervous system

Gliomas

Gliomas are tumors that arise from glial supportive tissue of brain. They are the most common primary brain tumors, accounting for 50% of all CNS tumors.

Astrocytoma

This is a glioma derived from astrocytes, and it is more common in children, usually occurring in the cerebellum. It accounts for 10% of all primary tumors in adults, usually in the cerebral hemispheres.

Common types of astrocytomas and their corresponding tumor grading:

- Benign juvenile pilocytic astrocytoma (grade I).
- Astrocytoma (grade I/II).
- Inaplastic astrocytoma (grade III).
- Glioblastoma multiforme (grade IV).

Prognosis depends on the degree of tumor differentiation and the size of the neoplasm. For example:

- Grade I: survival times of 20–30 years are possible.
- Grade IV: 20% survive for 1 year.

Oligodendrogliomas

These ill-defined, slow-growing tumors arise from oligodendrocytes in the white matter of the cerebral hemispheres, especially the temporal lobe. They account for 5% of all primary CNS neoplasms in adults, but they are rare in children.

The prognosis is relatively good.

Ependymoma

These tumors arise from the ependymal cells lining the ventricle and central canal of the spinal cord.

Consequences of excess ethanol intake on the central nervous system		
Disease	**Features**	**Mechanism**
Fetal alcohol syndrome	Cerebral malformations Facial and somatic malformations Growth retardation	Direct toxicity
Acute intoxication	Cerebral edema Petechial hemorrhages	Direct toxicity
Cerebral and cerebellar atrophy	Neuronal loss	Direct toxicity
Nutritional disorders	Wernicke's encephalopathy	Deficiency of vitamin B_1
Hepatocerebral syndromes	Hepatic encephalopathy Chronic hepatocerebral degeneration	Hepatic toxicity with secondary effects on CNS
Demyelinating disorders	Central pontine myelinolysis	Electrolyte disturbances

Fig. 14.14 Consequences of excess ethanol intake on the CNS. (Adapted from Underwood, 2000.)

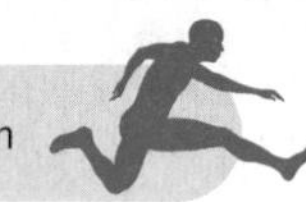

Ependymoma is the most common tumor of the spinal cord, accounting for 5% of all primary CNS neoplasms. It is common in children and young adults.

Medulloblastoma

This tumor of primitive neuroepithelial cells arises in the cerebellum in children, in whom it is the most common CNS tumor. It is malignant, with a rapid growth rate; obstruction of the fourth ventricle results in hydrocephalus.

Other tumors

Primary brain lymphomas

Associated with immunosuppression, especially AIDS, most primary brain lymphomas are high grade, non-Hodgkin's lymphomas of B cell type with a poor prognosis.

Germ cell tumors

These rare tumors are seen mainly in children; males more than females. Most arise near the pineal or pituitary gland, and they behave as malignant teratomas.

Meningiomas

These account for approximately 15% of adult intracranial tumors; females more than males. Tumors arise from the arachnoid mater, and they are usually benign but may invade adjacent bone resulting in erosion and hyperosteosis. Meningiomas produce symptoms by compression of brain tissue rather than by invasion.

Metastatic tumors

The CNS is a common site for metastasis, and tumors are usually multiple. They may arise from hematogenous or direct spread. The cerebellum is the preferred site, but they can affect any part of the brain as well as other intracranial structures, especially meninges (hence malignant meningitis). Metastases often occur at the boundary between grey and white matter.

The most common neoplasms to metastasize to the CNS are:

- Breast carcinomas.
- Bronchus carcinomas.
- Kidney carcinomas.
- Colon carcinomas.
- Malignant melanoma.

Disorders of the peripheral nervous system

Disorders of peripheral nerves are termed neuropathies, and they can be predominantly sensory, predominantly motor, or mixed depending on which nerves are affected.

Hereditary neuropathies

Hereditary motor and sensory neuropathies (HMSN)

Peroneal muscular atrophy (HMSN I + II; Charcot–Marie–Tooth disease)

This disorder is characterized by pronounced atrophy of the calf muscles with associated sensory deficits as a result of slowly progressive symmetric neuropathy. It is the commonest of the hereditary neuropathies, and it is usually autosomal dominant. It impedes ambulation and causes foot deformities (pes cavus), but it does not shorten the lifespan.

Fig. 14.15 provides a table of the different types of peroneal muscular atrophy and their characteristics.

Different types of peroneal muscular atrophy and their characteristics

	HMSN I	HMSN II
Type of neuropathy	Demyelinating neuropathy	Axonal neuropathy
Relative occurrence	75%	25%
Type of axonal loss	Large caliber axons	Large and small caliber axons
Nerve conduction velocity	Impaired (<30m/s)	Normal (>45m/s)
Time of onset	Early (first decade)	Later (second decade)
Effects	Severe distal wasting in legs	Weakness and wasting less marked

Fig. 14.15 Different types of peroneal muscular atrophy and their characteristics.

Dejerine–Sottas disease (HMSN III)

This severe, chronically progressive symmetric peripheral neuropathy is caused by hypertrophy of peripheral nerves, followed by gradual axon degeneration. There is delayed onset of motor skills (e.g., in walking) and gradual progression to wheelchair confinement in young adult life.

Hereditary sensory and autonomic neuropathies (HSAN)

This group of autosomal inherited diseases produce mainly sensory and autonomic neuropathies. There are three major types as described in Fig. 14.16.

Traumatic neuropathies

Lacerations

Laceration refers to a jagged tear of the peripheral nerve in which there is partial or complete loss of continuity of the nerve. It occurs most commonly from a penetrating injury such as a knife wound, or a misplaced intramuscular injection, or from bone fractures.

Note that:

- Disorders affecting many peripheral nerves are termed polyneuropathies, and they usually cause symmetrical deficits.
- Disorders affecting only one (mononeuropathy) or a few (multiple mononeuropathies) peripheral nerves typically cause asymmetrical deficits.
- Radiculopathies are disorders of nerve roots.

Avulsion

This is the tearing of nerve fibers from the surface of the spinal cord or from a muscle. It may be partial or complete depending on whether all or only some of the rootlets contributing to the spinal nerve are involved.

Nerve roots may be avulsed from the spinal cord in two ways:

- Tensile stresses from cervical plexus transmitted centrally can stretch and finally avulse the nerve roots.
- A spinal cord injury, such that displacement of the cord acts directly on the nerve roots between their attachment to the cord and their entry into the intravertebral foramen.

Both laceration and avulsion injuries cause the severed ends of the damaged nerve to retract and then to undergo Wallerian degeneration forming a traumatic neuroma. Subsequently, the proximal portion of the nerve develops neuritic sprouts which, if sited in proximity to the severed distal nerve, may reinnervate by regrowth along the nerve sheath.

If continuity of the nerve is completely interrupted, basal laminae sheaths no longer form continuous tubes to guide regeneration sprouts and so the potential for recovery is limited.

Compression/entrapment neuropathy

Compressed nerves undergo segmental demyelination with decreased nerve conduction velocity. If compression is prolonged or severe, axonal degeneration may occur. Symptoms of nerve compression are paresthesia, anesthesia, and loss of muscle strength.

Types of hereditary sensory and autonomic neuropathies (HSANs)

	HSAN I	HSAN II	HSAN III
Clinical syndrome	Ulcerative acropathy due to numbness	Congenital sensory neuropathy	Familial dysautonomia
Eponym	Morvan's	Giacci's	Riley–Day
Inheritance	Autosomal dominant	Autosomal recessive	Autosomal recessive
Affected neurons	Degeneration of large myelinated fibers of both peripheral nerves and posterior columns of spinal cord	Degeneration of large and small myelinated fibers	Degeneration of non-myelinated fibers with preservation of myelinated fibers Loss of neurons of autonomic ganglia

Fig. 14.16 Types of hereditary sensory and autonomic neuropathy.

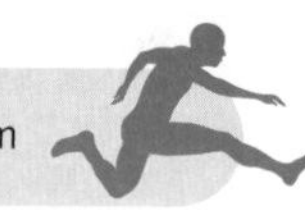

> Common sites of nerve compression are:
> - Nerve roots in the intervertebral foramina by prolapsed intervertebral discs or osteophytes due to osteoarthritis of the spine.
> - Median nerve in carpal tunnel at the wrist.
> - Ulnar nerve in flexor carpal tunnel at medial epicondyle of humerus.
> - Common peroneal nerve at the neck of the fibula.

Carpal tunnel syndrome

This is a disorder in which the size of the carpal tunnel is significantly reduced causing compression of the median nerve. Causes include inflammation of the flexor retinaculum, arthritic changes, etc.

Saturday night palsy

Radial nerve compression (in the middle of the arm), which may result from improper positioning of the upper limb during sleeping, especially in intoxicated persons.

Inflammatory neuropathies

Guillain–Barré syndrome (acute inflammatory demyelinating polyradiculopathy)

This is the most common form of acute neuropathy caused by immune-mediated demyelination of peripheral nerves, usually occurring 2–4 weeks after viral illness or vaccination.

Affected patients develop motor neuropathy with lesser sensory changes due to widespread demyelination of the peripheral nerves. Recovery (i.e., remyelination) occurs over 3–4 months and is usually complete.

Infectious neuropathies

Leprosy (Hansen's disease)

A chronic granulomatous disease caused by *Mycobacterium leprae*. It is the most common cause of peripheral neuritis worldwide, affecting about 10 million patients in total.

The clinicopathological features of leprosy are dependent on the host's response to infection, with a spectrum of disease ranging from tuberculoid to lepromatous form (Fig. 14.17).

Varicella-zoster virus (VZV)

An invasion of cutaneous sensory nerves during primary infection with VZV (chickenpox) leads to infection of the dorsal root ganglia where the virus

Comparison of peripheral nerve damage by lepromatous and tuberculoid forms of leprosy

	Lepromatous	Tuberculoid
Immune mechanism	Minimal immune response (occurs in patients with low cellular immunity)	Vigorous T cell mediated (delayed) hypersensitivity
Spread of organisms	Bacteremia occurs in peripheral sites	Bacteremia rare
Distribution in nerves	Widely disseminated diffuse nerve involvement	One or a few sites (asymmetrical)
Nerve enlargement and damage	Intense infiltration of nerves by vacuolated macrophages	Hallmark of nerve involvement is discrete, well-formed granulomas
Neurological deficit	Sensory and motor involvement Patchy loss of sensation	Sensory, motor, and autonomic involvement Peripheral nerve palsies Anesthetic areas prone to injury and secondary infection
Prognosis	Progressive and lethal	Progression slow, but immune response produces extensive destruction of tissue resulting in severe disfigurement Eventually heals spontaneously

Fig. 14.17 Comparison of peripheral nerve damage by lepromatous and tuberculoid forms of leprosy.

enters a latent state. Reactivation of VZV may occur years later causing shingles. The reason for reactivation is unknown, but there is increased incidence in the immunocompromised.

In shingles, VZV migrates down the nerves into the skin and causes vesicular lesions identical to those of chickenpox but confined to one or two adjacent dermatomes usually on the trunk.

Metabolic and toxic neuropathies

Peripheral neuropathy of diabetes mellitus

This occurs in both type 1 and 2 diabetes mellitus with a prevalence of 10–60% clinically, but up to 100% when evaluated by nerve conduction studies. There is increased prevalence with increased duration of the disease.

Pathogenesis

Vascular occlusion of the blood vessels supplying the nerves results in neuronal atrophy.

There are four types:

- Symmetrical and predominantly sensory polyneuropathy.
- Autonomic neuropathy.
- Proximal painful motor neuropathy.
- Cranial mononeuritis (mainly CN III, IV, and VI).

Metabolic and nutritional causes

Uremic neuropathy in renal failure

Approximately 60% of patients with chronic renal failure have symptoms of uremic neuropathy at onset of dialysis. It is expressed as pain and paresthesia with the lower extremities preferentially involved. Dialysis usually improves symptoms.

Thyroid dysfunction

Mild chronic sensorimotor neuropathy is sometimes seen in both hypothyroidism (more commonly) and hyperthyroidism.

Vitamin deficiencies

Vitamin deficiencies are important causes of peripheral neuropathies. Especially important are deficiencies of vitamins B_1 (thiamine), B_{12}, B_6 (pyridoxine), and E.

Toxic neuropathies

Many toxins cause damage to peripheral nerves. The most common toxins are:

- Drugs—isoniazides, sulphonamides, vinca alkaloids, dapsone, and chloroquine.
- Alcohol—in cases of chronic abuse.
- Industrial toxins—acrylamide, hexane, organophosphates, lead, arsenic, mercury.

Most toxins produce a "dying back" pattern of axonal damage resulting in a distal symmetric pattern of sensorimotor involvement. There is a "stocking-glove" distribution at onset, but continued exposure to the toxin extends the deficit to the lower calves and forearms.

Neuropathies associated with malignancy (metastatic neuropathy)

Cancer patients frequently have neurological symptoms caused by direct infiltration of individual nerves or plexuses.

Neoplasms of peripheral nerves

Peripheral nervous system tumors are illustrated in Fig. 14.18.

Peripheral nervous system tumors

Tumor	Features
Schwannoma	Benign tumor of Schwann cells of the nerve sheaths. Most common site is the vestibular branch of CN VIII
Neurofibroma	A tumor of the neural crest cells derived from the epineurium and endoneurium
Neurofibromatosis type I	An autosomal dominant neurocutaneous syndrome. Characterized by multiple neurofibromas
Neurofibromatosis type II	Autosomal dominant disorder affecting CN VIII
Tuberous sclerosis	Autosomal dominant disease causing epilepsy and mental retardation
Von Hippel–Lindau disease	Autosomal dominant disease characterized by multiple hemangiomas

Fig. 14.18 Peripheral nervous system tumors.

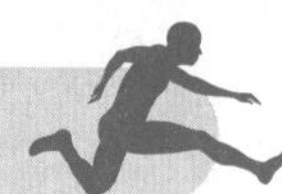

Disorders of the autonomic nervous system

Disorders of the sympathetic nervous system

Horner's syndrome

An uncommon condition caused by loss of sympathetic innervation to the eye. It is characterized by:

- Pupillary constriction (miosis) due to unopposed action of the pupillary constrictor.
- Partial ptosis (drooping) of the upper eyelid due to paralysis of smooth muscle fibers contained in the levator muscle of the upper eyelid.
- Enophthalmos (eye sunken into socket).
- Loss of sweating on affected side of the face.

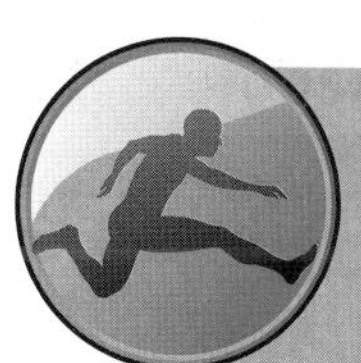

Lesions affecting any part of the sympathetic pathway (Fig. 14.19) may produce Horner's syndrome:

- Brainstem—tumors, vascular lesions, or syringobulbia.
- Cervical cord—tumors or syringomyelia.
- Cervical sympathetic chain—pancoast tumors (apical tumors of the lung) frequently invade adjacent sites; invasion of the superior cervical sympathetic ganglion often results in Horner's syndrome.

Trauma/surgical section of the sympathetic trunk

Surgical sympathectomies are sometimes performed for the relief of such conditions as:

- Raynaud's phenomenon—pallor, pain, and numbness of the fingers caused by vasospastic constriction of the digital arteries; sympathectomy is performed to improve limb perfusion.
- Causalgia—severe burning pain that occurs following injury to the major peripheral nerves of the limbs (e.g., median, ulnar, sciatic) due to disturbances of sympathetic reflexes.
- Hyperhidrosis—excessive sweating.

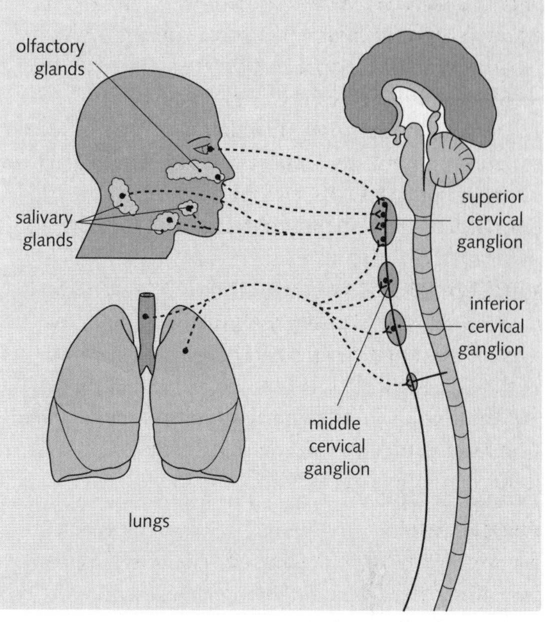

Fig. 14.19 Sympathetic innervation to the eye and face showing the relationship of the sympathetic trunk to the apex of the lungs.

The consequences of both traumatic or surgical section of the sympathetic chain depend on the level of the section, but may cause:

- Loss of blood pressure control → syncope (fainting).
- Impairment of sweating → hyperpyrexia.
- Impairment of bladder and bowel functions.
- Interruption of pathway to erectile tissue → impotence.

Pheochromocytoma

This is a rare tumor arising from chromaffin cells of the adrenal medulla, occurring in 1 in 1000 cases of hypertension. The majority are sporadic but about 10% are familial. Most are benign but about 5% are malignant.

Effects are those of hypersecretion of catecholamines (i.e., hypertension, hypermetabolism, and hyperglycemia). There is also pallor, headaches, sweating, and nervousness.

It may be associated with other endocrine neoplasias, namely:

- Multiple endocrine neoplasia syndrome (especially medullary carcinoma of the thyroid).
- Von Recklinghausen's disease.
- Von Hippel–Lindau syndrome.

It is diagnosed by increased amounts of urinary excretion of catecholamine metabolite vanillylmandelic acid (VMA).

Surgical removal of the tumor relieves hypertension and other effects.

Diseases of the parasympathetic nervous system

Effects of ablation of parasympathetic innervation

The commonest site of parasympathetic ablation is the vagus nerve (vagotomy) for treatment of duodenal ulcers. This is less common now due to the awareness of bacterial etiology (*Helicobacter pylori*) of intestinal ulcers.

Beneficial effects

Of benefit is the reduction of acid and pepsin secretion by abolishing direct vagal drive (and to a minor degree by reducing antral gastrin secretion).

Harmful effects

Impairment of antral motility is caused by abolishing receptive relaxation in the gastric corpus, and reducing the power of antral contractions.

The harmful effects of truncal vagotomy can now be largely overcome by performing a selective vagotomy instead, but this is less effective and it has a higher incidence of ulcer recurrence.

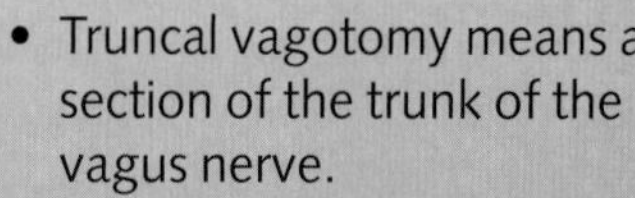

- Truncal vagotomy means a section of the trunk of the vagus nerve.
- Selective vagotomy means a vagotomy where only those vagal fibers that pass to the body of the stomach are divided, while those supplying the antrum, pylorus, and other abdominal viscera are spared.

- Describe the common pathological features of the CNS.
- What are the congenital malformations and developmental diseases of the CNS?
- Give examples of types of traumatic injury that affect the CNS.
- What is the pathogenesis of cerebrovascular disease?
- Name the infections of the CNS.
- Describe Creutzfeldt–Jakob disease.
- Give examples of diseases of demyelination and diseases of degeneration.
- Name the vitamin deficiencies and toxins that damage the CNS.
- What are the consequences of excess ethanol intake on the CNS?
- Name the neoplasms of the CNS.
- Name the different types of hereditary neuropathies.
- What are the causes and outcomes of traumatic neuropathies?
- Outline the pathology of Guillain–Barré syndrome (inflammatory neuropathy).
- Name infections that can cause neuropathies.
- Give types of metabolic and toxic neuropathies.
- Name the neoplasms of the peripheral nerves.
- What are the characteristics and causes of Horner's syndrome?
- Give indications for performing sympathectomies and describe their effects.
- Describe the pathology of pheochromocytomas.
- What are the effects of vagotomies?

Index

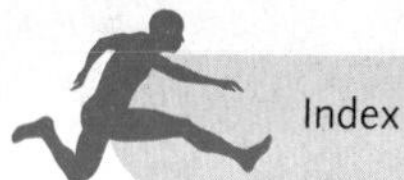

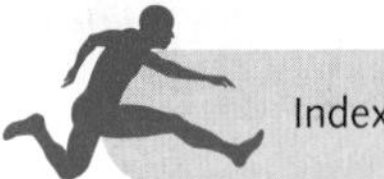

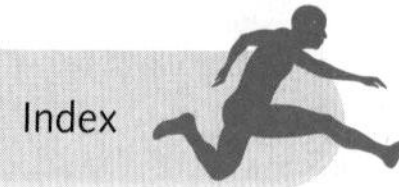

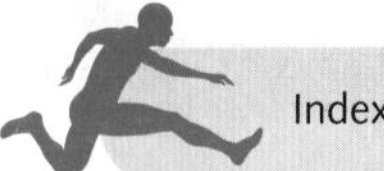

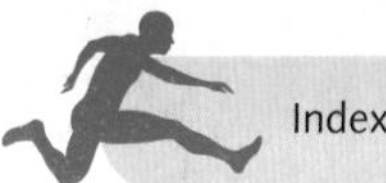

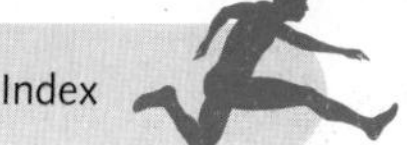

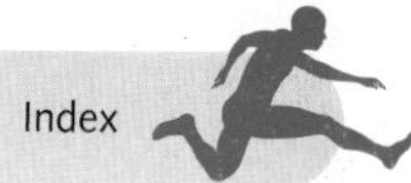